W9-CPF-181

Edited by

HERBERT K. COOPER, Sr.,
D.D.S., F.A.C.D., D.Sc.

ROBERT L. HARDING,
M.D., D.D.S., F.A.C.S.

WILTON M. KROGMAN,
Ph.D., LL.D., D.Sc., F.A.C.D.(hon.)

MOHAMMAD MAZAHERI,
D.D.S., M.Sc., F.A.C.D.

ROBERT T. MILLARD,
B.S., M.S.

H. K. Cooper Institute for Oral-Facial
Anomalies and Communicative Disorders,
Lancaster Cleft Palate Clinic,
Lancaster, Pennsylvania

STEVEN M. SPENCER
Editorial Consultant

W. B. SAUNDERS COMPANY
Philadelphia, London, Toronto

CLEFT PALATE

and CLEFT LIP:

A Team Approach to
Clinical Management
and Rehabilitation
of the Patient

1979

W. B. Saunders Company: West Washington Square
                          Philadelphia, PA 19105

                          1 St. Anne's Road
                          Eastbourne, East Sussex BN21 3UN, England

                          1 Goldthorne Avenue
                          Toronto, Ontario M8Z 5T9, Canada

Library of Congress Cataloging in Publication Data

Main entry under title:

Cleft palate and cleft lip.

1. Cleft palate.   2. Harelip.   1. Cooper, Herbert K.
II. Spencer, Steven M. [DNLM: 1. Cleft lip — Rehabilitation.
2. Cleft lip — Therapy.   3. Cleft palate — Rehabilitation.
4. Cleft palate — Therapy. WV440 C622]

RD525.C53   617'.522   76–41536

ISBN 0–7216–2687–4

Cleft Palate and Cleft Lip: A Team Approach to   ISBN   0-7216-2687-4
Clinical Management and Rehabilitation of the Patient

© 1979 by W. B. Saunders Company. Copyright under the International Copyright Union.
All rights reserved. This book is protected by copyright. No part of it may be reproduced,
stored in a retrieval system, or transmitted in any form or by any means, electronic, mechanical,
photocopying, recording or otherwise, without written permission from the publisher. Made
in the United States of America. Press of W. B. Saunders Company. Library of Congress
catalog card number 76-41536.

Last digit is the print number: 9   8   7   6   5   4   3   2   1

DEDICATION

We respectfully dedicate this book to the memory of Herbert Kurtz Cooper, Sr., Founder of the Lancaster Cleft Palate Clinic, who died April 17, 1978, at the age of 81 years.

ACKNOWLEDGMENT

The research at the Lancaster Cleft Palate Clinic was funded in large part by the National Institute for Dental Research, Program Grant DE-02172, 1964–1977.

We gratefully acknowledge the financial aid of the Gustavus and Louise Pfeiffer Foundation, which provided the furnishings for our Research Building and contributed to our research program.

CONTRIBUTORS

HERBERT K. COOPER, Sr. (Deceased), D.D.S., D.Sc., L.H.D., F.A.C.D., F.I.C.D., Orthodontist.

Founder and Director Emeritus of the Lancaster Cleft Palate Clinic; Clinical Professor of Surgery, Milton S. Hershey Medical Center, The Pennsylvania State University; Former Professor of Cleft Palate Therapy, School of Dental Medicine, University of Pennsylvania.
Historical Perspectives and Philosophy of Treatment

ROBERT L. HARDING, D.D.S., M.S., M.D., F.A.C.S., Plastic Surgery.

Plastic Surgeon, Harrisburg (PA) Hospital, and Harrisburg Polyclinic Hospital; Chief of Plastic Surgery of the Lancaster Cleft Palate Clinic; Clinical Professor of Surgery, Milton S. Hershey Medical Center, The Pennsylvania State University; Past President, American Cleft Palate Association; Past President, American Association of Plastic Surgeons; Former Chief of Plastic Surgery, Walter Reed Army Medical Center; and Former Editor of the *Cleft Palate Journal* of the American Cleft Palate Association.
Surgery

WILTON M. KROGMAN, Ph.D., LL.D., D.Sc., F.A.C.D. (hon.), Growth and Development.

Founder (1947) and Director Emeritus, Philadelphia Center for Research in Child Growth; Emeritus Professor of Physical Anthropology, School of Medicine, University of Pennsylvania; Adjunct Associate Professor of Pediatrics, Milton S. Hershey Medical Center, The Pennsylvania State University; Past President, American Association of Physical Anthropologists, Society for Research in Child Growth and Development, and International Society for Craniofacial Biology; Chief of Research, Lancaster Cleft Palate Clinic.
Craniofacial Growth; The Cleft Palate Team in Action

MOHAMMAD MAZAHERI, D.D.S., M.Sc., F.A.C.D. Prosthodontist.

Clinical Associate Professor of Surgery, Milton S. Hershey Medical Center, The Pennsylvania State University; Consultant to Dental Staff, Bethesda Naval Hospital, and to Veteran's Administration; Past President, American Cleft Palate Association; Chief of Dental Services, Lancaster Cleft Palate Clinic.
Prosthodontic Care

ROBERT T. MILLARD, B.S., M.A., Speech Pathology.

Chief of the Division of Speech at the Lancaster Cleft Palate Clinic.
Speech Evaluation and Treatment

HARRY E. CANTER, B.S., M.A., Biostatistics.

Associate Professor of Mathematics, The Millersville (PA) State College; Consultant in mathematical biostatistics to the Lancaster Cleft Palate Clinic.
Statistical Approach to Research

WILLIAM P. GRAHAM, III., B.A., M.D., Plastic Surgery.
Chief, Department of Plastic Surgery, Milton S. Hershey Medical Center, The Pennsylvania State University, and Clinical Staff of the Lancaster Cleft Palate Clinic.
Plastic Surgery

KITTY HEISERMAN (Deceased).
Case-Worker on Staff of Social Services Research of the Lancaster Cleft Palate Clinic.
The Social Worker in a Cleft Palate Clinic

ROSS E. LONG, SR., D.D.S., Orthodontist.
Private practice.
Orthodontics and Oral Orthopedics

ROSS E. LONG, JR., D.D.S., Orthodontist.
Chief of Orthodontics, Lancaster Cleft Palate Clinic; President, Lancaster Cleft Palate Clinic.
Orthodontics and Oral Orthopedics

JOSEPH A. MEIER, B.S., M.S.C., Ph.D., Biostatistics.
Professor of Mathematics, The Millersville (PA) State College; Consultant in mathematical biostatistics to the Lancaster Cleft Palate Clinic.
Statistical Approach to Research

SEISHI W. OKA, B.S., D.D.S., Ph.D., Genetics.
Chief of the Division of Genetics of the Lancaster Cleft Palate Clinic.
Epidemiology and Genetics of Clefting

J. MICHAEL PEPEK, D.D.S., Orthodontist.
Private practice.
Orthodontics and Oral Orthopedics

JOHN E. RISKI, M.S., Ph.D., Speech Pathology.
Formerly Speech Scientist, Lancaster Cleft Palate. Now at Duke Medical Center, Durham, North Carolina.
Speech Evaluation and Treatment

PAUL W. ROSS, B.E., M.E., D.E., Computer Analyst.
Associate Professor of Mathematics and Computer Science, The Millersville (Pa.) State College; Consultant in computing to the Lancaster Cleft Palate Clinic.
Computers in Analysis of Cleft Palate Clinic Data

STEVEN M. SPENCER,
Former Senior Editor (Science) of the *Saturday Evening Post*, Consultant to the Editorial Committee in the preparation of this book.
The Patient's Point of View

PHILIP STARR, B.A., M.S.W., Social Service.
Chief of the Division of Social Service Research at the Lancaster Cleft Palate Clinic.
The Social Worker in a Cleft Palate Clinic

ELCA T. SWIGART, B.S., M.A., Ph.D., Hearing.
Chief of Division of Audiology of the Lancaster Cleft Palate Clinic.
Hearing and Audiology

H. K. COOPER INSTITUTE FOR ORAL-FACIAL ANOMALIES AND COMMUNICATIVE DISORDERS AND THE LANCASTER CLEFT PALATE CLINIC

OFFICERS

GARY L. ELLIS
Executive Director

ROSS E. LONG, JR., D.M.D.
President

ROBERT L. HARDING, D.D.S., M.D.
Vice-President

BOARD OF DIRECTORS

MRS. WALTER W. POSEY, II — *Chairman*
LOUIS G. SHENK, JR. — *Vice-Chairman*
DR. THEODORE A. DISTLER — *Secretary*
ALBERT B. WOHLSEN, JR. — *Treasurer*
JOHN A. COOPER, D.D.S. — *Assistant Secretary*
VICTOR R. DESPARD, JR.
HOWE ATWATER
ELMER H. BOBST
SIMON A. CANTOR
JAMES P. COHO, ESQ.
H. K. COOPER, JR., M.D.
MRS. PAUL R. DILLER
RUFUS A. FULTON, JR.
WILLIAM C. HEYN
NORRIS J. KIRK, M.D.
C. PAUL MYERS

DIRECTORS EMERITUS

MRS. WALTER CARPENTER
ROSS E. LONG, D.D.S.
CLAIR R. McCOLLOUGH
HONORABLE JOSEPH B. WISSLER

PREFACE

The title of this volume, the breadth of its contents, and its close attention to the complex problems of patients as well as the concerns of teaching and research, all suggest the philosophy of the founder of the Lancaster Cleft Palate Clinic. Dr. Herbert Kurtz Cooper, Sr., has been persistently and consistently dedicated to the idea that scholarship and research are basic for successful habilitation and that all aspects of care and learning are augmented by a multidisciplinary approach.

Publication of the book comes after Dr. Cooper has completed the most active years of his professional work. But among the contributing authors are several who have been associated with him during the many years that he was building the Clinic, an institution that began on a modest basis in answer to what Herbert Cooper perceived as an acute need and which grew into what is now known as the H. K. Cooper Institute for Oral-Facial Anomalies and Communicative Disorders. So it is quite natural that the writer of this preface, who has known Dr. Cooper for 40 years and who worked with him during the early days of the Cleft Palate Clinic, should think back about the development of the project and the career of its founder. What were his contributions? What impact did they have on the field?

A possible view of the products of endeavor related to the habilitation of any group is that there is an on-going stream of knowledge, some of it obscure in origin. It is constantly amplified and modified by many individuals, each one a citizen in a scientific group. Among those interested in orofacial anomalies, Dr. Cooper is indeed a most distinguished and productive citizen.

The group at Lancaster was and continues to be a team in fact. Ideas of different members are sought out and considered carefully, so that the dividends of the interdisciplinary approach are exploited fully. This is probably why the team plan continues at Lancaster. The title of "team" was used quite generally throughout the country when the concept was becoming popular, but when the newness wore off, one heard statements to the effect that teams had made their contribution and were no longer necessary. This might imply that each discipline had acquired a static body of information that could be learned and then used independently. However, this is not true when a group really functions as a team. Interaction between members continues to shape ideas for research and treatment. In addition to advocating interdisciplinary study and clinical management, Dr. Cooper has set up a successful working model for his ideas that continues to demonstrate the soundness of his initial insights.

Written language cannot express the professional impact of a man com-

pletely. Personal qualities that are exceedingly important to successful habilitation and particularly important to the operation of a productive research and
treatment team are not projected in journals and books. The reader's insights
into the contents of this book might be enhanced by knowing that Dr. Cooper
is an unusually warm and sensitive man, whose great energy and enthusiasm
inspire both the patient and his professional associates, but never dominate
them. This explains the loyalty of those of us who were fortunate enough to
work with him, and the affection as well as the gratitude of his patients. With
his kind of leadership a team can and does work.

HAROLD WESTLAKE

RECOGNITION

This volume has in many ways been the result of a collaborative effort. Teamwork in the rehabilitation process described here has been its central theme. In the preparation of the various chapters the authors consulted one another to assure accuracy and balance where their presentations touched on their colleagues' specialties. For this interdisciplinary assistance the editors wish to express their appreciation.

Collaboration of a less deliberate but perhaps more pervasive kind has come from another source. Throughout the book, helping to make it the record of a closely knit organization for care, teaching, and research, one senses the role of the child patients and their parents. Over the years we of the Staff have come to consider them part of a large, devoted, and friendly family. Their cooperation with our treatment procedures and our research program, a co-operation expressed in a thorough understanding of our aims and in faithfully kept appointments, has contributed much to the Clinic's success in the management of communicative disorders. This close working relationship has helped us to convey the story of the Clinic's experience.

We should like to express special thanks to a number of these patients and former patients who graciously acceded to our request to relate their early experiences in living with their handicap and to reflect upon the changes brought about through rehabilitation. Their insightful statements appear in the last chapter of the book.

This book is veritably a team effort. The contributors are in a very real sense indebted to the Clinic Staff members — Beth Dreibelbis, Shelley Gitomer, Cathy Oehme, Deborah Schroll — for the gathering and tabulation of all our longitudinal data. Dr. Jeffrey Rubinstein provided dental care for the patients. In specific areas are Mary Jean Bechard (Social Service), Dorothy Biesecher (dental technician), Julia Fischel (Speech), Carol Fisher (Genetics), James Hecht (radiological technician), Carl Harding (dental technician), Dr. Isao Hayashi (photography), Linda McCullers (illustrator), Donna Steinmetz (Genetics), and Geraldine Sullenberger (Audiology). The various manuscripts were typed by Sherry Brinton, Isabelle Nicklaus, Gloria Nixdorf, and Linda Weaver.

We called upon colleagues in various universities: Dr. James Avery, Director, Institute for Dental Research, University of Michigan School of Dentistry, Ann Arbor (Embryology); Dr. William Williams, University of Florida, Gainesville (Speech); and Dr. Malcolm Johnston, Orthodontic Dept. and Dental Research Center, Dr. W. R. Posnick, Chief of Pedodontics, Cleft Palate Center, Ms. Roani Stott, Orthodontic Dept., and Dr. David J. Hall,

Orthodontics Dept., all at the University of North Carolina School of Dentistry, Chapel Hill. (These last four aided in preparing the chapter on Orthodontic care.)

All contributors to this book unite in thanking Steven Spencer for his unfailing aid in the editing of each chapter. His insight into the problems of presenting our ideas and our data in a meaningful fashion enabled each one of us to communicate more clearly and simply. His sense of humor and his "light touch" rendered the chores of writing and recasting less demanding and arduous than they might have been.

We are also indebted to Carroll C. Cann, Dental Editor of W. B. Saunders Company, for perceiving the possibilities in the book project when it was proposed to him, and for his wise and patient guidance as the work progressed.

A first and last acknowledgment is to our Founder and Director Emeritus, H. K. Cooper, Sr. In this we all join. . . .

CONTENTS

Chapter One

A basic assumption in our approach to rehabilitation has been that if an individual is to achieve something in life, that person should feel that he or she looks like a normal human being and should be able to speak easily and clearly. Nothing else is so necessary to one's social and educational development.[3]

Those of us who have an acceptable set of features with which to face the world, and a speech mechanism that keeps us in good contact with it, are apt to forget how vitally important these attributes are. The face is one area of the body seldom covered by clothing, the part by which others recognize us and, at first glance, react to us. When it is marred by congenital influences or by extrinsic causes, and when distorted speech issues from an imperfectly shaped vocal cavity, the result can be a cruel, at times overwhelming, handicap.

Clefts of the lip and palate all too often constitute such a handicap. They are the most common of facial, oral, and vocal defects. More than a quarter of a million people now living in the United States were born with a cleft of the lip, palate, or both. Almost every hour, somewhere in the United States, a child is born with an orofacial deformity. Among congenital anomalies of all kinds, clefts of the lip and palate are second only to clubfoot in frequency, occurring once in every 600 to 700 births in the white population, less frequently among blacks (one in every 2000 newborns.)

From the vantage point of close involvement with the lives of thousands of these scarred children and young adults for most of a long professional career, I have seen a steady improvement in their chances of realizing their full potential. Certainly those born in recent decades have far brighter prospects than those born before the middle of this century. Most of those who have received competent treatment during the past 30 or 40 years have acquired normal — or near normal — appearance and speech. The proportion obtaining good treatment has increased, thanks largely to a wider public awareness of what can be done for them and to a more conscientious attention to their problems on the part of the medical, dental, and other health professions.

HISTORICAL PERSPECTIVES AND PHILOSOPHY OF TREATMENT

HERBERT K. COOPER, SR.

> Speech is a mirror of the soul; as a man speaks, so is he.
> *Publilius Syrus, circa 42* B.C.

Unfortunately, not every child with a cleft has been able to enjoy completely satisfactory results. Often there have been delays in seeking qualified surgical and rehabilitative services. Sometimes the merits of all possible techniques, including a properly fitted speech appliance, have not been carefully weighed. Other failures can be blamed upon the baffling complexities of the cleft pathology itself, which have given rise to honest controversies over the best ways to correct the defect.

One must grant that the task all of us face can be exceedingly difficult. The troubles generated by the cleft condition can test the skills and patience of the most experienced clinician. Consider the picture drawn a few years ago by Maxine A. Schurter, plastic surgeon at George Washington University: "Few congenital deformities can lead to such a great variety of disabilities—pitiable looks, dental caries, poor dental occlusion, poor speech, middle ear infections, psychological aberrations, economic burdens, and fear of hereditary patterns. Few congenital anomalies have challenged the resources of more specialties and subspecialties."[9]

A CRIPPLING CONDITION

To this sorry list we at the Lancaster Cleft Palate Clinic would add still another descriptive term. We have never hesitated to call the cleft condition a *crippling* one, at least until it was satisfactorily corrected, but not everyone in the health professions and agencies has always regarded it as such. As a consequence, the child with a cleft has often had difficulty obtaining the assistance, especially the financial assistance, that he or she deserved and that those with more obvious and familiar disabilities were receiving. Although this discriminatory attitude is less prevalent today than it was in the past, it is a part of cleft palate history that I personally feel should not be overlooked, and I shall have more to say about it later in this introductory chapter.

The principal purpose of this volume as my colleagues and I have envisioned it is to share with others our thinking and our experience in carrying out our integrated, interdisciplinary approach to the complete rehabilitation of those with orofacial anomalies and communicative disorders. Most of the Lancaster Cleft Palate Clinic's efforts, as its name suggests, are focused on the problems of clefts. While this book will reflect that concentration, we shall also touch upon the surgical, prosthetic, and general rehabilitative services we provide for patients with other facial and speech defects, including those resulting from severe trauma or from cancer surgery.

The book has been written for everyone who is — or who may become — involved in the care of these patients, whether one's specialty is plastic surgery, pediatrics, dentistry (including particularly orthodontics and prosthodontics, but not excluding general dentistry), speech pathology, audiology or otology, social work, psychology, or physical anthropology and child growth. The author of each chapter covering research or clinical programs is, of course, a specialist in the subject he is writing about, and the attempt has been made to provide information that would be most relevant and most helpful to the research workers or clinicians dealing with their own phase of the problem. The state of the art may embrace different approaches to some aspects of cleft palate management. Our aim has been to explain our own methods at the Lancaster Cleft Palate Clinic — or the H. K. Cooper Institute for Oral-Facial Anomalies and Communicative Disorders, to use its full formal name.

We do not claim that our experience in the field is unique. It has been, however, unusually broad and for the most part gratifying, and it has extended over a considerable period of time. Established in 1938, ours was the first clinic in the country to devote itself full-time, on a day-by-day basis, to the diagnosis and treatment of cleft lip and palate and other facial anomalies. We have by now seen more than 30,000 cases and are examining and treating approximately 2,200 patients annually in 5,000 visits. Of this number about 230 are new patients every year.

Advances

In surveying the cleft palate scene as a whole, our attention is drawn to a number of solid developments that in recent decades have improved the condition of these patients and deepened our understanding of their personal problems. On the technical side, cineroentgenography, which we at the Lancaster Clinic were the first to employ in the examination of oral clefts, has made visible the speech mechanism at work. Sonography has given graphic form to the production of speech itself. These aids have permitted us to sharpen our diagnoses and improve the evaluation of our therapeutic methods. We have made better use of orthodontic and prosthodontic techniques, which in themselves have benefited from new refinements. We have gained new knowledge of — and respect for — the vulnerability of mid-facial growth centers, and in so doing have learned better how to avoid the deplorable results of some of the earlier surgical procedures. In this connection we at the Lancaster Clinic have combined the talents of the physical anthropologist, plastic surgeon, prosthodontist, and computer scientist in research on craniofacial growth, with conclusions that further demonstrate the advantages of conservative surgery. Our findings indicate that the child whose lip or palate is repaired according to conservative criteria, with meticulous heed to the growth centers, can expect at age six to have a dentofacial complex that is normal in structure, function, and esthetic appearance.

Finally, we have witnessed a much wider acceptance of the group or team approach, and believe that this has been a substantial factor in the improved standards of care. The problems confronting us are usually complicated, often frustrating, and nearly always require repeated observation over a long span of years—in many cases from infancy on into young adulthood. Their effective management can best be provided, we believe, through the closely coordinated wisdom and skills of several disciplines. Among the many authorities who have expressed agreement with this view are Parkins and Barbero, a pedodontist and pediatrician, respectively, who have written: "A *complete program of rehabilitation* for the child with a cleft lip or palate may require years of special medical, surgical, dental and speech treatment. Representatives of the specialties involved function more effectively on a team basis than individually."[7]

My own interest in the cleft palate problem arose out of my concern, as a young orthodontist in the 1920s, for those children whose teeth were so crooked as to give them a crooked face. Their malocclusion distorted not only their features but their speech. In many cases the underlying cause was cleft palate, sometimes so inexpertly repaired as to prolong if not compound the difficulty.

Exclusion from Programs

In 1928, during the administration of a Lancaster physician, the late Theodore Appel, as Secretary of Health, I became dental consultant to the new Pennsylvania Hospital for Crippled Children at Elizabethtown. I thought at the time that this might give me an opportunity to see and possibly to help more children with cleft palates, but I found that youngsters with this deformity were not considered "crippled." During my 12 years in the post I saw none of them at the hospital. They continued, however, to come to see me in my private practice in Lancaster, and I was bothered by the failure of the state crippled children's hospital to include these *facially* crippled youngsters in its responsibilities.

It was because of this experience that I began to ask the question in talks and in journal articles: "What is a crippled child?" The definition of the International Society for the Welfare of Cripples was "one whose activities may become so far restricted by loss, defect or deformity of bone or muscle as to reduce his or her normal capacity for education and self-support." By these criteria, I argued, the child whose oral and facial defects severely impaired the ability to communicate and thus diminished the "capacity for education and self-support" was most certainly crippled. Moreover, the physical defects, if not successfully treated, could lead to personality defects, social withdrawal, and other psychosocial problems. Still, this child was receiving much less than adequate consideration by the medical profession and the public health agencies traditionally charged with the care of crippled children.

Over the years I was to read many orthopedic textbooks and journals and I was struck by the fact that much space was taken up with the care and treatment of nearly every known deformity *except* those involving the face and mouth. In almost no instance was there reference in those general orthopedic publications to malformations of the jaws. Cleft lip and palate were omitted even from a volume, by an outstanding authority, devoted specifically to malformations of children.

Millions of dollars were being spent, and quite justifiably, on straightening legs and backs crippled by polio and other diseases, but comparatively little was being devoted, particularly through public institutions, to mending the crippled faces and voices resulting from the imperfect union of bone and flesh that we call cleft palate. We were fixing up one child's legs so that later he or she could walk in and ask for a job, but we were doing almost nothing for the next youngster, who could walk in for the job but couldn't ask for it with intelligible speech.

Consider the experiences of two mothers of handicapped children. Mrs. A's son has a clubfoot and she takes him to a hospital for crippled children, where he is readily admitted and treated—at public expense if she is in a low income bracket. Her neighbor Mrs. B has a boy with a cleft palate and an associated speech defect. She takes him to the same hospital but finds to her bewilderment and great disappointment that there is no provision there for treating this deformity. Which child is more seriously handicapped? Mrs. B regards the discrimination against her son as very strange, for she feels that if he had both a clubfoot and a cleft palate and could have only one defect corrected, she would certainly choose to have the palate repaired, and so would the boy if he could look into the future, because it would give him acceptable speech. In making such a decision Mrs. B might well have thought of Franklin D. Roosevelt, who during four elected terms as President could not walk to the platform, but once there could speak with persuasive eloquence.[4]

Need for a Clinic

In pleading the cause of the child with a cleft palate I had a staunch and effective ally in Robert H. Ivy, for many years professor of plastic surgery at the University of Pennsylvania and a member of our clinic staff until shortly before his death in 1974. Following his recommendation in 1938, the Secretary of Health of Pennsylvania appointed several surgeons in Philadelphia and Pittsburgh to perform operations on children whose families were financially limited. In 1949 a Cleft Palate Division was created in the state's Bureau of Maternal and Child Health with Dr. Ivy as chief, a position he held until 1966.

Meanwhile, as the only orthodontist between Philadelphia and Pittsburgh I was being called on to treat within my own specialty an increasing number of children with cleft palate. Often I was distressed at not being able to achieve better results in terms of speech, but in 1936 I gained fresh inspiration from a lecture I heard at the New York Society of Orthodontists delivered by a remarkable man, John J. Fitz-Gibbon of Holyoke, Massachusetts.

Born with a cleft palate, Fitz-Gibbon had taken up dentistry to learn how to overcome his own handicap as well as how to help others. He fashioned a speech appliance having a gold ball as the posterior element (the speech bulb), which served to complete the velopharyngeal valve action. With this prosthetic assistance he had developed such fine, clear speech that few would have suspected any anatomical impairment.

Others before Fitz-Gibbon had constructed speech appliances to help the individual with a cleft palate, notably Norman W. Kingsley (1850–1892), known as the "Father of Orthodontia," and Calvin S. Case (1871–1923).[5] I drew much inspiration from their writings also, but Fitz-Gibbon was the first person I had met who used such a device, and I seized upon the idea as just the thing I needed to help my own cleft palate patients.

At about this time a survey in the Lancaster public schools revealed a much higher incidence of cleft palate and other malformations of the face and jaws than had been suspected. The situation presented a challenge to orthodontists, for although the schools were employing a speech therapist, nothing was being done to correct the anatomical, physiological, and psychological factors that usually underlie or exacerbate the speech impairment. Often children with a cleft palate were seen whose speech so embarrassed them in the classroom or among friends that they would "clam up" and stop trying to speak. I recall a three-year-old girl who chattered happily to herself as long as she was not facing anyone, but the moment we engaged her in a game that required her to look up at an adult, she would stop talking and hide her face.

If the defect is inadequately corrected, it may erode the child's confidence. Actually the impediment itself may not greatly interfere with the ability to do things; it is the reaction it evokes in others that causes the damage.* Even some teachers and prospective employers have assumed that since the ability to speak is impaired, so is the ability to learn. They have failed to recognize that the defect is entirely in the mouth and not in the mind.

It became obvious to me that the best way to give the child with cleft palate the various kinds of help he or she needed — surgery, orthodontics, dentistry, speech — was through a clinic. I tried to get the Crippled Children's Hospital in Elizabethtown to set one up within its own walls, but I had no luck, even though I was on the hospital's staff and was also a member of the state's health advisory board. I was equally unpersuasive when I took my idea to the University of Pennsylvania, where I was a member of the School of Dentistry faculty. Such a clinic was later established there, but in the 1930s I could not bring about the necessary cooperation between the several divisions that would have been involved — medicine, dentistry, and speech (the last of which was in the College of Liberal Arts).

---

*One is reminded of the limerick by Anthony Euwer, often quoted by Woodrow Wilson:
As a beauty I'm not a great star.
Others are handsomer far;
But my face — I don't mind it
Because I'm behind it;
It's the folks out in front that I jar.

LANCASTER CLINIC

Defeated in my efforts to establish a clinic in what I thought were more logical places, I decided in 1938 to organize our own in Lancaster. We occupied, and still do, an old, red brick home converted for our use in a pleasant residential section near the center of town. We later added a two-story research building and a small laboratory unit. Assisting me in the orthodontic work were Eleanor Hallman, my son-in-law Ross E. Long, Robert Flowers, and later my son John A. Cooper. A speech therapist in the Lancaster school system, Genevieve Diller, joined me, first as a volunteer and then as a full-time staff member. Within the next few years we enlisted a speech pathologist, Robert T. Millard, who had just received his master's degree at The University of Iowa, and Mohammad Mazaheri, who had been taking special training in prosthodontics under my tutelage in a special program conducted jointly by the University of Pennsylvania School of Dentistry, where I was then professor of cleft palate therapy, and the Lancaster Clinic.

As demand for services increased, we added an x-ray specialist, a pediatrician, and a psychologist. The late George M. Dorrance, a well-known Philadelphia maxillofacial surgeon, was a consultant to the Lancaster Cleft Palate Clinic for many years and was succeeded by Dr. Ivy. Our present chief plastic surgeon is Robert L. Harding, chief of plastic surgery at the Harrisburg and Polyclinic Hospitals in Harrisburg and member of the Hahnemann Medical College faculty in Philadelphia, who also has a degree in dentistry. His associate on the clinic staff is William P. Graham, III, chief of plastic surgery at the Hershey Medical Center. Harold Westlake, one of the country's leading speech pathologists, was a member of our staff before he went to Northwestern University. Our research division is directed by Wilton M. Krogman, who retired several years ago as professor of physical anthropology at the University of Pennsylvania School of Medicine.

For several years during the 1940s the Clinic was sponsored by the Lancaster Rotary Club, which found our patients' needs similar to those of children they had long been helping through the National Association for Crippled Children and Adults. As a Rotarian I had taken crippled children to the Lancaster General Hospital for treatment and was an active fund raiser for the state's Easter Seal program. Our Clinic was never affiliated with the Easter Seal organization, but as a pioneer in the cleft palate field we became a model for other clinics set up in Pennsylvania (there are now 13). Many cleft palate facilities have since been established throughout the United States, a total of nearly 150 in the American Cleft Palate Association's "Team Directory." They are situated in nearly every state. By no means do all of them operate on a full-time basis, as ours does; many meet only once a week or less often.

In 1947, at the suggestion of Judge Joseph B. Wissler, the Lancaster Clinic was chartered as a nonprofit institution, with a board of 21 directors. With the added functions of research and professional training, and the increased scope of its clinical work, the name was later changed to the H. K. Cooper Institute for Oral-Facial Anomalies and Communicative Disorders, although the original Lancaster Cleft Palate Clinic designation is also retained.

In May 1974 the Clinic and Institute became affiliated with the College of Medicine of the Milton S. Hershey Medical Center, a unit of The Pennsylvania State University at Hershey. Several of our staff members who contribute significantly to the Clinic's joint program of cooperative patient care, education, and research hold academic appointments on the College of Medicine faculty, and students and residents from the College come to Lancaster for part of their training. A number of patients operated on for facial cancer at the Hershey Center come to Lancaster for construction of prostheses for cosmetic and speech purposes.

The National Institute of Dental Research has for a number of years provided grants for our research. We have also enjoyed the support of many private contributors from Lancaster and other parts of the country.

The True Team

Although the Lancaster Cleft Palate Clinic was the first of its kind in the country, it does not claim to have originated any miraculous methods of treatment. Its contribution has been rather to demonstrate the effectiveness of carefully planned teamwork in handling the multifaceted problems with which the cleft palate patient must struggle. Our staff at present numbers approximately 50 members and is drawn from many specialties. These include oral surgery, general dentistry, orthodontics and prosthodontics, plastic surgery, internal medicine, pediatrics, physical anthropology and anatomy, genetics, radiology, otolaryngology, speech pathology, audiology, and social work. We also employ the services of resident counselors and elementary and secondary school teachers in our summer residency program.

The word "teamwork" tends to fall glibly from the tongue of anyone involved in a joint approach to a problem, but the meaning differs with the context and the philosophy. There is the "vertical" team in which the decisions and the instructions originate at the top, with one person; the other members merely carry out their assigned duties. This works well on the football field, where the goal is a straight white line. In a clinic addressing itself to the complex and shifting ramifications of cleft lip and palate, however, it is our experience that a more even distribution of input, a wider sharing of ideas and opinions, among team members, achieves a better result.

I cannot emphasize too strongly the desirability of this balanced arrangement. Webster's definition of teamwork seems to apply most aptly to the clinic situation: "Work done by a number of associates, usually each doing a clearly defined portion, but all subordinating personal prominence to the efficiency of the whole." Individualism and initiative are to be respected, but a team can succeed only with smooth cooperation by men and women who, while feeling free and independent, are willing to do what is expected of them without friction. They must be motivated to act in the greatest interest of the patient, and in my opinion the only way to make this philosophy work is to follow the three "C's" — communication, cooperation, and coordination of effort.

We do not advocate a team without a leader, but we have found that major responsibility for decisions may logically shift from one member to another — or to two or three together — as different problems are met at different stages in the patient's continuing program of treatment and rehabilitation. (Dr. Krogman expands upon this time-table concept in his chapter, "The Cleft Palate Team in Action.") This principle, however, has not always been understood or appreciated. In many cleft palate clinics it is the plastic surgeon who is automatically the chief, with the other team members serving in strictly ancillary roles. We agree that during the first year or two of the patient's life, when initial repair of the lip and palate is of primary concern, the plastic surgeon is best qualified to decide on the type and extent of surgical intervention required and should be the "chairman of the team." In fact, the surgeon is so designated by our own Clinic in its by-laws, which emphasize the importance of "properly considered and well-timed surgery." But as the child's dentition and speech develop—or fail to develop properly—the expertise of others assumes equal or dominant importance. The orthodontist and prosthodontist, for example, and the speech pathologist and specialist in growth become vital to the child's development.

Alternatives to Repeated Operations

We particularly question the philosophy, so often followed in the past and perhaps pursued in some places even today, that relies on surgery as the only solution, allowing no alternative, even after earlier operations have failed to produce satisfactory results. We feel that before additional surgery is undertaken during adolescence or adulthood, there should be an interchange of views between members of the surgical, dental, and speech departments. A trained orthodontist is best able to assess malocclusion problems that could prejudice good surgical results. The speech pathologist can weigh the merits of different procedures as they may affect the physiology of speech. The group's final decision may be that a speech prosthesis will offer a better solution than another operation or may be effective as an adjunct to surgery in bringing about effective closure of the velopharyngeal valve. Although we prefer to correct the incompetency or insufficiency without a prosthesis if possible, we believe it is a disservice to patients to subject them to one operation after another without even considering the speech appliance as an alternative. It has been our experience that about 70 per cent of all cleft palate patients will require some type of fixed or removable prosthesis by 30 years of age.

Our own surgical colleagues and consultants, for whose skill and judgment we have had nothing but praise, have long been in accord with the policy of group action. We have, however, seen many referred patients—fewer in recent years than in the past—for whom repeated attempts to close the palatal gap had utterly failed to establish acceptable speech. Too often the surgeon had been content to evaluate the results solely from the anatomical appearance after the operation, neglecting to ascertain through follow-up studies whether the patient's speech mechanism had improved functionally, whether he or she could really speak better. Some surgeons have told me that they had never seen a cleft that couldn't be closed by surgery. This is true, and the same statement could be made by dentists with respect to closing the opening with an appliance, but no matter which method is used, merely closing the cleft does not guarantee good speech. The task is much more exacting than that. Nevertheless, we have seen instances in which, even though the first and second surgical attempts were obvious failures, the surgeon proceeded undeterred to a third, fourth, or even a fifth operation-—all without soliciting the opinion of experts in other disciplines or weighing the possible advantage of a prosthetic device—finally leaving the patient in worse condition than at the beginning of treatment. Actually we have seen individuals who have undergone as many as 30 operations.

I remember a girl of 16 who was referred to us after a series of 12 operations. The first had been carried out when she was six months old, the others at almost yearly intervals on into her sixteenth year. All of this surgery had failed to close the palatal defect adequately, and during most of those years she had been taking speech lessons with dishearteningly unsatisfactory results.

Through our team management, which in this case included the fitting of a speech appliance, we were able to help this girl to attain better speech and better social adjustment. She resumed her disrupted schooling, took a nurses' training course at St. Joseph's Hospital in Lancaster, and eventually became a supervisor of nurses in one of New York City's largest hospitals. She had succeeded; she had overcome her handicap, but years of frustrated communication and emotional stress could have been avoided had she received this comprehensive and integrated treatment beginning at age two or three, instead of at 16 years of age.

Early Failures

Happily, as we suggested at the opening of this chapter, the faces and voices of today's cleft palate population attest to the progress made in recent decades by surgeons and dentists with the indispensable help of the speech pathologists. This retrospective view of cleft palate management would not be complete, however, without touching upon a few factors I think may explain why the picture was often so discouraging.

Surgery

First, true expertise in oral and plastic surgery was late in developing; it was not until 1941 that plastic surgery became an American Board specialty. Meanwhile many of the cleft lip and palate operations were performed by general surgeons, who had little experience in working with the structures of the mouth. These structures constitute a highly demanding area of the body in which to operate, especially when growth has been interrupted and distorted as in the cleft anomalies. Surgical intervention undertaken at the wrong time with respect to centers of growth, or too extensively, can, as we now know, create more damage than it corrects. It can make the establishment of normal functions—mastication and swallowing, as well as speech—extremely difficult.

It must be said in defense of the surgeons that the vulnerability of the centers of facial growth and their potential for lasting damage if disturbed were not fully understood until around the 1940s. We had begun to suspect the cause of serious postsurgical distortions in some of the patients who came to us, and in 1949 Thomas A. Graber published a paper in which he concluded that surgery was indeed a principal cause of the more severe deformities he saw in a group of children with cleft lip and palate. This created considerable controversy, and as Ross and Johnston have pointed out, "The result has been a tremendous interest in facial growth and development."[8]

A major difficulty, of course, was that the results of a surgical mistake did not make themselves known until some years after the operation. Bauer, Trusler, and Tondra pointed out this lesson when, in discussing their own change of technique in the repositioning of the premaxilla in cleft cases, they stated: "Procedures that produce good initial results often fail to stand the test of time and growth. This fact makes mandatory the constant reevaluation of results so that errors can be discovered and remedied. This prevents succeeding patients from suffering the same fate."[1]

Medicine and Dentistry

Another situation that often prevented the child with a cleft palate from receiving prompt and effective care was the professional rift between physicians and dentists. This had a historical basis going back to around 1840, when the first formal dental schools were established in this country. The training of doctors and dentists became separated even though the schools were units of the same university. (Many dentists continued for some decades to learn their skills on a less formal basis.)

William J. Gies, a Columbia University professor of biological chemistry who became a leader in the dental education field, deplored this schism as he found it in a five-year survey of dental education in the United States and Canada that he made for the Carnegie Foundation for the Advancement of Teaching. In his 1926 report Gies, who was a good friend of mine, noted that few medical schools offered courses in oral hygiene, oral surgery, or dentistry, and he stated: "Owing to the failure of both physicians and dentists to recognize the fact that the primary objectives of dentistry and of medicine are identical—to keep people well—there has been very little practical cooperation between bodies representing the two professions." Arguing that dentistry "is quite as significant for the maintenance of health as some of the accredited specialties in medical practice," Gies recommended that it "should no longer be ignored in the medical schools and its main health service features should be given suitable attention in the training of general practitioners of medicine." He suggested that dentistry should either be made an accredited specialty in conventional medicine or made "fully equal" to such a specialty in grade of health service. "Antagonism between medicine and dentistry cannot be explained," he wrote, "on any basis of public interest or advantage and has no justification in any sentiments that are worthy of respect, for both professions are agencies for health service and cannot render it faithfully on any other conditions than those of earnest and effective cooperation."[6]

The antagonism has softened somewhat in the 50 years since Gies made his report, and the split has narrowed, but his recommendations regarding education have not been implemented. In spite of laudable efforts in a few university centers to develop programs to bring dentistry and medicine closer together, wholehearted and effective cooperation is still hard to find. Dental students still don't learn very much general medicine, and medical students don't learn enough about the teeth and their supporting tissues. As a consequence, certain health problems that require understanding and attention by both professions are often neglected.

School Health Examinations

Nowhere is this hiatus more obvious than in preparation for dealing with malocclusion and cleft palate. It is my opinion, after peering into thousands of mouths, that many oral conditions are overlooked and neglected by the existing methods of medical and health examinations, especially those offered in the public schools. Moreover, physical examinations in schools, no matter how thorough, can only improve the child's health if the findings are acted upon. As I observed in a paper a few years ago, we lack the power to enforce the health recommendations, though we can apparently command obedience to less important regulations. "A child with dirty hands or face may be sent home from school and told not to return until he is clean," I once commented. "However, that is not true so far as the mouth and teeth are concerned. Unfortunately, many of these children stay right on and are examined year after year while their mouths remain neglected, until the boys at least are eligible for the Armed Forces, where they are finally cared for, to the extent that it is possible under those circumstances."[3] A measure of the degree of early neglect was seen in records of World War II showing that 90.3 per cent of the Army, Navy, and Air Force inductees, men only a few years out of public school, had dental disease. Some 8000 dental treatments were required per 1000 men, including restorations, surgical procedures, and full or partial dentures.[3]

While such neglect is to be deplored on general health and esthetic grounds, it is even more lamentable if speech is impaired, as in some types of malocclusion and in cleft palate. It is strangely inconsistent, for example, that children, even in tax-supported programs for crippled children, are often receiving speech therapy while nothing is being done to correct the horrible conditions in their mouths. A typical case was a youngster I saw with a severe malocclusion, extensive caries, and aggravated periodontal disease, who was being given regular speech therapy. Providing speech lessons when such conditions are present—especially the malocclusion—is like giving a boy trumpet lessons on a trumpet whose valves are stuck.[3] We have also seen children taking speech lessons in a speech clinic when they were afflicted with a severe lateral lisp which should first have been treated by an orthodontist.

Prostheses and Benefits

There is still evidence that some government health units and third party payment groups do not understand or recognize the rehabilitative importance of certain dental services. Individuals with cleft palate or other facial defects—including those following cancer surgery—have great difficulty collecting reimbursement for prosthetic appliances that are essential to their normal function and appearance. The reason in most cases is simply that such appliances are usually provided by prosthodontists, who are members of the dental profession, whereas the insurance administrators and rule makers are apt to be medically oriented.

Your Medicare Handbook (1977), though directed to older people, contains passages typical of the kind of exclusion encountered by cleft palate patients, and since many facial cancer patients are in the over-sixty-five category, some of the Medicare rules apply directly to them. The *Handbook* states that "medical insurance can help pay for dental care only if it involved surgery of the jaw or related structures or setting fractures of the jaw or facial bones."[11] Since surgery of the palate does involve the jaw or related structures, it would be covered, but when it comes to paying for rehabilitation, the rules are different. Under the heading "Prosthetic Devices," the handbook has this to say: "Medical insurance helps pay for prosthetic devices needed to substitute for internal body organs. These include, for example, heart pacemakers, corrective lenses needed after cataract operations, and colostomy or ileostomy bags and certain related supplies. Medical insurance can also help pay for artificial limbs and eyes, and for arm, leg, back and neck braces. Orthopedic shoes are covered only when they are part of leg braces. *Dental plates or other dental devices are not covered.*"[11] (Emphasis mine.)

Speech appliances, designed and constructed by prosthodontists and laboratory technicians working under their direction, are usually classified as "dental devices," especially if they contain one or more teeth, and can therefore be ruled not compensable. In other words, these insurance groups will help you see and walk, but they won't help you talk.

Some of the insurance groups have broadened their coverage on these points within the last few years. Blue Cross authorities, asked about coverage of cleft palate rehabilitation, say that "it all depends on what type of contract the family has," but Blue Cross has in many cases refused to pay for speech appliances that were required following surgery for cleft palate or for facial or oral cancer. In my view it is utterly inconsistent and indefensible to allow payment to the surgeon for an operation that leaves a partially closed defect, and not permit payment for an appliance or restoration to complete the repair and restore function. (Patients at our Clinic are offered advice on insurance matters by our social service staff; this is discussed in the chapter on social work.)

H. K. COOPER INSTITUTE

Most of my attention, up to this point, has been devoted to developments and problems that have marked the recent history of cleft palate management in general, and to the history and philosophical approach of our own Clinic in particular. In the balance of this chapter I shall summarize briefly the Clinic's current pattern of operation. This will serve to introduce the much more thorough treatment of the various subjects, including not only clinical programs but growth, genetics, and research, to be presented by my colleagues in the chapters that follow.

Counseling at Birth

We have repeatedly emphasized the need to treat the whole child and not just a hole in the roof of his or her mouth. This is a philosophy that must be followed from the very moment of birth, and in its broadest sense, treatment must reach out to include the mother and the father, for unless cleft lip or palate is known to be present in the family background, the parents will be totally unprepared for it. No prenatal test is available to give a warning, as in certain other congenital conditions; the birth generally comes as a profound shock, especially to the mother. One minute her baby is inside her body, presumably healthy and normal; the next moment it is outside and she finds herself looking down at a pitifully deformed little face, or if the lip is not involved, she will soon be confronted by the palatal defect. It is at this time that she is most in need of psychological support from her obstetrician and pediatrician, and later from others. They must help her accept the child, while at the same time reassuring her that all is not as bad as it seems and that much can be done in due time to correct the defects and to minimize their consequences.

This is why, when I am asked what is the first thing to be done when a child is born with cleft palate, I reply: "Feed the child and treat the mother." Sucking is difficult, and the milk flows up into the nasal cavity and out the nose. In fact, a gush of milk from the nose may, in infants without a cleft lip, be the first signal that cleft palate is present. The feeding problems are usually less serious than the mother assumes, however, and much can be done through therapeutic counseling to alleviate her fears.

Breast-Feeding

She should be encouraged to breast-feed her baby if it is at all possible. This is desirable not only from the nutritional standpoint, but more important, it will strengthen the emotional bond between mother and child in a situation in which this bond is in danger of being impaired by the mother's ambivalent feeling toward her defective child.

If for some reason breast-feeding is not advisable and the bottle is employed instead, the mother is apt to be concerned that the infant will choke while taking it, but there is seldom need for alarm. When choking does occur, it is usually momentary and is the result of overfeeding, or of feeding too rapidly. It can also be caused by milk striking the back of the throat. All these causes can be avoided. The nipple opening should be just large enough to permit the milk to flow freely, but not so large that it will run out too fast when the bottle is inverted. Most infants with cleft lip and palate learn to hold the nipple against the side of the palate as they squeeze the milk out, and this prevents it from gushing against the back of the palate. Proper positioning of the child is important: the mother should cradle the baby in her arm in a semisitting posture, with the infant's body upright and tilted slightly backward.

In some instances it is helpful to use the Breck feeder, a bottle that permits the application of positive pressure. A nipple with attached flaps or wings to prevent leakage from the baby's cleft lip is also available. In our experience we have seen little need for the latter device, except on rare occasions when the defect is very large or there has been an accompanying nerve disorder. For the most part the early management of nourishment is focused on getting enough calories into the baby, who may be a slow nurser, without tiring the child or the mother.

Surgery of the Palate

Repair of the hard and soft palate defects is usually not undertaken until the child is 12 or 18 months old. Three goals are kept in mind: first, to help the child speak clearly (this requires a soft palate that is movable and long enough); second, to reestablish the palatal-eustachian tube muscle function, as it is related to normal hearing; and third, to bring about normal dental function and appearance.[10] These multiple aims make it highly important that the team approach be employed in planning the surgery and the subsequent treatment program.

In the Lancaster Clinic many of the specialists are resident staff members on a full- or part-time basis. This makes it easy for the surgeon, orthodontist, and speech pathologist, for example, to exchange views in an informal face-to-face situation. Usually the conference is held after each one has made an examination of the patient, and full use is made of such preliminary studies as x-rays, cineroentgenography, dental casts and face masks, and various speech and hearing tests (see chapter on audiology).

Dr. Harding discusses in his chapter the principles of conservative surgery that have played an important part in achieving good results, and in that connection I would like to call attention to the fact that some of these principles are grounded in Wolff's law of the transformation of bone. About a hundred years ago Julius Wolff, a German anatomist, having observed how the bones of fowl and other animals responded to abnormal pressure, concluded: "Every change in the form or function of a bone or of its function alone is followed by changes in its internal architecture and no less definite alterations in its external conformation in accordance with mathematical laws." Stated more succinctly in Dorland's Illustrated Medical Dictionary: "a bone, normal or abnormal, develops the structure most suited to resist the forces acting upon it." As applied to the cleft lip and cleft palate, especially if the cleft involves the maxilla, this means that a properly repaired lip may help mold the underlying cartilage and bone. The muscles, in other words, may assist by acting as living orthopedic appliances.

Cineroentgenography

One of the most useful technical adjuncts in the evaluation process is cineroentgenography, which for the first time permits thorough observation of the lips, tongue, soft palate, and throat wall during speech and swallowing. Our Clinic was the first, in the mid-1950s, to adapt the newly developed image intensification fluoroscopy to the orofacial area.[10] The Philips tube, patented in 1934, produces an image 1000 times brighter than that of the conventional fluoroscope screen, with only a fraction of the radiation dose. It is therefore possible to take 100 feet of 16-mm. film with no more exposure than is needed to make one four-second x-ray of a single tooth with the average dental x-ray machine.[2]

With the cineradiography equipment we can photograph the dynamic interrelationships of the speech organs on x-ray film, while simultaneously recording the sounds on tape. This enables us to assess with great precision the patient's status and functional progress over a period of time. We can also use the instrument to analyze the development of speech in normal children. In the cleft palate patient and in those with other orofacial anomalies, the technique has helped in determining the kind of surgery required in the velopharyngeal region, as well as in assisting in the design and placing of obturators when these are indicated.

Intimately linked with the assessment of the individual's speech and voice mechanisms is a careful examination of his or her ears and hearing. A person who does not hear all speech sounds is unlikely to reproduce all the sounds, as anyone is aware who has heard a profoundly deaf person talk. We therefore give high priority to the contributions of the audiologist and the otolaryngologist and we make sure that every patient is examined by them. It is well recognized that the child with a cleft of the palate is unusually susceptible to middle ear infections, which if not cleared up can cause temporary and sometimes permanent hearing loss. Since we believe that the diagnosis of speech and hearing disorders must not be limited to the perceptive range of the human ear, we employ electronic aids to help us.

Summer Residence Program

Frequently a patient will come to the Clinic from a long distance, seeking evaluation and advice, and will not be able to remain in Lancaster for extended treatments. It is then our practice to carry out the necessary studies and examinations and refer the patient, with written recommendations, back to specialists in his or her home community. In many instances, however, we suggest periodic return visits to the Clinic for a checkup or for an adjustment of a prosthesis as the child grows.

Much of the Clinic's therapy is administered in the usual outpatient pattern, except for the surgery, which is performed in Harrisburg or Hershey. For those who live too far away for Clinic visits, we have been providing a summer residence program of eight weeks, another innovation in the cleft palate program for which our Clinic can claim credit. The children live in a dormitory next door to the Clinic and are supervised by resident counselors. My mother, the late Caroline Amanda Cooper, was housemother for the first 10 years. Speech lessons are arranged on both an individual and class basis, the groups being organized according to age and ability. Also offered are school subjects, taught by certified teachers, and various enrichment activities, such as games, sports, and other recreation. The children may spend weekends at home or receive visits from their parents. Not only do they benefit in terms of improved speech, but they also become much more comfortable in social situations, including the normal boy-girl relationships so many had missed in school. Many have progressed so rapidly in eight weeks that upon their return to regular school they have been at the head of their class. (Further details on the residency program appear in the chapter on communication.)

Rehabilitation of Cancer Patients

Our major attention has been on cleft lip and palate and upon velopharyngeal insufficiency, but our oral and plastic surgeons have also been correcting mandibular dystrophies to bring about more acceptable appearance, dental occlusion, and speech. And many older people who have undergone mutilating operations for orofacial cancer have been fitted at the Clinic with prosthetic replacements to cover the defect. When needed, speech appliances and speech lessons have also been provided. I recall one of the first patients referred to us with this problem, a woman whose facial cancer had been removed five years before we saw her. The defect was so extensive and disfiguring that she had refused to leave her house all that time. She practically lived in her kitchen. But there were two things she wanted to do: go to the five-and-ten-cent store and attend Sunday school. We prepared a prosthesis that filled in the facial defect and made her presentable, and she was overjoyed to be able to go out in the neighborhood again. More recently a middle-aged secretary underwent surgery that removed much of the left side of her face, including the orbit. A restoration was made, including an artificial eye, and she was able to return to her job.

The Clinic assists in the rehabilitation of those who have had the larynx removed for cancer and who as a result have become voiceless. Some 9000 men and women experience this misfortune every year, according to the International Association of Laryngectomees, which is associated with the American Cancer Society. A laryngectomee, Walter C. Herr, certified as an instructor by the Association, is employed at our Clinic to teach esophageal speech. Those who cannot master this method or who find it unacceptable are offered a choice of pneumatic or electronic speech aids, including the Cooper-Rand electronic instrument that I developed some years ago.

Interdisciplinary Research

Much of our research program, directed by Dr. Krogman, is, like our clinical program, interdisciplinary in nature. Krogman, a specialist in growth, has been working with Harding, a plastic surgeon, and Mazaheri, a prosthodontist, in analyzing the effect of surgical intervention on the growth curve of children. In short, they have concluded that conservative surgery, as contrasted with earlier procedures that disturbed the centers of facial growth, permits the child to attain a normal dentofacial complex by the time he or she is six years old. Other growth studies have measured the effect of the surgical insertion of a pharyngeal flap, at different ages, upon the child's spontaneous speech. They determined that it is preferable to delay the operation until the age of six.

In the field of genetics Seishi W. Oka, who is also a dentist, now has a computer terminal in his laboratory that permits him to exchange genetic data with scientists in other centers. His studies will aid him in testing the "multifactorial hypothesis" of the genetics of clefts, and in the all-important genetic counseling that he provides to patients and their families at the Clinic. Research that has immediate clinical significance is also being conducted by Elca T. Swigart in audiology and by Philip Starr and Kitty Heiserman in the social service department.

In all of these projects the cooperation of patients is essential. Over the years we have enlisted some five hundred patients in what we call a longitudinal series that permits examination and specific studies at regular intervals. In nearly four decades of helping men, women, and children with speech problems, the Clinic has accumulated a large file of patient records—and recollections. The records are in the form of diagnostic and progress notes, details of operations, photographs, x-rays, dental casts, cineroentgenography and sonography films, disc or tape recordings of voices before and after speech rehabilitation, and letters from patients and parents.

Many of these records extend back over 20 or 30 years in the life of an individual. Combined with the continuity within our own staff, these contacts with people we have come to know well have imparted, I believe, a high degree of reliability to our observations. Such contacts have helped afford us the privilege of seeing how well these individuals have overcome their physical and behavioral handicaps and how they have grown to become well-integrated personalities, able to hold their own in a highly communicative world.

We do not claim to have achieved 100 per cent perfection in all of our endeavors, but we believe our score has been a good one, and we hope this account of our philosophy and our program will prove valuable to others facing the same challenges.

References

1. Bauer, T. B., H. M. Trusler, and J. M. Tondra. *In* Grabb, W. C., S. W. Rosenstein, and K. R. Bzoch (eds.): Cleft Lip and Palate: Surgical, Dental, and Speech Aspects, Boston, Little, Brown, p. 311, 1971.
2. Cooper, H. K.: Cinefluorography with image intensification as an aid in treatment planning for some cleft lip and/or palate cases. Am. J. Orthod., *42*:819, 1956.
3. Cooper, H. K.: Recent trends in the management of oral-facial and speech handicaps. Am. J. Orthod., *49*:683, 1963.
4. Cooper, H. K.: Ministry of service. Am. J. Orthod., *52*:606, 1966.
5. Eby, J. D.: Maximum improvement in congenital orofacial clefts, Editorial. Am. J. Orthod., *42*:867, 1956.
6. Gies, W. J.: Dental Education in the United States and Canada, New York, The Carnegie Foundation for the Advancement of Teaching, pp. 5–10, 1926.
7. Parkins, F. M., and G. J. Barbero. *In* Vaughan, V. C., and R. J. McKay (eds.): Nelson Textbook of Pediatrics, Philadelphia, W. B. Saunders Co., p. 762, 1969.
8. Ross, R. B., and M. C. Johnston: Cleft Lip and Palate, Baltimore, Williams & Wilkins, p. 158, 1972.
9. Schurter, M.: Foreword to special issue on clefts of lip and palate. J. Am. Med. Wom. Assoc., *21*:895, 1966.
10. Team Management for the Cleft Lip and Palate Patient, Lancaster, Pa., Lancaster Cleft Palate Clinic, pp. 11, 26, 38–39, 1974.
11. Your Medicare Handbook. Department of Health, Education, and Welfare, Pub. No. (SSA) 76–10050, Washington, D.C., Government Printing Office, pp. 26 and 32, 1976.

Chapter Two

CRANIOFACIAL EMBRYOGENESIS

EVOLUTIONARY BACKGROUND

The cleft palate has a history—or better, a potential—extending back at least 200 million years to the evolutionary transition from the Reptilia to the Mammalia. At this time a bony partition arose to separate the oral and nasal cavities and to keep distinct the functions of food ingestion and respiration. The reptiles had an incomplete hard palate which was fenestrated, but the mammals achieved a solid and complete hard palate, one that would become vulnerable to the incomplete closure that we call a cleft. Today this embryological defect occurs in a number of orders of Mammalia.

If we are to trace the origin of cleft palate to the development of bone, we must go back at least 570 million years, at which time a mineralized skeleton first appeared in a number of different forms of life, and the basic vertebrate skeletal pattern was begun. The primary structural and functional vertebrate axes or gradients were head to tail (cephalocaudad), back to front (dorsoventral), and midline to side (mediolateral). There was a long, flexible vertebral column built around a primitive axial stiffening (the notochord) and the body was bilaterally symmetrical and segmented, though such segmentation was not clearly discernible in the head region, which was located at the anterior end of the body as a housing for functional sensorimotor coordination. In the fishes the body was organized posteriorly for the propulsive tail. The brain was housed in the head, with the spinal cord dorsal in position and surrounded by neural (vertebral) arches. The gut was ventral in position, anterior to the vertebral column, and ran from oral opening to anus. The total oropharyngeal region was housed within the rigid bars of the gill arches, and there were at first no jaws as such, for feeding was via filtering through the gills.

In this discussion our area of concern is the head, which may be logically considered as an integral and interrelated part of the total organism, and which will adapt, as circumstances dictate, to all functional changes in body structure or form.

The foregoing, then, is the functional and structural organization of all vertebrate life from the fishes and reptiles and on into the mammals—a "basic patent" in nature, to use William King Gregory's term. It is the framework inherited and adapted by all Mammals, including Man. Within the total "basic patent" was another and lesser one, the vertebrate skull, giving support to the brain and its special sense organ systems. The oral cavity was at first a small prepharyngeal vestibule. In the pharynx were the laterally placed

CRANIOFACIAL GROWTH: PRENATAL AND POSTNATAL

WILTON M. KROGMAN

gill pouches (gill clefts), which were oval in shape and braced by gill arch struts that developed independently from the central axial skeleton. The entire ororespiratory complex was shaped like a horizontal "V," i.e., the V was on its side with its wide part opening anteriorly. The surrounding musculature acted as pumps, carrying water through the gills and serving the dual functions of respiration and feeding: oxygenated water flowed over the gills and particles of food were withheld in the foregut.

The gill arch musculature gave rise to the cranial base–branchial arch joint at the apex of the V. As the most anterior gill arches, which bordered the "mouth," grasped larger food particles, grabbing "jaws" arose, so that the upper arm of the horizontal V became an upper jaw, the lower arm a lower jaw. In time a toughened skin invaginated the two arms of the V-shaped jaws and formed teeth.

The earliest rigid support for the head structures was cartilaginous bone. This bone had been preformed in deeply placed cartilage which arose near the axial skeleton and gave support to the anterior viscera. These curved sup-

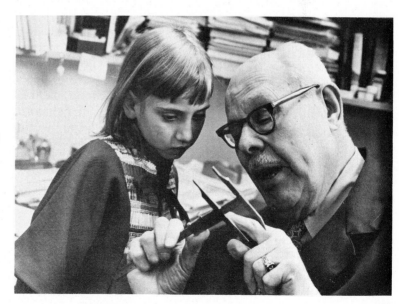

Dr. Krogman explaining use of calipers to a child.

porting structures are called visceral, branchial, or gill arches. Soon there appeared intramembranous bone of dermal origin, which was always near the surface. The earliest fishes, for example, had a craniofacial carapace made up of many dermal bones. In this way there was achieved a vertebrate craniofacial complex formed by the two solid units of a brain case with an enclosed upper jaw joined to a compound lower jaw. This resulted in an outer dermal bone covering and an inner cartilaginous foundation. The cartilage element for the upper jaw was derived from the reptilian structure that related the palatal complex to the jaw joint: the palatoquadrate cartilage. The cartilage element for the lower jaw was Meckel's cartilage.

We may view the bony development in the skull of the Reptilia (the immediate precursors of the Mammalia) as a helmet-like dermal carapace which extended down the sides of the skull to the upper jaw edges, where it housed marginal rows of teeth. There were openings only for the nostrils and eyes, and a notch at the back of the ear opening. The dermal bones extended anteriorly to the roof of the mouth, covering the cartilage bones of the brain case and the upper jaw to form the early elements of the primary palate, i.e., that anterior portion of the palate (the premaxilla) which housed the upper incisors; the lower jaw was also housed in dermal bones. The posterior part of the palate (maxilla and palatine bones) formed what may be called the secondary palate, which would contain the canine, premolar, and molar teeth of mammals. At first the reptilian teeth were simple interlocking cones held in the premaxillary and maxillary bones of the upper jaw, and the dentary bone of the lower jaw. The jaw joint was formed by bones of cartilaginous origin: in the upper jaw the hind end of the palatoquadrate cartilage ossified as the quadrate; in the lower jaw the hind end of Meckel's cartilage ossified as the articulare. From the muscle mass lodged in the temporal fossae under the cranial roof, the movers of the joint developed.

The evolution of the reptilian skull to the mammalian skull entailed certain logical and adaptive changes: the posterior portion of the palate, or secondary palate, developed to completely separate the oral and nasal cavities; the premolars and molars became multicusped, replacing the single-cusped reptilian teeth; the zygomatic arches enlarged, bowing outward, to serve larger adductor muscles of the jaw; many dermal bones disappeared, and the dentary bone dominated the lower jaw, establishing articular contact with the squamous portion of the temporal bone to give rise to the temporomandibular joint (TMJ); and the older jaw joint formed by the quadrate and articulare bones persisted as the auditory ossicles, the malleus and the incus. This evolution of the skull involved not only the development of a hard palate, but a far-reaching series of changes in the dentition and the entire jaw, face, and skull architecture. It is important to realize that all these adaptive changes were interrelated, so that the evolution of the mammalian craniofacial complex was a "package deal."

There is a maxim that to a degree "ontogeny recapitulates phylogeny" — more popularly, "every form climbs its own family tree." This is not the place to argue the potency of the evolutionary adaptive thrust, but it *is* the place to note that there are certain basic structural and functional elements or complexes that *must* be taken as part of a common vertebrate-mammalian heritage when we consider human craniofacial development. In considering palatal clefts, we may argue that palatal closure (or completeness) is an age-old heritage, a *norm* that has persisted for over 200 million years. We may permit ourselves to observe that in man palatal closure is epigenetic, in the sense that such closure is genetically governed by an age-old mammalian gene complex. Man's palate closes not because he is human, but because of his mammalian ancestry.

EMBRYOGENESIS IN MAN

When this book was first planned, we had no doubt that the inclusion of a discussion of embryonic development was necessary in order to understand the phenomena of clefts. Moreover, such a discussion was necessary for the interpretation of our genetic data and the understanding of the processes of structural and functional development, both in the circumstances of clefting and in normal craniofacial development. Because we have no professional embryologist on the Cooper Institute staff, we must rely completely upon the research of others. In presenting this part of our book we acknowledge our indebtedness to Avery,[1] Burdi,[4, 5] Humphrey,[11] Johnston,[15] Patten,[24] Ross and Johnston,[25] and Stark.[31] In essence, we shall present a synthesis of the concepts and data provided by these researchers.

Fourth to Sixth Week

Avery has provided a summary of the human face and neck area at the fourth week after conception.[1] The areas under the forebrain are segmented and the five branchial arches are seen as tubular enlargements, bounded and defined by clefts and grooves. In part, the mid- and lower face arise from the first (mandibular) and second (hyoid) arches, while the third arch will contribute to the base of the tongue. Within each branchial arch there will develop skeletal, muscular, vascular, connective tissue, epithelial, and neural elements.

In his study of amphibian embryos Johnston has made certain observations that he feels are applicable to mammalian development as well.[15] Facial processes and visceral arches are formed principally from mesenchyme, which is loosely organized embryonic tissue from which skeletal and connective tissues are formed. Mesenchyme is formed by migrating cells derived from the ectoderm of neural crest cells which are found in folds at the margins of the neural plate. The importance of this finding is that for most of the body the mesenchyme is derived from mesoderm, whereas in the head region most of it is derived from ectoderm. The crest mesenchyme initially forms all tissues between the overlying epithelium and the underlying forebrain and eye in the upper facial region, i.e., the frontonasal and maxillary processes.

In the sixth week two small oval elevations appear, above and lateral to the future mouth; within 48 hours the elevations become depressions which will be the nostrils, and the tissue around them will form the bridge and wings of the nose. Between the nasal pits or potential nostrils arises the medial nasal process, and lateral to the nasal pits arise the lateral nasal processes. The tissue below each nostril represents the first separation of the oral and nasal cavities and is the primary palate. This very early-formed structure includes the prolabium, the premaxilla and its four incisor teeth, and the cartilaginous septum. In mammals the primary palate is formed in two phases. First, the epithelium of the olfactory pit tunnels back through the mesenchyme to make contact with the roof of the primitive oral cavity, and spaces within this epithelium form the initial nasal passage: in this manner an isthmus of epithelially covered mesenchyme bridges the medial and lateral nasal processes. Second, there is a migration of mesenchymal cells, mostly from the maxillary process, that enlarges the isthmus and consolidates the primary palate.

Cleft Lip. In this two-phase process, failure of the lining of the olfactory pits to make contact with that of the oral cavity may lead to a form of choanal atresia or failure of the nasal passages to open posteriorly into the throat, and failures of mesenchymal consolidation of the isthmus will result in a cleft lip (with or without cleft palate). The sixth week is the critical time for lip cleft-ing. It is thought that complete cleft lip arises when the epithelial fusion of the swellings around the nasal pocket does not occur and a primary cleft formation arises in the embryonic face. A simple cleft lip is developed when the epithe-lial fusion process ceases prematurely and the epithelial wall is too short as it comes into the nasal cavity. In this sense, such a cleft is an early-arrested phase in epithelial fusion. A cleft lip with bridges occurs when the epithelial wall is laid down defectively and remains beyond the normal time. In this set of circumstances persistence of the isthmus or tissue bridge in the cleft lip could account for an epithelial remnant known as Simonart's band.

According to Stark, absence of mesoderm in the lip and premaxilla is a factor in the development of a cleft in these structures: "Lack or even diminu-tion in mesoderm will lead to the formation of a cleft in the area that is meso-derm-poor."[31] There is an initial epithelial anlage in the region that is to be-come the lip, within which are one central and two lateral masses of meso-derm, and if any of this is absent or deficient, the epithelial wall will be thinned and a cleft will develop.

The role of the premaxilla is an important one. Stark calls it the "anterior keystone of the hard palate,"[31] with the nasal airway as its superior limit. In the fourth week the nose begins as a pair of concave ectodermal plates just above the epithelial wall of the lip, and deepening occurs to form blind nasal pits, which rupture in the fifth week to form the posterior nasal choanae. Lip and premaxilla develop concurrently, and by the seventh week form a single unit that gives rise, in part, to the primary palate.

In the fourth week there occurs a bending in the region of the future neck, with the ultimate effect that the head is more erect with reference to the total body. The brain has a ventral and a dorsal flexure, and in man this is basically a reflection of our evolution as a biped, which brought with it a bending of the cranial base, a balancing of the skull on the vertebral column, and a steadied horizontal gaze. More local craniofacial adjustments include vaulting of the back of the skull, a bending of the cranial base at sella (which we shall later discuss as the sellar angle), downward and forward movement of the nuchal plane of the occipital bone, forward movement of the foramen magnum and occipital condyles, and backward movement of the entire orofacial complex.

Seventh to Eighth Week

At about the seventh week, subsequent to the development of the nasal pits, facial proportions change, mainly owing to growth lateral to the pits. The forepart of the brain is also expanding, so that the laterally placed maxillary regions move centrally and forward, i.e., the eyes and adjacent cheek tissues are rotated 90 degrees to the front of the face. As a result the medial nasal area forms only a small part of the midportion of the upper lip and is between the maxillary processes; later it will become the philtrum. Now the embryonic face is recognizable as human: the eyes are frontal; the nose is differentiated; and the mandible is a larger entity. With increased facial height the nostrils are no longer on the same horizontal level with the eyes. The furrows (clefts) separating the nasal, mandibular, and maxillary areas are less distinct. External ears are visible and they will be fully formed by the sixteenth week.

At this point in embryogenic time the anterior facial and palatal structures are pretty well differentiated: the lip and primary palate are an integral unit; and the nasal structures for olfaction, the optic area for vision, the maxillary-zygomatic complex for muscular buttressing, and the mandible for reciprocal action with the maxilla are all structurally and functionally interrelated. The tongue also has a place in the facial-palatal complex. Early in the fourth week the tongue had developed from occipital muscular segments and had then grown forward as two major portions: the body, or oral part, from the first branchial arch; and the base, or pharyngeal part, from the second, third, and fourth branchial arches. By the seventh week the body to base proportions are such that the central area is relatively small and the lateral lingual swellings relatively large. The lateral border of the tongue is now separated from the developing alveolar ridges and the tongue is a fast-growing unit, pushing into the nasal cavity and between the two laterally placed palatal shelves. By the eighth to ninth weeks the tongue muscles are differentiated.

In Figure 2–1 is shown a summation up to this point. Patten offers a series of more or less schematic drawings showing, in frontal view, what he calls "some of the important steps" in the development of the human prenatal face. The period covered is four to eight weeks (3.5 mm. to 28 mm.), and by the eighth week the face is recognizably human.

The stage is now set for the completion of the drama of the bony palate: the primary palate is to be joined by the secondary palate so that oral and nasal cavities are completely separated. In a sense, therefore, in the seventh to eighth weeks of embryogenesis (ontogeny) we are at the reptile to mammal evolutionary stage (phylogeny). The human palatal-oral complex will achieve its mammalian destiny!

As noted earlier, the tongue, in enlarging, had pushed between bilaterally placed palatal shelves, which are the medial portions of the bilateral maxillary processes and, according to Stark,[31] are composed of mesoderm surfaced by ectoderm. In early growth the tongue positions itself in the oronasal cavity prior to the growth spurt of the laterally positioned palatal shelves. The shelves must then necessarily grow toward the floor of the oral cavity, where, owing to limited space, they become oriented in a vertical position on either side of the tongue.

Then in the seventh and eighth weeks several coordinated and time-linked things happen: the tongue recedes from the oronasal cavity and the palatal shelves rotate or roll over the tongue, moving from the position beside it to one above it. The shelves become horizontal above the tongue and immediately begin to grow toward the midline and one another, as though two horizontal sliding doors were closing at the center. (See Figures 2–2 and 2–3.)

Palatal Closure. It is probable that the initiation of palatal closure occurs when the fetus is 29 to 33 mm. crown-rump length and 47 to 49 days of ovulational age. Some hold that "closure" means the touching of the palatal plates at any place along the palatal plane, but others define complete closure as ac-

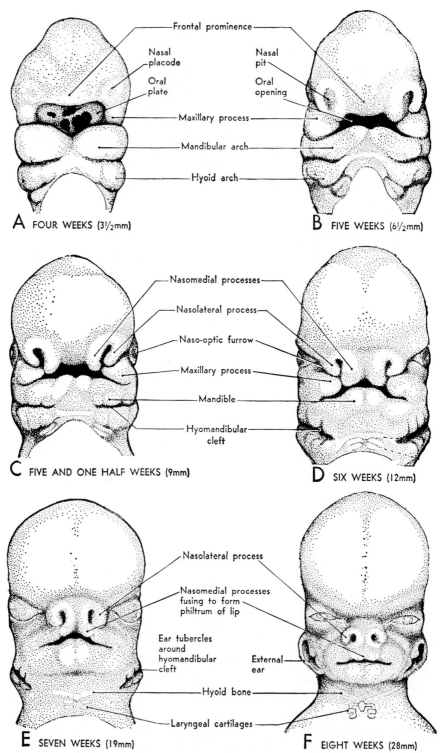

FIGURE 2–1 Frontal aspect, major steps in the formation of the face. (From Morris: Morris' Human Anatomy. *In* Patten, B. M.: Human Embryology, 3rd ed. Copyright © 1968 by McGraw-Hill, Inc. Used by permission of McGraw-Hill Book Company.)

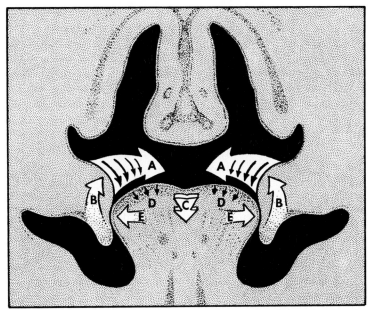

FIGURE 2–2 Movements of palatal shelves and tongue during palatal closure. Tongue moves anteriorly (C), depressing downward (D), and laterally (E), as the palatal shelves slide from B to A over the tongue and below the nasal septum. (From Avery, J. K.: Prenatal facial growth. *In* Moyers, R. E.: Handbook of Orthodontics, 3rd ed., Chicago, Year Book Medical Publishers, 1973.)

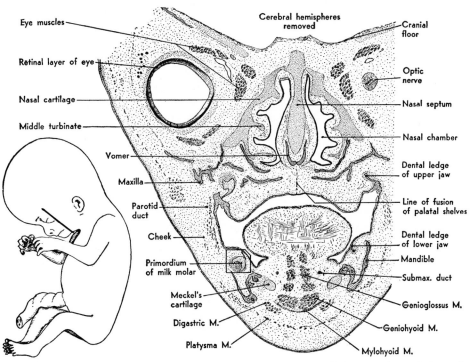

FIGURE 2–3 Projection drawing (×10) of section through jaws of human embryo of eleventh week, crown-rump length (CRL) 58 mm. Left outline shows actual size of embryo, with line across jaws showing location of section. (Small polygon around milk molar delineates area of higher magnification, not shown here.) (From University of Michigan Collection, EH198. *In* Patten, B. M.: Human Embryology, 3rd ed. Copyright © 1968 by McGraw-Hill, Inc. Used by permission of McGraw-Hill Book Company.)

tual fusion of the shelves to one another along their entire length. In some fetuses it was found that interpalatal shelf space was open posteriorly as late as the tenth week. It seems that the movement of the palatal processes generally occurs within the short period of a few days, and that fusion proceeds rapidly once the shelves are elevated.

According to Stark,[31] there is a very interesting reversal of direction in this development: elevation of the shelves begins at the back and proceeds toward the front (dorsoventral) of the oronasal cavity; fusion, complete by the twelfth week, begins at the front and proceeds toward the back (ventrodorsal).* The result is, of course, a completed bony palate and a 100 per cent separation of the oral and nasal cavities – in essence, the true mammalian condition has been achieved.

The statement just made suggests a teleological explanation of normal palatal fusion as part of a mammalian phylogenetic heritage. One could argue that the palatal shelves were destined to meet and fuse in the midline. Stark hints at this when he uses the term "shelf force," implying an intrinsic medialward movement, whether by growth at free shelf margins or by a medialward directive or compressive force of the entire maxillary process of which the shelf is the medial part.

It has been suggested on the basis of studies on mice that there may be an inherent tissue factor in shelf elevation, a developing network of fibers that act as a directive force as they are placed under tension by growth within the shelves themselves. It has been pointed out, however, that in general embryonic development elastic fibers appear later than do collagen fibers (sixteenth and eleventh weeks, respectively); hence, there are no differentiated fibers in the embryo at the time of palatal shelf movement, i.e., at the time of secondary palate formation.

Sensorimotor Stimulus and Response.   Apart from arguing for an epigenetic closure coding, we may look to a more evident set of factors, such as an early sensorimotor stimulus-response complex. The earliest reflex to develop in the facial area is the opening of the mouth at eight to nine weeks; initially this mouth reflex is part of the total head and trunk lateral flexion reflex pattern. It is important to note that the mandibular movements involved in the opening of the mouth do not depend on the presence of the temporomandibular joint. On this point Humphrey avers that the differentiation of the joint after jaw reflexes begin "indicates that the movement of the mandible contributes to the normal development of this joint."[11]

It may be argued that the response of the paraoral structures to stimuli will begin related structural and functional movements. Thus, tongue pressure exerted in a reflex swallowing action may facilitate a medialward movement of the palatal shelves, i.e., a neurological cheek and tongue reciprocal relationship may be brought into play. There are other, more gross movements that may have a trigger effect, such as the bringing of the head and neck region into a more vertical alignment with the body. At about the same time the descent of the heart into the thorax provides room for a lowered tongue in a less crowded oral cavity (at this time our heart was literally in our mouth). Head

---

*There is a suggestive analogy in the development of the neurophysiological function gradient in human limbs, proximal to distal (cephalocaudad). However, in terms of bony epiphyseal union – which is maturation – the gradient is distal to proximal (caudocephalad).[23] This seems to indicate an intriguing contrast between the potential of function and its achievement and use. It is interesting that this is found in the craniofacial and in the appendicular complexes.

and mouth movements, especially the elevation of the mandible, may have played a role in this repositioning.

Another factor affecting the palatal area is the vascular supply. In the seventh and eighth weeks branchial arch vessels give rise to the external and internal carotid arteries. During the sixth week the stapedial artery, arising from the internal carotid, supplies the midface, but in the seventh week it is cut off from the internal carotid. At the same time the branches to the maxilla and mandible of the internal carotid join with adjacent facial branches of the external carotid. Obviously, the timing of this transition in blood supply is critical, and the processes of palatal shelf closure must be related to the change.

The entire palate does not unite simultaneously. In the secondary palate, posterior to the primary palate, closure results in the disappearance of the mid-line space between the right and left palate shelves. The anterior palatine foramen and the maxillary and premaxillary contact margins will persist as the boundary between primary and secondary palates. As bone forms in the palate, sutures will come into being, providing for important growth expansion of the palate.

Bony Supporting Structures. Johnston points out that the dual origin of skeletal tissues in the craniofacial region may explain certain unusual developmental phenomena.[15] As an example, he cites a family showing defective formation of crest-derived (ectodermal) bone while the mesodermally derived bone is relatively normal. This suggests a specific induction mechanism in bone formation from neural crest cells, while the induction of other crest derivatives (e.g., portions of the teeth) and induction of bone derived from the mesoderm appear to be normal. We might add that bone preformed in cartilage and bone of dermal origin appear to be under differential and selective genetic and endocrinic control. Examples of genetic control may be seen in Down's syndrome, achondroplasia, and cleidocranial dysostosis (the clavicle and cranium are *both* of intramembranous origin). An example of endocrinic control is seen in the growth inhibition of bone of cartilaginous origin in congenital hypothyroidism.

The basic bony elements in the developing skull are truly craniofacial, for they arise to support first the brain, then the face. The elements are all on the midline, and have been referred to as "a bar of cartilage" extending from the nasal area to the foramen magnum. This bar is the major element in the chondrocranium. The anterior portion supports the anterior facial area and is a factor in its growth; it has an early fibrous attachment to the premaxilla. It has been said that this cartilaginous bar doubles its size by 10 to 14 weeks, triples it by 17 weeks, and is six times as large by 36 weeks. Anteriorly it forms the nasal capsule, which has a medial septal component (perpendicular plate) and two lateral cartilaginous wings; posteriorly this bar forms the sella turcica, and most posteriorly the occipital cartilage, from which portions of the sphenoid, temporal, and occipital bones will arise. The cranial base will begin to ossify by the eighth week, and the ethmoid will arise from the nasal capsule. The several skeletal elements of the chondrocranium are separated by synchondroses which will provide for growth and expansion of the cranial base.

Humphrey states that after the eighth week, i.e., after the palatal shelves have come together to form the secondary palate, the mandible grows more rapidly than does the maxilla, and as a result the previously retrognathic mandible becomes, for a while, orthognathic or even mildly prognathic. This situation may be related to one or a combination of time-linked developments: (1) the repositioning of the tongue in the floor of the mouth; (2) the appearance of the cranial flexure; and (3) the movements of the jaw and the contact of the tongue with the oral mucosa, which may lead to an increased blood supply in the mandibular area as the condyle reaches the glenoid fossa (though the evidence is inconclusive).

Pharynx and Soft Palate.   Along with the cartilaginous and bony supporting structures must be considered the pharynx, which is located within the nasopharyngeal area of the craniofacial complex. The embryonic evidence suggests that the pharynx grows differentially and that it elongates with the caudal displacement of its branchial skeletal supports. The pharyngeal airway maintains a fairly constant form that is related to the relative stability of the mandible and the relative mobility of the thyroid cartilage and hyoid bone (with development the latter move progressively lower in relation to the cranial base and the mandible). It is enlarged anteroposteriorly via the adjustive balancing of the head and neck on the vertebral column.

The soft palate develops from the displacement of epithelium by mesenchyme, and not as a result of the epithelial fusion of the processes of secondary palatal fusion; therefore, it arises relatively independently of the hard palate.[6]

Overview of Cleft Factors

In the development of clefts there are two major sets of possible factors, which may be termed structural and functional. The former category has to do mainly with the interrelated *form* of the parts of the cranial-facial-palatal complex, the latter with the *manner* in which the palatal processes behave as they move together. If we were to put into schematic form the various etiological data for clefts, they might be organized somewhat like this:

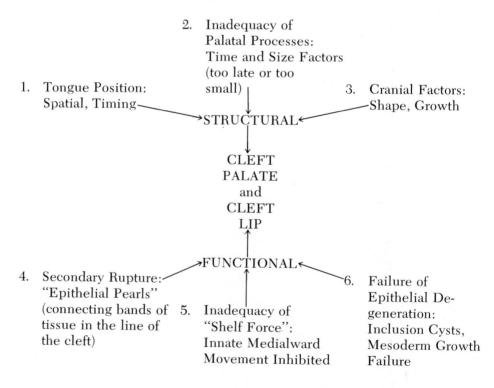

2. Inadequacy of
    Palatal Processes:
    Time and Size Factors
    (too late or too
    small)

1. Tongue Position:
    Spatial, Timing

3. Cranial Factors:
    Shape, Growth

STRUCTURAL

CLEFT
PALATE
and
CLEFT
LIP

FUNCTIONAL

4. Secondary Rupture:
    "Epithelial Pearls"
    (connecting bands of
    tissue in the line of
    the cleft)

5. Inadequacy of
    "Shelf Force":
    Innate Medialward
    Movement Inhibited

6. Failure of
    Epithelial De-
    generation:
    Inclusion Cysts,
    Mesoderm Growth
    Failure

1. The tongue may play a part in a delaying action, i.e., a failure of synchrony between descent of the tongue and elevation of the palatal shelf. A delay between cranial flexion and the palatal closure sequence may result in a crowded condition in the oral cavity so that the tongue cannot be sufficiently lowered from between the palatal shelves.

2. It may be argued that the right and left palatal shelves must be wide enough to bridge the mid-line gap they are destined to close. If they are diminished in size, it is possible that the shelves may not have a mid-line meeting, or that they may close too late. Since their origin is in the laterally positioned maxillary processes, which are growing laterally, late closure results in insufficient tissue with which to meet at the midline.

3. It is possible that basal cranial growth, transversely oriented, may increase the mid-line space to be taken up by the opposing shelves. This could happen if the elevation of the shelves were delayed, and during this delay basal cranial growth spread the palatal shelves (or the maxillary processes) apart.

4. The presence of "epithelial pearls" (epithelial remnants) at the margins of the cleft palate has been interpreted as evidence of a secondary rupture after closure has occurred. In this sense such "pearls" are a result, not a cause, of failure to close.

5. The failure of "shelf force" may be causative, and it may be epigenetic since the innate nature of the shelves is to come together. The failure also may be due to the differential tension of the connective tissues within the shelves themselves. The tension could be differential fiber growth, or it could be innate functional stress set up by the types of connective tissue, per se, which may inhibit an inherent medial-ward directive force.

6. In the formation of a lip cleft a causative factor may be inclusion cysts that are caused by buried ectoderm at the potential fusion site. In turn, this problem may be construed as failure of epithelium to degenerate, causing mesoderm to penetrate the preexisting epithelial structure.

This breakdown should be considered a provisional and schematic summary, for just as the genetic background is said to be multifactorial, so is the etiological background multicausative.

The embryogenesis of the craniofacial complex is a "fearful and wonderful" phenomenon: there are factors of timing, form, function, and organ system, all of which must relate to one another with the greatest precision. Think of all the vital areas this complex must serve: the brain (sensorimotor responses); the eye (vision); the ear (hearing and balance); the nose (respiration and olfaction); the oropharyngeal area (ingestion, taste, and speech); the skeletal framework (structure) and its attached muscles (neuromuscular function); and the entire arteriovenous organization (nourishment).

Size, dimension, proportion, rate, and direction—all of these factors combine successfully in a normal craniofacial complex. The parts come neatly together, each contributing to the achievement of an integrated whole. This terse statement, in fine, may well serve as a summary of craniofacial embryogenesis. It is estimated that in every 700 viable births, one has a cleft lip, cleft palate, or both. The other 699 are miraculously free of this birth defect.

PRENATAL GROWTH OF NORMAL CRANIOFACIAL STRUCTURES (WITH SPECIAL REFERENCE TO THE PALATE)

Just as normal (non-cleft) embryogenesis has been outlined, so will normal pre- and postnatal growth be discussed for the structures comprising the total craniofacial-dental complex. It is our feeling that non-cleft structural and functional growth patterns must be established in order to set up norms or standards that provide frameworks of reference and comparison. If we regard clefts as an interference with a normal growth process, then we must evaluate that interference. This means considerations of inhibited or deviated growth, distorted amount, rates, times of interference, and the manner in which these factors relate in kind, degree, and severity to cleft type. To put it simply, if the craniofacial complex is not growing as it should, how can this be assessed in both absolute and relative terms?

Once more we must have recourse to data derived from the literature, for at the Institute we have done no basic research in palatal growth in the fetus. Therefore, the following discussion is based on Burdi,[4, 5, 6] Freiband,[8] Ingham,[12] Inoue,[13] and Stark.[31] Note that emphasis has been placed upon mid-facial growth, i.e., growth of the palatal and dental arch.

The term mid-facial does not tell the whole story; rather, one should say mid-craniofacial or mid-sagittal. The midline of the cranium involves a veritable chain of synchondrosal and sutural interrelationships (see Figure 2–4), which merit recognition as a basicranial-facial continuum. The major cartilaginous synchondrosis is the occipitosphenoid in the cranial base, an important site of adjustive craniofacial development. The sutures are those between the several bones of the facial skeleton.

One of the most illuminating studies of prenatal craniofacial growth is that of Burdi.[4] His study is based upon the parasagittal section (just lateral to the nasal septum) of the heads of 24 white human fetuses of 70 to 227 mm. crown-rump length (CRL) and 12 to 24 weeks of age (the second trimester). Measurements were made on the cranial base: anterior, N–S; posterior, S–Ba; basicranial axis, N–Ba; total cranial base, N–S–Ba; and cranial base angle or sellar angle, N–S–Ba.* Measurements of the septum yielded anterior, middle, and posterior heights and anterior, middle, and posterior lengths.

---

*In the final section of this chapter, "Measurement of Form and Function," all commonly used endopoints, dimensions, planes, lines, and angles are defined and illustrated.

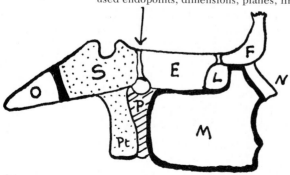

FIGURE 2–4 Position of sphenoethmoid suture (arrow) relative to retromaxillary sutures in pterygopalatine upper facial view. (O = basiocciput, S = sphenoid, E = ethmoid, L = lacrimal, F = frontal, N = nasal, M = maxilla, P = palatine, Pt = lateral pterygoid plate.) The cartilage between O and S is that of the occipitosphenoid synchondrosis. (From Scott, J. H.: Am. J. Phys. Anthropol., 16:319, 1958.)

In the second trimester the anterior cranial base uniformly contributed to more than half of the total cranial base length: 54 per cent at 70 mm. CRL, and 60 per cent at 227 mm. CRL. All cranial base lengths were correlated at the 0.01 level of significance with the growth in CRL, and this is of note, for it affirms very early that linear bodily growth is synchronous with growth timing in the jaws and face. The angular relationship between the anterior and posterior cranial base lengths (the cranial base angle, N–S–Ba) showed minor fluctuations, but a noticeable overall stability (Figure 2–5).

Nasal Septum

The role of the nasal septum in mid-facial growth has been universally accepted as of major importance; partial or total extirpation of the septum in the experimental animal has resulted in inhibited or deviated mid-facial development. Burdi noted that "the entire nasal septum, as well as individual regions," demonstrated a significant correlation between increasing septal height and CRL in the human fetus. Figure 2–6 presents data on anterior, middle, and posterior septal heights. The anterior height grew faster than did the posterior when both were compared by unit increase to the CRL. There were no such differences between anterior and middle heights. During growth from 70 to 227 mm. CRL, anterior height increased 157 per cent, middle 156 per cent, and posterior 148 per cent.

Growth in septal length was also significantly correlated with CRL. Compared to growth in septal height, that of septal length showed a very different pattern: the greatest relative increase in length was in the posterior septum and the least in the anterior septum (Figure 2–7). In the 70 to 227 mm. CRL period, posterior septal height increased 181 per cent, middle 168 per cent, and anterior 124 per cent.

If septal lengths and heights are related in a schematic polygon (S–N–SP–

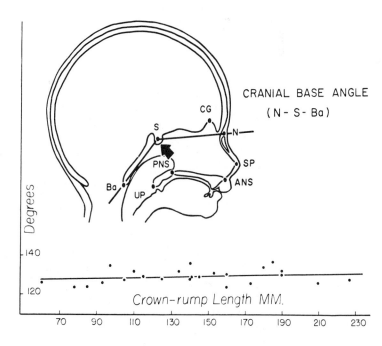

FIGURE 2–5 Cranial base angle (N-S-Ba) in second prenatal trimester. (ANS = anterior nasal spine, Ba = basion, CG = crista galli, N = nasion, PNS = posterior nasal spine, S = sella, SP = septal point, UP = uvular point.) (From Burdi, A. R.: J. Dent. Res., 44: 112, 1965.)

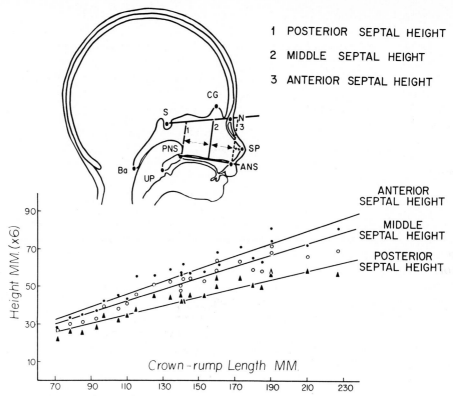

1 POSTERIOR SEPTAL HEIGHT

2 MIDDLE SEPTAL HEIGHT

3 ANTERIOR SEPTAL HEIGHT

FIGURE 2–6 Nasal septum heights in second prenatal trimester. (From Burdi, A. R.: J. Dent. Res., *44*:112, 1965.)

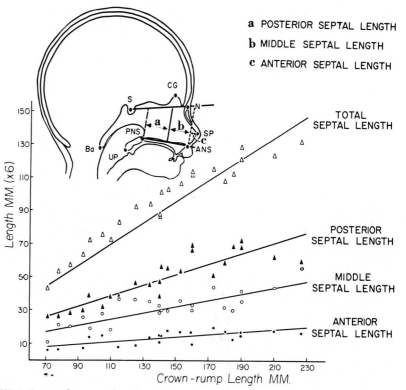

a POSTERIOR SEPTAL LENGTH

b MIDDLE SEPTAL LENGTH

c ANTERIOR SEPTAL LENGTH

FIGURE 2–7 Nasal septum lengths in second prenatal trimester. (From Burdi, A. R.: J. Dent. Res., *44*:112, 1965.)

ANS–PNS, with S registered on the baseline S–N), a very intriguing pattern of growth is suggested (Figure 2–8). The bony palate (PNS–ANS) shows a downward and forward inclination, i.e., there is not only increase in palatal length, but also movement of the whole. One cannot help being impressed by the apparent regularity of the septal polygon, for in a compensatory manner it combines a relatively greater gain in anterior height and a relatively greater gain in posterior length. This reflects a similarly patterned growth in the entire mid-facial complex, of which the nasal septum is a vital component.

In the palatal area both hard (ANS–PNS) and soft (PNS–U) palates grew in length at a rate significantly correlated with CRL. In the 70 to 227 mm. CRL period the hard palate increased 157 per cent, and at 70 mm. CRL the soft palate was 33 per cent of the total length of the palate, while at 227 mm. CRL it was 31 per cent. Hard palate to soft palate ratios, therefore, held constant in the second prenatal trimester (Figure 2–9).

The stability of the growth patterns of nasal septum and hard and soft palates is enhanced by the angular relationship of the palatal plane to the anterior cranial base, posterior cranial base, and basicranial axis (Figure 2–10).

Three fairly clear patterns of growth in the craniofacial complex may be recognized during the second prenatal trimester: (1) angular relationships within the complex show no real change with increasing CRL; (2) linear dimensions of cranial base, nasal septum, and palate correlate with CRL increase; and (3) upper and mid-face grow downward and forward, away from the cranial base and the sella turcica.

Growth in Craniofacial Height and Depth

Inoue investigated the morphological development of the craniofacial complex in Japanese fetuses with the aim of analyzing the dimensional and proportional changes with age in the fetal period.[13] To achieve this he employed tracings of lateral x-ray head films of 242 male and female fetuses, ages

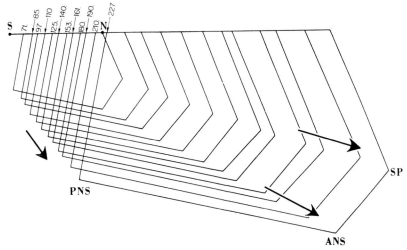

FIGURE 2–8 Septal polygons showing pattern of growth in fetuses of 70 to 227 mm. crown-rump length (CRL). (From Burdi, A. R.: J. Dent. Res., 44:112, 1965.)

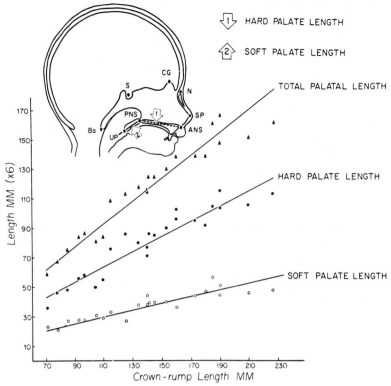

FIGURE 2–9 Growth of hard and soft palates in second prenatal trimester. (From Burdi, A. R.: J. Dent. Res., *44*:112, 1965.)

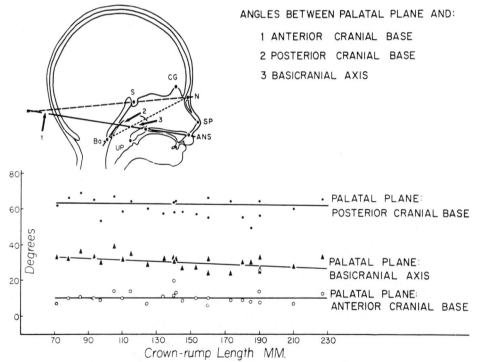

FIGURE 2–10 Angular relationships of palatal plane and anterior cranial base, posterior cranial base, and basicranial axis, in second prenatal trimester. (From Burdi, A. R.: J. Dent. Res., *44*:112, 1965.)

three to 10 lunar months (the last 6 calendrical months of pregnancy). In such lateral head films two sets of measurements can be taken: anterior to posterior (depth), and superior to inferior (height). These are sagittal and vertical measurements, respectively.

In his study Inoue set up two axes or coordinates, the X and the Y. The Y axis* was established as the Frankfort horizontal or eye-ear plane, and a number of lines parallel to the FH were drawn through critical end points. The X axis was established as a perpendicular to the Y axis through sella (S), the midpoint of the sella turcica, and a number of lines parallel to the X axis were drawn through critical endpoints. In this way a number of vertical (height) and horizontal (depth) dimensions, at right angles to one another, could be taken.

Inoue introduced two useful indexes: (1) the Growth Index, wherein each fetal facial dimension of height and depth, for each lunar month, was expressed as a percentage of a corresponding Japanese adult value, based on a 1959 study by Sakamoto; and (2) the S–N Index, wherein each depth dimension, measured to the Y axis, was expressed as a percentage of the measurement of N (nasion) to the Y axis.

The important finding that emerged from Inoue's material is that the dentofacial growth in the prenatal period covered was basically similar in pattern to that of Burdi's white fetuses, i.e., sizes and proportions established at four lunar months held fairly evenly through 10 months while dimensions increased 2.1 to 2.5 times. There was some differential growth—e.g., height growth was a bit more than depth growth, lower facial height increased a bit more than did upper—but the total dentofacial configuration as seen in the lateral view remained quite similar. Even when the fetal measurements were compared percentagewise to adult measurements, change in size was proportionate.

The size of the normal (non-cleft) fetal face and jaws doubles or triples in lunar months three through 10, but such size increase is uniform in height and depth so that proportions remain quite constant. This is what is meant by "pattern growth." The studies by Burdi for the second trimester and by Inoue for the entire period of fetal growth unite in proclaiming a uniformity in normal (non-cleft) craniofacial growth.

Growth in Craniofacial Length and Breadth

Freiband took a number of palatal length and breadth measurements of 102 white fetuses, three to 10 lunar months of age.[8] In Figure 2–11 anterior, middle, and posterior lengths are graphed in relation to maximum palatal length. Anterior palatal length is from the incisive point to a line connecting the right and left lateral sulci; middle palatal length is from the bisulcal line to a line connecting the right and left molar points; posterior palatal length is from the bimolar line to a line connecting the right and left postgingival points; and maximum palatal length is from the incisive point to the bi-postgingival line.

In Figure 2–11 note that anterior and middle palatal lengths make a uni-

---

*In the orthodontic literature involving craniofacial growth the Y axis of Downs is from sella turcica to gnathion (S–Gn). This axis is presumed to portray the downward and forward growth of the face.

form contribution to total palatal length; on the other hand, posterior palatal length makes the greatest contribution, relatively and absolutely. This suggests that the maximum growth in palatal length is posteriorly directed. This fact is in direct agreement with what has been noted of posterior septal length growth; both palate and septum grow lengthwise in synchrony.

Figure 2–12 throws light on changes of form in the fetal palate. Maximum breadth (bimolar) and maximum length (incisive point to bi-postgingival line) are plotted against age in fetal months, and it is seen that rate of breadth increase exceeds that of length increase.

Here we pose an interpretation: palatal length increase is greatest in the posterior section, and palatal breadth increase, overall, exceeds that of palatal length. This suggests that such differential palatal growth has a functional import, i.e., it is related to the length of dentition in that dental development has an anteroposterior gradient and a breadth gradient because dentoalveolar growth is appositional, in order to accommodate the housing of the teeth.

The changes of shape in the palate, which are due to differential rates and amounts of growth in breadth and length, may be expressed by a craniometric palatal index: maximum breadth ÷ maximum length × 100. Index values and classifications are:

Dolichuranic	<110	long, narrow palate
Mesuranic	110–114.9	moderately long palate
Brachyuranic	≥115	broad palate

In prenatal life the consistent trend is from a long and narrow palate to a broad palate, with the anterior segment of the arch—the premaxillary area—the most variable.

At this point we may sum up that in terms of absolute growth, the dimen-

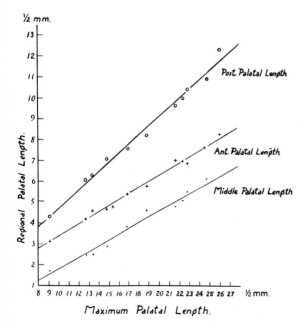

FIGURE 2–11 Growth rate of anterior, middle, and posterior palatal divisions related to maximum palatal length. Anterior and middle grow at uniform rate, with posterior greatest. Overall, palate is growing in posterior direction. (From Freiband, B.: J. Dent. Res., 15:103, 1937.)

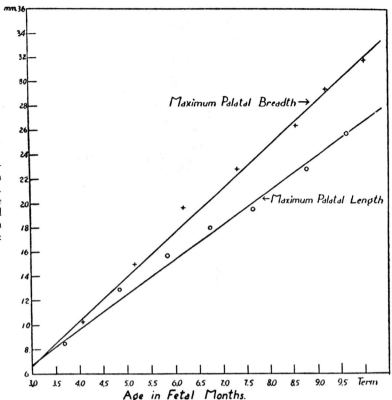

FIGURE 2–12 Relation of maximum palatal length and breadth from third fetal month to term. Breadth growth is more rapid, due to growth of the alveolar arch and its developing dentition. (From Freiband, B.: J. Dent. Res., *15*: 103, 1937.)

sions of palatal length, breadth, and height all show interrelated rates of growth in terms of velocity, with breadth increasing faster than length. As regards length, growth occurs more rapidly posteriorly than midmost or anteriorly, i.e., there is apparently an early growth provision for the elongation of the dental arch as dental elements are added to the hind end of the arch. The palate has a flat roof in early fetal life, but with differential increase in breadth and length, the palatal arch becomes progressively more vaulted.

Maxillary and Mandibular Arches

Burdi and Lillie undertook an analysis of morphological changes in the shape of the maxillary dental arch using 15 Caucasian embryos six and one-half to 12 weeks of age.[5] Quite apart from the craniometric palatal breadth to length ratio quoted earlier, the shape of the palate has been variously described as semiellipsoid, paraboloid, U-shaped, oval or rounded, and horseshoe-shaped. Employing occlusal-dental contact points it was accepted that the occlusal-dental arch line could be described by a catenary curve, which is a geometric curve resembling a multi-linked chain suspended by its ends and hanging freely. The shape of the curve is related to the transverse distance between the two end-point suspensions and the projected length of the arch being compared.

It was found that from six and one-half to eight weeks the arch was wide and flattened anteroposteriorly and did not conform to the catenary curve.

From seven and one-half to nine weeks the C-shaped arch showed elongation and increasing depth. Not until nine and one-half to 12 weeks did arch growth proceed to the point of conformity to the catenary curve. Burdi and Lillie suggest that "the catenary curvature of the postnatal dental arch can be first recognized as early as 9.5 weeks of development."[5]

The important fact emerges that change in the shape of the embryonic palatal arch is due to "a carefully coordinated pattern of dimensional as well as directional growth of all the tissues which surround the dental arch." These tissues, as factors, must include the oropharyngeal environment, the cartilaginous nasal capsule, and the supportive craniofacial skeleton.

Ingham studied the growth of the prenatal mandible in 20 Caucasian fetuses at ages 10.8 to 38.0 weeks with a 46 to 253 mm. crown-rump length.[12] Bigonial width (at jaw angles), total mandibular width (bicoronoid), alveolar (dental) arch width and length, mandibular ramal height, and mandibular corporal length were measured. In the mandible may be seen a reflection of the pattern of growth of the maxillopalatine area. The ratio of alveolar arch length to mandibular length and the ratio of bigonial width to bicoronoid width are both constant. Alveolar arch length increases more rapidly than does ramal height, and alveolar arch width increases more rapidly than does bicoronoid width (Figure 2–13).

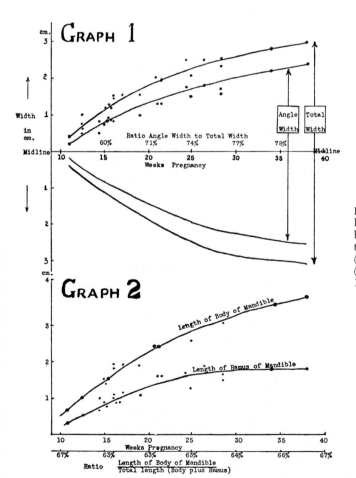

FIGURE 2–13   Graph 1: Ratio of mandibular arch width at angles (bigonial width) to bicoronoid width, or total width in Ingham's terminology. Graph 2: Ratio of alveolar plate (mandibular body) length to ramal length. (From Ingham, T. R.: J. Dent. Res., 7:647, 1932.)

Up to this point in our discussion the data and their interpretation have been rather localized and particulate, as though the dental arches, upper and lower, and their supporting bones (maxilla and mandible), were more or less isolated and independent. This is not so, and could be misleading. To be sure, reference has been made to "pattern growth," to "coordinated growth," and so on, but it is important to observe that "dentofacial" is not enough, for more than teeth, arches, and facial bones are involved. What is really involved is *craniofacial*, the total cranial base and total facial construct. There is a reciprocal relationship that must be evaluated with respect to possible feedback mechanisms. If there is a deviant or disturbed growth in the cranial base, is it reflected in a malrelationship within the facial structure? Conversely, if there is a growth insult in the facial skeleton, is this shadowed in how the cranial base grows? These questions are not rhetorical, for they strike at the heart of the problem, which will be considered in a later section of this book: How does clefting affect the growth potential of the cranial base palatal arch mid-facial skeleton complex?

What this detailed analysis is leading up to is this: If fetal craniofacial growth is patterned, i.e., is consistent in dimensional velocity and proportionate change, then a disturbance *within* that pattern may have repercussions within the whole anatomical area. For example, a mid-line palatal cleft may have an effect elsewhere in the midface. It is like the ripple effect of a stone thrown into a pool of water; the waves radiate in all directions and are deflected only where they meet certain boundaries.

During fetal life there is a remarkable overall stability. The geometric form of the upper face is a stable entity. The hard and soft palate vary somewhat in their contribution to the total palate length, though relative soft palate length remains constant. And by the end of the third month the external nose has taken on a definite profile, which remains relatively unchanged throughout fetal life.

An important growth relationship is that in which cranial base, septum, and palate are all correlated with growth in crown-rump length. This has great interpretive and evaluative import, for, as was stated earlier, it links general bodily growth to craniofacial growth. As crown-rump length goes, so go head and face, in terms of growth-time and in terms of dimensionality or growth-size. But, since dimensions are so interrelated, angular relationships do not change. There is an overall configurational unity, and as a result the directional growth of the upper and midface is downward and forward.

The Cleft Variable

Normal prenatal growth of the craniofacial complex has an inherent stability and regularity about it that is of import when we begin to look at the ramified effects of clefts. We know reasonably well what to expect in the second and third prenatal trimesters of normal fetal palatal growth in terms of rate, increment, direction, and timing. Clefts occur in the first prenatal trimester, before attainment of the patterned growth noted earlier, and it may be logically assumed, therefore, that any inhibition, aberrancy, or deviation that shows up in the second and third trimesters *may be* attributed to or associated with the cleft. We might put this in algebraic terms: postcleft craniofacial-dental growth $= x + y$, where x is the expected growth pattern and y is the disturbance of that pattern by clefting. We may even say more, namely, that x is an acceptable, almost predictable constant and that y is a variable to be factored for in the cleft palate dentofacial assemblage.

Teratogens

It is apropos at this point to note that clefts may be environmentally caused, i.e., that the variable y may be introduced via a teratogen. As a rule the term "teratogen" is applied to an environmental agent that causes congenital malformation. In a very broad sense abnormal genes and chromosomes might be considered teratogens. A great number of teratogens have been identified, and a logical grouping adapted from Stark[31] and from Warkany,[32] can be found in Table 2–1 (not all are specific for clefts). These teratogenic substances act in a number of different ways, some rather general, others more or less specific. Some of their effects are as follows:

TABLE 2–1 Teratogens

VIRAL DISEASES	**ENDOCRINIC FACTORS**
German measles (rubella)	Steroid hormones (adrenal)
Toxoplasmosis	cortisone
Rat virus (RV)	glucocorticoids
Cytomegalic inclusion disease	hydrocortisone
	prednisolone
TOXIC FACTORS	adrenocorticotropic hormone (ACTH) (?)
Nitrogen mustards	Sex hormones (steroid)
Thalidomide (few cases CL[P])	testosterone
Alkylating agents	progesterone
chlorambucil	diethylstilbestrol
thiotepa	Thyroid
colchicine	maternal thyroidectomy
selenium	propylthiouracil
triethylenemelamine (TEM)	iodine compounds
boric acid	trypan blue
salicylic acid	Pancreatic
chlorcyclizine	tolbutamide (Orinase)
	maternal diabetes
DEFICIENCY FACTORS	Maternal adrenalectomy
Metabolites	
vitamin A (hypo, hyper)	**PHYSICAL AND MECHANICAL FACTORS**
vitamin E	Hypoxia
riboflavin	Hydramnios
folic acid	Radiation
magnesium	Oligohydramnios
pantothenic acid	
Antimetabolites	
aminopterin	
galactoflavin	
6-mercaptopurine	
azaserine	
5-fluorodeoxyuridine	
aminonicotinic acid	

(Adapted from Stark, R. H. (ed.): Cleft Palate, A Multi-Discipline Approach, New York, Harper and Row, 1968; and Warkany, J.: Congenital Malformations: Notes and Comments, Chicago, Year Book Medical Publishers, 1971.)

1. In overall organogenesis riboflavin is necessary. During organogenesis radiation may cause chromosomal aberrations. The alkylating agents may affect DNA in a manner similar to radiation.

2. The antimetabolites block enzyme or inductor factors, inhibit the substrate, and form foreign nuclear proteins—all of which interferes with DNA synthesis.

3. Hypoxia may give rise to a vascular deficiency.

4. Cortisone may give rise to an inhibition of palatal shelf elevation. In addition it may have the following effects: inhibition of synthesis of sulfomucopolysaccharides; decrease in amniotic fluid; increase in water retention; inhibition of RNA synthesis; inhibition of mitosis; stabilization of lysosomal membranes; myopathy; and perhaps other effects.

5. Tolbutamide inhibits the uptake of glucose.

6. Oligohydramnios may cause hyperflexion of the head fold, resulting in micrognathia. The small jaw pushes the tongue up between the palatal shelves. The head is turned to the right by the enlarging heart; as a result the lip is inferior in position on the left side and pressed against the chest wall. This may result in a left-side cleft lip.

There are two observations to be made about this detailed listing of teratogens: (1) they are, overall, experimental substances; and (2) very few of them act on human subjects. The goal in the experimental administration of a teratogen in the first trimester of pregnancy (the organogenic phase) is to see which of the effects of a given teratogen correlates the most highly with the induced cleft palate. For example, one may administer a teratogenic substance to several different strains of an experimental animal and then determine the process or processes that correlate highly with a palatal cleft.

It is pretty well established that the Primates, including *Homo sapiens*, are relatively immune to the effects of most teratogenic agents. For example, the monkey (macaque) is affected (in terms of producing a palatal cleft) only by trypan blue and thalidomide. This immunity to other teratogens may be due, in part, to the fact that most often in infra-Primate experimental animals the doses are relatively great. There is also the possibility that Primate immunity to most teratogens (other than hypoxia, radiation, and other mechanical and environmental factors) is an evolutionary selective acquisition. With the increased specialization of the central nervous system has come an equally specialized susceptibility to disturbances in metabolism at the cellular level in the biochemistry of the more highly evolved organism from its DNA-RNA stages through organogenesis. Over evolutionary time the Primates, leading to man, have been selected for an ever-increasing resistance to the effects of teratogens. This implies both an absolute (kind) and a relative (amount) teratogenic immunity.

Teratogens do serve an experimental purpose: they highlight, often step-by-step, the processes leading to a given type of congenital defect and often pinpoint what "goes wrong" in a given developmental sequence or stage. In this way they have given us a clearer understanding of why cleft lips and palates develop.

POSTNATAL GROWTH—
NORMAL AND CLEFT

In preceding pages we have noted the embryological origin of palatal clefts and the normal or non-cleft growth of the fetal craniofacial complex, i.e., the cranial base and the palatal-maxillary-facial complex. This has given us a picture of normative prenatal craniofacial growth and development. We are ready, therefore, to appraise postnatal craniofacial growth. This we will do from two major aspects: (1) normal (non-cleft) postnatal growth; and (2) the postnatal growth of the craniofacial complex as it may reflect, or be affected by, a cleft palate and/or lip. The first aspect will focus upon the use of normative growth standards as *frameworks of comparison* for cleft palate and lip growth. The second aspect will focus upon the pattern of growth in patients with a cleft and *how* it may differ from the non-cleft norm; it is here that we shall present our own clinical research data. Postnatal growth generally is considered as extending from birth to 20 years of age. We may assume that by the age of 20 years craniofacial growth has reached 100 per cent adult values.

NORMAL GROWTH

Over the years I have calculated an overall perspective of postnatal growth in face and jaws. There are two assumptions: (1) facial growth in its entirety occurs in three planes or sets of dimensions, which are sagittal or depth (D), transverse or breadth (B), and vertical or height (H); and (2) as noted, these three sets of dimensions have reached 100 per cent adult values at age 20 years. At birth breadth dimensions are 55 to 60 per cent of their adult value, height 40 to 45 per cent, and depth 30 to 35 per cent.[*] This gives a formula of 6 to 4½ to 3 (B, H, and D, respectively). Now this means that there must remain, postnatally, 40 to 45 per cent in breadth growth, 55 to 60 per cent in height, and 65 to 70 per cent in depth. The formula now becomes 4 to 5½ to 7 (B, H, and D, respectively).

This 4 to 5½ to 7 ratio represents the relative distances of the three main "avenues" of facial growth to be traversed: breadth is the shortest, height in between, and depth the longest. The face will grow most in a forward direction, next in an up and down direction, and least in a side to side direction. This development is of paramount importance in watching the pre- and postoperative facial growth of the child with a cleft, because the palatal cleft, essentially a mid-line failure, is oriented mainly to depth growth, the major avenue of growth, and hence the most liable to be inhibited or deviated.

While it is true that B, H, and D dimensions will all gain their 100 per cent adult value at about 20 years, the three sets of dimensions will not all proceed toward that goal at the same rates of speed or at the same times during that

[*]These percentages are in sharp contrast to cranial growth as exemplified by postnatal head length: In the first six months the rate of increase is 50 per cent, second six months 20 per cent, second year 10 per cent, third year 4 per cent, and then on to 18 years at 2 to 1 per cent. If adult value is 100 per cent, then 64 per cent of head length is attained at birth, 75 per cent in the first six months, 83 per cent in the second six months, 88 per cent in the second year, 92 to 95 per cent by five years, and 100 per cent at 18 years.

period. In a way the B, H, and D "runners" will all breast the tape together at age 20, but during the "race" the lead will change quite a few times.

Facial growth is extremely complex. It must serve vision (orbits); hearing (ears); olfaction and breathing (nasal aperture); mastication, deglutition, and speech (oropharyngeal structures); the dynamics of functional movements (bone and muscle); and finally, it must provide a balance with cranial growth, so that a true craniofacial complex is involved.

Facial Growth and Tooth Eruption

Palatal clefts are so involved with dentofacial growth that it is useful at this point to relate facial growth in breadth, height, and depth to tooth eruption stages. The teeth in their arches are, in a sense, the arbiters of depth growth (arch length) and breadth growth (arch breadth). While this situation relates mainly to upper (palatal) arch, it also applies (perhaps reciprocally) to the lower (mandibular) arch, and the growth of both arches is registered in total facial growth.

In the discussion that follows we shall establish five dental stages with ages approximated[*]:

I. Deciduous dentition $\dfrac{\text{m2 m1 c i2 i1} \mid \text{i1 i2 c m1 m2}}{\text{m2 m1 c i2 i1} \mid \text{i1 i2 c m1 m2}}$ (by 3 years)

II. Beginning replacement by permanent teeth $\dfrac{\text{I2 I1} \mid \text{I1 I2}}{\text{I2 I1} \mid \text{I1 I2}}$ and eruption $\dfrac{\text{M1} \mid \text{M1}}{\text{M1} \mid \text{M1}}$, respectively (by 6 years)

III. Replacement $\dfrac{\text{P2 P1} \mid \text{P1 P2}}{\text{P2 P1} \mid \text{P1 P2}}$ (by 10 years)

IV. Replacement $\dfrac{\text{C} \mid \text{C}}{\text{C} \mid \text{C}}$ and eruption $\dfrac{\text{M2} \mid \text{M2}}{\text{M2} \mid \text{M2}}$ (by 12 years)

V. Eruption $\dfrac{\text{M3} \mid \text{M3}}{\text{M3} \mid \text{M3}}$ (by 18–20 years)

---

[*]The deciduous dentition is given in small letters, the permanent in capital letters: i1–2 or I1–2 = central and lateral incisors; c or C = canine; m1–2 = first and second molars; P1–2 = first and second premolars, M1–2–3 = first, second, and third molars. Upper and lower are given, e.g., $\underline{\text{M1}}$ = upper, $\overline{\text{M1}}$ = lower. The premolars are the successors of the deciduous molars. The deciduous teeth total 20, the permanent teeth total 32. M1–2–3 have no deciduous predecessors.

for another. Size, as has been said, is increased basically through sutural growth, while shape is basically changed through remodeling. Experimental studies on various animals, especially primates, have employed vital dyes and metallic markers to demonstrate the processes of growth and remodeling. In essence the change in the shape of a bone or of a bony complex is accomplished by an interplay of bone added (deposition, apposition) and bone taken away (resorption). This interplay is differential in both amount and time, that is, amounts added or removed and the times of change in different facial bones and areas are variable. If the deposition and resorption cycle was absolutely uniform in amount and time in the first 20 postnatal years, then a small baby face would become only a large baby face.

For our purposes we shall note remodeling changes only in certain facial areas: (1) the *upper dental arch*, with deposition on the inner (lingual) side and at the maxillary tuberosity, and resorption on the outer (buccal and labial) side; (2) the *hard palate*, with deposition on the palatal surface and resorption on the nasal floor and maxillary sinus floor (thus, the hard palate, separating the oral and nasal cavities, actually becomes lower in the remodeling that occurs); (3) the *zygomatic arch*, with resorption on its outer facial surface and on its inner mid- and posterior temporal fossa surface, and deposition in the most anterior part of its temporal fossa surface and along its entire lower lateral surface; (4) the *ascending ramus* of the mandible, with deposition in the upper two-thirds of the outer surface, resorption in the lower one-third, and a remodeling process on the inner surface just about the reverse of that on the outer surface; and (5) the *condylar area* of the mandible, with deposition at its inner surface and on the head, and resorption along the outer surface.

Palatal Dimensions

In our careful watch over the development of the child with a cleft, assessing the changes in size and conformation that we have been discussing, we find that periodic measurement of the dental arches is of particular importance. It helps us in determining whether or not the child is progressing at the proper rate and in the proper direction toward the desired norms. It also guides us in planning some of our treatment strategies. Fortunately, there is a rich store of mensurational data based on normal individuals to provide standards against which to compare the children under our care.

The dental arches in the newborn non-cleft infant have been measured in English children by Clinch on 70 sets of dental casts, upper and lower.[7] The *upper alveolar arch* has a "dental groove" which divides it into two parts: a lateral labiobuccal where the teeth later erupt, and a linguobuccal. The gum pad is more or less horseshoe-shaped and is divided into 10 segments: i1–2, c, and m1–2 (right and left). The i1 and c segments are about equal in size, the i2 segment very small, the m1 segment larger, and the m2 segment indistinct. The *lower alveolar arch* is divided similarly, though the segments are not as distinct, and it is U-shaped or tends to be rectangular. The following measurements were taken: height of palate at highest point of m1 segment; arch length, upper and lower, from labial crest of i1–2 ridge to most distal part of

TABLE 2–3   Dental Arch Measurements in Non-Cleft Infants
(in mm.)

DIMENSION	AVERAGE	RANGE	DIFF. OF RANGE
Palate H	7.49	6.73–8.75	2.02
Arch L, upper	21.16	20.50–21.60	1.10
Arch B, upper, bi-c	24.75	23.50–25.58	2.08
Arch B, upper, bi-m1	30.17	29.50–31.21	1.71
Arch L, lower	17.05	15.48–18.63	3.15
Arch B, lower, bi-c	21.70	19.50–23.23	3.73
Arch B, lower, bi-m1	25.96	22.75–26.77	4.02

(Adapted from Clinch, L.: Int. J. Orthod., *20*:359, 1934.)

m2 segment; arch breadth, upper and lower, bicanine, at buccal side of the distal c groove; and arch breadth, upper and lower, bi-first molar, at widest part on buccal side of m1 segment. The averages and ranges of these measurements are shown in Table 2–3. It is worth noting that palatal height at birth is relatively the most variable dimension, with a range difference of 2.02 mm. compared to its average of 7.49 mm. Maxillary arch breadth at the m1 level is relatively the least variable, closely followed by upper arch length. On the whole, however, maxillary (palatal) breadth and length at birth vary little, while palatal height is highly variable.

For the first postnatal year we may turn to the data on palatal growth of Bakwin and Bakwin for New York children.[2] The following dimensions were taken: maximum palatal breadth at the m1–2 level; posterior palatal breadth between right and left postgingivae; maximum palatal length from incisivum (between i1–2) to posterior breadth chord; anterior palatal length from incisivum to maximum palatal breadth chord; and maximum palatal height, taken as maximum height above surface of the gingivae. Their data are given in Table 2–4. In this period (birth to 55 weeks) the absolute growth increment is as follows:

DIMENSION	MALE	FEMALE
Maximum palatal length	5.2 mm.	4.5 mm.
Anterior palatal length	5.5 mm.	6.2 mm.
Posterior palatal breadth	5.3 mm.	2.4 mm.
Maximum palatal breadth	5.7 mm.	4.0 mm.
Maximum palatal height	2.6 mm.	1.9 mm.

(From Bakwin, H. and R. M. Bakwin: Int. J. Orthod., *22*:1018, 1936.)

TABLE 2–4   Palatal Growth in the First Postnatal Year (in mm.)

Age in Weeks		Maximum Palatal Length Mean	S.D.	Anterior Palatal Length Mean	S.D.	Posterior Palatal Breadth Mean	S.D.	Maximum Palatal Breadth Mean	S.D.	Maximum Palatal Height Mean	S.D.
Males											
Birth	(89)°	25.6	1.60	–	–	25.5	1.20	30.6	1.50	7.6	2.00
0–3	(42)	25.6	1.65	13.2	1.34	26.2	1.53	31.1	1.75	7.8	1.72
4–7	(28)	26.5	2.04	14.2	1.52	26.7	1.80	32.0	2.46	8.8	1.09
8–15	(36)	27.2	2.28	14.6	1.82	27.7	2.36	32.6	2.68	9.5	1.24
16–23	(31)	28.5	2.18	16.3	2.12	28.5	2.06	33.3	2.44	9.7	0.92
24–31	(36)	29.1	2.08	16.2	2.48	30.2	2.12	35.4	2.50	10.3	1.03
32–39	(17)	30.2	2.27	17.2	2.56	29.7	1.80	34.5	2.50	10.3	1.12
40–47	(13)	30.4	2.02	17.9	1.73	32.1	2.06	36.8	2.65	10.5	1.13
48–55	(12)	30.8	2.24	18.7	2.82	30.8	1.54	36.3	2.50	10.2	1.38
Females											
0–3	(22)	25.8	1.51	13.8	1.17	26.1	1.46	30.5	1.73	8.1	1.12
4–7	(16)	25.8	1.82	13.4	1.20	26.1	1.46	30.5	1.58	8.3	0.85
8–15	(26)	26.6	2.28	14.0	1.63	26.4	1.50	30.5	2.04	9.0	1.15
16–23	(20)	26.8	2.75	14.3	1.70	27.4	1.88	31.4	1.91	9.3	1.09
24–31	(10)	28.5	1.69	16.5	2.02	28.1	1.70	33.6	2.16	9.6	1.01
32–39	(17)	29.7	2.02	17.4	1.88	29.2	1.78	34.1	2.17	9.2	0.96
40–47	(8)	30.9	–	18.1	–	28.8	–	33.9	–	10.4	–
48–55	(4)	30.3	–	20.0	–	28.5	–	34.5	–	10.0	–

°Numbers in parentheses are number of casts measured. (From Bakwin, H. and R. M. Bakwin: Int. J. Orthod., 22:1018, 1936.)

Anterior palatal length increases absolutely just as much as does total palatal length, so that it becomes relatively greater: it is about 50 per cent of maximum palatal length at 0 to 3 weeks, and 60 per cent at 48 to 55 weeks. In both males and females posterior palatal breadth does not keep pace with maximum palatal breadth, i.e., the palate becomes relatively narrow posteriorly. Palatal height increases steadily but slightly, a bit more in males than in females.

The Sillman Data

In our experience the most reliable longitudinal data on postnatal dental arch growth are those of Sillman.[27, 28, 29] In 1966 Sillman presented his collection to the Philadelphia Growth Center and the University of Pennsylvania Department of Anthropology. The original casts are now at the University of Pennsylvania School of Dental Medicine, and duplicate study casts were made at the H. K. Cooper Institute for both the Department of Anthropology and the Institute. The collection is of 750 dental casts of 65 Caucasian New Yorkers taken from birth to 25 years. There is an average of 35 casts for each age group and an average of 12 casts per individual. The 65 persons are not represented by annual casts over the entire age span, i.e., this is a "mixed" longitudinal series. In his total material[29] Sillman set up the six dental stages shown in Table 2–5.

TABLE 2–5 The Sillman Dental Stages (in years)

| | MALE | | FEMALE | |
STAGES	Average	Range	Average	Range
1. edentulous	0.18	0.0–0.38	0.08	0.0–0.24
2. deciduous (complete)	3.27	2.47–4.07	3.33	2.59–4.07
3. I1–M1	8.04	7.07–9.02	8.03	7.08–8.99
4. P1–2	11.73	10.54–12.93	11.22	9.87–12.57
5. M2	13.64	12.61–14.67	13.60	12.51–14.69
6. M3	21.40	19.81–22.98	21.54	19.75–23.34

(Adapted from Sillman, J. H.: Am. J. Orthod., 37:481, 1951.)

Sillman's outstanding 1947 study[27] can be usefully compared with our present Research Series at the Institute, for it focuses on the first postnatal decade. His data on the growth of arch breadths, upper and lower, were serially based on 38 Caucasian children from birth to nine years of age. He reported an interesting, almost rhythmic alternation between periods of noticeable increase and periods of very slight increase:

1. First, most marked increase, birth to 0.34 yr
2. Very slight increase, 0.34 to 1.06 yr
3. Second increase, 1.06 to 1.92 yr
4. Very slight increase, 1.92 to 5.08 yr
5. Third increase, 5.08 to 7.80 yr
6. Very slight increase, 7.80 to 9.50 yr

We can schematize these data as we did for facial growth in breadth, height, and depth. In the following table we have rounded off the time periods to the nearest year where practicable:

AGE	VELOCITY OF GROWTH	
Birth to 3 mo	++	most marked
3 mo to 1 yr	(+)	very slight
1 yr to 2 yr	+ (++?)	moderate to (?) marked
2 yr to 5 yr	(+)	very slight
5 yr to 8 yr	+	moderate
8 yr to 9½ yr	(+)	very slight

Dental growth, as interpreted above, increases most vigorously in the first three months, followed by growth accelerations in the second year and in late childhood. This timing-picture suggests that growth is oriented to the eruption of the deciduous teeth (by about two and a half to three years) and the crypt formation of the $\frac{M1}{M1}$ (first permanent molar), for when this tooth is erupted palatal breadth at M1 level is 90 to 95 per cent of its adult value.

In his 1964 study[29] Sillman presents curves of arch growth in length and breadth that are useful for normative comparisons. The curves cover a period from birth to 27 years. Sillman bases his length and breadth dimensions on four endpoints on the maxillary arch. He defines these points as follows (Figure 2–14):

Point I. In the maxillary edentulous infant this point is located by the inter-

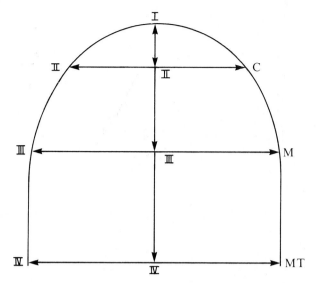

FIGURE 2-14   The Sillman graph for dental arch dimensions.

section of the (mid) sagittal plane with the everted ridge. . . . As the dentition unfolds this point is always located by a line drawn through the center of the first incisal edges intersecting the median line.

Point II.   In the edentulous infant this point is located by the intersection of the lateral sulcus with the crest of the gum pad. . . . With the eruption of the dentition the lateral sulcus becomes the interdental papilla. In order to locate Point II . . . the relationship must be noted between the midpoint of the distal border of the canine and the mesial groove of the first deciduous molar, or the first premolar. . . .

Point III.   This point cannot be determined in the edentulous infant. It is first located at the distal groove of the second deciduous molar. In order to locate this point during the changing dentition, its relationship to the first permanent molar must be noted.

Point IV.   This point is the posterior limit of the dental arches. [In the maxillary arch of the infant one may] have the gingival groove on the buccal and lingual aspects, plus the pterygomandibular raphe, which is slightly lingual to Point IV [as a guide. Also useful is the posterolateral sulcus.] MT = maxillary tuberosity, which marks the posterior limit of the maxillary dental arch.

There is only one Point I, at the front center of the arch, as defined above. But Points II, III, and IV, identifying the canine, molar, and posterior positions, respectively, are of course paired, one set along the right arm of the arch, the corresponding set along the left arm. Arch breadth can thus be measured at each of three positions: between the two canine points, between the two molar points, or between the two posterior points. Total arch length is measured along the midline, projected from Point I to a transverse line connecting the two Points IV (posterior). The canine section of arch length is from Point I to the transverse line joining the two Points II (canine), and the molar section measures from Point I to the transverse line between the two Points III (molar).

In Figures 2-15A and 2-15B Sillman graphs the lengths of the maxillary and mandibular arches for males and females, respectively. Absolute lengths do not differ significantly between males and females, but total length is 4 to 5 mm. greater in males. Maxillary arch lengths uniformly exceed mandibular arch lengths. The slope of the curves demonstrates an early velocity

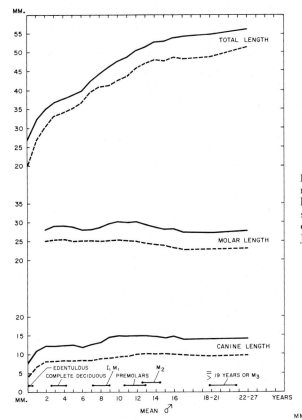

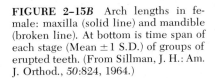

FIGURE 2–15A Arch lengths in male: maxilla (solid line) and mandible (broken line). At bottom is time span of each stage (Mean ± 1 S.D.) of groups of erupted teeth. (From Sillman, J. H.: Am. J. Orthod., *50*:824, 1964.)

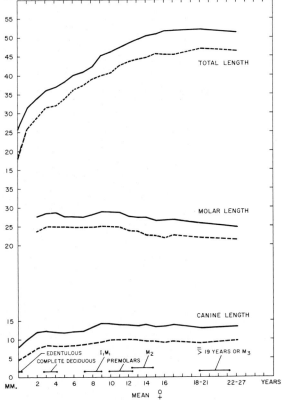

FIGURE 2–15B Arch lengths in female: maxilla (solid line) and mandible (broken line). At bottom is time span of each stage (Mean ±1 S.D.) of groups of erupted teeth. (From Sillman, J. H.: Am. J. Orthod., *50*:824, 1964.)

in the growth of canine length in the first two years, with a secondary upsweep at about eight to 10 years. The curve for total length sweeps with a quite uniform velocity, but the molar length curve is virtually a plateau.

If we accept the canine curve as representing the most anterior transverse segment of the arch, there is an early accommodation for growth of $\dfrac{i2-i1\,|\,i1-i2}{i2-i1\,|\,i1-i2}$ and $\dfrac{c}{c}$. The molar length is a midlength from $\dfrac{c\,|\,c}{c\,|\,c}$ through $\dfrac{m2-m1\,|\,m1-m2}{m2-m1\,|\,m1-m2}$ and $\dfrac{M1\,|\,M1}{M1\,|\,M1}$ and is very stable. Since I–IV increases and I–III does not, we must conclude that the growth of arch length occurs basically in its posterior segment, III–IV. It is noteworthy that the slopes of the curves of total arch length and width continue in males to ages 25 to 27, whereas these curves in females reach a plateau by this age. The stability of growth in the anterior half of the arches and the vigor of growth in the posterior half are of great moment in the evaluation of adjustive growth in cases of operated palatal clefts.

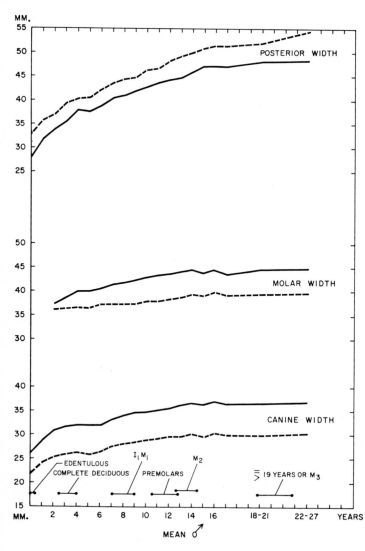

FIGURE 2–16 Arch widths in male: maxilla (solid line) and mandible (broken line). At bottom is time span of each stage (Mean ± 1 S.D.) of groups of erupted teeth. (From Sillman, J. H.: Am. J. Orthod., *50*:824, 1964.)

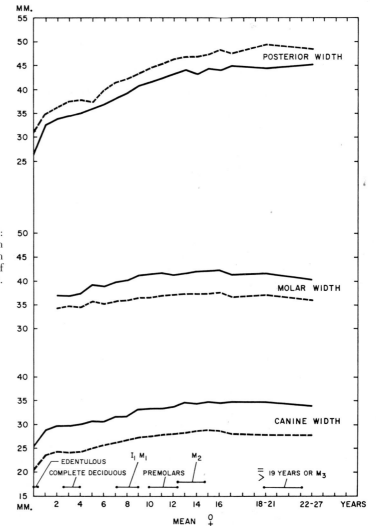

FIGURE 2–17 Arch widths in female: maxilla (solid line) and mandible (broken line). At bottom is time span of each stage (Mean ± 1 S.D.) of groups of erupted teeth. (From Sillman, J. H.: Am. J. Orthod., *50:*824, 1964.)

Figures 2–16 and 2–17 are curves of breadths of the maxillary and mandibular arches in males and females, respectively. Again the slope of the curve of the canine width represents an initial velocity at $\frac{c\mid c}{c\mid c}$ level, with a slight suggestion of an increase at 10 to 12 years for $\frac{C\mid C}{C\mid C}$ more noticeable in males. The curve of molar width has only a slight upward slope, i.e., growth of bimolar breadth is moderate to slight. Posterior width shows a steady increase, with a greater velocity in the first several years. Consideration of these widths suggests that the dental arches become broader posteriorly, i.e., after the first year the arches "open out" posteriorly, becoming more divergent. Mandibular posterior width exceeds its maxillary counterpart at all ages. As is the case with arch lengths, male arch breadths are 4 to 5 mm. greater than female arch breadths.

The Philadelphia Data

It is not possible (nor is it necessary) in this portion of the book to give an additional and exhaustive presentation of the mensurational data on growth in palate, dental arches, and face. The normative data gathered from 1948 to 1971 by the Philadelphia Center for Research in Child Growth and Development is basic.*

Palatal breadths, taken as outer or buccal dimensions, may be given at several levels for the birth to five years, 10 years, and 15 years age stages. These dimensions in males, along with female (F) size relationships, are as follows:

Breadth Dimension	Birth–5 yr	10 yr	15 yr
Upper bi–m1, bi–P1	36–40 mm. F 1 mm. less	44 mm. F 2–3 mm. less	46 mm.
Lower bi–m1, bi–P1	32–36 mm. F 1 mm. less	39 mm. F 1–2 mm. less	41 mm.
Upper bi–M1	50 mm. (6 yr) F 1–2 mm. less	55 mm. F 1–2 mm. less	57 mm.
Lower bi–M1	49 mm. (6 yr) F 1–2 mm. less	53 mm. F 1–2 mm. less	55 mm.

Upper arch length as measured forward from a line tangent to the posterior part of the molar segment (M1) to the lingual aspect of the incisor segment is approximately 27 to 28 mm. during the birth to five years period, 39 mm. at 10 years, and 37 mm. at 15 years, male and female. Lower arch length measured the same way is 24 to 25 mm. in the birth to five years period, 35 mm. at 10 years, and 32 mm. at 15 years, male and female.

In the Philadelphia material the growth of palatal breadth for the period of transition from deciduous to permanent teeth was measured. The breadths at six years of age and at 12 years were as follows (in mm.):

Breadth Dimension	Male	Female
bi–c or bi–C (lingual midpoint, mesiodistal)	24–25†	23 to 25
bi–m1 or bi–P1 (mid mesiodistal cusp at neck)	26 to 27	25 to 26
bi–m2 or bi–P2 (mid mesiodistal cusp at neck)	31 to 33.5	30 to 32.5
bi–M1 (mid mesiodistal cusp at neck)	31 to 33	30 to 32

†The dimensions 24 to 25 mean that the breadth at the level mentioned has gone from 24 mm. at 6 yr to 25 mm. at 12 yr. It is obvious that palatal breadths are virtually definitive by 6 yr.

Also in the Philadelphia data covering six to 12 years, palatal length (lingual aspect neck of I1 | I1 to posterior nasal spine) increased from 41.5 mm. to 45.5 mm. in males, and 41 mm. to 43.5 mm. in females. Similarly, arch length (a line tangent to posterior M1 to lingual aspect neck of I1|I1) increased from 38 mm. to 39 mm. in males, and 37 mm. to 38 mm. in females.

---

*The data are "modified longitudinal," i.e., one sample is birth to eight years, the other six to 17½ years. Subjects were non-cleft. The Center, now at the Children's Hospital of Philadelphia, has been renamed the Krogman Center for Research in Child Growth and Development.

Cranial Base and Upper Face

Attention must be paid to several mid-line dimensions other than palatal and dental arch growth, but mainly to sagittal (anteroposterior) rather than transverse (breadth) growth. These dimensions are found in the cranial base and in the upper face (breadth) and in the following the male and female averages are pooled (see Appendix for definitions):

CRANIAL BASE	2½ YR (Decid. teeth)	6 YR (M1)	12 YR (M2)
Clival length (Ba–S)	25.8 mm.	33.4 mm.	38.0 mm.
Basifacial length (Ba–N)	72.0 mm.	80.0 mm.	90.0 mm.
Anterior cranial base length (S–N)	41.4 mm.	49.8 mm.	54.6 mm.
S to foramen caecum	36.5 mm.	43.0 mm.	45.5 mm.
Foramen caecum to N	4.9 mm.	6.8 mm.	9.1 mm.
Upper Face Breadth, Mid			
Interorbital (bidacryon)	13.1 mm.	17.3 mm.	20.6 mm.

The periodicity of growth of the cranial base—a very important adjustment zone in craniofacial growth—is noteworthy. The following are incremental data (in mm.) for each cranial base dimension:

DIMENSION	INCREASE 2 YR, 6 MO TO 6 YR	INCREASE 6 YR TO 12 YR
Clival length (Ba–S)	7.6	4.6
Basifacial length (Ba–N)*	8.0	10.0
Anterior cranial base length (S–N)	8.4	4.8
S to foramen caecum	6.5	2.5
Foramen caecum to N	1.9	2.3

*On an annual basis the percentage increase for Ba–N in the first 10 years is as follows:

B–1 yr	14.8%	4–5 yr	2.5%	7–8 yr	3.5%
1–2 yr	4.8%	5–6 yr	3.9%	8–9 yr	2.3%
2–3 yr	2.8%	6–7 yr	3.7%	9–10 yr	2.2%
3–4 yr	2.7%				

This breakdown covers the period between the eruptions of M1 and M2 and points to the conclusion that cranial base growth has achieved by the age of six years about 66 to 75 per cent of its 12-year values. The 2 years, 3 months to 6 years period pretty well covers a time which includes palatal closure, while the 6 years to 12 years period covers growth up to the beginning of the circumpubertal acceleration.

It should be pointed out that the anterior cranial base is divided into two parts: (1) sella to foramen caecum,† and (2) foramen caecum to nasion. This division recognizes the fact that the sella to foramen caecum region is cartilaginous in origin, while the foramen caecum to nasion region is intramembranous. The slight increase in this dimension is in the frontal bone (sinus?).

†The sella to foramen caecum dimension is craniometric. On the lateral x-ray head film the foramen caecum can be approximately fixed on the S–N line at the base of the posterior shadow of the crista galli.

As far as facial breadths and heights are concerned, it is sufficient to note two dimensions in each category:

FACIAL BREADTHS	BIRTH TO 5 YR	10 YR	15 YR
Bizygomatic (Zy–Zy)	110–115 mm. F 2–3 mm. less	120 mm. F 3–5 mm. less	126 mm. F 3–5 mm. less
Bigonial (Go–Go)	78–88 mm. F 2–3 mm. less	98 mm. F 2–3 mm. less	101 mm. F 3–5 mm. less
FACIAL HEIGHTS	BIRTH TO 5 YR	10 YR	15 YR
Total (Na–Gn)	75–85 mm. F 3–4 mm. less	102 mm. F 5 mm. less	107 mm. F 5 mm. less
Upper (N–Ss)	28–36 mm. F 1–2 mm. less	43 mm. F 2 mm. less	45 mm. F 2 mm. less

Methods of Measurement

The data tabulated up to this point are based on three major investigative procedures: craniometry, cephalometry, and dental models. With the exception of the Philadelphia serial material, the data are cross-sectional. The only data strictly craniometric (on skulls) are the measurements that subdivide the anterior cranial base (S–N). Other facial dimensions are cephalometric, i.e., taken directly on the head and face of the subject. Palatal and dental arch data are based on serial dental models. Another stricture to be noted is that only averages are given. In our own researches, to be discussed later, we shall take up the theme of variability.

A short digression into historical perspective will be helpful at this point, for I have participated in the threefold methodological progress in craniofacial research: from skull (craniometry), to head (cephalometry), to x-ray head film (roentgenographic cephalometry). Craniometry not only was basic, but still is, since the great majority of landmarks and measurements picked up in the x-ray head film, both lateral and anteroposterior, involve the bones of the cranium and facial skeleton.

It is possible, of course, to pick up soft tissue details in x-ray head films. These details are of two kinds: (1) tissue overlying the bony substructure—these endpoints and measurements are cephalometric; and (2) the soft tissues of the oropharyngeal areas, oriented to the functional space of the area and to the bony support of the pharyngeal tissues.

Accordingly, we can measure bony craniofacial growth, cephalometric growth of tissue, and tissue form and function in oropharyngeal growth. All these structures and systems have definable landmarks and dimensions (see Appendix).

Over and above the available craniometric and cephalometric normative mensurational data, we may have recourse to standard roentgenographic cephalometric head films. These are standard tracings on a serial basis of head films taken in two views: lateral and posteroanterior or facial. The former are the most widely used by far. At the Institute we use two sets of radiographic norms, both covering a birth to 18 years period: the Broadbent-Bolton Cleveland Standards,[3] and the Philadelphia Standards (unpublished data). The Cleveland Standards are for lateral and anteroposterior views, the Philadelphia Standards for lateral views only. Both are based on middle-class (socioeconomic) Caucasian children.

GROWTH OF THE CLP FACE

Before turning to the growth of the CLP face, based upon our own clinical and research data at the Institute, it will be profitable to review our discussions of normal embryogenesis, normal fetal craniofacial growth, and normal postnatal craniofacial growth. The fact emerges that a cleft palate is not an isolated event. A cleft lip is even less isolated. The timing of a CP or a CL in embryonic development strongly hints that the total craniofacial complex, especially along the midline, may be involved; adjacent bony elements may, as it were, register the "shock waves" of the mid-palatal cleft. If this is so, then we may look back to the second trimester patterning we saw in Burdi's data and venture an opinion—almost a prediction—that whatever dysplasia clefting may induce will be similarly patterned in the sense that growth may, to a degree, perpetuate the dysplastic craniofacial complex. Such a warped complex—if it *is* warped—will continue its pattern to term, and we shall see it and evaluate it at birth.

Rehabilitation

Step 1 is to evaluate as soon after birth as possible the degree to which a given cleft-type has introduced an inhibited or dysplastic fetal cranio-facial pattern. Step 2, still in a growth sense, follows after lip surgery at about three months. In the same vein Step 3 follows after palatal surgery at 18 months (± 2 months). We thus pose for interpretation and evaluation two major growth circumstances essentially oriented to the palate: pre- and postoperative craniofacial growth and development.

This brings our focus to a subteam in the corrective process: the plastic surgeon, dental specialist, radiographic technician, researcher in growth and development, and research orthodontist. Our principal surgeon is Robert L. Harding, and most of the lip and palate operations are performed by him. This in itself is an important factor in our evaluation of the repaired lip and palate because insofar as it is possible (allowing for individual patient responses) technique is a constant, and decisions of type of repair are mainly made by one man. This arrangement, which assures unified surgical choices and consistency of technique, is most important where the problems themselves are so variable. Mohammad Mazaheri is the Institute's dental specialist, and under his direction all basic morphological and dental data are gathered both pre- and postoperatively that have a direct bearing on the evaluation of cranial, facial, and dental relationships. He takes all infant dental casts, and his dental residents continue to do so after the patient is two years old. Under Mazaheri's direction James Hecht takes all x-ray head films (roentgenographic cephalometric and cineradiographic) and careful records are kept of all dental conditions, including anomalies. W. M. Krogman is the researcher in growth and development. With data made available by Harding and Mazaheri, the dental models, x-ray head films, and other materials are studied and analyzed correlatively; the lateral and anteroposterior x-ray head films are traced by Mr. Hecht, who also digitizes them according to the methods of Walker (skeletal framework) and Mazaheri (soft tissues of face and oropharynx). Tracings are also made for special studies by the research orthodontist* and by John Riski, speech pathologist and researcher. The digitized tracings are coded and punched via the Optical Chart Reader and Scanner (OSCAR) by Cathy Zimmerman. Added to this subteam (and to *all* similar subteams) are the skills of the biostatisticians Joseph Meier and Harry Canter, and the computer expertise of Paul Ross. These men advise concerning research design and analysis of data.

The Research Series

We shall now report on the studies based on our *Research Series*, established in 1964 under N.I.D.R. Program Grant DE–02172 (currently DE–02172 [13]). This Series comprises some 350 children with clefts, seen regularly from birth. We are not yet prepared to report on all data gathered over the 1964 to 1976 period. In the following pages we shall report in detail on the birth to six years period, which in itself will necessitate some qualifying evaluation at the end of this discussion.

In 1961 Mazaheri discussed the general prosthetic care of closed vertical dimensions in cleft palate patients. At that time he made the following statement: "Lack of lateral and vertical growth of the maxilla and overclosure of vertical dimensions are often seen in cleft palate patients. Complete dentures supported by natural teeth are the ideal treatment for these patients."[19] Implicit in this statement are two inferences: palatal clefts may have repercussions in contiguous maxillary and maxillofacial structures; and such relatively widespread relationships may necessitate the additional remedial aid of a prosthesis.

In 1967 Mazaheri, Harding, and Nanda reported on the effect of surgery on maxillary growth and cleft width.[21] There were six males and six females with UCLP, and the same number with CP (hard and soft) in their study. All were seen on four consecutive visits between the ages of 23 days and two years, four months. Four groups of dental casts and x-ray head films were established at the following times: (1) prior to lip surgery (average age one month, 26 days); (2) after lip surgery (average age three months, two days); (3) after anterior palate closure via a vomer flap (one year, one month); and (4) after soft palate closure via a median sagittal suture (one year, five months). Several significant dimensions are reported in Table 2–6.

Note the striking reduction of 7.76 mm. in cleft width with lip repair. Possible causative factors are muscle function and inherent growth potential. A properly repaired lip restores the function of the M. orbicularis oris and its associated facial muscles (almost certainly MM. quadratus labii superioris and inferioris). This group forms, in essence, a vertically placed sphincter. Then, with the circumlabial muscles as a functional unit (also called a functional matrix), a horizontally placed buccal sphincter-like muscle may come into

*Since 1971, in arrangement with Fujio Miura, D.D.S., Ph.D., Chairman of Orthodontics, Tokyo Medical and Dental School, we have had the excellent clinical and research aid of his graduate students in orthodontics, all with the D.D.S. and the Ph.D.: Drs. Keiichi Ishiguro, Kooji Hanada, Gakuji Ito, Nobuo Suzuki, Hajime Ohyama, Tetsuya Kamegai, and Isao Hayashi.

TABLE 2-6   Widths (in mm.) Before and After Repair

TIME	BITUBEROSITY W		CLEFT W		BIMAXILLARY W	
	$\overline{X}$	S.D.	$\overline{X}$	S.D.	$\overline{X}$	S.D.
Before lip repair	30.5	2.65	10.1	5.5	45.0	4.59
After lip repair	30.3	2.99	2.34	2.26	44.4	4.87
After palate repair	–	–	–	–	48.1	1.28

(Adapted from Mazaheri, M., R. L. Harding, and S. Nanda: Plast. Reconstr. Surg., *40*:22, 1967.)

play, the M. buccinator, right and left. Along with the greatly improved function of the facial musculature lateral to medial compressive forces may arise, acting on right and left palatal segments.

We cannot overlook the fact that the free mid-margins of the cleft may have an inherent tendency to grow medialward; after all, had the palatal shelves united they would have formed a mid-line sutural system—itself an area of growth.

The lip and palatal surgery had no effect upon the bimaxillary and bituberosity dimensional growth. The width of the latter, however, was smaller than in our Sillman data, and it is possible that, overall, there was a slight growth inhibition in the posterior palatal area still registered at two years, four months.

Changes in Arch Form

In a closely related study Harding and Mazaheri studied 80 children with bilateral cleft lip and palate with the use of maxillary and mandibular dental casts.[10] The study focused on growth and spatial changes in arch form in these BCLP patients. The period covered was through the ages of changing dentition, and casts were available at one and one-half months, six months, one year, one year and six months, two years, and three years. The BCLP data were compared with unilateral cleft lip and palate (UCLP) and with non-cleft (Normal). It was found that differences in maxillary widths between BCLP and UCLP "although great at birth, became less significant after repair of the lip." Again, as in the preceding study which went up to two years, 4 months, these BCLP and UCLP patients at three years had maxillary widths less than those in the Sillman data. There was, nevertheless, another positive reaction, for by the age of three years an initial segmental asymmetry had been corrected to an end-to-end relationship.

A study by Mazaheri and colleagues throws additional light upon changes in arch form and dimensions in cleft patients.[20] Dental casts of 30 UCLP and 40 CP (hard and soft palate) patients from birth to five years were studied. The longitudinal data were taken one and one-half months before surgery; and six months, one year, one and one-half, two, three, four, and five years after lip surgery. The numbers of dental casts studied were as follows:

CLEFT-TYPE	MAXILLARY	MANDIBULAR
UCLP	194	171
CP	225	203
Normal	194	194

In the dimensional data "a significant pattern of antero-posterior and lateral dimension retardation was noted immediately after surgical treatment." By the age of four years this retardation was no longer registered. Once more, widths were more affected than were lengths: at five years widths were smaller than in the Sillman norms, but lengths had caught up.

There were constant and uniformly progressive changes in the relationship between the greater and lesser segments of the cleft arch. In most cases in which the larger segment overlapped the lesser even up to two years, an end-to-end relationship had been established. It was observed in this study that mandibular arch lengths and widths were reduced in CP patients as compared to UCLP and Normal. This, concluded the authors, "appears to suggest a definite tendency toward mandibular (relative) hypoplasia in CP subjects."[20]

In Figures 2–18 and 2–19 are shown changes in segmental relationships and palatal heights. Both figures show palatal casts cut transversely, Figure 2–18 at the posterior palatal plane (bituberosity) and Figure 2–19 at the bicanine plane.

Increments in Maxillary Growth

In 1974 Mapes and coworkers published a longitudinal study of maxillary growth in 40 UCLP patients (23 male, 17 female).[18] In these patients

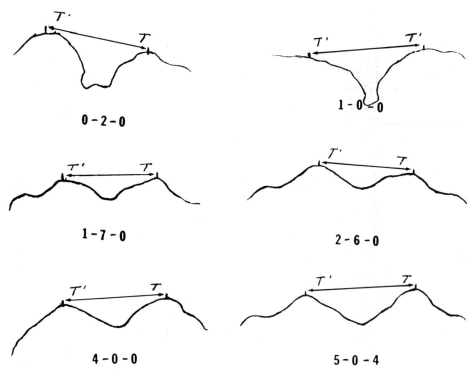

FIGURE 2–18 Segmental relationship changes and palatal heights from two months to five years of age, with casts cut transversely at plane of posterior palatal tuberosities (T–T'). (From Mazaheri, M., et al.: Am. J. Orthod., 60:19, 1971.)

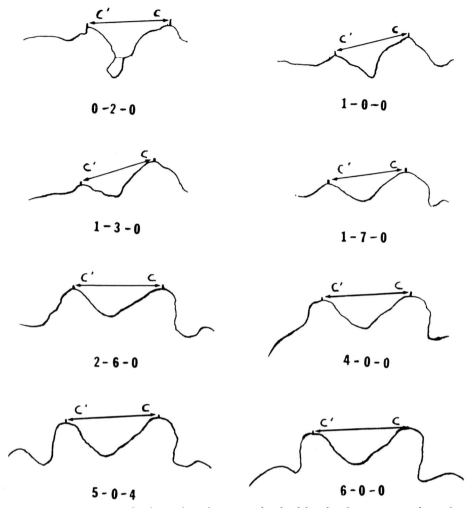

FIGURE 2–19 Segmental relationship changes and palatal heights from two months to five years of age, with casts cut transversely at canine plane (C–C′). (From Mazaheri, M., et al.: Am. J. Orthod., *60*:19, 1971.)

the lip was closed by a triangular flap at 3.3 months, the hard palate was closed via a vomer flap to the incisive foramen at 13.7 months, and the soft palate was closed by a simple median suture at 16.6 months. Casts were taken at two months, six months, one year, one and one-half, two, three, four, five, and six years.

In Figure 2–20 a photocopy of a maxillary cast is shown with the following endpoints located (see Appendix):

I = crest of ridge on line from labial frenum to incisive papilla.

L = anterior end of lesser segment

G = anterior end of greater segment

C and C′ = canine points = intersection of the groove of the lateral labial frenum and the crest of the ridge that coincides with the interproximal point between c and m1.

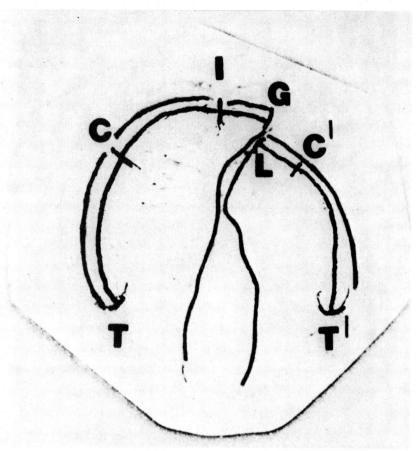

FIGURE 2–20   Photocopy of maxillary cast. Shown are crest of ridge, mesial and distal borders of the cleft. See text for definition of points. (From Mapes, A. M., et al.: Cleft Palate J., *11*:450, 1974.)

T and T′ = tuberosity points = junction of the crest of the ridge with the outline of the tuberosity.

The following measurements were taken:

I–G = anterior portion of clefted segment

L–C′ = posterior portion of clefted segment up through distal c.

I–C′ = il–c length of affected side (= I–G + L–G).

I–C = il–c length of unaffected side.

C′–T′ = canine to tuberosity length on affected side.

C–T = canine to tuberosity length on unaffected side.

I–T′ = incisor to tuberosity length on affected side (= I–C′ + C′–T).

I–T = incisor to tuberosity length on unaffected side.

In Figure 2–21 is shown the growth rate of the I–C and I–C′ segments with lip surgery noted at two to six months and palatal surgery at one to two years. In this anterior segment of the arch there is noted a growth rate (incremental) below normal at the times of lip and palatal surgery. By three to four years, however, the incremental growth rate on both affected and unaffected sides approaches that of the Normal.

In Figure 2–22 the incremental growth of the posterior arch segments

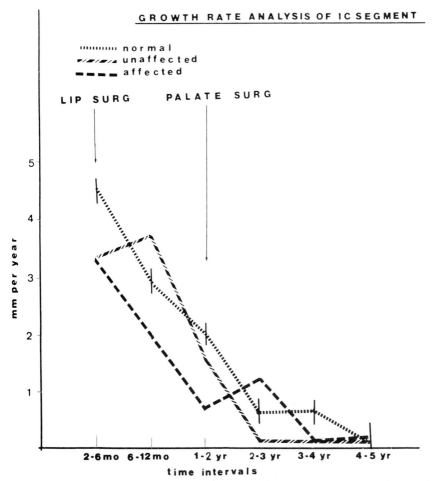

FIGURE 2-21 Growth rate of the I–C and I–C′ segments of normal children and of unaffected and affected sides of palates of children with clefts, as related to surgical procedures. (From Mapes, A. M., et al.: Cleft Palate J., *11*:450, 1974.)

(C–T and C–T′) is shown with lip and palatal surgery noted. The affected side grew more slowly than Normal during the period of lip surgery, but from six to 12 months after lip closure an incremental growth rate of 1.62 mm. per annum approximated the Normal 1.2 mm. per annum rate.

In Figure 2–23 the growth of the entire side is shown (I–T and I–T′). Again there are incremental growth lags, compared to Normal, at lip surgery and at palatal surgery, but by three years the rates verge upon those of the Normal.

In this study the authors found an asymmetry between affected and un-affected segments, basically in the I–C and I–C′ areas, that persisted through the sixth year (P < 0.05). The posterior segment length C–T was shorter than the C′–T′ segment by 0.9 mm. at birth, but by four years they were equal. The authors feel that the C′–T′ incremental growth was probably accelerated ("hyperplastic"), since C–T is about the same length as in the Normal.

To summarize, there seems to have occurred a compensatory catch-up growth: "both the anterior and posterior segments have a combined length

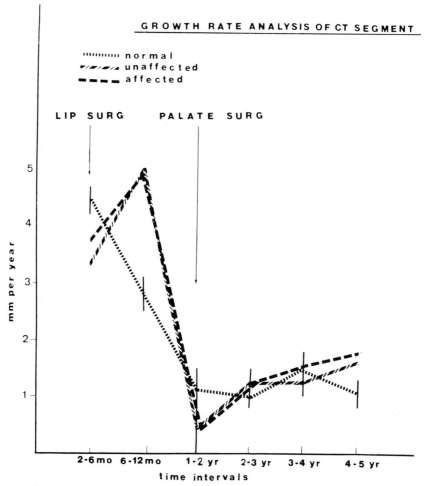

FIGURE 2–22   Growth rate of the C–T and C–T′ segments of normal children and of unaffected and affected sides of palates of children with clefts, as related to surgical procedures. (From Mapes, A. M., et al.: Cleft Palate J., *11*:450, 1974.)

(which) yields an alveolar length on the affected side which is not significantly asymmetrical from the unaffected side by the sixth year."[18]

Cleft and Non-cleft Growth

In 1975 Krogman and colleagues reported on a longitudinal study of the craniofacial growth of children with clefts as compared with non-cleft children.[17] The period covered was birth to six years. The study involved 59 isolated CP cases and 43 CL(P) cases and was based on serial lateral x-ray head films with the Normal derived from the Cleveland Roentgenographic Cephalometric Standards for one to six years of age. In this study the cranial base was found to be an area of adjustment and adjustive growth to clefting, as determined by the behavior of the point basion (Ba) on the anterior margin of the foramen magnum. In the Normal the growth trajectory at Ba is downward and backward; in CL(P) and CP it is downward and forward. The total cranial base complex (Ba–S–N) seems to be more affected in CL(P) than in

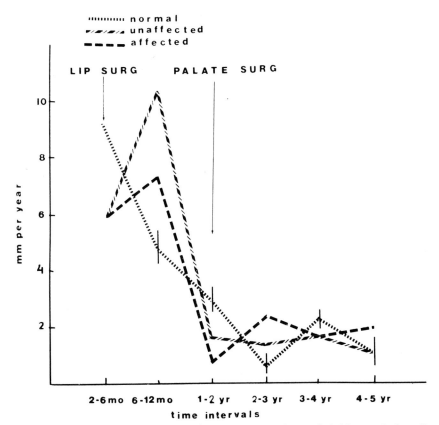

FIGURE 2–23 Growth rate of the I–T and I–T′ segments of normal children and of unaffected and affected sides of palates of children with clefts, as related to surgical procedures. (From Mapes, A. M., et al.: Cleft Palate J., *11*:450, 1974.)

CP, for the former is more divergent from the Normal. The sellar angle (cranial base flexion angle) Ba–S–N, however, decreases uniformly in the six-year period much as does the Normal.

This study was important not only for its indication of catch-up growth by six years, but for the analysis of mandibular growth. We found no hypoplasia (no micrognathic tendency) at all. In Figure 2–24 are shown growth in corporal length (Go–Gn), ramal height (Ar–Go), and overall mandibular length (Ar–Gn). In none of these dimensions do the CP and CL(P) differ from the Normal. The gonial angle (Ar–Go–Gn, or ramal-corporal) is more obtuse in CP and CL(P), compared with Normal, and as a result the lower border of the mandible forms a steeper angle with the Frankfort horizontal, and the anterior end of the mandibular body (at Gn) is depressed downward and backward (Figure 2–25). It is this circumstance that gives the face in clefting an appearance of lower facial retrusion.

In Figure 2–26 we illustrate what appears to be a positional growth change in the mandible. On the tracing of lateral x-ray head film the S–N (anterior cranial base) line was drawn, and a vertical to S–N through S was drawn. Then, in successive head films, tracings were superimposed on the

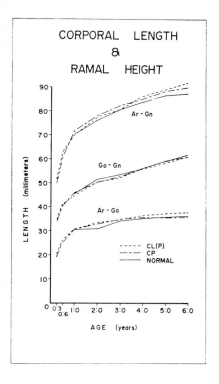

FIGURE 2-24 Growth of corporal length (Go–Gn) and ramal height (Ar-Go) from birth to six years in CL(P), CP, and Normal. (From Krogman, W. M., et al.: Cleft Palate J., *12*:59, 1975.)

FIGURE 2-25 Gonial angle (ramal-corporal), birth to six years in CL(P), CP, and Normal. (From Krogman, W. M., et al.: Cleft Palate J., *12*:59, 1975.)

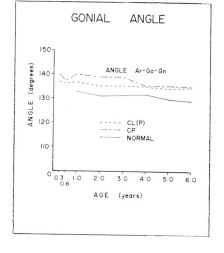

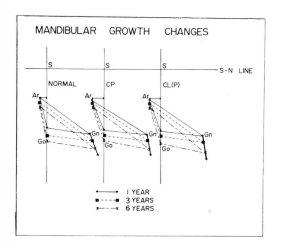

FIGURE 2-26 Growth changes, birth to six years of age in the mandible of CL(P), CP, and Normal. (From Krogman, W. M., et al.: Cleft Palate J., *12*:59, 1975.)

S–N line with Go registered on the vertical to S–N through S. This comparison was done at one, three, and six years. Two conditions became apparent: (1) in CP and CL(P) the mandibular condyle is slightly retropositioned, as judged by the relation of Ar to the constructed vertical line; and (2) the anterior position of the mandible at Gn tends to grow more directly downward in clefts than in the Normal. The data here complement that of Figures 2–24 and 2–25. In patients with palatal clefts the mandible in our longitudinal series of CL(P) and CP is not smaller than in Normal; its gonial angle and its slight retropositioning combine to give a slight appearance of retrognathism.

In 1976 Ishiguro and colleagues summarized an analysis of 140 posteroanterior x-ray head films, serially studied from birth to six years.[14] They were taken from the same Lancaster Research Series as the lateral head films discussed above. Represented were 51 UCLP, 27 BCLP, and 62 CP. In the study of these posteroanterior x-ray head films, the X axis was established as the *Standard Line* (S–Line), connecting the right and left Zf points (orbital points of the zygo-frontal suture). The Y axis was drawn perpendicularly to the S–Line from a point bisecting that line. All vertical (height) measurements were to the right and left of the Y axis. On the posteroanterior x-ray head films 18 endpoints were located, from which nine breadth measurements and eight height measurements were derived. A further refinement was to designate the side of the UCLP: right side was UCLP (1) and left side was UCLP (2).

As in the analysis of postoperative growth in the lateral x-ray head film, it was concluded from the posteroanterior x-ray head films that catch-up growth was such that by the age of six years, breadth and height dimensions were within the normal range of variation. One finding, however, was suggestive: BCLP breadth dimensions were, on the whole, greater than those in UCLP and CP, a possible indication of a slight hyperteloric tendency in BCLP.

For those of us who have worked with both the cephalometry of the living head and tracings of x-ray head films, there is no doubt that the soft tissues of the facial profile reflect quite closely the subjacent bony framework of the face. With this in mind Hanada and Krogman undertook a longitudinal study of postoperative changes in the soft tissue profile in bilateral cleft lip and palate patients from birth to six years.[9] The study was based on 25 cases, 16 male and nine female, in which the lip was closed at three to six months, the hard palate at 12 months, and the soft palate at 16 months. In Figure 2–27 the profile of the BCLP cases (both sexes pooled) is compared with that of the Normal at one year and at six years. The nose as a whole is slightly retrusive, the upper lip is retrusive relative to the cranial base, and the lower lip is slightly protrusive relative to the upper. The maxillomandibular relationship is normal by the age of six years. At both one year and six years the BCLP profile as a whole is slightly retrusive relative to the Normal, though less so at the latter time, and at six years the BCLP profile is functionally, structurally, and esthetically harmonious. As a result it was concluded "that early 'dentofacial orthopedics' is not a necessary precursor to lip and palate closure in BCLP" for achievement of normal incremental facial growth and balanced, proportional growth as well.

In 1967 Mazaheri, Nanda, and Sassouni undertook a pilot study, with small samples, of the mid-facial growth of children with clefts (UCLP, BCLP)

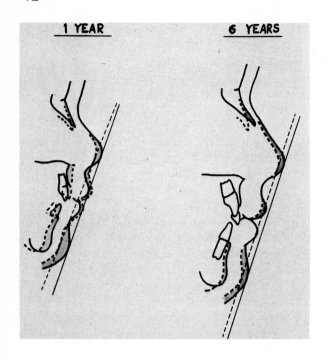

FIGURE 2–27   Soft tissue profile in bilateral cleft lip and palate (BCLP) (broken line) at one and six years of age, compared to non-cleft Normal (solid line). (From Hanada, K., and W. M. Krogman: Am. J. Orthod., 67:363, 1975.)

compared with their non-cleft siblings.[22] In this study there were 54 lateral x-ray head films, 27 cleft cases, and 27 normal siblings. Two age groups were established as follows:

Cleft-type	Younger 7 Yr (6–9 Yr)	Older 11 Yr (10–14 Yr)
UCLP	8	8
BCLP	4	7
Total	12	15

The data were cross-sectional, and all patients with a cleft had received surgery. The younger and the older sibling groups were first compared to give an idea of normal (non-cleft) changes in growth (Figure 2–28). In the tracings at seven and 11 years the palatal plane (ANS–PNS) remains directly comparable in that ANS has grown downward and forward while PNS has grown downward. The resultant palatal slope is patterned in the seven years and 11 years control groups.

Next the tracing of the UCLP sample was compared with that of the Normal at seven and one-half years (Figure 2–29). At this age no real difference was evident in either the cranial base or the palatal areas, and at 11 years the cranial base and palate in UCLP are still much the same as in Normal, though there may be a slight reduction in vertical dimensions in the 11 years UCLP (Figure 2–30).

When the BCLP sample is compared with the Normal at 11 years, the story is a bit different (Figure 2–31). PNS in both the BCLP and the Normal is at the same anteroposterior level; ANS, on the other hand, is 6 mm. behind the Normal in BCLP. As a result the entire palatal plane has an upward tilt at PNS.

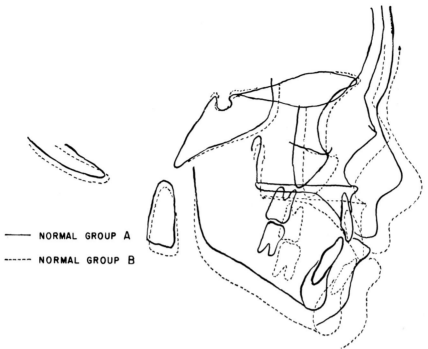

FIGURE 2–28 Growth changes in Normal control (A) at seven and (B) 11 years of age in siblings of children with unilateral (type III) cleft lip and palate. Palatal planes parallel, ANS down and forward, PNS down. (From Mazaheri, M., et al.: Cleft Palate J., 4:334, 1967.)

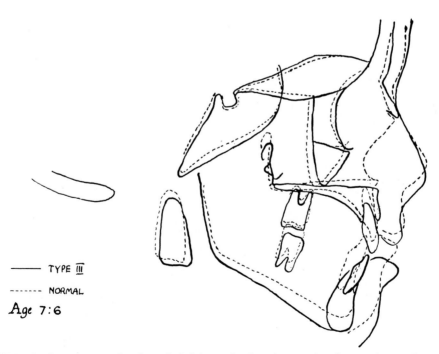

FIGURE 2–29 Comparison of unilateral cleft lip and palate (type III) and Normal control at seven years, six months. No real difference in cranial base, or palatal size and position. (From Mazaheri, M., et al.: Cleft Palate J., 4:334, 1967.)

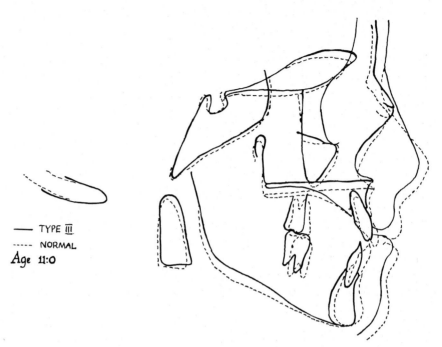

FIGURE 2–30 Comparison of UCLP (type III) and Normal control at 11 years. Palate has same size and anteroposterior position in both. UCLP may show slight vertical underdevelopment. (From Mazaheri, M., et al.: Cleft Palate J., 4:334, 1967.)

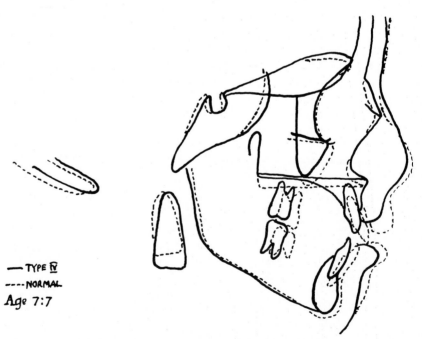

FIGURE 2–31 Comparison of BCLP (type IV) and Normal control at 11 years. PNS at same anteroposterior level, with ANS retrusive approximately 6 mm. Palatal plane tipped up posteriorly at PNS. (From Mazaheri, M., et al.: Cleft Palate J., 4:334, 1967.)

It should be noted that no individual measurements were used in this study; the tracings of the UCLP, BCLP, and siblings at seven and 11 years were done via the composite method, i.e., the tracings in Figures 2–28 through 2–31 were, in a sense, averaged. The authors note that "the growth pattern of the midfacial region was ... subjectively evaluated."[22] While no obvious growth retardation was found in the UCLP sample when compared with the Normal, it was stated that in the BCLP sample "there is a major growth retardation." The authors conclude, and we concur, that longitudinal (as opposed to cross-sectional) studies of non-cleft and cleft siblings are sorely needed.

The analysis of the longitudinal craniofacial growth data of the Institute's Research Series very obviously covers the early phase of postnatal growth, embracing infancy and early childhood, i.e., from birth to six years of age. This has taken us through the initial high velocity of growth from birth to two years and into the relative deceleration of the early childhood to mid-childhood transition period. In mid-childhood growth, velocity is relatively slow, except in late midchildhood when the incipience of the pre- and circum-pubertal acceleration in growth is manifest.

SUMMARY

In the analyses of our Research Series that have been presented in the preceding pages we have stated that there is postoperative (both lip and palate) catch-up growth, so that by the age of six years the maxillofacial complex, both hard and soft (profile) tissues, is acceptably normal. According to the mensurational data of non-cleft controls and the careful comparison of x-ray head film standards, the craniofacial complex in repaired CL(P) patients is within the normal range of variation. In saying this we are prepared to recognize that the position of these patients in a normal distribution may be "below the average" in the sense of $\overline{X} - S.D.$ (mean minus one standard deviation). We must insist, however, that this possibility of below-the-mean size is *not* a measure of dysplasia, for the maxillofacial and maxillomandibular relationships are, as we stated earlier, structurally, functionally, and esthetically harmonious. The palate, the mandible, and the total profile ensemble are "good" — taken as a total group there are no "crippled faces" as stigmata of a congenital failure and of surgical intervention.

In our dimensional curves of the growth of the maxillofacial complex we have quite consistently noted an interruption — a slight lag — in the velocity of growth after lip repair (three months) and after palate repair (14 to 20 months). This is understandable and, indeed, to be expected. The intervention of the surgeon's knife is traumatic — it is a shock to the hard and soft tissues involved. There may occur short periods of insufficient blood supply or even of interrupted innervation; the metabolic gradient of orderly cellular growth and replacement may be inhibited and slowed down. For a time all structures involved in corrective surgery may, through insult and shock, go into a temporary stasis, but the innate resiliency of vigorously growing tissues (hard and soft) will assert itself and the processes of orderly development will take over — indeed, they may accelerate a bit. This, somewhat simplistically stated, is what we mean by "catch-up growth."

This reassuring situation has not always existed, for many clinicians and researchers have pointed in the past to the "irremediable damage" caused by operative procedures. The "irreversible trauma of the knife" was formerly a byword in the cleft palate field. As late as 1972 Ross and Johnston stated that surgery "introduces morphological changes and new growth factors which almost invariably have a deleterious effect on facial development" (p. 165) and that "surgery produces residual scar tissue which inhibits and distorts growth [to produce] abnormal facial development in cleft lip and palate" (p. 196). They feel that there will result a "mild, long term inhibition of the necessary forward movement of the entire nasomaxillary complex."[25]

The issue is thus joined, because our Research Series longitudinal data for the first six years of postnatal growth in the CLP patient have shown neither "abnormal facial development" nor any marked or dysplastic "inhibition" of growth. In looking at this apparent contradiction two major sets of circumstances must be considered. In the hard palate, growth occurs by apposition on the palatal surface of the maxilla and at the maxillary tuberosity; thus palatal vaulting and palatal (dental arch) length are remodeled and in the process increased in size and changed in proportion. The dental arch, per se, is also a partner in the remodeling process with resorption lingually and apposition labially (anterior) and bucally (posterior). These, let us emphasize, are *growth processes* and, hence, *growth loci.* If these areas are traumatized to the extent of producing relatively widespread masses of scar tissue, then we can envision a scar tissue rigidity that will be inhibitory or distortive in its effect.

In 1974 we set out to test the following hypothesis: "Operative intervention in cleft palate cases which *minimally involves* (emphasis added) bone-growth potential will guide and facilitate maxillofacial growth . . . so that post-operative growth, in a *catch-up* manner, will provide for the achievement of an acceptably normal cranio-facio-dental growth pattern."[17] In a longitudinal study of 59 CP and 43 combined UCLP and BCLP cases from birth to six years, employing lateral x-ray head films, we stated: "We have observed that there is a general post-operative *catch-up growth in both cleft types* (CP and CLP), more so in CP. It is our conclusion that conservative surgery [minimally involving periosteal tissues] has facilitated rather than inhibited or deviated growth in both the maxillofacial skeletal complex and the soft tissues of the labio-facial complex. In the data presented . . . our hypothesis has been substantiated." The noninvolvement (or the minimal involvement) of growth areas or growth loci, and the minimal production of scar tissue, are almost certainly part of the answer to successful postoperative growth. Heightened surgical awareness of the need to interfere least with growth potentials is the key, for it seems that areas of proliferating growth are the most prone to the production of scar tissue.

The issue is still moot because it can be argued that catch-up statements made for the first six years of growth will not hold true for later growth, especially for the vigorous growth tempos of the period of pubertal changes from 10 to 15 years of age. Strictly speaking we cannot answer that type of argument until we have gone over our postsixth year longitudinal material in the same manner as our birth to six years data. The problem centers around the following question: "Will differential growth rates occur after six years in the maxillofacial complex in clefting that may lead to a dysplastic condition?" This practically involves the possibility of a latency that will be evoked by the growth velocities of the circumpubertal period—a sort of delayed reaction situation. On the basis of sheer logic we hold this possibility to be conceptually incorrect.

From the prenatal period and on into the postnatal period we have noticed in the normative non-cleft data cited as controls a well-defined tendency toward patterned growth. There is an orderliness in differential rates, sites, and timing that almost seems genetically entrenched. Will this hold true in cleft patients with a craniofacial pattern that is acceptably "normal" by six years? We think so, and we argue by analogy. In 1970 Krogman published a monograph on the cephalofacial and somatic growth of Caucasian and black children in Philadelphia from six to 17 years of age.[16] The data were longitudinal and the children were non-cleft, i.e., they had normal heads, faces, and jaws. As the term "cephalofacial" implies, the living head and face were measured. There were no significant changes in growth in the facial area between six years and about 12 to 14 years (Figure 2–32). The average facial configuration (pattern) held. The face was bigger, but proportionately so; differential growth in the mandibular corpus at the chin may have conduced to a relative prognathism, more marked in males.

This development suggests prediction — an overall pattern-oriented prediction, rather than one for specifics of regional areas or structures. It certainly applies to a normal growth process untrammeled by any trauma. Will it apply to the cleft maxillofacial complex which has achieved "normality" by six years? We hope so — we even venture to think so!

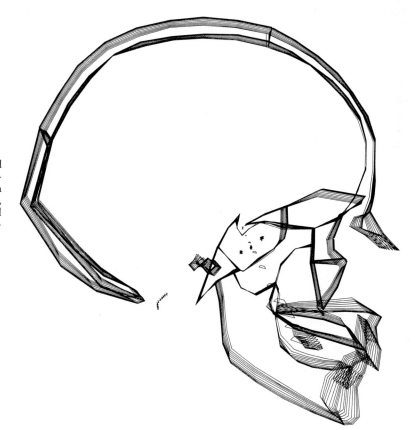

FIGURE 2–32 Computerized tracings of the average craniofacial growth of Philadelphia white males (non-cleft Normal), eight to 15 years of age, based on serial observations. (Krogman, 1949 to 1969.)

APPENDIX: _____
THE MEASUREMENT OF
FORM AND FUNCTION
(With John E. Riski)

Size, proportion, and angular relationships are of relevance to a number of major areas concerned with clefts: surgery, dentistry, growth and development, and speech. The involved regions are, of course, the head and face of the cleft patient, i.e., the skeletal framework and the associated soft tissues of the craniofacial area. The skeletal framework embraces the bones of the cranium and the bones of the face. The associated soft tissues embrace first, the soft tissue overlay (the soft tissues of the external head and face) and second, the deeper soft tissues of the nose and throat (the naso-oro-pharyngeal complex). All of these measurements can be taken on x-ray head films of the cleft subject (roentgenographic and cineradiographic).

Basically the measurements of the skeletal structures of the cranium and face are those that have been employed for many years by physical anthropologists. They have been used and adapted by researchers in dentistry (especially orthodontics) and in the cleft palate field. There is an interesting and meaningful succession of technique in anthropological methodology: (1) craniometry, or the measurement of the skull; (2) cephalometry, or the measurement of the head; and (3) roentgenographic cephalometry, or the measurement of the tracing of the x-ray head film. Method 1 resulted in only cross-sectional data; methods 2 and 3 permitted the gathering of serial or longitudinal data. In our present discussion we shall consider the x-ray head film mainly in its lateral view (norma lateralis sinistra). The facial x-ray head film (norma facialis) has not been fully explored, but we shall include some data derived from the facial (posteroanterior) head film.

In the presentation that follows we shall define endpoints, dimensions, proportions or ratios, and angular relationships for both hard parts (bone) and soft parts (tissues). To anyone who has surveyed the literature of morphology and function in the cleft palate field it must be obvious that the number of points, etc., is limited only by the creative imagination of the researcher. We have index files on literally hundreds of such mensurational details, but we shall present only those that we have used for their constructive and enlightening nature. Most of them we have devised ourselves; some we have adapted from the studies of other researchers. Often the same points have been named differently by individual researchers, and in some instances endpoints have been arbitrarily defined alphabetically, as A, B, C, and so on. We have consistently redefined these latter points in relation to the structure(s) being measured.

In principle we have accepted the prevailing rule that all named points are given in alphabetical order, followed by an appropriate abbreviation: Basion (Ba). However, there are many points, especially for soft tissues, that are not named but are designated only by letters. An example is AA, which is on the anterior aspect of the first cervical vertebra but is not given a name. These alphabetically designated points also have been listed in alphabetical order.

We are setting up five major categories of measurement: (1) craniometric; (2) facial soft tissue; (3) oropharyngeal; (4) velopharyngeal; and (5) palatal, including the dental arch. Categories 1, 2, 3, and 4 relate to both the x-ray head film (mainly lateral) and cineradiographic frames, while 5 relates to the dental model. In each category the definitions will be given in alphabetical order.

In the definitions which will follow certain conventions are employed that refer mainly to notations of the dentition and require clarification. There are two sets of teeth, deciduous (milk) and permanent, with 20 in the former and 32 in the latter. The deciduous teeth are one central and one lateral incisor, one canine, and two molars (right and left, upper and lower); the permanent teeth are central and lateral incisors, canine, first and second premolars, and first, second, and third molars. The deciduous teeth are noted in lower case letters (for example i1–2, c, m1–2); the permanent teeth are noted in upper case letters (I1–2, C, P1–2, M1–3). In indicating a single tooth or a group of teeth the uppers are underlined, the lowers overlined—thus $\overline{m1}$ and $\overline{M2}$ are a lower deciduous first molar and a lower second permanent molar, respectively, while the corresponding upper tooth designations would be $\underline{m1}$ and $\underline{M2}$. The underline and overline may be thought of as the line of occlusal contact between upper and lower teeth.

There is another convention to be noted, i.e., some of the endpoints and other markings are on the lateral head film, while some are on the facial head film. We shall use (L) to designate the former and (F) to designate the latter. Several markings are on both lateral and facial head films and will be designated as (L) (F).

CRANIOMETRIC

Craniometric Points (Figure 2–33)

Anterior nasal spine (ANS): the tip of the anterior nasal spine.   (L)

Articulare (Ar): point determined in the lateral head film where the posterior margin of the ascending ramus of the mandible intersects the shadow of the cranial base.   (L)

Basion (Ba): the most anterior point on the anterior margin of the foramen magnum.   (L)

Biorbitale (Biorb): the most lateral point on the lateral margin of the bony orbit, right and left.   (F)

Crista galli (CG): located as the highest point on the superior contour of the crista galli.   (L)

Ectomolare (Ecto–M): junction of buccal alveolus of upper $\underline{M1}$ with neck of $\underline{M1}$, right and left ($\underline{M1}|\underline{M1}$ ecto.).   (F)

Endomolare (Endo–M): junction of lingual alveolus of upper $\underline{M1}$ with neck of $\underline{M1}$, right and left ($\underline{M1}|\underline{M1}$ endo.).   (F)

Ethmoidale (SE): upper margin of sphenoethmoid synchondrosis (also called Sphenoethmoidale).   (L)

Gnathion (Gn): the lowest point on the mandibular symphysis in the midline, where the anterior surface becomes confluent with the base of the mandibular body.   (L)   (F)

Gonion (Go): the point (right and left) on the mandibular angle determined

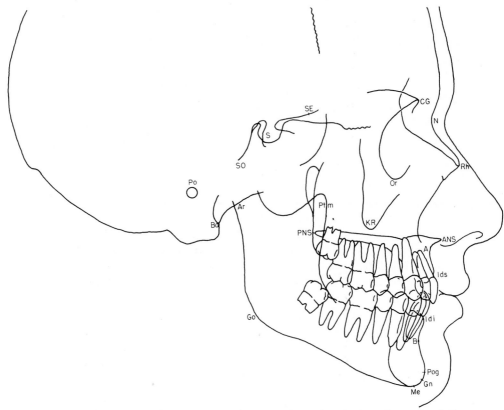

FIGURE 2–33   Craniometric endpoints as located in the lateral x-ray head film.

by the bisection of the angle formed by the intersection of the mandibular
and ramal lines. In the lateral head films if right and left Go are not superimposed, the point Go′ is taken as the mean between the two.   (L)

Inferior alveolar point (see *Intradentale inferius*).

Infradentale (see *Intradentale inferius*).

Interorbitale (Inorb): point marking the most medial margin of the bony orbit,
right and left.   (F)

Intradentale inferius (Idi): the tip of the alveolar septum between right and
left lower incisor teeth ($\overline{i1}|\overline{i1}$ or $\overline{I1}|\overline{I1}$) on the labial aspect. Idi is also known
as the inferior alveolar point and the infradentale.   (L)   (F)

Intradentale superius (Ids): the tip of the alveolar septum between right and
left upper central incisors ($\underline{i1}|\underline{i1}$ or $\underline{I1}|\underline{I1}$) on the labial aspect. Ids is also
known as the upper alveolar point and the supradentale.   (L)   (F)

Key-ridge (KR): seen in the lateral head film as the lowest point on the zygomaxillary abutment.   (L)

Menton (Me): the lowest point on the shadow of the mandibular symphysis,
seen in the lateral head film.   (L)

Nasale (Na): points on right and left lateral borders of the nasal aperture marking maximum breadth of the aperture.   (F)

Nasion (N): the most anterior point of the nasofrontal suture as seen in the
lateral head film.   (L)

Nasospinale (Nsp): the lowest point on the lower margin of the nasal (pyriform) aperture; usually taken as mean between right and left Nsp points.   (F)

Orbitale (Or): right and left, the lowest point on the lower margin of the bony orbit. In the lateral head film if right and left Or are not superimposed, the point Or' is taken as the mean between them.   (L)

Pogonion (Pog): the most anterior point on the symphyseal mandibular contour of the lateral head film; may be abbreviated as P.   (L)

Point A (Subspinale, Ss): seen on the lateral head film as the most posterior point (or the "deepest point") of the concavity below the anterior nasal spine.   (L)

Point B (Supramentale, Sm): seen on the lateral head film as the most posterior point (or the "deepest point") on the concavity on the mandibular symphysis above the mental prominence of the chin.   (L)

Porion (Po): the uppermost point (right and left) of the bony external auditory meatus; in the lateral head film it may be determined as the uppermost point of the ear-rod of the cephalostat.   (L)

Posterior nasal spine (PNS): the tip of the posterior nasal spine; PNS may be obscured by the shadow of <u>M2</u>, or it may be absent due to a cleft. Under these circumstances Ptm may be projected to the PP where its intersection is Ptm', which now may be accepted as a close approximation to PNS.   (L)

Pterygomaxillary fissure (Ptm): the lowest point in the space between the maxillary tuberosity and the pterygoid processes of the sphenoid.   (L)

Rhinion (Rh): tip of the nasal bones.   (L)

Sella (S): the midpoint, seen laterally, of the sella turcica; located by inspection.   (L)

Septal point (SP): located as the most anterior point on the nasal septum, seen from lateral view.   (L)

Sphenoethmoidale (see *Ethmoidale*).

Spheno-occipitale (SO): the uppermost point, endocranially, of the spheno-occipital synchondrosis.   (L)

Subspinale (see *Point A*).

Supradentale (see *Intradentale superius*).

Supramentale (see *Point B*).

Upper alveolar point (see *Intradentale superius*).

Zygion (Zy): point (right and left) on the zygomatic arch marking maximum bizygomatic breadth.   (F)

Zygofrontale (Zf): the inner or orbital aspect of the zygofrontal suture, right and left.   (F)

Zygomaxillare (Zm): lowest point on the zygomaxillary suture, right and left.   (F)

Craniometric Dimensions (Figure 2–34)

Anterior cranial base length (ACBL): S–N; it may be subdivided into S–CG and CG–N. It is often referred to as cranial base length (CBL). S–N is c. 95 per cent of its adult length at c. 7 years. It is often used as a plane of superimposition in serial data, with S registered on S.

Anterior facial height (AFH): N–Gn or N–Me; most often termed total facial height (TFH).

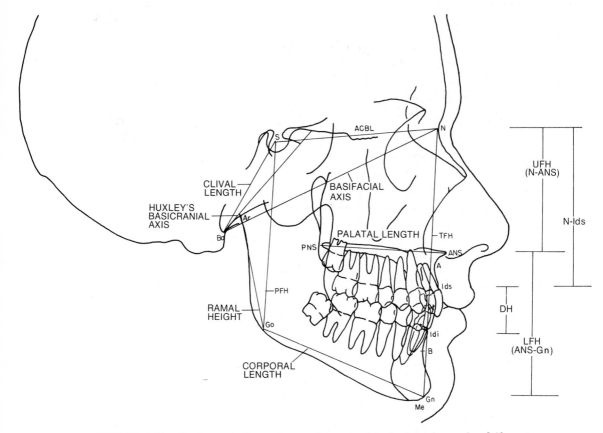

FIGURE 2-34 Craniometric dimensions as determined in the lateral x-ray head film.

Basicranial length (BCL): Huxley's original definition is Ba–SE; it is most often now Ba–N. (More functionally it is an axis and should be called basifacial axis, a line of demarcation between cranial and facial skeletons).

Biorbital breadth (BOB): between right and left Biorb.

Cranial base length (CBL) (see ACBL).

Clival length (CL): posterior cranial base length; Ba–S. It may be subdivided into Ba–SO and SO–S.

Dental height (DH): Ids–Idi when jaws are in occlusion.

Interorbital breadth (IOB): between right and left Inorb.

Lower facial height (LFH): ANS–Gn or ANS–Me; also may be given as Idi–Gn, or Idi–Me, which is mandibular symphysis height.

Mandibular corporal length (ML): most often Gn–Go, but may be Me–Go or Pog–Go; taken parallel to the lower border of the body of the mandible.

Mandibular ramal height (RH): Ar–Go.

Nasal breadth (NB): Na–Na'.

Nasal height (NH): N–Nsp.

Palatal arch length (PAL): from line tangent to posterior margin of crown of m2|m2 (deciduous arch) or posterior margin of crown of M1|M1 to lingual aspect of Ids.

Palatal breadth (PB): inner is between right and left endo–M, outer is between right and left ecto–M.

Palatal length (PL): from the lingual aspect of Ids to PNS. Where PNS is absent due to a cleft, the axis of Ptm projected to the palatal plane approximates PNS at the point of intersection, Ptm'. In the lateral head film PL = ANS–PNS, which also constitutes the palatal plane (PP).

Posterior facial height (PFH): S–Go; this is only roughly comparable to AFH (TFH).

Septal heights (SH) (on fetal head)

Anterior: a perpendicular to the palatal plane through ANS is erected; its intersection with the S–N line is the upper endpoint; the distance ANS to this intersection is the anterior SH.

Mid: similar perpendicular through CG is erected; its intersection with S–N is the upper endpoint; the distance along this perpendicular is the mid SH.

Posterior: similar perpendicular at PNS is erected; its intersection with S–N is the upper endpoint; distance PNS to S–N intersection is posterior SH.

Septal lengths (SL) (on fetal head)

Anterior: line drawn parallel to palatal plane through SP; anterior SL is distance from SP to the perpendicular of anterior palatal height.

Mid: similar parallel drawn; mid SL is distance between perpendiculars of anterior and mid SH.

Posterior: similar parallel drawn; posterior SL is distance between perpendiculars of mid and posterior SH.

TFH (see AFH).

Upper face height (UFH): N–ANS or N–Ids.

Craniometric Planes (Figure 2–35)

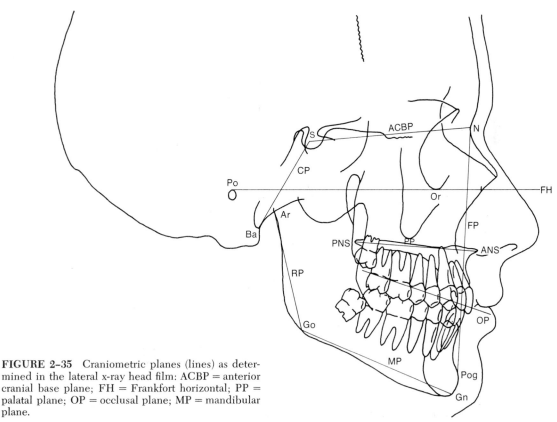

FIGURE 2-35 Craniometric planes (lines) as determined in the lateral x-ray head film: ACBP = anterior cranial base plane; FH = Frankfort horizontal; PP = palatal plane; OP = occlusal plane; MP = mandibular plane.

Strictly speaking there are no *planes* in either the lateral or facial head films; there are only *lines*. Yet, the use of "planes" is so entrenched in the literature that we bow to usage.

Anterior cranial base plane (ACBP): S–N.

Clival plane (CP): Ba–S.

Facial plane (FP): N–Pog.

Frankfort horizontal (FH): horizontal plane established by right and left Po and left Or. All roentgenograms are taken with the subject's head oriented in the FH. This is a true plane.

Mandibular plane (MP): Gn–Go; occasionally Me–Go; lower border of the body of the mandible.

Occlusal plane (OP): plane established by half the over-bite of $\frac{I1 \mid I1}{I1 \mid I1}$ and half the cuspal overlap of $\frac{M1 \mid M1}{M1 \mid M1}$, as seen in the lateral head film.

Palatal plane (PP): plane of ANS–PNS.

Ramal plane (RP): Ar–Go; posterior border of mandibular ascending ramus.

Craniometric Angles (Figure 2–36)

Angle N–Pog to FH (facial angle): this angle is a measure of total facial prognathism (protrusion).

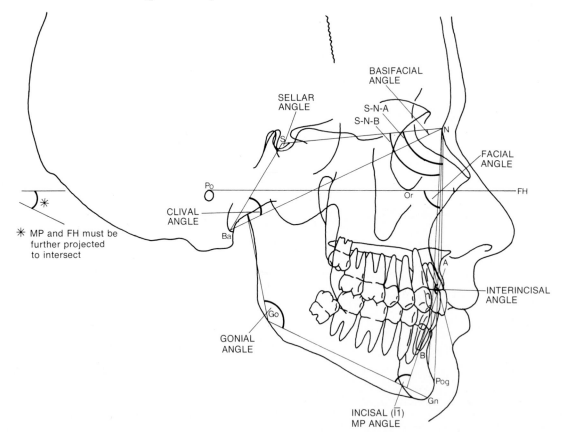

FIGURE 2–36 Craniometric angles as measured in the lateral x-ray head film.

Angle S–N–A: drawn from sella to nasion to Point A. This angle relates the anteroposterior position of the midface to the cranial base.

Angle S–N–B: drawn from sella to nasion to Point B. This angle relates the anteroposterior position of the mandible to the cranial base.

Angular relationships of OP: OP to ACBP, OP to FH, OP to MP, OP to FP.

Basifacial angle: S–N–Ba.

Clival angle: N–Ba–S.

Gonial angle: angle formed by intersection of ramal plane (Ar–Go) with mandibular plane (Go–Gn).

Incisor–MP angle: angle formed by intersection of axis of $\overline{\text{II}}$ with MP.

Interincisal angle: angle formed by intersection of the axes of $\overline{\text{I1}}$ and $\underline{\text{11}}$. The axes of $\underline{\text{I1}}$ and $\overline{\text{II}}$ are lines from the root apex to the incisal margin.

Mandibular plane angle: angle formed by intersection of projection of MP with FH.

Sellar angle: Ba–S–N; angle of flexion of cranial base; also called saddle angle.

S–N–A/S–N–B difference: the difference in degrees between these two angles is a measure of maxillomandibular relationship.

Traditionally the abstraction of data from x-ray films has required a method of hand measurement using rules, calipers, and protractors. This system is relatively simple and does not use sophisticated equipment, but it is time-consuming and introduces the possibility of human error at several levels of analysis.

In the early sixties, while working with W. M. Krogman at the Philadelphia Growth Center, Geoffrey F. Walker developed the Walker digitization of the lateral x-ray head film (Figure 2–37). This method takes advantage of the qualities of head films that lend themselves to computerization, increases the accuracy of the analysis of cephalometric data, and reduces the amount of professional supervision that is required during collection and analysis of data. This system enables the researcher to code, store, retrieve, and analyze large amounts of data most efficiently.

Digitization converts a cephalometric tracing into a series of points. Initially, the standard craniometric points are located and plotted, and the intervening distance between any two of the standard points is then evenly subdivided. For example, Gnathion (Gn) and Gonion (Go) are located on the inferior border of the body of the mandible. The distance between Gn and Go is then subdivided into equal fourths so that the Gn–Go, or the inferior border of the mandible, is represented by a total of five digitized points. In a similar manner a total of 177 "landmark points" are plotted onto the lateral head film tracing.

Once these points have been plotted, the subsequent step is to "read" them onto punch cards. This step utilizes a scanning device (the Optical Chart Reader and Scanner or OSCAR*) that is capable of reading each point as described by two coordinates: the distance along an X axis and the distance

---

*Manufactured by the Bensen-Lehner Corporation.

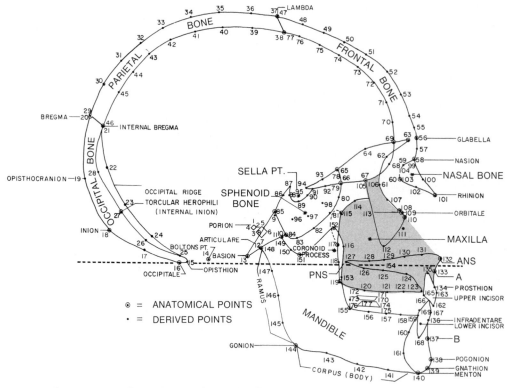

FIGURE 2–37 The Walker model of the digitization of the craniometric outline seen in the lateral x-ray head film. (Courtesy of G. F. Walker, B.D.S., Dept. of Orthodontics, School of Dentistry, University of Michigan.)

along a Y axis. The distance of any point from the origin is read as the length of a hypotenuse of a right angle triangle and can be computed from the Pythagorean theorem.

After the digitized points are read onto punch cards and the data stored in the computer, programs may be written to determine any dimensions, angles, and ratios or to reproduce the traced contour.

FACIAL SOFT TISSUE

Facial Soft Tissue Points* (Figure 2–38)

> *A':* soft tissue counterpart of Point A.
> *Alare* (Al): the point (right and left) across the "wings" of the nose establishing maximum nasal breadth.   (CE)
> *B':* soft tissue counterpart of Point B.
> *Cheilion* (Ch): the most lateral aspect of the vermilion of the mouth, right and left.   (CE)

---

*In the definitions here given those marked (CE) are taken cephalometrically rather than on the facial x-ray head film.

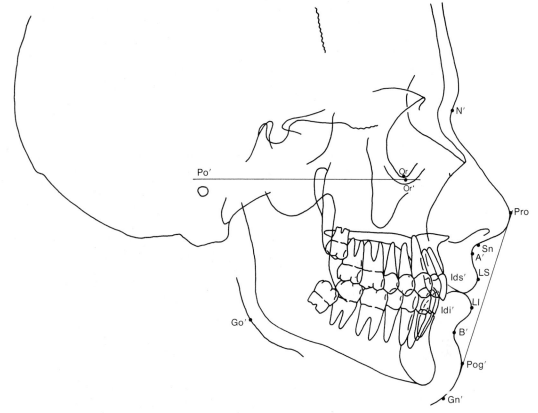

FIGURE 2–38 Facial soft tissue endpoints as located in the lateral x-ray head film.

Ectocanthion (Ectocanth.): the most lateral aspect of the orbital fissure (the lateral corner of the eye-slit).   (CE)

Endocanthion (Endocanth.): the most medial aspect of the orbital fissure (the medial corner of the eye-slit).   (CE)

Esthetic line: Pro–Pog'; this profile line is used to evaluate the esthetic appearance of the mouth. Ideally the line should be roughly tangent to the anterior contour of the upper and lower lips (Lab. sup. and Lab. inf., respectively).

Gn': soft tissue counterpart of Gn.

Go': soft tissue counterpart of Go.

Intradentale inferius (Idi'): tip of the intradental papilla between $\overline{i1|i1}$ or $\overline{I1|I1}$.

Intradentale superius (Ids'): tip of the intradental papilla between $\underline{i1|i1}$ or $\underline{I1|I1}$.

Labrale inferius (LI): the most anterior point on the convexity of the lower lip.

Labrale superius (LS): the most anterior point on the convexity of the upper lip.

N': soft tissue counterpart of N.

Or': soft tissue counterpart of (left) Or.

Po': the most lateral point on the roof of the cartilaginous external auditory meatus. Po' is functionally the soft tissue counterpart of Po. In practice Po' is usually located as the contact point of the ear-rod of the cephalostat with the external auditory meatus (ear-hole).

Pog': soft tissue counterpart of Pog; may be abbreviated as Pg.

Pronasale (Pro): tip of the cartilaginous (soft tissue) nose; the tip of the nose has also been designated as No.

Pupillare (Pup): the midpoint (right and left) determined by inspection of the pupil of the eye when the subject is looking straight ahead. (CE)

Stomion (Sto): the mid-line contact point of the upper and lower lips.

Subnasale (Sn): mid-line point of junction of external inferior aspect of the cartilaginous nasal septum (columella) with the skin of the upper lip.

Zy': soft tissue counterpart of Zy.

Facial Soft Tissue Dimension (Figure 2–39)

> *Bigonial (mandibular) breadth* (BB): Go'–Go', right and left.
> *Biocular breadth* (Bioc B): ectocanth.–ectocanth., right and left.   (CE)
> *Corporal length* (mandible) (CL): Gn'–Go'; may be taken on each right and left mandibular corpus.   (CE)
> *Dental height* (DH): Ids'–Idi'.
> *Facial breadth* (FB): Zy'–Zy', right and left.

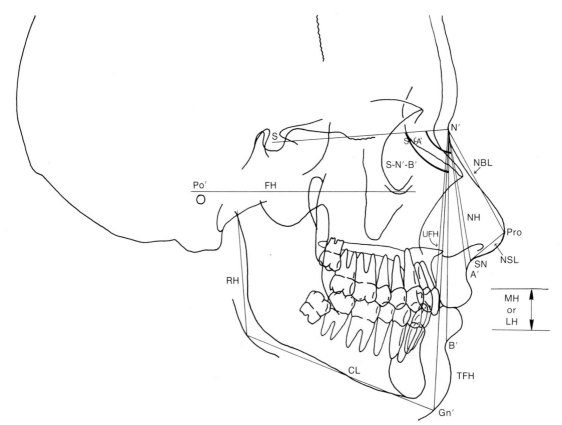

FIGURE 2–39   Facial soft tissue dimensions as determined in the lateral x-ray head film.

Interocular breadth (IB): endocanth.–endocanth., right and left.   (CE)
Interpupillary breadth (IPB): Pup–Pup, right and left.   (CE)
Lower facial height (LFH): Idi'–Gn'.
Mouth breadth (MB): Ch–Ch, right and left.   (CE)
Mouth (lip) height (MH or LH): mid-line vertical dimension of the margin of the upper and lower lips (LI–LS).   (CE)
Nasal breadth (NB): A1–A1, right and left.   (CE)
Nasal bridge length (NBL): N'–Pro.
Nasal height (NH): N'–SN.
Nasal septal length (NSL): Pro–SN.
Ramal height (mandibular) (RH): measured by Go' to a point at the base of the tragus of the ear. This upper point can be located by palpation, opening and closing the mandible; it is thought by some to be on a level with the top of the mandibular condyle.   (CE)
Total facial height (TFH): N'–Gn'.
Upper facial height (UFH): N'–Ids'.

OROPHARYNX

In a sense the foregoing are basically data that delineate the soft tissue profile as seen from norma lateralis. We have included, however, some points and dimensions in the posteroanterior x-ray head film tracing (norma facialis). The ones we have included are oriented mostly to the mid-line breadth dimensions at upper face level to elucidate the possibility or the extent of hypertelorism (excessive interocular breadth due to laterally placed orbits).

Speech researchers have followed closely the efforts of workers in the fields of physical anthropology and dentistry in the use of standard cephalometric procedures. Speech physiologists have applied many of these standardized landmarks, planes, and angles to the study of the positioning and movements of the speech articulators. Frequently it has been necessary to add new points for the purpose of studying speech physiology, such as the estimated point of the insertion of the levator muscles into the velum (LV). Some of the points and measurements used early in the study of speech were discarded as it was learned that they were not meaningful. As pointed out earlier, the system has been confused by investigators who have used different terms and abbreviations for the same point, and by those who have developed and used alphabetical abbreviations. The following is a compilation of those points, dimensions, and angular and areal measures which have been found useful to the study of the oropharyngeal structures in speech function. As in the preceding sections, an attempt has been made to use roentgenographic cephalometric abbreviations where they exist and to logically abbreviate other names that have been added to the literature by researchers. These points and dimensions are those observed in a lateral view of the oropharynx. Some have been defined in earlier sections but have been duplicated here for convenience and to demonstrate their applicability to the study of speech physiology. Most of the points and dimensions are applicable to the evaluation of both still roentgenograms and cineradiographic film.

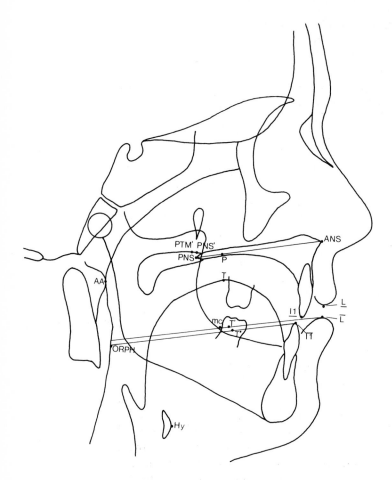

FIGURE 2-40 The oropharyngeal points as located in a lateral cineradiographic frame.

Oropharyngeal Points (Figure 2–40)

Atlas (AA): the most anterior point on the tubercle of the arch of C1, the first cervical vertebra or atlas.

Anterior nasal spine (ANS): the tip of the anterior nasal spine.

Hyoid (Hy): the most anterior point on the body of the hyoid bone at the junction of the anterior and superior surfaces.

Incisor points

Mandibular central incisor ($\overline{\text{il}}$ or $\overline{\text{Il}}$): the tip of the mandibular central incisor.

Maxillary central incisor ($\underline{\text{il}}$ or $\underline{\text{Il}}$): the tip of the maxillary central incisor.

Lip Points

Lower lip ($\overline{\text{L}}$): the most superior point on the lower lip.

Upper lip ($\underline{\text{L}}$): the most inferior point on the upper lip.

Stomion (Sto): the midline of contact between the upper and lower lips while in quiet closure.

Midpoint of oral cavity (MC): the point of the bisection of the $\overline{\text{L}}$ line.

Oropharynx point (Orph): the intersection of the incisal reference line (IRL) with the posterior pharyngeal wall (PPW).

Point P: The intersection of the palatal plane (PP) and a line drawn perpendicular to the palatal plane through the highest point of the tongue (T).

Posterior nasal spine (PNS): the tip of the posterior nasal spine.

(PNS'): the point on the nasal side of the velum nearest to PNS.

Pterygomaxillary fissure' (Ptm'): the projection of the lowest point in the space between the maxillary tuberosity and the pterygoid process of the sphenoid (Ptm) to the palatal plane (PP) via a perpendicular.

Tongue points

Tongue high point (T): the highest point of the tongue by visual inspection.

Tongue anterior (Ta): the most anterior point of the tongue by visual inspection.

Tongue posterior (Tp): the most posterior point of the tongue by visual inspection.

T': the highest point of the tongue (T) projected onto the $\overline{\text{L}}$ line.

T'': the highest point of the tongue (T) projected onto the incisal reference line (IRL).

Oropharyngeal Planes and Lines (Figure 2–41)

Hyopharyngeal plane: a plane constructed parallel to the palatal plane (PP) through the most anterior point of the hyoid (Hy).

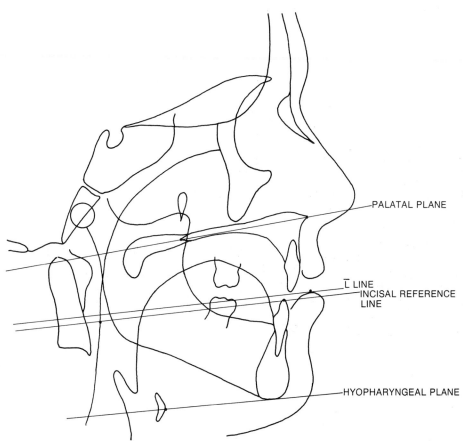

PALATAL PLANE

$\overline{\text{L}}$ LINE
INCISAL REFERENCE LINE

HYOPHARYNGEAL PLANE

FIGURE 2–41 The oropharyngeal planes and lines established to approximate a horizontal plane.

Incisal reference line (IRL): a line constructed parallel to the palatal plane (PP) through the tip of the lower central incisor ($\overline{\overline{I1}}$) ($\overline{i1}$). This line also may be constructed parallel to the Frankfort horizontal.

$\overline{L}$ line: a line constructed parallel to the palatal plane through the tip of the lower lip.

Palatal plane: a line drawn through the anterior and posterior nasal spines (ANS–PNS).

Oral Cavity Dimensions (Figure 2–42)

Anterior oral cavity lengths

The anterior half bisection (B) of the incisal reference line.

MC–$\overline{L}$: the anterior half bisection of the line drawn from the superior tip of the lower lip ($\overline{L}$) to the posterior pharyngeal wall (PPW).

$\overline{I1}$–T″: the distance measured between the tip of the mandibular central incisor ($\overline{\overline{I1}}$) ($\overline{i1}$) and the projection of the highest point of the tongue (T″) onto the incisal reference line (IRL).

Oral cavity lengths

$\overline{I1}$–Orph: the distance along the incisal reference line from the tip of the lower central incisor ($\overline{\overline{I1}}$) ($\overline{i1}$) to point Orph.

$\overline{L}$–PPW: the distance along the line (constructed parallel to the palatal

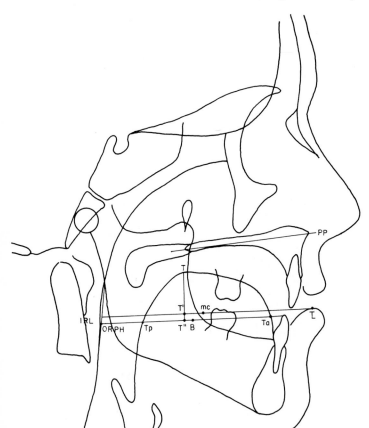

FIGURE 2–42 Lines and points for determining the height and length dimensions of the oral cavity.

plane) from the tip of the lower lip to the intersection of the line with the posterior pharyngeal wall (PPW).

Posterior oral cavity lengths

The posterior half bisection of the incisal reference line (IRL).

MC–PPW: the posterior half bisection of the line drawn from the superior tip of the lower lip ($\overline{L}$) to the posterior pharyngeal wall (PPW). This distance is measured from the midcavity point (MC) to the posterior pharyngeal wall.

Orph–T": the distance measured between the point of intersection of the incisal reference line (IRL) with the posterior pharyngeal wall (PPW) and the projection of the highest point of the tongue (T") onto the incisal reference line.

Tongue dimensions

Tongue length (Ta–Tp): the distance measured along the incisal reference line (IRL) from the point where it intersects the anterior aspect of the tongue (Ta) to the point where the IRL intersects the posterior aspect of the tongue (Tp).

Tongue height (T–IRL): the distance measured perpendicularly from the highest point of the tongue (T) to the incisal reference line (IRL).

Oropharyngeal Apertures and Minimal Distances (Figure 2–43)

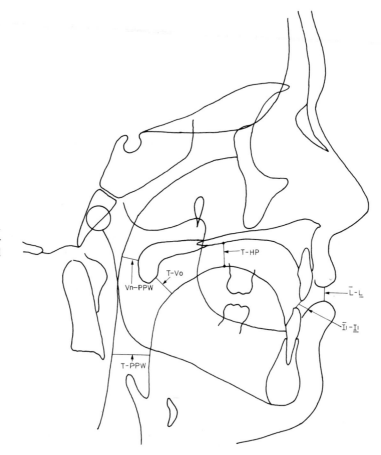

FIGURE 2-43 Measures for determining oropharyngeal apertures or minimal distances within the oral cavity.

Incisor opening ($\overline{\text{I1}}$–$\underline{\text{I1}}$): the minimal distance measured between the tip of the mandibular central incisor ($\overline{\text{I1}}$) and the maxillary central incisor ($\underline{\text{I1}}$) at rest or during function. (Also $\overline{\text{i1}}$ and $\underline{\text{i1}}$).

Lip aperture ($\overline{\text{L}}$–$\underline{\text{L}}$): the minimal distance measured between the lower ($\overline{\text{L}}$) and upper ($\underline{\text{L}}$) lips at rest or during function.

Tongue–hard palate aperture (T–HP): the least distance measured between the tongue (T) and the hard palate (HP) at rest or during function.

Tongue–pharynx aperture (T–PPW): the least distance measured between the tongue (T) and the posterior pharyngeal wall (PPW) at rest or during function.

Tongue–velum aperture (T–Vo): the least distance measured between the tongue (T) and the velum (Vo) at rest or during function.

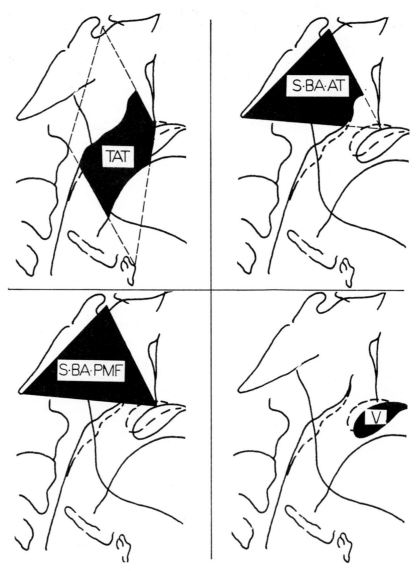

FIGURE 2–44 Areal measures of the oropharynx, nasopharynx, and associated structures. (After Wildman, A. J.: Am. J. Orthod., 47:439, 1961.)

Velopharyngeal aperture (Vn–PPW): the least distance measured between the velum (Vn) and the posterior pharyngeal wall (PPW) at rest or during function.

Oropharyngeal Areas (Figure 2–44)

Adenoid tissue area (S–Ba–PPW or S–BA–PMF, as in Fig. 2–44): the amount of adenoid tissue determined planimetrically.
Nasopharyngeal areas
   S–Ba–Ptm' or S–BA–AT as in Fig. 2–44: the amount of nasopharyngeal area within the lines demarked by sella (S), basion (Ba), and Ptm'.
   TAT: the amount of nasopharyngeal area bounded by the (1) tongue; (2) adenoid tissues (AT) (actually this is the posterior pharyngeal wall); (3) a line connecting the anterior point on the tubercle of the atlas (AA) and the anterior point of the hyoid (Hy); and (4) a line connecting sella (S), Ptm', and the anterior point of the hyoid (Hy).
Velar area (V): the sagittal outline of the velum.

Oropharyngeal Angles (Figure 2–45)

Angles AA–S–Ptm', Ba–S–Ptm': the degree of interspace between AA and Ba and Ptm'.
Angles N–S–AA, N–S–Hy, and N–S–Ptm': the relative anteroposterior position of AA, Hy, and Ptm'.
Angles S–Ba–ANS, S–Ba–PNS, and S–Ba–Ptm': the relative superoinferior position of ANS, PNS, and Ptm'.
Angle S–Ptm'–Hy: the relative anteroposterior position of the body of the hyoid bone.
Angles S–N–AA, S–N–ANS, S–N–Hy, and S–N–PNS: the relative anteroposterior position of AA, ANS, Hy, and PNS.

VELOPHARYNGEAL

Velopharyngeal Points (Figure 2–46)

Height of velar elevation (HVE): the highest point of velar elevation on the nasal side of the velum during maximum function.
Height of velar contact (HVC): the highest point of velar contact with the posterior pharyngeal wall.
Levator insertion (LV): the most outward point on the convexity of the velum. This point is arbitrarily taken as the insertion of the levator into the velum.
LVf: LV during function.
LVr: LV at rest.
Lowest velar contact (LVC): the lowest point of velar contact with the posterior pharyngeal wall.
Midpoint of velar contact (MVC): the midpoint of velar contact with the posterior pharyngeal wall. It is measured as the midpoint between the highest point of velar contact (HVC) and the lowest point of velar contact (LVC).

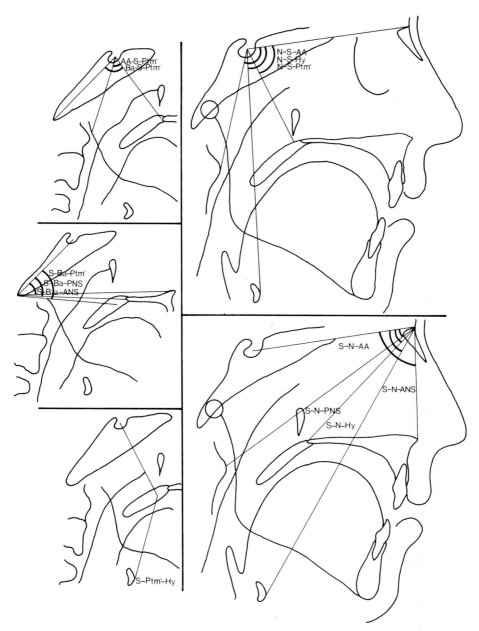

FIGURE 2–45 Angular measures for determining the positional relationship between structures.

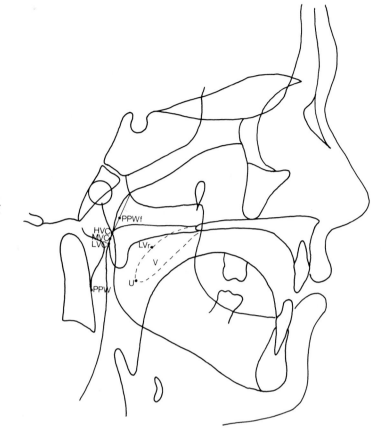

FIGURE 2–46 Points in the naso-pharynx for defining parameters of velopharyngeal movement and closure.

Posterior pharyngeal wall (PPW): the margin of the posterior pharyngeal wall.
PPWf: the point of the most forward excursion of the posterior pharyngeal wall during function.
Uvula (U): the tip of the uvula.
Velum (V): the cross-section outline of the velum.
Vn: the nasal side of the velum.
Vo: the oral side of the velum.

Velopharyngeal Dimensions (Figure 2–47)

Height of velopharyngeal closure (HVC–PP): the distance measured from the highest point of velar contact (HVC) to the palatal plane (PP).
Height of velar elevation (HVE–PP): the distance measured from the highest point of velar elevation (HVE) to the palatal plane (PP).
Nasopharyngeal depth
   AA–Ptm′: the distance measured from the anterior tubercle of the first cervical vertebra (AA) to the projection of Ptm (Ptm′) onto the palatal plane (PP).
   AA–S′: the distance measured from the anterior tubercle of the first cervical vertebra (AA) to the projection of S (S′) onto the palatal plane (PP).

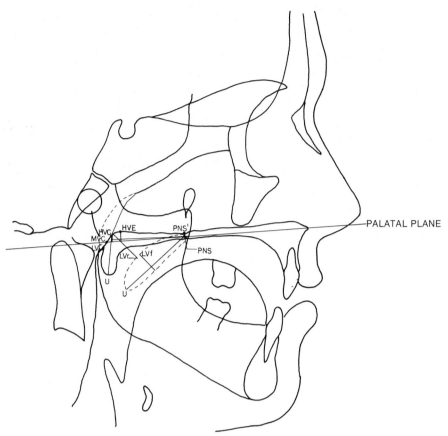

FIGURE 2–47 Measures for determining parameters of velar elevation and velopharyngeal closure.

PNS–HVC: the distance measured from the highest point of velar contact (HVC) with the posterior pharyngeal wall to the posterior nasal spine (PNS).

PNS–MVC: the distance measured from the midpoint of velar contact (MVC) with the posterior pharyngeal wall to the posterior nasal spine (PNS).

PNS–PPW: the distance measured along the palatal plane from the posterior pharyngeal wall (PPW) to the posterior nasal spine (PNS).

Ptm'–PPW: the distance measured along the palatal plane from the projection onto the plane of Ptm (Ptm') to the posterior pharyngeal wall (PPW).

Nasopharyngeal height (PNS–cranial base): the distance measured from the posterior nasal spine to the cranial base (Ba–N). The distance is measured perpendicular to the palatal plane.

Pharyngeal wall movement

PPWr–PPWf: the distance measured from the most forward excursion of the pharyngeal wall in function (PPWf) to that same point at rest (PPWr). The measure is taken parallel to the palatal plane.

PPWf–PP: the distance measured perpendicularly from the most forward excursion of the pharyngeal wall in function (PPWf) to the palatal plane.

This is the relationship of the posterior pharyngeal wall movement to the palatal plane.

Pharyngeal wall thickness (AA–PPW): the thickness of the posterior pharyngeal wall at the level of the atlas (AA). This is measured as the closest distance from AA to the PPW.

Velar lengths

PNS–U: the distance measured from the posterior nasal spine (PNS) to the tip of the uvula (U). This measure should be made while the velum is in a rest position.

PNS'–U along Vn: the distance measured from the projection of the posterior nasal spine (PNS') to the tip of the uvula (U) along the nasal side of the velum (Vn). This measurement can be made at any time during rest or during function.

Velar thickness at rest

The maximum thickness of the velum measured at a right angle to the PNS–U line.

The thickness of the velum measured at a right angle at the bisection of the PNS–U line.

Velar thickness during function (PNS'–U): the thickness of the velum measured at the midpoint of velar length. Velar length is measured PNS'–U for this measure of velar thickness.

Velar movement (LVr–LVf): the distance measured from the point of levator insertion at rest (LVr) to the point of levator insertion during function (LVf).

Velopharyngeal seal: (HVC–LVC): the distance measured between the highest (HVC) and lowest (LVC) points of contact of the velum with the posterior pharyngeal wall.

Velopharyngeal Ratios

Vnr to Vnf/PPWr to Vnr: the amount of velar movement during function relative to the velopharyngeal aperture at rest.

PPWr to PPWf/PPWr to Vnr: the amount of posterior pharyngeal wall movement during function relative to the velopharyngeal aperture at rest.

PPWr to PPWf + Vnr to Vnf/PPWr to Vnr: the amount of velar and pharyngeal wall movement during function relative to the velopharyngeal aperture at rest.

Velopharyngeal Angles (Figure 2–48)

Angle V to PP: the angle measured at the PNS–U (posterior nasal spine–uvula) axis with the palatal plane (PP). The angle can be measured at any time from rest through functional changes in the position of the velum.

Angle LVr–LVf: the angle of velar movement. This is measured as the angle of the intersection of a line LVr–LVf (levator insertion at rest and the levator insertion during function) with the palatal plane.

Angle PNS–HVC–U: the angle of the velum (V) in functional contact with the posterior pharyngeal wall (PPW).

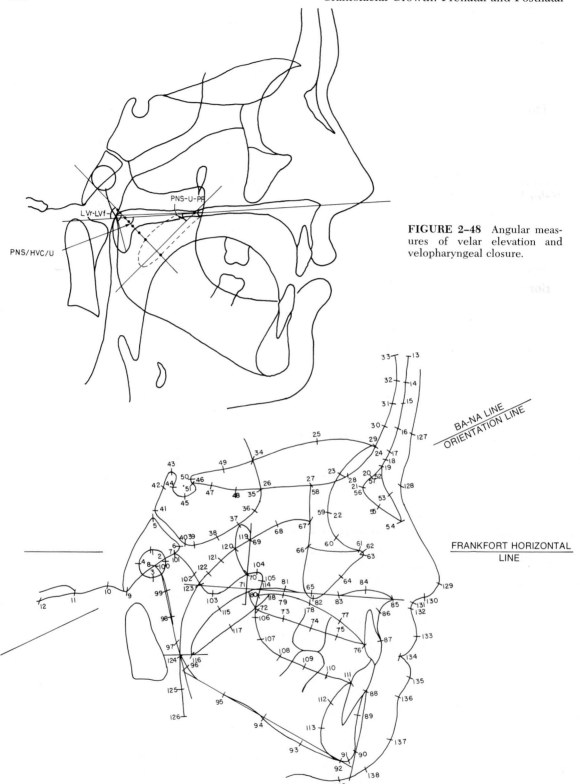

FIGURE 2–48 Angular measures of velar elevation and velopharyngeal closure.

FIGURE 2–49 The Mazaheri adaptation of the Walker model (see Figure 2–37) in the lateral x-ray head film to locate orofacial skeletal and soft tissue endpoints.

The Walker digitizing method, described earlier, has been developed and utilized for measuring and describing in quantitative terms the human cranium as portrayed on an x-ray film. Cleft palate research necessitates the measurement of all cleft structures including hard parts (bone, or in this case parts of the skull) and soft parts (tissue). To meet this need, Mazaheri adapted the Walker digitizing method by adding digitized points on the facial soft tissue profile and on the soft palate (Figure 2–49).

Analysis of these data provides information on the growth of cleft structures and the effects of surgery and physical management procedures. Programs have been developed which allow correlation of the points utilized by Walker and those utilized by Mazaheri.

Further adaptations of the digitizing procedure have been developed by Riski for the purpose of analyzing cineradiographic films of the oropharyngeal structures during speech function (Figure 2–50). He has added points to those used by Mazaheri. Structures digitized for cine analysis include the posterior pharyngeal wall, velum, hard palate, tongue, maxillary and mandibular incisors, and selected points on the mandible.

Recently speech researchers at the Clinic have been studying the application of digitizing procedures to the study of the oropharyngeal structures in speech function. The advantages of digitizing described earlier also apply here. The ability of the digitizing procedure to handle large amounts of data

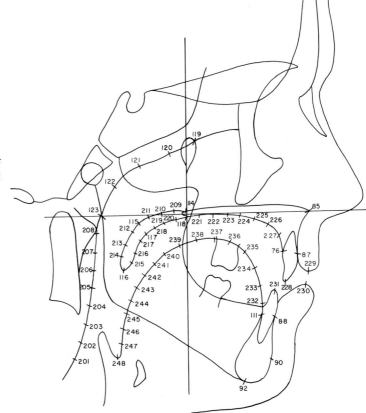

FIGURE 2–50 The Riski model of digitization for plotting the positioning and movement of the speech structures.

efficiently is important when analyzing cineradiographic films. Filming speeds of 24, 60, or even 100 frames per second can result in exceedingly large amounts of data to code, store, retrieve, and analyze. Further, once the data are coded and stored there is no need to go back to the tracings to make additional measurements; it is a simple matter of retrieving the stored data for additional analysis. A more detailed discussion of the clinical and research applications of cineradiography appears in Chapter 8.

PALATE AND UPPER DENTAL ARCH

In 1971 Mazaheri and coworkers reported on changes in arch form and dimensions of cleft patients.[20] The method of measurement employed was based on a Xerox reproduction of the maxillary dental model. Certain endpoints were marked on the casts prior to photocopying.

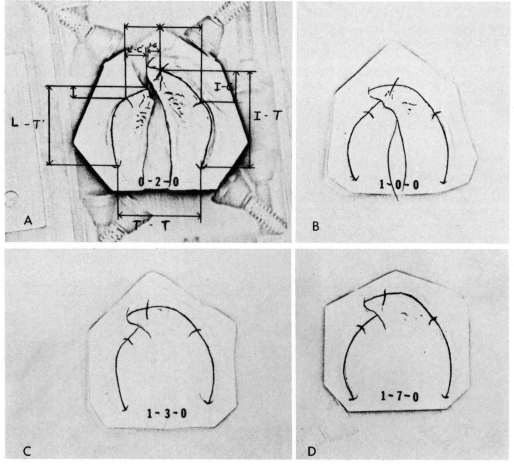

FIGURE 2–51   Photocopy of maxillary casts. Prior to photocopying, crest of ridge, mesial border of cleft tuberosities, canines, and incisive points are marked on casts. Transverse and anteroposterior measurements are made on photocopy. Note segmental relationship before lip and after palate closure. (From Mazaheri, M., et al.: Am. J. Orthod., 60:19, 1971.)

Endpoints and Lines on Dental Models
(Figures 2–51, 2–52, and 2–53)

Crest of the ridge: in older patients the teeth were carefully removed from the ridge and the midportion of the ridge was established as the crest.
Margin of the cleft.
Tuberosity points: the tuberosity and the crest of the ridge were outlined on the casts, and the junction of these lines was called T, T'.
Canine points: the intersection of the groove of the lateral labial frenum and the crest of the ridge was called C, C'. In all casts with teeth the C, C' coincided with the mid-interproximal point between the canine and first deciduous molar.
L: the anterior endpoint of the lesser segment.
G: the anterior endpoint of the greater segment.
I: the point at the crest of the ridge on the line drawn from the labial frenum to the incisive papilla.
R, R': the points at the intersection of the crest of the ridge and the lower posterior limit of the mandibular ridge.

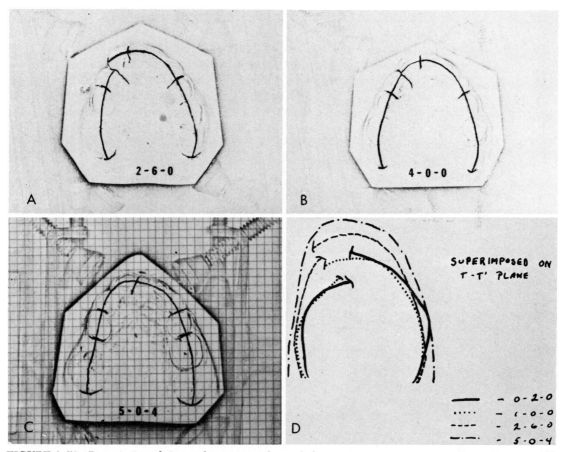

FIGURE 2–52 Parts *A, B,* and *C* are photocopies of casts belonging to same patient as in Fig. 2–51. Noticeable change in segmental relationship began in this patient at age two years six months, and at age three segments were in end-to-end relationship without any early orthopedic or orthodontic treatment. *D* is photocopy superimposed at T–T' at ages indicated. Note change in segmental relationship of arch form and dimension and pattern of maxillary growth. (From Mazaheri, M., et al.: Am. J. Orthod., *60:*19, 1971.)

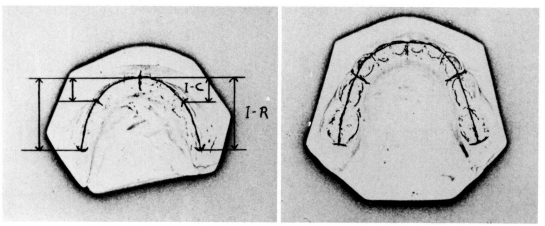

FIGURE 2–53   Photocopies showing method of measurement of mandibular casts. (From Mazaheri, M., et al.: Am. J. Orthod., *60*:19, 1971.)

T–T': this line is called the intertuberosity or the base line.

t–t': the points at which the intertuberosity line T–T' intersects the lines that outline the mesial borders of the cleft.

M–M': to locate these points a perpendicular was erected from the base line (T–T') to the incisal point (I); at the level of the bisection of this distance (I–T–T') a line parallel to the base line was drawn, reaching the crest of the alveolar ridges of both segments. The intersections of this transverse line with the outlines of the alveolar crest on both sides were labeled points M and M', respectively.

C–C': the line connecting C, C'.

X: intersection of the transverse line from L (parallel to the base line T–T') with the perpendicular from the base line to point G.

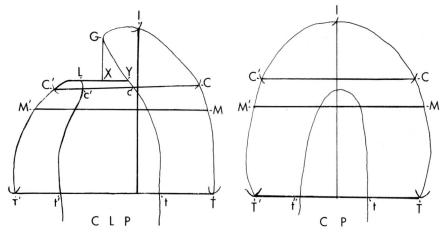

FIGURE 2–54   Graphic view of photostat of maxillary cast of cleft lip and palate (CLP) and cleft palate (CP) subjects, demonstrating points from which lines are drawn and measurements are made. (From Mazaheri, M., et al.: Am. J. Orthod., *60*:19, 1971.)

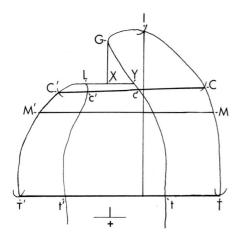
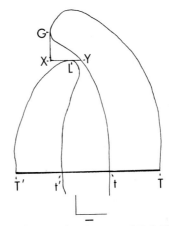

FIGURE 2–55 When segments are separated in alveolar area and L is farther from Y and X, L–X reading is positive; in situation in which greater segment overlaps lesser segment, X is farther from Y than L; therefore, L–X reading is negative. (From Mazaheri, M., et al.: Am. J. Orthod., *60*:19, 1971.)

Y: intersection of the transverse line from L (parallel to the base line T–T′) with the outline of the mesial border of the greater segment.

Dimensions* (Figures 2–54 and 2–55)

Width dimensions
 T–T′: intertuberosity width or upper posterior arch width.
 M–M′: middle arch width.
 C–C′: canine width (anterior arch width)
 R–R′: lower posterior arch width.
 t–t′: posterior cleft width.
 c–c′: cleft width at area of canine crypt.
 G–L: alveolar cleft width.
Length dimensions
 I–T: anteroposterior length of greater segment.
 I–C: incisor-to-canine length.
 C–T: canine-to-tuberosity length.
 I–G: anterior portion of cleft segment.
 IG–LT′: total anteroposterior length of cleft segments.
 L–T′: posterior portion of cleft segment; called "lesser segment."
Transverse and anteroposterior dimensions (in the region of the alveolar cleft)
 L–Y and L–G: transverse and oblique width of anterior cleft.
 L–X: transverse relation of lesser to greater segment. When segments are separated at alveolar cleft and L is farther from Y than X, reading is positive. In situations in which greater segment overlaps lesser segment, that is X is farther from Y than L, reading is negative.
 G–X: anteroposterior relation of lesser to greater segment. If alveolar border of lesser segment is positioned anterior to greater segment (very rare),

---

*Measured in horizontal view, i.e., looking down on the models.

this measurement is negative; otherwise, positive measurement should be anticipated.

L–X and G–X: combined reading that provides immediate information about the spatial relationship of the greater and lesser segments at the alveolar cleft in both unilateral and bilateral clefts.

References

1. Avery, J. K.: Prenatal facial growth. *In* Moyers, R. E.: Handbook of Orthodontics, 3rd ed., Chicago, Year Book Medical Publishers, pp. 27–50, 1973.
2. Bakwin, H., and R. M. Bakwin: Form and dimensions of the palate during the first year of life. Int. J. Orthod. Oral Surg., *22*:1018, 1936.
3. Broadbent, B. H., Sr., B. H. Broadbent, Jr., and W. H. Golden: Bolton Standards of Dentofacial Development and Growth, St. Louis, C. V. Mosby, 1975.
4. Burdi, A. R.: Sagittal growth of the nasomaxillary complex during the second trimester of human prenatal development. J. Dent. Res., *44*:112, 1965.
5. Burdi, A. R., and J. H. Lillie: A catenary analysis of the maxillary dental arch during human embryogenesis. Anat. Rec., *154*:13, 1966.
6. Burdi, A. R., M. Feingold, K. S. Larsson, et al.: Etiology and pathogenesis of congenital cleft lip and cleft palate, an N.I.D.R. state of the art report. Teratology, *6*:255, 1973.
7. Clinch, L.: Variations in the mutual relationships of the maxillary and mandibular gum pads in the newborn child. Int. J. Orthod. Dent. Child., *20*:359, 1934.
8. Freiband, B.: Growth of the palate in the fetus. J. Dent. Res., *15*:103, 1937.
9. Hanada, K., and W. M. Krogman: Longitudinal study of post-operative changes in the soft tissue profile in bilateral cleft lip and palate, birth to six years. Am. J. Orthod., *67*:363, 1975.
10. Harding, R. L., and M. Mazaheri: Growth and spatial changes in the arch form in unilateral cleft palate and lip patients. Plast. Reconstr. Surg., *50*:591, 1972.
11. Humphrey, T.: Development of oral and facial motor mechanisms in human fetuses and their relation to human craniofacial growth. J. Dent. Res., *50*(6), Part I:1428, 1971.
12. Ingham, T. R.: Study of the human fetal mandible. I, Nature of its change in shape. J. Dent. Res., *7*:647, 1932.
13. Inoue, N.: A study of the developmental changes of the dentofacial complex during the fetal period by means of roentgenographic cephalometrics. Bull. Tokyo Med. Univ., *8*:205, 1961.
14. Ishiguro, K., W. M. Krogman, M. Mazaheri, and R. L. Harding: Longitudinal study of morphological craniofacial patterns via p-a X-ray head films in cleft patients from birth to six years of age. Cleft Palate J., *13*:104, 1976.
15. Johnston, M. C.: The neural crest in abnormalities of the face and brain. *In* Bergsma, D. (ed.): Morphogenesis and Malformation of Face and Brain, New York, Alan R. Liss, pp. 1–18, 1975.
16. Krogman, W. M.: Growth of head, face, trunk, and limbs in Philadelphia white and Negro children of elementary and high school age. Monogr. Soc. Res. Child Dev., *35*:1, 1970.
17. Krogman, W. M., M. Mazaheri, R. L. Harding, et al.: A longitudinal study of craniofacial growth in children with clefts as compared to normal, birth to six years. Cleft Palate J., *12*:59, 1975.
18. Mapes, A. M., M. Mazaheri, R. L. Harding, et al.: A longitudinal analysis of the maxillary growth increments of cleft lip and palate patients. Cleft Palate J., *11*:450, 1974.
19. Mazaheri, M.: Prosthetic treatment of closed vertical dimensions in the cleft palate patient. J. Prosthet. Dent., *11*:187, 1961.
20. Mazaheri, M., R. L. Harding, J. A. Cooper, et al.: Changes in arch form and dimensions of cleft patients. Am. J. Orthod., *60*:19, 1971.
21. Mazaheri, M., R. L. Harding, and S. Nanda: The effect of surgery on maxillary growth and cleft width. Plast. Reconstr. Surg., *40*:22, 1967.
22. Mazaheri, M., S. Nanda, and V. Sassouni: Comparison of midfacial development of children with clefts and their siblings. Cleft Palate J., *4*:334, 1967.
23. Moore, J. C.: The developing nervous system in relationship to techniques in treating physical dysfunction. *In* Zamir, L. J.: Expanding Dimensions in Rehabilitation, Springfield, Ill., Charles C Thomas, pp. 3–20, 1969.
24. Patten, B. M.: Human Embryology, 3rd ed., New York, McGraw-Hill, 1968.
25. Ross, R. B., and M. C. Johnston: Cleft Lip and Palate, Baltimore, Williams and Wilkins, 1972.
26. Scott, J. H.: The cranial base. Am. J. Phys. Anthropol., *16*:319, 1958.

27. Sillman, J. H.: Serial studies of changes in dimensions of the dental arches from birth to nine years. Child Deve., *18*:106, 1947.
28. Sillman, J. H.: Serial study of good occlusion from birth to 12 years of age. Am. J. Orthod., *37*: 481, 1951.
29. Sillman, J. H.: Dimensional changes of the dental arches: a longitudinal study from birth to 25 years. Am. J. Orthod., *50*:824, 1964.
30. Sparrow, S. S., B. G. Brogdon, and K. R. Bzoch: The effect of filming rate and frame selection in cinefluorographic velopharyngeal analysis. Cleft Palate J., *1*:419, 1964.
31. Stark, R. B.: Congenital defects. *In* Stark, R. B. (ed.): Cleft Palate: A Multi-Discipline Approach, New York, Harper & Row, pp. 45–59, 1968.
32. Warkany, J.: Congenital Malformations: Notes and Comments, Chicago, Year Book Medical Publishers, 1971.

Chapter Three ────────────────────────────────

Total habilitation of the child born with an orofacial cleft is the goal of the Lancaster Cleft Palate Clinic and the theme of this volume. Yet in one sense habilitation of the individual is only the immediate aim, only one phase of a broader purpose. The long-range view reaches to a far wider horizon, one that encompasses the whole human population and looks to the day when causes will be fully understood and these congenital anomalies can be eliminated as a major threat to health and happiness.

That time, of course, is still in the distant future. And considering the subtlety and complexity of the forces that impinge upon the developing human organism, it may never be reached. But the goal is sufficiently challenging to engage the concerted efforts of the total cleft palate team, clinicians and researchers alike. As a member of that team, the geneticist finds himself fully involved in evaluating the growing store of knowledge in the expanding field of genetic diseases, contributing to it, and seeking ways to apply relevant segments of that information to the problems of orofacial clefting that now occur.

Recognizing that an overall attack upon the problem of facial clefts should include attention to the causative factors, insofar as they are known, the Lancaster Cleft Palate Clinic in 1969 organized a Department of Genetic Services, with a full-time geneticist. The geneticist's role embraces the following duties: First, as a counselor, he imparts to parents and other concerned family members information about the suspected causes, he dispels myths and superstitions that so often surround the birth of a congenitally malformed child, and he interprets the tabulated risks of recurrence of the defect in subsequent children. Second, he devotes a part of the time to research into those elements, either genetic or environmental, that may figure in the etiology of orofacial clefting. And finally, as he is trained in the nosology (classification) of genetic diseases, he aids in the diagnosis of the patient's condition. Here the geneticist may assist in the identification of a syndrome with multiple associated anomalies. These particulars bear not only upon the treatment of the affected child but also upon the counseling of the parents.

Everyone who participates in the treatment of a child with a cleft is asked at one time or another: "What caused this?" "Why did it happen?"

EPIDEMIOLOGY AND GENETICS OF CLEFTING:
With Implications for Etiology

SEISHI W. OKA

and "Why did it happen to my child?" None of us has all the answers. Even if we did, we would find it difficult to give replies that would fully satisfy distraught parents, for an explanation itself cannot make the problem disappear. Nevertheless, knowledge and understanding do assist the patient and the family to live with a situation that, with skilled clinical help, will become more acceptable as time goes on. Providing this information in clinics that do not have access to a geneticist is sometimes difficult. Published sources of information, often contradictory or inconclusive, may be difficult to interpret; incorrectly interpreted information can be worse than no information at all.

It will be the purpose of this chapter, therefore, to survey relevant data on the subject, including the many reports on the epidemiology of orofacial clefts. This is one of the commonest congenital disorders in a list that numbers more than 1700 anatomical and biochemical faults.[72] It is the responsibility of each of us who is engaged in the habilitative process to be familiar with what is currently known about the possible causative factors, both hereditary and environmental, and about how they interrelate. In this connection we shall look again at the age-old question of whether a congenital condition results from heredity or environment. The nature and degree of interaction of the two in each case are important in understanding the risks. Long-term studies of families known to be at high risk may well enable us to identify some environmental factors that turn risk into a congenital maldevelopment. By controlling these factors, for example, by optimizing the environment, we may eventually reduce the incidence of this malformation in the population.

It is our hope that, from the accumulated research reports, we can distill information useful to those concerned with the causes of orofacial clefting. Some of the information can serve as a reference in deriving recurrence risk figures, important in genetic counseling. Such figures cannot, however, constitute a specific guide for the counseling of each patient. Each individual is unique and requires the interpretation, by a trained geneticist, of family and medical histories as these relate to the defect.

It may be helpful, therefore, to touch upon the basic principles of counseling, with hints on how and when the risk factors can best be presented to families, who are often under considerable stress and anxiety. This we shall do later in the chapter.

EPIDEMIOLOGY OF CLEFT LIP, CLEFT LIP AND PALATE, AND CLEFT PALATE

Basic to the study of the genetics of any anomaly or disorder is its epidemiology, or the "study of the laws and factors governing the occurrence and distribution of a disease and disorder in a population. These factors include the characteristics of the population, the causative agencies and the biological, social, and physical environment."[32]

The relationship of epidemiology to human genetics is illustrated by the fact that as the geneticist seeks common factors in the population that may be implicated in the etiology of orofacial clefting, he is working in the realm of the epidemiologist. Conversely, as the epidemiologist looks more toward family aggregates of a disease, he is involved in genetic problems. Thus, both the geneticist and the epidemiologist find areas of overlap, and they have traditionally approached the problems of diseases in a population on a fully cooperative and interactive basis.

Collecting data specifically on the incidence of clefts should be relatively simple, partly because the defect is usually a highly visible one. But interpreting these data in a way that will reflect what is actually occurring in the population under study may be difficult. In the first place, information gathered from hospitals and clinics will be biased toward the more severe cleft types or those with associated malformations. There will even be a certain amount of bias toward the segment of the population able to attend a specific clinic or hospital. An affected individual who dies prior to treatment, for example, will usually be missed in the tabulation.

Nor is information from birth certificates and maternity record entirely reliable. One study showed that among patients seen in a large university cleft palate clinic the fact that they were born with facial clefts of one type or another had been omitted from their birth certificates in 29.4 per cent of the cases.[74] This study also noted that the frequency of underreporting increased with the more covert cleft types; more than 50 per cent of the clefts of the palate only were not recorded on the birth certificates. Ivy[53] recognized these errors of omission by adjusting the incidence of all cleft types to allow for 20 per cent underreporting.

It is virtually impossible to avoid all bias and error. And perhaps the most reliable course of action one can take to counteract such shortcomings in estimating frequency of clefts in the population is to use figures derived from several large consecutive series of studies of infants.[33]

Even these, as well as other large bodies of data that must be utilized, are susceptible to a certain degree of bias. Many good studies on the incidence of orofacial clefts have been produced, however, and additions are continually being made to the registers. The point is that one must carefully assess all his sources as he pursues the main purposes of epidemiological studies, namely, to detect any causal relationship between a disease (in this case orofacial clefts) and one or more associated factors and to verify any suspected correlation by adequate statistical methods.

Racial Variation

In clefting, as in many other disorders that affect the human species, clues to etiology, genetic or otherwise, have been sought in the variations by race, sex, and geographical area. The incidence of clefts reported in the literature does vary widely among these categories, and there are also differences among some of these groups with respect to cleft type. But here, as we have just warned, the data must be examined critically, for the counts do not always agree within the same population group. Reliability may depend in part on how thoroughly and impartially the investigators looked for cases, a factor called *ascertainment*. Ross and Johnston,[91] reviewing several surveys and selecting only those that they felt had been adequately ascertained, recorded a distinct gradient in the incidence of cleft lip and cleft palate CL(P) among various racial groups. The lowest incidence was among American blacks, ranging from 0.21 to 0.41 per 1000 live births. The highest was found among Orientals, Japanese being the most thoroughly studied, with a range among several surveys from 1.14 to 2.13 per 1000 births. American and Western European Caucasians fell in an intermediate position, with an incidence between 0.77 and 1.40 per 1000

TABLE 3–1 Incidence of Cleft Lip±Palate and Cleft Palate Per Thousand Births by Race and Years Investigated

AUTHOR(S)	YEAR	COUNTRY AND RACIAL GROUP	DATA YEARS	TOTAL BIRTHS	NUMBER AND INCIDENCE (PER THOUSAND)		
					CL±P	CP	All Clefts
Fogh-Andersen	1942	Denmark: Caucasian	1910–1940	128,306	149 (1.16)	44 (0.34)	(1.50)
MacMahon and McKeown	1953	England: Caucasian	1940–1950	218,693	168 (0.77)	108 (0.49)	(1.26)
Leck, et al.	1968	England: Caucasian	1950–1959	186,046	249 (1.34)	105 (0.56)	(1.90)
Hay	1971	USA: Caucasian	1963	58,686	94 (1.60)	36 (0.61)	(2.22)
Czeizel and Tusnadi	1971	Hungary: Caucasian	1962–1967	110,229	114 (1.03)	30 (0.27)	(1.30)
Czeizel and Tusnadi	1971	Hungary: Caucasian	1962–1967	714,091	455 (0.64)	137 (0.19)	(0.83)
Higgins and O'Brien	1974	Ireland: Caucasian	1966–1973	43,817	44 (1.00)	38 (0.87)	(1.87)
Myrianthopoulos and Chung	1974	USA: Caucasian	1973–1974	24,153	35 (1.45)	30 (1.24)	(2.69)
Chung and Ching	1974	USA: Caucasian	1948–1966	77,013	151 (1.96)	33 (0.43)	(2.39)
Saxen	1975	Finland: Caucasian	1972–1973	116,407	85 (0.73)	105 (0.90)	(1.63)
Oka	1975	USA: Caucasian	1960–1972	2,324,535	1,865 (0.80)	876 (0.38)	(1.17)
Greene, et al.	1964	USA: Black–mothers	1956–1960	271,327	92 (0.34)	57 (0.21)	(0.54)
Altemus and Ferguson	1965	USA: Black	1952–1962	79,842	19 (0.24)	17 (0.21)	(0.45)
Myrianthopoulos and Chung	1974	USA: Black	1973–1974	25,126	18 (0.72)	24 (0.96)	(1.67)
Oka	1975	USA: (Non-Caucasian)*	1960–1972	318,839	88 (0.28)	60 (0.19)	(0.46)
Mitani	1943	Japan: Japanese	1922–1940	49,645	58 (1.17)	36 (0.73)	(1.90)
Neel	1958	Japan: Japanese	1948–1954	64,569	136 (2.11)	35 (0.54)	(2.64)
Chung and Ching	1974	USA: Japanese	1948–1956	67,608	123 (1.82)	44 (0.65)	(2.47)
Tretsven	1963	USA: Amerindian	1955–1961	7,461	18 (2.41)	9 (1.20)	(3.62)
Lowry and Renwick	1969	Canada: Indian	1952–1964	20,196	55 (2.72)	9 (0.45)	(3.16)
Niswander and Adams	1967	USA: Amerindian	1963–1968	25,341	35 (1.38)	15 (0.59)	(1.97)
Niswander, et al.	1975	USA: Amerindian	1964–1969	43,409	74 (1.70)	26 (0.60)	(2.30)

*Includes Orientals and Hispanics, but population is predominantly black.

live births. The racial gradient conforms fairly well to figures reported in the past.[43, 62, 81]

Examining in more detail the extensive literature on incidence of clefting throughout the world, we find a wide range for both cleft palate and cleft lip and for cleft palate alone (Table 3–1). For Caucasians the rate of CL(P) ranged from a low of 0.64 per 1000 in Hungary[23] to a high of 1.96 per 1000 in Hawaii.[19] However, the studies in Hungary show discrepancies that may reflect differences in ascertainment. The 0.64 figure just cited was derived from records of populations living outside of Budapest. During the same period these authors personally recorded the incidence of malformations from several hospitals in Budapest and found a higher incidence for both CL(P) and CP, 1.03 and 0.27 per 1000 live births, respectively. It can be assumed that the investigators were able to make a more complete count of cases in the Budapest hospitals than had been made in the population outside of the city. But here another problem of interpretation arises, one to which we have previously alluded, namely, the actual differences between the clients of clinics and the nonclinic or nonhospital populations.

Still another source of error must be kept in mind. Many reports do not define the base population, failing to state, for example, whether the incidence was recorded among live births only or whether stillbirths were included. Clefts associated with other malformations will also affect the estimate of incidence for all types of clefts. Myrianthopoulos and Chung[80] extracted data from approximately 56,000 pregnancies followed from the first month through labor and delivery in 12 institutions. They recorded malformations of all types and reported that for 24,153 live births of Caucasian children there were 35 cases of clefts of the lip with or without cleft palate and 30 cases of isolated cleft palates. These rates, 1.45 and 1.21 respectively per 1000 live births, included clefts associated with other malformations (possible syndromes) and are therefore high. Clefts without associated malformations totaled 11 for CL(P), or 0.45 per 1000, and 2 CP, or 0.08 per 1000. Although these data are from a large population group, they illustrate one source of bias in figures reported in the literature.

The next largest group of studies on the incidence of clefts covers Orientals, specifically Japanese. Generally the ascertainment in Japan is good, as reflected in the similarities of CL(P) rates reported by the various authors. Neel's[81] report of 2.11 per 1000 for CL(P) is highest. The incidence of CP alone varies from a low of 0.23 to a high of 0.73 per 1000.[63, 78]

Among four studies of American blacks (Table 3–1) the incidence was highest in the report by Myrianthopoulos and Chung.[80] This again reflects the total number of clefts, including those associated with other malformations. In general, however, the incidence for both cleft types, i.e., CL(P) and CP, is lower in blacks, with CL(P) much lower than CP in comparison with both Caucasians and Orientals. In the analysis by Oka[86] the incidence by race and year was graphed (Figure 3–1). For both male and female non-Caucasians, it increased from the year 1969 to a high incidence during 1971, especially for females. This appears to be a period of real increase, although it may reflect better reporting after 1968. There was also a period of high incidence in 1962 for both male and female non-Caucasians. Further information is needed to explain the fluctuation

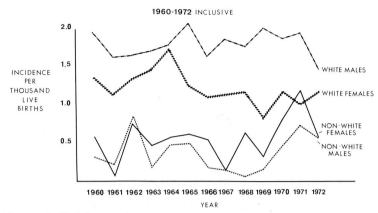

1960-1972 INCLUSIVE

INCIDENCE
PER
THOUSAND
LIVE
BIRTHS

WHITE MALES

WHITE FEMALES

NON-WHITE
FEMALES

NON-WHITE
MALES

1960 1961 1962 1963 1964 1965 1966 1967 1968 1969 1970 1971 1972

YEAR

FIGURE 3–1 Incidence of all clefts per thousand live births in Pennsylvania for Caucasian (white) and non-Caucasian (non-white) males and females—corrected for 20 per cent underreporting. (Data from Oka, 1975.)

for both Caucasians and non-Caucasians during the 13 years reported in Pennsylvania.

Recently reports have come in from previously unreported areas. In France the incidence of CL(P) was found to be 1.06 per 1000 and for CP it was 0.46 per 1000.[8] Klásková-Burianova[58, 59] derived incidence figures for CL(P) and CP in Bohemia, Czechoslovakia, from 1964 to 1972. The incidence of CL(P) was 1.3 per 1000 and CP only was 0.6. Ascertainment in this study was nearly 100 per cent. The epidemiology of clefts in Romania from the records of two maternity hospitals in Bucharest between the years 1960 and 1971 was 1:1215 live births for all types of clefts among 50,344 newborns.[15] Unfortunately the cleft types were not separated. These results are comparable to those reported for Caucasians in previous studies.

A Mexican study reports an incidence of 0.91 per 1000 for CL(P) and 0.12 per 1000 for CP.[1] These figures are lower, especially for CP, than those reported for Caucasians. This is interesting in view of the fact that the Mexican population has an admixture of Mexican Indian. This difference in the incidence may be due to the type of population from which the cases were selected. All were patients being treated at a major medical center in Mexico City. Lutz and Moor[69] found the incidence of CL(P) among infants born to Mexican-American mothers in a maternity hospital in southern California to be 1.24 per 1000, a figure closer to the Oriental and Amerindian rates.

It is interesting to speculate on the study by Ching and Chung,[19] who found that in Hawaii offspring of racial admixture have an intermediate frequency. It was suggested by them that underlying genetic factors may act additively.

Overall, after reviewing the extensive body of epidemiological studies, it can be said that there is a distinct racial gradient in the incidence of CL(P) with a minor difference in the incidence of isolated CP. The Orientals (Japanese) are the highest for CL(P) (1.61 per 1000), Caucasians are intermediate (0.90 per 1000), and American blacks are the lowest (0.31 per 1000) (Figure 3–2).

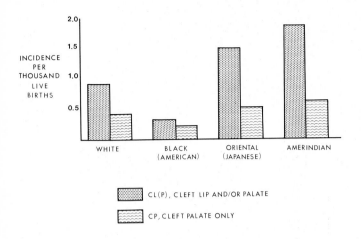

INCIDENCE PER THOUSAND LIVE BIRTHS

2.0
1.5
1.0
0.5

WHITE   BLACK (AMERICAN)   ORIENTAL (JAPANESE)   AMERINDIAN

CL(P), CLEFT LIP AND/OR PALATE

CP, CLEFT PALATE ONLY

FIGURE 3–2 Incidence of CL(P) and CP in the major racial groups. (Data from Table 3–1 and unpublished research, Oka, 1977.)

Trend in Incidence

Next we may examine the reports of changes in incidence over time. Has the rate of orofacial clefts been increasing or not? Some studies suggest it has, and a few reasons have been offered. But the reports in our opinion are inconclusive, and if there has been an actual increase, the reasons for it have yet to be proved. One of the most respected authorities, Fogh-Andersen,[31] reviewed previously published reports, which reflected an increased incidence of cleft palate. And in his own detailed study in Denmark he found a rise from 1.31 per 1000 during the period from 1938 through 1942 to 1.64 per 1000 from 1953 through 1957, a difference he considers to be statistically significant. To account for the greater numbers, he suggests a possible increase in fertility among cleft individuals as a result of better surgical techniques, with fewer surgical deaths and improved cosmesis and function. We have ourselves found that adults who have benefited from improved cleft palate team care consider their defects less serious than many viewed these in the past. They are therefore less concerned about having children who may be similarly affected. As one of them (who has an unaffected daughter) put it, "Cleft palate can be corrected so early and so well today that we consider it more of a nuisance than a real handicap."

However, it should be pointed out that Fogh-Andersen's data are based only on the number of cleft patients reporting for surgery and not on the number of infants with clefts among all newborns. His figures may therefore reflect a bias in selection. Tünte[101] reported an increase in cleft cases in Germany of 50 per cent from 1915 to 1962. But Tünte observes that if a change from total sterility to normal, effective fertility took place during this time period for the cleft population, it would account for only a 2 per cent increase in the total number of cleft-affected infants born in 1962. He therefore concluded that the cause of the observed increase in the frequency of cleft cases in Germany must be due to some unknown factors.

On the other hand, Brogan and Woodings[13] found a decline in the incidence of cleft lip and palate in Western Australia during a 10 year period. Higgins[50] found a similar trend in Ireland. In both of these studies, the incidence of isolated cleft palate fluctuated during the years examined.

When we add up the evidence, then, we are still faced with the question: "Are these apparent changes in the incidence of clefts real?" The question remains unanswered. It seems obvious that other populations must be carefully studied to determine whether or not a real increase, attributable to a change in some etiological pressure, is occurring, especially in areas where advanced medical, surgical, and habilitative care is available.

Seasonal Variation

Another question that has been posed in the hope of throwing light on causative factors concerns the possible seasonal variation among births of children with clefts. A number of investigators have sought evidence regarding this point, and a few appear to have seen peaks of cleft births during certain months. But there is a discouraging lack of consistency. For example, Edwards[27] reported a higher birth rate in March for infants with cleft lip in Birmingham, England. Charlton,[17] using Edwards' method for determining cyclical trends, also found that March was a high incidence month for isolated clefts of the lip in Australia. But maximum months for all types of clefts were April and August. Others found March and May to be high months for cleft lip and palate and for isolated cleft palate but could perceive no seasonal trend for cleft lip alone. While a study in the United States showed the highest incidence of CL(P) for January births,[105] a study of more than 2000 cleft cases in Japan found that the incidence of CL(P) was lower from December to February and high during March through May.[38] Isolated cleft of the palate did not show a seasonal trend in either of these two studies.

In Finland, Saxen[92] reported that an earlier study showed a seasonal trend, but the trend was not evident when using a large volume of data. The later study, however, did show some evidence of an association of cleft births with peak periods of fever and influenza outbreaks. It is not clear whether causative organisms (viruses) or therapeutic drugs are related to these births.

It is obvious, merely from the references just cited, that it would be difficult to trace a clear pattern of parallelism between the birth of children with clefts and any particular season of the year. In fact, many authors, including Fogh-Andersen,[30] have reported that they could not discern any such time relationship. Many of the studies have suffered from the same problems that beset many other epidemiological surveys. And taken as a whole the evidence does not seem to support any explicit seasonal trend.

Sex Differences in the Incidence of Clefts

While seasonal variation studies are distinguished by their inconclusiveness, the evidence is quite strong in the matter of sex differences in the incidence of orofacial clefts. The ratios differ, however, with different types of clefts. A number of studies show similarities among three main points: (1) more males are born with the combination of cleft lip and/or palate, CL(P); (2) of all CL(P) cases, male and female, the males have the more severe defects; and (3) more females are affected with isolated clefts of the palate.

The first and third points are amply supported by the material in Table 3–2, which is drawn from 26 studies made in the United States, Canada, Great Britain, Australia, Denmark, Israel, and Japan. It embraces 10,885 individuals with CL(P). In all but one study the proportion of male to female children among those with CL(P) was given, and the total count in all groups was 6736 males and 4149 females, a proportion of 62 per cent to 38 per cent. The percentage of males ranged as high as 72.3 per cent in a West Australian study, 71.8 per cent in the state of Montana, and 71.7 per cent in Scotland. In most groups the male proportion was about 55 to 65 per cent, and in only two of these studies did the females have more CL(P) than the males, namely, in a group of 18 Israeli hospital cases, in which the ratio was 11 females to 7 males, or 61.1 per cent versus 38.9 per cent, and in a group of 88 non-Caucasians (predominantly blacks) tabulated by Oka[86] from Pennsylvania birth records. Here 42 per cent of the clefts occurred in males and 58 per cent in females.

Most of these studies were made among Caucasian infants, although there were four Japanese studies, with a total of 4289 individuals. But the sex ratio among the Japanese did not differ appreciably from that in the Caucasian populations.

When isolated cleft palate was studied, the sex ratio was completely reversed in a large majority of the groups. Of the 4004 cases reviewed in the 26 studies, 2294 or 57.3 per cent were females and 1710 or 42.7 per cent were males. In only four groups did males with isolated cleft palate outnumber females (Table 3–2).

If we accept this evidence that a definite difference does exist between the sexes as far as the incidence of clefts is concerned — and the evidence seems pretty solid — our next question is why? How does one account for the greater vulnerability of the male fetus to the attack upon his developing lip and palate? How does one explain the higher susceptibility of the female fetus to forces that produce an isolated cleft of the palate without harming the lip and other anterior structures? Fogh-Andersen[30] long ago proposed a theory that the two cleft types, CL(P) and isolated CP, may be genetically independent. But the question still remains: "What is it in the genetic matrix or the developmental schedule of the two sexes that can account for this independence or these differences?"

An interesting explanation is offered in a hypothesis presented by Meskin and his group.[76] They suggest that there is a difference in the developmental time sequence between males and females and that at any given moment during embryogenesis the male is more advanced in orofacial growth than the female. In other words, there may be a sexual dimorphism in the rate of lip and palate development. Consequently, if this is true, a teratogenic insult upon the organism at a particular point in embryogenesis will inflict its damage upon the structure undergoing change at that time, such as palate closure and fusion. (See Chapter 2 on craniofacial embryology.)

In the male the interruption occurs during closure and fusion of the lip and primary palate, which therefore suffer damage. However, the secondary palate has already closed and thus escapes the growth interruption that we call clefting. At this same date in the developmental calendar—or chronological age—the female fetus is less advanced. Closure of the secondary palate is taking place, and this structure is therefore vulnerable to attack. The teratogenic interruption is apparently transient. It disappears and, in the majority of cases, leaves the subsequent closing of the female lip and primary palate unaffected.

Support for the Meskin hypothesis is seen in the work of Burdi and Silvey,[14] who examined histological sections of 46 human embryos at varying gestational ages and found a significant difference between the sexes in temporal development of the lip and palate. Females were retarded in palatal closure by almost a week in comparison with males. However, further studies, using larger samples of each sex, will be required to determine whether the phenomenon reported in this initial study is real. The developmental time difference between the sexes is contrary to development in other parameters, especially postnatally.

Laterality of Clefts

Another peculiarity of the cleft situation, which may eventually be a clue to the cause of the condition, is that more instances of unilateral cleft lip or cleft lip and palate occur on the left side.[109] However, cleft palate is itself more often associated with bilateral than with unilateral cleft of the lip—86 per cent are bilateral compared with 68 per cent that are unilateral.[33] This finding appears to support the idea first promoted by Fogh-Andersen[30] that cleft palate associated with cleft lip is secondary to the lip defect and that the more severe the lip defect the greater the likelihood that defects of the palate will occur.

Clefts and Associated Abnormalities

All too often human orofacial clefting has been considered a distinct pathological entity without regard to the possibility that clefts of both the lip and the palate, singly or in combination, may frequently be associated with other malformations. Because cleft cases with additional malformations may have a different etiological basis, they must be differentiated from those in which orofacial clefting is the sole malformation. Many of the cases with additional malformations are syndromes associated with chromosomal aberrations; others are not so clearly definable. Nevertheless, although it has been estimated that these cases account for approximately 3 per cent of all cleft cases, they are clearly distinct from those cases in which orofacial clefting is the sole malformation.

The extent to which clefting is associated with other malformations is illustrated by several surveys. In a review by Gorlin and Pindborg[41] of several cleft palate populations, it was reported by Curtis[22] that associated abnormalities occur with isolated cleft of the palate with a frequency 30 times that of these same malformations in the non-cleft general population. This underscores the fact that CP often does not occur alone and is liable

TABLE 3–2   Sex Ratio of Cleft Type by Race: Percentage in Brackets

Author(s)	Year	Country: Source of Sample and Race	CL(P) Male Per Cent	CL(P) Female Per Cent	CL(P) Total	CP Male Per Cent	CP Female Per Cent	CP Total	Sample Total
Hixon	1951	Canada: Ontario: Hospitals Caucasians	326 (63.8)	185 (36.2)	511	55 (45.0)	69 (55.0)	123	634
Mazaheri	1958	USA: Clinic Caucasian	286 (66.7)	143 (33.3)	429	103 (42.6)	139 (57.4)	242	671
Rank and Thompson	1960	Australia: New South Wales: Caucasian	85 (62.5)	51 (37.5)	136	26 (46.4)	30 (53.6)	56	192
Knox and Braithwaite	1962	England: Several sources Caucasian	252 (65.2)	134 (34.8)	386	77 (41.0)	111 (59.0)	188	574
Drillien, et al.	1966	Scotland: Surgical records Caucasian	66 (71.7)	26 (28.3)	92	27 (36.5)	47 (63.5)	74	166
Iyer	1967	England: Hospital cases Caucasian	– –	– –	–	44 (50.0)	44 (50.0)	88	88
Meskin, et al.	1968	Illinois: Cleft clinic Caucasian	204 (67.8)	97 (32.2)	301	67 (38.0)	109 (62.0)	176	477
Bear	1973	England: Hospital cases Caucasian	143 (61.6)	89 (38.4)	232	30 (30.9)	67 (69.1)	97	329
Lowry and Renwick	1969	British Columbia: Handicapped registry Caucasian	322 (65.3)	171 (34.7)	493	120 (49.2)	124 (50.8)	244	737
Bardanouve	1969	Montana: Birth records Caucasian	242 (71.8)	95 (28.2)	337	121 (63.4)	70 (36.6)	191	528
Bixler, et al.	1971°	Denmark: Hospital records Caucasian	281 (63.9)	159 (36.1)	440	61 (40.7)	89 (59.3)	150	590
Brogan and Woodings	1974	West Australia: Surgical Cases Caucasian	146 (72.3)	56 (27.7)	202	68 (52.3)	62 (47.7)	130	332
Spry and Nugent	1975	South Australia: Hospital records Caucasian	252 (65.8)	126 (34.2)	368	43 (27.9)	111 (72.1)	154	522
Chi	1974	New South Wales: Australia: Hospital records Caucasian	85 (62.5)	51 (37.5)	136	26 (46.6)	30 (53.6)	56	192
Tal, et al.	1974	Israel: Hospital cases Caucasian	80 (61.5)	50 (38.5)	130	25 (55.6)	20 (44.6)	45	175

TABLE 3–2 Sex Ratio of Cleft Type by Race: Percentage in Brackets *(Continued)*

Author(s)	Year	Country: Source of Sample and Race	CL(P) Male Per Cent	CL(P) Female Per Cent	CL(P) Total	CP Male Per Cent	CP Female Per Cent	CP Total	Sample Total
Myrianthopoulos and Chung	1974	USA: 12 institutions: birth records Caucasian	20 (57.1)	15 (42.9)	35	19 (63.3)	11 (36.7)	30	65
Bear	1976	England: Various hospitals Caucasian	198 (61.1)	126 (38.9)	324	50 (34.0)	97 (65.9)	147	471
Oka	1975	USA: Penna. birth records Caucasian	1,241 (66.5)	624 (33.5)	1,865	407 (46.5)	469 (53.5)	876	2,741
TOTAL		CAUCASIAN	4,219 (65.7)	2,198 (34.3)	6,417	1,369 (44.6)	1,698 (55.4)	3,067	9,484
Kobayashi	1958	Japan: Hospital cases Japanese	51 (60.7)	33 (39.3)	84	5 (29.4)	12 (70.6)	17	101
Kobayashi	1958	Japan: Clinic cases Japanese	263 (61.0)	168 (39.0)	431	52 (35.0)	98 (65.0)	150	581
Fujino, et al.	1963	Japan: Surgical records Japanese	1,319 (55.6)	1,053 (44.0)	2,372	157 (34.5)	298 (65.5)	455	2,827
Fujino et al.	1967	Japan: Surgical records Japanese	794 (56.6)	608 (43.4)	1,402	79 (36.9)	135 (63.1)	214	1,616
TOTAL		JAPANESE	2,427 (56.6)	1,862 (43.4)	4,289	293 (35.0)	543 (65.0)	836	5,125
Azaz and Kaye	1967	Israel: Hospital cases Various races?	7 (38.9)	11 (61.1)	18	6 (75.0)	2 (25.0)	8	26
Myrianthopoulos and Chung	1974	USA: 12 institutions, birth records Black	12 (66.7)	6 (33.3)	18	15 (62.5)	9 (37.5)	24	42
Oka	1975	USA: Penna. birth records, non-Caucasian, predominantly black	37 (42.0)	51 (58.0)	88	22 (36.6)	38 (63.3)	60	148
TOTAL		BLACK	49 (46.2)	57 (53.8)	106	37 (44.0)	47 (56.0)	84	190
Lowry and Renwick	1969	British Columbia: Handicapped registry Amerindian	34 (61.8)	21 (38.2)	55	5 (55.6)	4 (44.4)	9	64
TOTAL		ALL GROUPS	6,736 (62.0)	4,149 (38.0)	10,885	1,710 (42.7)	2,294 (57.3)	4,004	14,889

°Updated data originally reported by Fogh-Andersen, 1942.

to be associated with other abnormalities. For cleft lip and palate, between 10 and 25 per cent of the cases had abnormalities in other organs. Similar results were found for CP and CLP by other workers. For CP, the abnormalities most commonly found were umbilical hernia and deformities of the limbs and ear.[52] For CLP, Beder and associates[7] listed mental retardation, congenital heart disease, and abnormalities of the fingers and toes. In a more recent survey of several authors by Gorlin and associates,[40] there was a consistent finding of a differential malformation rate between isolated cleft palate and cleft lip with or without cleft palate. In all cases, isolated cleft palate was more often associated with additional malformations in comparison with isolated cleft lip or cleft lip in combination with cleft palate.

Sexual and racial differences in the rate of associated malformations for both CLP and CP in more than 50,000 consecutive live births were studied by Myrianthopoulos and Chung.[80] For the total sample, both males and females of all races, 71 per cent of CL(P) cases and 85 per cent of CP cases were affected with multiple malformations. The data broken down by sex and race revealed that 80 per cent of Caucasian males with CL(P) and 95 per cent with CP had other malformations, whereas 51 per cent of the Caucasian females with CL(P) and 91 per cent with CP were affected with additional abnormalities. Black males with CL(P) and CP had additional malformation rates of 75 per cent and 87 per cent respectively. Black females were affected with rates of 83 per cent and 78 per cent for CL(P) and CP respectively. In an earlier survey Meskin and Pruzansky[75] tabulated the malformation profile of 372 probands and found that regardless of cleft types females were more likely to be affected with additional malformations than were males. This finding contradicts the results of Myrianthopoulos and Chung for both black and Caucasian male and female cleft cases. They observed that black females with CL(P) had a higher rate of associated malformations than either black or Caucasian CL(P) males. This discrepancy can probably be explained by a difference in the populations studied. Meskin and Pruzansky gathered their data from records at a cleft palate clinic. Myrianthopoulos and Chung obtained their data from records of consecutive live births and may therefore have included severe multiple malformed children, who may die prior to surgical correction of the cleft. As such, the data may reflect a differential in mortality between male cleft cases with additional malformations and their female counterparts, with male cases having a higher mortality rate.

Rather than tabulating cleft cases with additional malformations, let us look instead at developmental anomalies that are associated in varying degrees with orofacial clefts. Some of these defects are so well known as to constitute definite syndromes. Some are inherited in mendelian form, and some are gross chromosomal defects. Gorlin, Červenka, and Pruzansky[40] have compiled a list of syndromes that have clefts in their nosology. They list 17 autosomal dominant, 18 autosomal recessive, 4 X-linked, and 18 nongenetic syndromes. Fifteen chromosomal anomalies are also described. The chromosomal aberrations that sometimes involve orofacial clefts as part of the somatic feature include trisomy D (Patau's syndrome), which almost always has a cleft of the lip and palate. The other chromosomal defects are not so frequently associated. For the autosomal dominant trait, the best known is the dominant lip syndrome, in which bilateral fistulas on the vermilion of the lower lip are usually present. These depressions are sinuses that communicate with minor salivary glands and often exude viscid saliva spontaneously or with pressure.

Parental Age and Birth Rank

Among the variables examined in an epidemiological survey are parental age and birth rank. Both of these variables are closely related, for older mothers in a sample will obviously tend to have a large sibship and thus will have more children of higher birth order. Parental age usually is focused on maternal age, as witnessed by the increased risk of Down's syndrome in children born to mothers over 40 years of age. For such a clear-cut syndrome involving an extra chromosome, a mechanism for etiology based upon maternal age can be postulated. This is for the "age-dependent" trisomy of chromosome 21, which involves an incorrect segregation or migration (nondisjunction) of the chromosomes into the daughter cells during the first or second meiotic division. The causal relationship is not clearly known, but perhaps it may be due to an overaged ovum prior to the first meiotic division at ovulation or to an overaged ovum postovulation that suffers a nondisjunction at the second meiotic division. The "age-independent" Down's syndrome cases, which can occur to children of young mothers, are due to another mechanism, *translocation*. The reader who is interested in pursuing the subject further will find it extensively covered in any medical genetics text.

For parents of children with clefts of the lip and/or palate such a clear-cut relationship between maternal or paternal age, birth rank, and incidence is not evident. The dilemma of interpreting the information can be illustrated as follows: If a child in a later birth rank is born with a cleft, it may be caused by some phenomenon associated with increased maternal age, or it may be completely independent of maternal age but due to some adverse effect of multiparity. Nevertheless, several studies have incorporated these variables in these analyses (see survey by Greene[42]) and have found no significant relationship between maternal age, birth rank, and the incidence of a child born with a cleft. Several of the studies cited suffered from various methodological shortcomings. More recent studies in Finland[92] and in Sweden[49] did not reveal any significant maternal or paternal age effect, nor did the distribution of the probands according to birth rank show any significant difference from expected values.

Among those recent studies that did note a positive relationship between parental age and cleft defects are those by Czeizel and Tusnadi[23, 24] in Hungary, who reported a positive association between advanced maternal age and the birth of children with cleft lip, with or without cleft palate. They found significantly more CL(P) children born to mothers above the age of 35. This association, however, was not perceived for isolated cleft palate cases. Birth rank itself was not related to either CL(P) or CP. Woolf and his coworkers[108] presented data collected in Utah relating to parental age. A significant positive relationship was seen between maternal age and the birth of children with clefts of the lip, with or without palatal involvement. Here again, birth order did not have any effect on the occurrence of clefts of all types. A later study by Woolf[106] suggested that the effect of parental age on the incidence of CL(P) may be a function of paternal age.

The interpretation of the relationship between the effect of parental age and birth rank influencing the incidence of orofacial clefts is presently difficult to establish. The procedures of data collection and analysis differ in the various studies and comparisons are thus difficult to make. A slight influence of parental age may exist for CL(P), but the exact nature of this association is not known at present.

Twin Studies

Twin studies are a good source of information about the relative influence of genetic and environmental factors in human orofacial clefting. The one major drawback, however, is the low frequency of monozygotic twins born with a particular malformation. Hay and Wehrung,[48] using the figure of 1 per 50 for the incidence of twin births and 1 per 800 live births for the incidence of clefts, calculated that 40,000 births would have to be studied in order to detect one twin with a cleft. This is assuming that both orofacial clefting and the birth of twins are independent phenomena. It is obvious then that in order to accumulate sufficient twin data, previously published studies must be utilized. The immediate shortcoming in following this procedure is that the methods used by the various investigators to determine zygosity vary widely; some use only morphological similarity, while others will resort to more stringent criteria, such as matching blood groups or the use of skin homografts.

Fogh-Andersen[30] surveyed published data and added 28 twin pairs from his own sample. He found a significant difference in the concordance rate for CL(P) between monozygotic (MZ) and dizygotic (DZ) twins. This difference was not found for isolated CP. Metrakos, Metrakos, and Baxter[77] reported ten twin pairs with clefts, two or which were monozygotic pairs. They surveyed published case histories to supplement their data and selected only those cases in which zygosity was reported. From a total of 29 MZ and 29 DZ pairs they found a concordance rate of 31.0 per cent for MZ and 6.3 per cent for DZ twins for clefts of the lip and/or palate. The concordance rate for the MZ twins was much higher for cleft lip and cleft lip and palate than for cleft palate alone. Their conclusions agree with Fogh-Andersen in that heredity appears to play an important role in the etiology of CL(P) and a less important one in CP.

Hay and Wehrung[48] analyzed 214 twins with clefts recorded on birth certificates. This study did not show the higher incidence of clefts among twins as compared with singletons that was found in an earlier study.[43] The incidence rate was found to be similar between like and unlike-sexed twins, whereas isolated cleft palate was observed more often among male twins than among unlike-sexed twins or single births. This is a reversal from the usual female preponderance in CP. The investigators thus postulated that there may be: (1) higher fetal mortality among female MZ twins or (2) a positive association between the malformations, male sex, and MZ twinning.

Because of the rarity of twins born with congenital malformation, the problem of zygosity determination, the required criteria for concordance, and so forth, twin studies are less attractive as a source of genetic data than one could wish. Edwards[28] states that the value of twin studies is rather limited, since the extra information that they convey does not compensate for the trouble of finding the affected twins. We know that, a priori, MZ twins resemble each other more than sibs who are not cotwins. The degree of resemblance is difficult to interpret, and a common error of interpretation arises from the fact that any difference between MZ twins is due solely to environment. Nevertheless, twin studies have shown that both genetic and environmental factors are involved in the etiology of cleft defects. The relative importance of the two factors cannot be determined by this method, however, nor can we conclude that there is a clear-cut difference in the relative proportion of genetic and environmental factors in cleft lip and palate versus isolated cleft of the palate.

Family Studies

Several studies have indicated there are familial predispositions to clefting. In 1909, Rischbeth concluded that one in five patients with cleft lip and palate had at least one relative similarly affected.[26] Bhatia[8] summarized results from various familial and population surveys in several different countries and concluded that overall about a third of the cases of cleft lip and palate have a positive family history. He determined that this positive family history is present one and a half times as frequently in cleft lip with or without cleft palate (40 per cent) as in isolated cleft palate (28 per cent). Data from the Lancaster Cleft Palate Clinic substantiate the greater number of positive family histories in the cleft lip and/or palate probands (Table 3–3). A positive family history is present in CL(P) probands 1.24 times as frequently as in isolated CP probands. This difference in the incidence of positive family history between the two cleft types suggests a stronger genetic influence in the former. Embryological evidence also indicates that these cleft types are etiologically distinct.[99] Such evidence shows that clefts of the secondary palate can be induced by teratogens administered after the primary palate has closed and that the

TABLE 3–3   Total Number of Probands and Number of Probands and Percentage with a Positive Family History at the Lancaster Cleft Palate Clinic (By Sex and Cleft Type)

	TOTAL SAMPLE			POSITIVE FAMILY HISTORY					
CLEFT TYPE	Male	Female	Total	Male	Per Cent	Female	Per Cent	Total	Per Cent
CLP	205	117	322	68	33.0	40	34.0	108	34.0
CL	58	33	91	13	22.0	5	15.0	18	20.0
CP	114	146	260	31	27.0	34	23.0	65	25.0
TOTAL	377	293	673	112	30.0	79	27.0	191	28.0

failure of secondary palate closure in mouse embryos with a cleft of the lip and primary palate can be a developmental consequence of the first malformation. It appears then that the factors involved in the formation of CL(P) are distinct from those involved in forming clefts of the secondary palate alone. This also would indicate that any studies of families with CL(P) or CP should separate these two varieties of defects.

The genetic difference between the two major cleft types in humans was determined by family studies. Several investigators[6, 30, 34, 106, 108] have presented evidence that close relatives (siblings) of patients with CL(P) have a significantly increased incidence of CL(P) but not of CP, whereas siblings of patients with CP have an increased incidence of CP but not of CL(P). In addition, it was found that when an affected parent-child relationship existed, the type of cleft found in the parent, whether CL(P) or CP, was the same type most frequently occurring in the child.[107] A similar pattern was seen in a Japanese population and in a Danish population.[9] An exception to this similarity of cleft types within families is the dominant lip pit syndrome. This syndrome has been thoroughly investigated by van der Woude.[102] In families in which clefts occur with lower lip fistulas, concordance of cleft types between parent and offspring may not occur. Van der Woude has shown that the mode of inheritance for this syndrome is autosomal dominant and that the dominant gene causing this syndrome occurs in about one in 200 cleft cases.

One of the most comprehensive family studies was conducted by Woolf.[106] He combined data from Arizona and Utah and analyzed the families of 496 propositi to determine the frequencies of CL(P) in their relatives. A significant decrease in the frequency of affected relatives was found as the degree of relationship diminished (more distant relatives). This conspicuous decrease in the frequency as one proceeds from first degree to second degree to third degree relatives is one criterion for polygenic inheritance and clearly distinguishes it from dominant inheritance. This was shown by Carter[16] for several malformations including CL(P). Using a population incidence of 1.2 per 1000 live births in Utah, Woolf and coworkers[108] determined frequencies of CL(P) in first degree relatives to be 33 times, for second degree relatives 5 times, and for third degree relatives 3 times the incidence in the general population.

Woolf[108] also demonstrated the polygenic nature of CL(P) by determining the influences of family history on the frequency of this malformation in the sibs of the propositi. This comparison is to mendelian modes of inheritance. If CL(P) is recessive, all sibs born subsequent to a CL(P) child should have a 25 per cent chance of having the malformation. In dominant inheritance, the frequency of affected individuals in each successive group of relatives will decrease by only one half. These risk figures should hold regardless of the presence of the anomaly in other relatives. In polygenic inheritance, a threshold is assumed, and an affected child will vary as to the number of genes he possesses above the threshold number. Normal parents of the propositus will vary in the number of genes they possess below the threshold. The obvious rule is that the larger the number of cleft-predisposing genes possessed by the parents, the greater the probability that they will have an affected child. This rule can be extended to other relatives, so that a propositus who has a close affected relative probably has more of the genes than a propositus who has a more distant affected relative or who has a negative family history. Thus, the greater the number of genes possessed by the propositus, the higher the probability he will have an affected sib. This was demonstrated when it was found that the overall frequency of CL(P) in the sibs of the propositi increased with the number of family members affected from the distant to closer relatives.[108]

In family studies, the ascertainment of information about affected relatives, especially after second degree relatives (grandparents, uncles, aunts), becomes more difficult. A prospective study of families that uses stringent criteria both for gathering information and follow-up on relatives is desirable. Since many of the studies have indicated a genetic influence in human orofacial clefting, further family studies of a cross-sectional nature will not add much to our existing knowledge. What is lacking is a concerted effort to determine which of the cleft cases have a stronger genetic etiology. This can be done initially only by extracting information from those cases that have multiple affected relatives, preferably only to third degree relatives.

Clefts and Environmental Agents

The environmental variables known to cause clefts were discovered through experimental teratology. A comprehensive list of these teratogens and a possible mechanism by which they may cause the malformation were covered in detail in the previous chapter (Chapter 2). In this section a more generalized approach to the developmental mechanism in orofacial clefting will be taken, with more emphasis placed on historical aspects. It will be seen that experimental production of clefts in animals is relatively recent in the time scale of historical preoccupation with the total problem of congenital malformations.

Clefts of the palate can be produced by many methods. The pioneering work by Hale,[45, 46] who induced blindness in pigs by restricting vitamin A in pregnant sows, also produced cleft lip and cleft palate in some of the blind littermates. It was not certain, however, whether these facial clefts could be attributed entirely to materal vitamin A deficiency. An occasional cleft lip and palate was also obtained in a later study with vitamin A deficient sows. It was concluded, however, that these oral manifestations should not be considered regular components of the deficiency syndrome.[87] Vitamin A deficiency in rats produced a variety of malformations, but facial clefts were not a part of them. Then in 1943 regular experimental production of facial clefts in this animal became possible when Warkany and associates[104] showed that cleft palate appeared in a syndrome of skeletal defects induced by maternal riboflavin deficiency. Posterior palatal clefts were found in 15 per cent of the offspring of pregnant rats deficient in riboflavin. Cleft lip and clefts of the primary palate were only occasionally found. The incidence of palatal clefts in rat litters was increased by the use of a combination of riboflavin deficiency and the antimetabolite galactoflavin.[83] This combination increased the incidence to 39 per cent.

Similar results were found for mice, using the same treatment, but it appeared that the effect was specific for a particular strain of mice. Kalter and Warkany[56] using the DBA mouse strain, were able to induce cleft palate in 41 per cent of the offspring of treated pregnant mice. When they used other strains, the results were much lower. The withholding of another vitamin, folic acid, from pregnant rats can also cause cleft palate. Folic acid deficiency induced by an antimetabolite during days 10 to 13 of gestation resulted in cleft palate in 100 per cent of the offspring. Induction of folic acid deficiency during days 9 to 11 resulted in 86 per cent cleft palate and 93 per cent cleft lip.[82] This study illustrates the importance of timing when administering the agent in relation to the type and amount of congenital malformation produced in the offspring of treated animals.

Aside from a deficiency, induction of cleft palate was attempted by the addition of a factor in pregnant animals. In 1951, Fraser and Fainstadt[35] successfully produced cleft palate by injecting large doses of cortisone into pregnant females of the A/JAX mouse strain. This fundamental experiment provided a basis for succeeding experiments designed to search for embryological and genetic factors that might be implicated in the causation of clefts. Fraser and coworkers[36] and Kalter[55] found that the injection of cortisone during a specific time of gestation (10 days) and the duration of injections (4 days) produced clefts in 100 per cent of the offspring of the A/JAX animals. When the experiment was duplicated using the C57BL mouse strain, only 18 per cent of the offspring were affected. Thus, a difference between the two strains in sensitivity to the teratogenic action of cortisone was demonstrated. Embryological factors could now be studied, taking account of the fact that under certain conditions cleft palate could be induced in almost 100 per cent of the offspring. This provided a method of experimentally pinpointing deviations during the developmental sequence in palatal development. It was postulated that cortisone caused cleft palate in mice by interfering with the normal alignment of the palatine shelves from the vertical to the horizontal plane. Conceivably, delay in shelf movement, inability of the shelves to grow without fusion, increase in head width without increase in palatal width, or a combination of these, could result in a palatal cleft, since the shelves are too far apart to come together and fuse when they attain their horizontal position. The differences in the incidence of induced cleft palate between the C57BL embryos and the A/JAX strain caused by administration of cortisone was found to be partially due to the difference in the time of closing of the palatal shelves, as between these two strains, the C57BL embryos exhibited earlier palatal closing.

It was also found that the shelf movement in the C57BL strains was less inhibited by cortisone in comparison with the A/JAX embryos. The complex interaction of the many factors, both intrinsic (genetic strain difference) and extrinsic (exogenous teratological agents), contributing to the formation of palatal clefts could now be studied. Several studies were then undertaken to determine the role of the tongue position, tongue movement, shelf force, mandibular development, and synthesis of mucopolysaccharides in the production of cleft palate.

Although there is now an experimental model available to study the basic mechanisms that could be implicated in palatal clefting, translation of these results to the human experience remains obscure. Cortisone, which has been mentioned as a successful agent for producing palatal clefts in mice, is often given to women during pregnancy. Although occasional reports of a child born with a cleft after such treatment have been published,[25, 47] a causal relationship between maternal cortisone treatment and offspring with cleft palate cannot be established, since the overwhelming majority of children born to treated mothers are normal.[103]

It was earlier demonstrated that timing of the administration of teratogens was important in producing clefts in experimental animals. This is of no less importance in humans, but here the exact time of maximum sensitivity to a teratogen cannot be determined experimentally. It can only be inferred from human embryo and fetal data pertaining to the time of morphodifferentiation, closure, and fusion of the orofacial structures. This period spans almost the whole of the first trimester of pregnancy. Although the critical stages for lip and palate fusion can be located between the sixth and ninth week postimplantation, any insult prior to this period can conceivably influence development to cause lip and/or palatal defects. To further compound the difficulty in determining the nature and action of suspected teratogens, there are other interrelated factors, such as the genetic susceptibility of the embryo and the physiological and pathological status of the mother. The latter factor is of importance in drawing conclusions about the role of cortisone or other therapeutic drugs as the mediator of clefts in human offspring. Since only women with a pathological condition are treated with cortisone, it would be difficult to establish a definite correlation between cortisone and clefting in humans. This was stated succinctly by Saxen,[92] who tried to establish a relationship between maternal influenza, drug consumption, and oral clefts. In epidemiological studies that attempt to establish linkage between different potential teratogens taken by pregnant women "confounding is created by the pathological conditions for which the drugs were taken and also by other drugs which were taken simultaneously." Examples given were linkages between hormone intake and maternal bleeding, between antiemetics and vomiting, and between epilepsy and anticonvulsant therapy. Because of this confounding effect, retrospective studies based on maternal pregnancy histories are difficult to interpret. Thus, conclusion based solely upon drug intake and frequency of congenital anomalies should be approached with caution.

Genetic susceptibility of the embryo was demonstrated by the strain difference in the sensitivity of mice to the action of cortisone in the production of clefts. Species difference is even greater and is exemplified by the sensitivity of animals to the action of thalidomide on the developing embryo. It is a powerful teratogen in rabbits but relatively safe in rats. Although this drug served to alert the medical and lay public alike to the potential danger of indiscriminate medication in early pregnancy, it did not, however, produce malformed children in all women who took the drug during the critical period of organogenesis. Because of the strain difference in the susceptibility to thalidomide in experimental animals, this drug illustrated the difficulty in extrapolating results from experimental animals to man. The first studies were performed in rats and mice, with no typical limb anomalies resulting. Large doses (more than 200 times the human dosage) caused fetal death and anomalies in the sternum and vertebral columns of these animals. Then rabbits were used, and the typical leg anomalies comparable to those that developed in man were produced.[93] It is of interest, however, that when thalidomide was tested on rats deficient in the vitamin pantothenic acid, the deficiency intensified the effect on the fetuses and produced limb anomalies that were not produced when the drug was used alone.[37] This illustrates the possibility of synergistic action of various drugs or various deficiencies, or both, that further complicates extrapolation of retrospective studies in humans.

Nevertheless, the thalidomide disaster naturally focused attention on the potential danger of all medication used during pregnancy. Meclizine, an antihistamine used to combat nausea and vomiting, came under suspicion for two reasons. First, in addition to its action as an antiemetic, it produces a mild sedative effect; therefore, its indication for use during pregnancy was similar to thalidomide. Second, meclizine in large doses was found to cause cleft palate in rats.[57] However, several retrospective studies using large populations of women found that the incidence of malformations in the children of mothers who had taken meclizine was no higher than in those who had not taken the drug.[67, 73, 93, 109]

Other drugs suspected of causing a cleft in humans include phenmetrazine (a CNS stimulant) and aminopterin (an abortifacient). But the cases reported are isolated and are single associations, and thus do not prove causation.

Although the list of drugs and other agents found to be effective in causing clefts in experimental animals is large, there is very little known about agents that could mediate the prevention of such malformations. As with causative agents, attempts at prophylaxis against orofacial clefting utilized experimental animals. Reduction of cleft palate in the litter of cortisone-treated mice by the administration of pyridoxine (vitamin B_6) was reported by some investigators,[88] although others did not find such an effect.[64] The administration of either riboflavin or pyridoxine to mice was found to reduce the incidence of cortisone-induced cleft palate.[110]

The fact that cortisone induces clefts in mice and that vitamins appear to reduce the number of cleft offspring in litters of mothers treated with cortisone led investigators to attempt to find a causal relationship between maternal stress and cleft incidence and to assess the efficacy of supplements of vitamins to reduce the incidence. In humans, retrospective studies were attempted by reviewing maternal pregnancy histories. In one study the family and pregnancy histories of 400 mothers were evaluated.[89] Three hundred and six women had no positive family history for clefting. Two hundred and seventy-five of the mothers were reported not to have taken vitamin supplements, or if they did, they took them late in pregnancy. Eighty-seven mothers who had given birth to a child with a cleft and who had subsequent pregnancies were evaluated for vitamin intake. Forty-eight mothers did not receive vitamin therapy during 78 subsequent pregnancies in this group. Four of their offspring had clefts of various types, and there was one case of epilepsy. Of the 39 mothers who were given vitamin supplements, no cases or clefts or other congenital anomalies were reported. Although the results seem to indicate an effect of the vitamin in the right direction, they are not conclusive, since the data were obtained via mailed questionnaires and did not include a control group.

In conclusion, reviews of environmental factors of human orofacial clefts have shown that: (1) studies purporting to establish a relationship between a specific exogenous factor and clefts rely on isolated cases and are inconclusive and (2) retrospective studies that show a lower frequency of orofacial clefts in mothers who have taken vitamin supplements during their pregnancies show only small differences and are inconclusive. It appears then that no single factor can be described that is of major importance in human orofacial clefting; nevertheless, there is still the hope that preventive measures can be established for this malformation. Prospective studies are currently being planned using more stringent criteria. At the present time, however, no known universal teratogen for clefts in humans can be blamed. Environmental factors are undoubtedly important, and possible prevention of this malformation presently may result from two measures: (1) establishing an optimum in-utero environment, specifically during the first trimester, and (2) genetic counseling. The first measure will include the maternal as well as the fetal environment. The second measure will be discussed in more detail later in the chapter.

GENETICS OF CLEFTING

In the previous section it was seen that several agents have been successfully used in the production of cleft lip and cleft palate in litters of experimental animals. The effectiveness of these cleft-causing agents was found to be dependent upon several factors, one of which was the strain within a particular species of experimental animal. Clearly, there are differences in the susceptibility of different strains to the action of teratogenic drugs, and since the teratological reaction to the agents within each strain is consistent, we can conclude that the differences reflect dissimilarities in the genetic constitution of the various strains. How does this relate to clefts in the human population? In reviewing the literature on the epidemiology of cleft lip and palate, several salient points were brought out. We found, for example, that the incidence for clefts varied consistently among different racial groups. And it was also reported that populations that emigrated to another country more or less maintained the incidence of their parental generation.[65] We also discovered that in studies of populations with racial crosses, the incidence of clefts in their offspring was intermediate to that of the parental races. Twin studies also indicate that monozygotic twins have a higher concordance rate for this defect. That is to say, if one twin has a cleft, the chance that the other twin will also have a cleft is much higher in monozygotic than in dizygotic twins. Finally, family studies indicate that overall about a third of all index cases have a positive family history for this malformation, i.e., it is a condition that appears to "run in families" but one that has no clearly definable mode of inheritance.

Therefore, cleft of the lip and palate is a malformation that has a genetic basis but also can be caused by exogenous agents. It thus requires a complex interaction of both environmental and genetic factors. The old nature-nurture controversy, i.e., whether clefting is due to heredity or to environment, therefore becomes meaningless. Those investigators who attempted to show that genetic factors predominate developed simple mendelian genetic models in an attempt to establish a strict genetic relationship, and those who favored an environmental explanation resorted to experimental teratology.

Multifactorial Inheritance

By far the most accepted genetic model for cleft lip and palate is the multifactorial model. This model has been described and touted in several publications and is now almost a catch phrase for all phenomena that have a complex basis, ranging from genetic disease to behavioral profiles. There is a danger that the term "multifactorial" may become a "wastebasket" explanation for any phenomenon requiring input from a wide range of factors. It is true that the multifactorial model stresses the complex interaction of environmental and genetic components in the development of a trait. The point, however, is that the multifactorial theory is a broad descriptive one, attempting to incorporate in one term the concept that several factors are involved in the development of a trait, be it genetic disease or not. As such, both normal and abnormal traits are within the purview of the concept. What has not been emphasized is the fact that the idea propounded by the multifactorial theory is based on experimental evidence and that the concept and the method of analysis were first developed by geneticists around the turn of this century.

An analogy to the multifactorial threshold model will be presented to describe the overall concept and to clarify certain terms that have sometimes been used synonymously with the multifactorial model.* These terms are *polygenic* and *quasi-continuous.*

Let us imagine that a vessel is partially filled with fluid and that there is no way to view the level of the fluid in the vessel. This vessel represents the developing individual, and the level of the fluid represents the genotype, or the total genetic endowment (genome) received from both parents, plus intrinsic environmental factors and interaction between genes. The fluid level is raised through physical displacement by objects put into the vessel. We can use pebbles of various shapes and sizes in our example. The larger the objects, the more fluid will be displaced. We can designate the pebbles as environmental agents and/or conditions that contribute to a trait (e.g., clefting); therefore, they represent exogenous factors. As more and more pebbles are dropped into the vessel, the more fluid will be displaced until after a given period, which we equate to the intrauterine developmental time, the fluid may either spill over the lip, or it may come close to the lip and not spill over.

Since several genes are involved, the fluid is a polygenic system, the exact number of genes being unknown. In this system, then, the more genes inherited from either or both parents, the higher the level of the fluid. There-

---

*This model is adapted from one used by Dr. Roger Ladda in his presentation of multifactorial inheritance to the medical students at the Milton S. Hershey Medical Center, the Pennsylvania State University.

fore, in a "high risk" family more of the genes contributing to clefting will be passed from one generation to the next. It can be seen that as we drop in the environmental agents (pebbles) the fluid level will rise proportionately and overflow. The vessel with a higher initial fluid level will overflow much sooner with fewer added pebbles. If during a given period of time the same quantity of pebbles is dropped into an equal-sized vessel with a lower fluid level, the amount of fluid spilled will be less for this vessel than for the one with the higher initial level.

Two important concepts are illustrated here. First, when the fluid begins to overflow down the side of the vessel, the threshold has been crossed. And second, depending upon the initial volume of the fluid, the amount of overflow caused by an equal number of pebbles will differ; the vessel with more fluid will exhibit greater overflow. This phenomenon can be equated to the severity of the defect. Severity can therefore be determined by increased input of environmental agents or by input of a given quantity of environmental agents into an equal-sized vessel containing a greater initial volume of fluid. The point illustrated here is that the lip of the vessel is the threshold beyond which the malformation can be recognized. The level of fluid and the mass of pebbles are quantitative and therefore continuous, whereas the spilling over of the fluid is discontinuous and qualitative since it is an "either-or" phenomenon. Once there is an overflow, the amount of fluid spilled is again quantitative and relates to severity. Thus this illustrates what has been termed quasi-continuous variation[44] in that we have a continuous gradient that approaches a threshold and when once it passes the threshold the distribution becomes discontinuous. The underlying continuous distribution has been referred to as the underlying liability to a disease.[28, 29]

In this model, unaffected individuals are those who did not initially have a sufficient volume of fluid, so that regardless of the amount of input of pebbles it was not enough to reach the threshold. Relatives will have varying amounts of genes contributing to orofacial clefting. The closer the relationship, the greater the number of genes shared in common, and consequently the closer the degree of relationship to the affected individual, the greater the number of genes responsible for clefting carried by the relative.

In our model three factors are critical. First, we equated the initial fluid level with the quantity of genes possessed by the individual at the start of development that contributes to clefting, plus the interaction between the genes and inherent unknown environmental factors. Second, this level, although unknown for each case, can be assumed to have a graded or continuously distributed value for a large population. We thus assumed that the distribution would approximate a normal curve. And finally, we did not make any distinction between the various vessels and assumed that all vessels were of the same size and shape.

Going from our descriptive model, we will attempt to explain the multifactorial-threshold model as applied to human population. The assumption that we established for the vessel model is transferred as follows: Since it is assumed that a large number of independent genetic and environmental variables are involved, their distribution in a population will be described by a normal (bell-shaped) distribution.

The rationale for this assumption comes mainly from two sources. In breeding experiments with plants or animals in which a large sample in any particular generation may be analyzed and any trait studied (such as sugar content in corn), the trait in question approximates a normal or gaussian distribution. Likewise, when a large sample of people are measured for a particular trait (for example, height), we have a wide range represented, from the shortest to the tallest, which also closely approximates a normal distribution. Note that these traits are continuous.

For clefts of the lip and palate, the underlying normally distributed variable is considered as the *liability*, which includes several genetic loci interacting with each other and acted upon by several environmental agents. The total liability is multifactorial and is produced by the genetic liability and the environmental liability. The trait in question (orofacial clefts) occurs when an individual's total liability lies beyond a particular threshold. This threshold is determined by the population incidence. Thus all those who are affected constitute the proportion of the population beyond the threshold. The majority of the population who are unaffected will be in the midrange of the distribution. In considering the first degree relatives of those who are affected (sibs, parents, and offspring), we note that, on the average, they share 50 per cent of their genes in common. They will, therefore, have more of the genes that predispose them to a greater "risk" or liability to clefting than will the general population, but less than those who are affected. The average number of genes contributing toward clefting will be one half the distance between the average of the general population and the average of the affected individuals. The distribution of the first degree relatives (also assumed to be normally distributed) will thus be shifted toward the threshold, with the mean halfway between the general population mean and the mean of those who are affected.

Second degree relatives who, on the average, share 25 per cent of the genes in common with the proband will thus have their mean shifted one quarter the distance toward the affected mean. Third degree relatives will be toward the affected mean by an eighth, and by the time fourth degree relatives are reached the incidence begins to approach that of the general population. The first assumption of a normal distribution of liability is still maintained for all degrees of relationship. This assumption allows the use of some of the properties of the normal or bell-shaped curve, which is a member of a family of frequency curves. The area under the normal curve has been determined as relative cumulative frequencies for this family of frequency curves, therefore for any given value of a mean, the relative frequency (a probability) can be obtained. Thus for first degree relatives a shift of the mean to the right by one half will more than double the proportion at risk. A second assumption that allows the comparisons of the distributions of the relatives is that the variances are equal; therefore, the shape and size of the curves will be equal. This assumption is rather questionable, since the distributions of the relatives are derived from the population distribution. Nevertheless, it has been accepted to permit the determination of the proportion of relatives affected by using standard deviation units to locate areas under the normal curve.

Although this reasoning may appear to be on unsubstantial foundations, it has fortuitously granted a method of testing several predictions of incidences under the multifactorial model. These predictions are testable from family and epidemiological data and are:

1. The risk to relatives of the proband decreases the more distant the

TABLE 3–4 Comparative Frequencies of Clefts in Relatives of Proband with Similar Cleft Types*

	CL±P	CP
Population	0.0014	0.0004
First degree relatives (parents, sibs, offspring)	0.0334	0.0269
Second degree relatives (grandparents, aunts, uncles, nieces, and nephews)	0.0062	0.0058
Third degree relatives (first cousins)	0.0035	0.0038

*Adapted from Stewart, R. E., and G. H. Prescott (eds.): Oral Facial Genetics. St. Louis, The C. V. Mosby Co., 1976. From several sources.

relationship. Table 3–4 shows incidence figures in relatives of CL ± P and CP probands combined from several sources. The incidence (empirical risk) decreases sharply from the first degree relatives to second degree relatives and declines less abruptly from the second to third degree relatives.

2. In a multifactorial condition, the risk will vary from one family to another depending upon the number of affected individuals in the pedigree. This is in contrast to a single gene condition in which the risk remains the same regardless of whether there was a previously affected child. In an autosomal dominant condition the risk to subsequent offspring will remain at 50 per cent and for an autosomal recessive condition 25 per cent. In cleft lip and palate the risk increases with the number of affected relatives. The calculated empirical risk figure for the second child of unaffected parents with one child affected with CL ± P is between 4.5 and 5 per cent. If one parent and one child are affected, the risk figure increases to between 10.5 and 17.4 per cent.[98]

3. When there is a sex difference in the incidence of a multifactorial trait, the risk to relatives should depend on the sex of the proband. The less affected sex presumably will have a higher threshold, so that those who are affected must carry more cleft-predisposing genes. Therefore, the relatives will be proportionately at greater risk. Table 3–2, which is derived from 26 sources, gives the total number of male and female probands by cleft types for all races. There is a total of 10,885 probands for CL ± P, 6736 of them males and 4,149 females, for a ratio of 1.62 males to each female for this cleft type. For isolated cleft palate 4004 cases are listed, showing an excess of females

TABLE 3–5 Sex of Proband and Frequency of Affected First Degree Relatives*

	CL±P PROBAND		CP PROBAND	
	Male	Female	Male	Female
Number of relatives	1936	1157	269	481
Number affected	63	52	15	17
Percent affected	0.033	0.050	0.056	0.035

*Adapted from Stewart, R. E., and G. H. Prescott (eds.): Oral Facial Genetics. St. Louis, The C. V. Mosby Co., 1976. From various sources.

over male probands, with 2294 and 1710 cases respectively, for a female to male ratio of 1.34. Clearly more males are affected with CL ± P and more females with CP. We would, therefore, expect a higher proportion of affected relatives for female CL ± P probands and likewise an excess of affected relatives for male CP probands. Table 3–5, which is adapted from several sources, shows such a trend. The frequency of affected first degree relatives of female CL ± P probands is 5 per cent, whereas for relatives of male CL ± P probands the frequency is lower, at 3.3 per cent. For CP probands, the percentages are reversed; 5.6 per cent for males and 3.5 per cent for females.

4. An increase in the severity of the cleft type under the multifactorial model would indicate that more genes predisposing to clefting have segregated to the affected individual. Consequently there would be greater risk to relatives of those probands who are more severely affected. In the quantification of severity in orofacial clefts, bilateral cleft lip and palate will be classified as the most severe expression, with unilateral clefts of the lip as the mildest. Isolated cleft palate will not be considered, since there are not enough data available to test this hypothesis.[96] If a child has a cleft lip, the risk to subsequent sibs is approximately 2.6 per cent. If the child has a unilateral cleft of the lip and cleft palate, the risk increases to 4.1 per cent. With the most severe manifestation, bilateral cleft of the lip and cleft palate, the risk to subsequent siblings increases to 5.6 per cent.[33]

The predictions generated by the multifactorial-threshold theory appear to be confirmed by the accumulated data for CL(P) and slightly less for isolated CP. The ratiocination underlying the model, however, depends a great deal upon the empirical data concerning risks to relatives of affected individuals. Fitting the data to the model may appear tautological, yet with the severe limitation imposed upon genetic studies of human populations, it may never be possible to clearly delineate the genetic component of orofacial cleftings. Thus estimation of heritability is at best only an approximation, with no direct method presently available for verification. Nevertheless, the multifactorial-threshold model has some utility in predicting recurrence risk, and at the very least it has tempered the approach of those seeking the etiology of human orofacial clefting by avoiding looking for purely environmental or for simple and exclusively genetic explanations.

Recurrence Risk and Genetic Counseling

Although epidemiological, experimental, and family studies have uncovered data on the complexity of the etiology of orofacial clefting, the value of these studies is in developing capabilities of predicting and therefore preventing a recurrence of the malformation. Epidemiological data tell us that for any given conception in a population the chance of having a child with a cleft will be the incidence in the particular population. Experimental data alert us to the possible teratogens that can be implicated in causing a malformation, including clefts of the lip and/or the palate. Family data reveal that the risk of having an affected child increases with a positive family history. The multifactorial-threshold model describes the amount of risk to a potential newborn according to the degree of relationship of an affected relative. We have yet to take into consideration, however, the sex, type, and severity of the cleft of the affected relative. We have seen that these factors have some effect on the risk to the unborn child. Although there are published family data, extensive information, including the factors just mentioned, for all possible pedigrees is not available.

Before discussing the risk of re-occurrence of cleft lip and palate, it may be well to define the phrase "empirical risk" as applied to orofacial clefts. It simply means a prediction of re-occurrence of a cleft in a family based upon a prior observation in a similar family under similar circumstances. Empirical risks for orofacial clefts, therefore, are derived from family studies tabulating the number of affected relatives of the index case. It is apparent that a large population of families must be ascertained in order to establish empirical risk figures for all possible families with different patterns of affected relatives. The available risk figures based upon empirical data are thus mostly concentrated for first degree relatives. Tables 3–4 and 3–5 are therefore crude empirical risk figures tabulated for first degree relatives, which are grouped rather than identified with specific relationships. The risk of re-occurrence (recurrence risk) for subsequent births, as derived from these tables, cannot be applied to specific families except in a general way. These data, however, confirm one observable consequence of multifactorial inheritance that differs from single factor inheritance, i.e., the risk to the unborn child increases with an affected relative and the increase is directly related to the degree of relationship of the affected relative. Predicted recurrence risk based upon the type of first degree relatives affected by cleft type is tabulated in Table 3–6. It is evident from this table that there is an increase in the risk to subsequent children when more than one first degree relative is affected, which is also consistent with the multifactorial theory.

These figures may be used for counseling, for the majority of the cases seen in an exclusively cleft treatment clinic, such as we have at the Lancaster

TABLE 3–6 Empirical Risk Figures By Cleft Type, Number, and Type of Affected First Degree Relatives*

PARENTS	SIBS +	SIBS −	PER CENT CL±P	PER CENT CP
Normal	1	0	4.0	3.5
	1	1	4.0	3.0
	2	0	14.0	13.0
One affected	0	0	4.0	3.5
	1	0	12.0	10.0
	1	1	10.0	9.0
	2	0	25.0	24.0
Both affected	0	0	35.0	25.0
	1	0	45.0	4.0
	1	1	40.0	35.0
	2	0	50.0	45.0

+ Affected
− Unaffected
*From Tolarova, M.: Empirical recurrence risk figures for genetic counseling of clefts. Acta Chir. Plast. (Praha), 14:234–235, 1972.

Cleft Palate Clinic, will be sporadic cases. However, for intensive counseling, it is evident that a complete and accurate family pedigree is essential, for it has been our experience that upon questioning, many of the ostensibly sporadic cases actually turn out to have a positive family history. This finding can substantially change the risk figure. In addition, the presence of additional malformations in the proband or affected relatives will alter the recurrence risk figure. Therefore, adequate diagnosis is imperative.

Empirical risk figures play another role in genetic research. Segregation analysis requires observing the proportion of affected and unaffected individuals in families. These observations are used to test a series of genetic hypotheses. The most basic segregation values (frequencies) for single gene inheritance are 1/2 and 1/4, for autosomal dominant and autosomal recessive respectively. However, these frequencies are modified by other factors that influence the partial manifestation of a trait. It is neither within the scope nor the intent of this chapter to attempt to explain the analytical method of segregation analysis, except to state that the method developed by Morton[79] to test alternative modes of inheritance has been applied to cleft lip and cleft palate data.[20, 98] Although segregation analysis did not clearly discriminate between a single locus two allele, and multifactorial models, recurrence risk was, however, extended to families with different numbers of affected sibs and parents and also took into consideration the number of unaffected sibs. This is much more preferable than relying on purely empirical risk figures, which do not take into account the unaffected relatives. Extension of segregation analysis can conceivably predict recurrence risk in more remote relatives, although with less power than for first degree relatives.[79] For recurrence risks involving more distant affected relatives, simulation of the multifactorial model for a variety of possible sibships has been developed.[94] Thus the effect of remote affected relatives is taken into consideration and permits the calculation of exact recurrence risk in sibships and approximate risk in complex families. This method is available as a computer program, and since the results vary with population incidence and heritability estimates, it will be tailored for particular family samples.

It may be argued that such complex efforts are not necessary, since the majority of cleft cases are sporadic, and that an estimate derived from purely empirical data will be sufficient. It may be further argued that estimated risks derived by the methods just cited are based upon populational, genetic, and theoretical mathematical assumptions and are therefore not infallible. But these methods are useful tools for arriving at approximate risk figures when empirical data are not available for individuals who have a complex familial pattern. For those not versed in the complexity of deriving risk figures, there is a great temptation to disregard the effects of an irregular pattern of affected relatives in the pedigree and to concentrate on the immediate sibship for empirical figures. Although in most cases an approximate risk figure may be sufficient, disregarding other affected relatives may in some cases result in a wide disparity between the empirical and the estimated recurrence risk figures. Tables for estimated recurrence risk for complex families are available, and the interested reader is referred to them.[10, 94]

What we have just covered is directly applicable to genetic counseling. The qualifications of a genetic counselor will not be discussed here, except that ideally the person should have both a clinical background and some additional training in genetics. Since the patient is first seen by a physician, usually the pediatrician, initial questions concerning etiology and recurrence risk will be directed to him. In most cases he will have some medical genetic training, and these inquiries may be satisfactorily answered at that time. For more in-depth counseling, however, the parents should be referred to a qualified clinical geneticist. In genetic counseling, a mere repetition of recurrence risk figures will not be adequate, for although all parents of children with clefts may not seek genetic counseling, those who do usually want more information than just numbers. They are concerned with the how's and why's of the occurrence of a cleft in either themselves or their child. In addition, these risk figures must be translated for them into probability statements that they can understand.

In effect, the role of a genetic counselor is exactly that of a translator who can explain the known etiological factors involved in clefting, and who can also clarify estimated recurrence risk figures. His role is analogous to that of someone confronted by a patient or family with an actual language barrier. Imagine a couple who has a child with a cleft coming to a clinic from a foreign country. Neither the parents nor the child can speak English, and furthermore, no one on the clinical staff is able to speak their language. Let us assume then that the diagnosis and treatment plan are complicated by consideration of alternative methods of treatment. Let us assume in this hypothetical case that the width of the cleft precludes a definite choice of a treatment modality, for example, a prosthesis or surgical closure. Perhaps a prosthetic appliance would be more acceptable, but dental development or the condition of oral health may not be optimum to fabricate the appliance. Moreover, close follow-up of the patient for periodic replacement of the appliance to accommodate growth changes or for repair in the event of breakage is impossible, since the expense of periodic return trips for the patient will be prohibitive. To further complicate the situation, suppose that the parents assumed that a simple prosthesis was to be constructed, with no surgery contemplated. Under these circumstances, the surgeon, who incidentally also does not speak their language, elects to close the cleft surgically.

Now to translate the treatment procedure to the parents is obviously very difficult, requiring diplomacy, sensitivity, basic knowledge of the surgical procedure, and the ability to explain why in this situation surgery is preferable. A direct word-for-word translation by an interpreter will not be sufficient. So it is with genetic counseling, for the counselor too must be able to translate, but in his case he must translate current epidemiological and experimental data relating to cleft etiology, as well as interpret recurrence risk estimated from a complex genetic model, and apply them to a particular family history. It is therefore apparent that resorting to simple empirical risk tables will not be sufficient.

In the face of the foregoing, it is obvious that each counseling case is different. In our setting here in which the major portion of the case load consists of orofacial cleft patients, we do occasionally see children with multiple congenital anomalies. Many of these cases are definite syndromes. Provisional diagnoses are usually available, although often the diagnosis may be questioned, and the patient and the family may have been specifically referred to the clinic for identification of a syndrome. Under these circumstances, additional diagnostic tests, including cytogenetic and bio-chemical evaluation, may be necessary. A clinic providing genetic services should therefore be part of a medical genetics unit or should have ready access to one. Those of our patients who require additional diagnostic tests, such as karyotyping, are referred to the Division of Medical Genetics at the Milton S. Hershey Medical Center, a short distance from Lancaster. Through this affiliation, expert consultation in other branches of medicine is also available. The counselor should be aware of genetic heterogeneity, and expert consultants are necessary to validate a diagnosis.

In counseling orofacial cleft patients with no additional complications such as a syndrome or additional malformations, or in counseling the families of such patients, a most important requisite is a detailed and accurate family history. At the time of the initial interview, data on the immediate family are gathered. A medical as well as a pregnancy history of the mother is ob-tained, with close attention given to any unusual illness or any medication, especially during the first trimester of pregnancy with the affected child. Culturo-familial information is also gathered. This is usually available in the files from Social Services. Although we attempt to obtain as comprehensive a family history as possible, it usually becomes unreliable beyond the third degree relatives. All of the relatives are recorded by name. Affected relatives are recorded, together with names of hospitals in which they were patients and attending physicians if available. Release forms are also obtained at this time to obtain birth and surgical records of the propositus. After all pertinent data are in hand, a pedigree of the family is constructed. This pedigree is essential in genetic counseling, for not only is it valuable to the counselor in determining the pattern of affected relatives but it also aids those counseled in visualizing genetic relationships.

In a straightforward sporadic case, recurrence risk may be conveyed during the first interview. For some patients an estimate of recurrence risk is sufficient, but often questions as to etiology of clefting must be answered. A second interview is sometimes necessary when estimation of recurrence risk requires further investigation. Parental attitude will also dictate whether subsequent sessions are required. Those who harbor feelings of guilt or who are under familial or social pressures or those who have difficulty in comprehending recurrence risk as a probability will require additional sessions. Often the impact of a child born with a cleft will have affected the family so much that the subject of etiology will be the prime topic for discussion. This is especially so when a child is affected with additional malformations or when his condition represents a syndrome. At this time recurrence risk figures may be presented, but usually parental concern is still centered around the birth of their affected child and thoughts of re-occurrence of the condition in subsequent children may not be apparent. Appointments for further sessions can be made, but under these circumstances the parents will usually make the request.

The parents' interpretation of recurrence risk for subsequent children can be greatly influenced by the counselor. It is important then that the presentation of risk figures be geared to the individual and that any bias by the counselor be avoided. The decision of parents to have or not to have additional children should be their own. The role of the counselor is to present facts, as far as they are known, about the medico-genetic aspects of orofacial clefting, and not to get involved directly in the decision-making process. Should a couple elect to have another child, the counselor has the responsibility of promoting adequate prenatal care. Although preventive measures against human orofacial clefting have not been substantiated, vitamin supplements, especially folic acid and pyridoxine, have been suggested as a possible prophylaxis.[12, 21, 88] Information regarding the recommended dosage of 5 mg. of folic acid, 10 mg. of pyridoxine hydrochloride, and a Stress Formula vitamin tablet used in one ongoing study,[12] together with pertinent literature, is forwarded to the patient's obstetrician. This daily dose is taken from the first suspicion of pregnancy until at least the fifth month. Prescription of the supplement is with the approval and guidance of the obstetrician.

All records of the interview, pedigree, and counseling sessions are forwarded to the referring physician. Generally, following the counseling session a letter is sent to the counseled family, and provision for future appointments, if desired, is provided. Genetic counseling is not limited to the immediate family, but is extended to other family members. If there are any questions regarding the risk to other relatives, counseling services are provided for them. We have found this to be of concern to those families who have several affected members, the so-called "high risk" families.

In conclusion, it is hoped that this chapter provides information useful to those working in the many professions involved in the habilitative care of children with orofacial clefts, so that when they are questioned about the etiology or recurrence risk, they will be able to reply with knowledgeable answers.

References

1. Altemus, L. A., and A. D. Ferguson: Comparative incidence of birth defects in Negro and White children. Pediatrics, 36:56, 1965.
2. Armendares, S., and R. Lisker: Genetic analysis of cleft lip with or without cleft palate and cleft palate alone in a Mexican group (author's transl.). Rev. Invest. Clin., 26(4):317, 1974.
3. Azaz, B., and E. Koyoumondjisky-Kaye: Incidence of clefts in Israel. Cleft Palate J., 4:227, July, 1967.
4. Bardanouve, V. T.: Cleft palate in Montana. Cleft Palate J., 6:213, July, 1969.
5. Bear, J. C.: The association of fetal wastage with facial cleft conditions. Cleft Palate J., 10:346, 1973.
6. Bear, J. C.: A genetic study of facial clefting in Northern England. Clin. Genet., 9:277, 1976.
7. Beder, O. E., H. E. Coe, R. P. Brafladt, and J. D. Houle: Factors associated with congenital cleft lip and palate in the Pacific Northwest. Oral. Surg., 9:1267, 1956.
8. Bhatia, S. N.: Genetics of cleft lip and palate. Brit. Dent. J., 132:95, 1972.
9. Bixler, D., P. Fogh-Andersen, and P. M. Conneally: Incidence of cleft lip and palate in the offspring of cleft parents. Clin. Genet., 2:155, 1971.
10. Bonaiti-Pellié, C., and C. Smith: Risk tables for genetic counseling in some common congenital malformations. J. Med. Genet., 11:374, 1974.
11. Briard, M. L., C. Bonaiti-Pellié, J. Feingold, B. Pavy, J. Kaplan, and E. Bois: Genetics and epidemiology of cleft lip and cleft palate. Ann. Chir. Plast., 19(2):87, 1974.
12. Briggs, R. M.: Vitamin supplementation as a possible factor in the incidence of cleft lip palate deformities in humans. Clin. Plast. Surg., 3:647, 1976.
13. Brogan, W. F., and T. L. Woodings: A decline in the incidence of cleft lip and palate in Western Australia, 1963 to 1972. Med. J. Aust., 2(1):8, 1974.
14. Burdi, A. R., and R. G. Silvey: Sexual differences in closure of the human palatal shelves. Cleft Palate J., 6:1, 1969.

15. Canavea, I., and V. Chiriac: Incidence of congenital cleft lip and cleft palate in newborn infants. Stomatologia (Bucur.), 20(4): 347, 1973.
16. Carter, C. O.: Genetics of common disorders. Br. Med. Bull., 25:52, 1969.
17. Charlton, P. J.: Seasonal variation in incidence of some congenital malformations in two Australian samples. Med. J. Aust., 7:833, Oct., 1966.
18. Chi, S. C.: Cleft lip and cleft palate in New South Wales. Aust. Dent. J., 19(2):111, 1974.
19. Ching, G. H. S., and C. S. Chung: A genetic study of cleft lip and palate in Hawaii. I. Interracial crosses. Am. J. Hum. Genet., 26(2):162, 1974.
20. Chung, C. S., G. H. S. Ching, and N. E. Morton: A genetic study of cleft lip and palate in Hawaii. II. Complex segregation analysis and genetic risks. Am. J. Hum. Genet., 26(2):177, 1974.
21. Conway, H.: Effects of supplemental vitamin therapy on the limitations of incidence of cleft lip and palate in humans. Plast. Reconstr. Surg., 22:450, 1958.
22. Curtis, E. J.: Genetical and environmental factors in the etiology of cleft lip and cleft palate. J. Can. Dent. Assoc., 23:576, 1957.
23. Czeizel, A., and G. Tusnadi: An epidemiological study of cleft lip with or without cleft palate in Hungary. Hum. Hered., 21:17, 1971.
24. Czeizel, A., and G. Tusnadi: A family study of cleft lip with or without cleft palate and posterior cleft palate in Hungary. Hum. Hered., 22:405, 1972.
25. Doig, R. K., and O. M. Coltman: Cleft palate following cortisone therapy in early pregnancy. Lancet, 2:270, 1956.
26. Drillien, C. M., T. T. S. Ingram, and E. M. Wilkinson: The Causes and Natural History of Cleft Lip and Palate. Baltimore, The Williams and Wilkins Co., 1966.
27. Edwards, J. H.: Seasonal incidence of congenital disease in Birmingham. Ann. Hum. Genet., 25:89, 1961.
28. Edwards, J. H.: Familial predisposition in man. Br. Med. Bull., 25:58, 1969.
29. Falconer, D. S.: Inheritance of liability to certain diseases estimated from the incidence among relatives. Ann. Hum. Genet., 29:51, 1965.
30. Fogh-Andersen, P.: The Inheritance of Cleft Lip and Cleft Palate. Copenhagen, A. Busck, 1942.
31. Fogh-Andersen, P.: Recent statistics of facial clefts frequency, heredity, mortality. In Hotz, R. (ed.): Early Treatment of Cleft Lip and Palate. Berne and Stuttgart, Hans Huber, 1964.
32. Francis, T.: Genetics and epidemiology—Opening comments. In Neel, J. V., M. W. Shaw, and W. J. Schull. (eds.): Genetics and Epidemiology of Chronic Diseases. Symposium sponsored by U. S. Public Health Service, Publication No. 1163, Feb., 1965.
33. Fraser, F. C.: The genetics of cleft lip and cleft palate. Am. J. Hum. Genet., 22:336, 1970.
34. Fraser, F. C., and H. Baxter: The familial distribution of congenital clefts of the lip and palate. Am. J. Surg., 87:656, 1954.
35. Fraser, F. C., and T. D. Fainstadt: Production of congenital defects in the offspring of pregnant mice treated with cortisone. Pediatrics, 8:527, 1951.
36. Fraser, F. C., T. D. Fainstadt, and H. Kalter: The experimental production of congenital defects with particular reference to cleft palate. Études Néo-Nat., 2:43, 1953.
37. Fratta, I. D., E. B. Sigg, and K. Maiorana: Teratogenic effects of thalidomide in rabbits, rats, hamsters and mice. Toxicol. Appl. Pharmacol., 7:268, 1965.
38. Fujino, H., K. Tanaka, and Y. Sanui: Genetic study of cleft-lips and cleft-palates based upon 2,828 Japanese cases. Kyushu J. Med. Sci., 14:317, 1963.
39. Fujino, H., H. Tashiro, and Y. Sanui: Empirical genetic risk among offspring of cleft lip and cleft palate patients. Jap. J. Hum. Genet., 12(2):62, 1967.
40. Gorlin, R. J., J. Červenka, and S. Pruzansky: Facial clefting and its syndromes. Birth Defects: Original Article Series, 7:3, June, 1971.
41. Gorlin, R. J., and J. J. Pindborg: Syndromes of the Head and Neck. New York, McGraw-Hill Book Co., 1964.
42. Greene, J. C.: Epidemiology of congenital cleft of lip and palate. Public Health Rep., 78:589, 1963.
43. Greene, J. C., J. R. Vermillion, S. F. Hay, S. F. Gibbens, and S. Kerschbaum: Epidemiologic study of cleft lip and cleft palate in four states. J. Am. Dent. Assoc., 68:387, 1964.
44. Grüneberg, H.: Genetical studies on the skeleton of the mouse. IV. Quasi-continuous variation. J. Genet., 51:95, 1952.
45. Hale, F.: Pigs born without eyeballs. J. Hered., 24:105, 1933.
46. Hale, F.: Relation of maternal vitamin A deficiency to microphthalmia in pigs. Texas J. Med., 33:228, 1937.
47. Harris, J. W. S., and I. P. Ross: Cortisone therapy in early pregnancy. Lancet, 1:1045, 1956.
48. Hay, S., and D. A. Wehrung: Twins with cleft: A descriptive statistical analysis of selected variables. Cleft Palate J., 8:397, 1971.
49. Henriksson, T. G.: Cleft Lip and Palate in Sweden: A Genetic and Clinical Investigation. Univ. of Uppsala, Sweden, Inst. for Med. Genet., 1971.

50. Higgins, T. A., and N. G. O'Brien: Cleft lip and palate in the Newborn. Ir. Med. J., 67(21):559, 1974.
51. Hixon, E. H.: A study of the incidence of cleft lip and cleft palate in Ontario. Can. J. Public Health, 42:508, 1951.
52. Ingalls, T. H., I. E. Taub, and M. A. Klingberg: Cleft lip and cleft palate: Epidemiologic considerations. Plast. Reconstr. Surg., 34:1, 1964.
53. Ivy, R. H.: Congenital anomalies as recorded on birth certificates in the division of vital statistics of the Pa. Dept. of Health, for the period, 1951–1955, inclusive. Plast. Reconstr. Surg., 20:400, 1957.
54. Iyer, V. S.: Isolated cleft palate. Cleft Palate J., 4:124, 1967.
55. Kalter, H.: The inheritance of susceptibility to the teratogenic action of cortisone in mice. Genetics, 39:185, 1954.
56. Kalter, H., and J. Warkany: Congenital malformations in inbred strains of mice induced by riboflavin deficient, galactoflavin containing diets. J. Exp. Zool., 136:531, 1957.
57. Kendrick, F. J., and C. T. G. King: Oral anomalies induced in the rat by meclizine hydrochloride. Oral Surg., 18:690, 1964.
58. Kláskova-Burianová, O.: An epidemiological study of cleft lip and palate in Bohemia. Acta Chir. Plast. (Praha), 15(4):258, 1973.
59. Kláskova-Burianová, O.: Incidence of cleft lip and palate in Bohemia. Rozl. Chir., 53(3):147, 1974.
60. Knox, G., and F. Braithwaite: Cleft lips and palates in Northumberland and Durham. Arch. Dis. Child., 38:66, 1963.
61. Kobayashi, J.: A genetic study of harelip and cleft palate. Jap. J. Hum. Genet., 3:73, 1958.
62. Krantz, H., and F. Henderson: Relationship between maternal ancestry and incidence of cleft palate in children. J. Speech Hear. Disord., 5:285, May, 1947.
63. Kurozomi, S., H. Okazaki, N. Kosaka, M., Kido, T. Tanaka, Y. Nazakowa, K. Fujiwara, K. Yasukara, and N. Okura: A genetic study of harelip and cleft palate. Jap. J. Hum. Genet., 8:120, 1963.
64. Larsson, K. S.: Closure of the secondary palate and its relations to sulpho-mucopoly-saccharides. Acta Odont. Scand., 20(Suppl. 31):5, 1962.
65. Leck, I.: Ethnic differences in the incidence of malformations following migration. Br. J. Prev. Soc. Med., 23:166, 1969.
66. Leck, I., R. G. Record, T. McKeon, and J. H. Edwards: The incidence of malformations in Birmingham, England, 1950–1959. Teratology, 1:263, 1968.
67. Lenz, W.: How can the teratogenic action of a factor be established in man? South. Med. J., 64(suppl. 1):41, 1971.
68. Lowry, R. B., and D. H. G. Renwick: Incidence of cleft lip and palate in British Columbia Indians. J. Med. Genet., 6:67, 1969.
69. Lutz, K. R., and F. B. Moor: A study of factors in the occurrence of cleft palate. J. Speech Hear. Dis., 20:271, Sept., 1955.
70. MacMahon, B., and T. McKeown: The incidence of harelip and cleft palate related to birth rank and maternal age. Am. J. Hum. Gen., 5:176, 1953.
71. Mazaheri, M.: Statistical analysis of patients with congenital cleft lip and/or palate at the Lancaster Cleft Palate Clinic. Plast. Reconstr. Surg., 21(3):193, 1958.
72. McKusick, V. A.: Mendelian Inheritance in Man. 3rd Ed. Baltimore, Johns Hopkins Press, 1971.
73. Mellin, G. W., and M. Katzenstein. Meclizine and foetal abnormalities. Lancet, 1:222, 1963.
74. Meskin, L., and S. Pruzansky: Validity of the birth certificate in the epidemiological assessment of facial clefts. J. Dent. Res., 46:1456, 1967.
75. Meskin, L. H., and S. Pruzansky: A malformation profile of facial cleft patients and their siblings. Cleft Palate J., 6:309, July, 1969.
76. Meskin, L. H., S. Pruzansky, and W. H. Gullen: An epidemiological investigation of factors related to the extent of facial clefts. I. Sex of patient. Cleft Palate J., 5:23, Jan., 1968.
77. Metrakos, J., K. Metrakos, and H. Baxter: Clefts of the lip and palate in twins (including a discordant pair whose monozygosity was confirmed by skin transplant). Plast. Reconstr. Surg., 22:109, August, 1958.
78. Mitani, S.: Malformations of newborns. Sankato Fujinka, 11:345, 1943.
79. Morton, N. E., S. Yee, and R. Lew: Complex segregation analysis. Am. J. Hum. Genet., 23:602, 1971.
80. Myrianthopoulos, N. C., and C. S. Chung: Congenital malformations in singletons: Epidemiologic survey. Report from the Collaborative Perinatal Project, Stratton, Intercont. New York and London, Medical Book Corp., 1974.
81. Neel, J. V.: A study of major congenital defects in Japanese infants. Am. J. Hum. Genet., 10:398, 1958.
82. Nelson, M. M., H. V. Wright, C. W. Asling, and H. M. Evans: Multiple congenital abnormalities resulting from transitory deficiency of pteroylglutamic acid during gestation in the rat. J. Nutr., 56:349, 1955.

83. Nelson, M. M., H. V. Wright, C. D. C. Baird, and H. M. Evans: Effect of 36-hour period of pteroylglutamic acid deficiency on fetal development in rat. Proc. Soc. Exp. Biol. Med., 92:554, 1956.

84. Niswander, J. D., and Adams, M. S.: Oral clefts in the American Indians. Public Health Rep., 82(9):807, 1967.

85. Niswander, J. D., M. V. Barrow, and G. J. Bingle: Congenital malformations in the American Indians. Soc. Biol., 22(3):203, 1975.

86. Oka, S. W.: Oralfacial clefts in Pennsylvania, 1969–1972. Unpublished data, 1975.

87. Pallundan, B.: A-Avitaminosis in Swine. Copenhagen, Munksgaard, 1966.

88. Peer, L. A., H. Gordon, and W. Bernhard: Effects of vitamins on human teratology. Plast. Reconstr. Surg., 34:358, 1964.

89. Peer, L. A., L. P. Strean, J. C. Walker, W. G. Bernhard, and G. C. Peck: Study of 400 pregnancies with birth of cleft lip/palate infants. Plast. Reconstr. Surg., 22:442, 1958.

90. Rank, B. K., and J. A. Thomson: Cleft lip and palate in Tasmania. Med. J. Aust., 2:681, Oct., 1960.

91. Ross, R. B., and M. C. Johnston: Cleft Lip and Palate. Baltimore, The Williams and Wilkins Co., 1972.

92. Saxen, I.: Epidemiology of cleft lip and palate. An attempt to rule out chance correlations. Br. J. Prev. Soc. Med., 29(2):103, 1975.

93. Saxen, L., and J. Rapola: Congenital Defects. New York, Holt, Rinehart and Winston, Inc., 1969.

94. Smith, C.: Recurrence risk for multifactorial inheritance. Am. J. Hum. Gen., 23:578, 1971.

95. Spry, C. C., and M. A. Nugent: Some epidemiological aspects of clefts of the primary and secondary palate in South Australia, 1949–68. Aust. Dent. J., 20(4):250, 1975.

96. Stewart, R. E., and G. H. Prescott (eds.): Oral Facial Genetics. St. Louis, The C. V. Mosby Co., 1976.

97. Tal, Y., H. Dar, S. T. Winter, and G. Bar-Joseph: Frequency of cleft lip and palate in Northern Israel. Isr. J. Med. Sci., 10(5):515, 1974.

98. Tolarova, M., and N. E. Morton: Cleft lip and palate—recurrence risk and genetic counseling. Acta Univ. Carol., (Med. Monogr.) (Praha), 56:83, 1973.

99. Trasler, D. G., and F. C. Fraser: Role of the tongue in producing cleft palate in mice with spontaneous cleft lip. Develop. Biol., 6:45, 1963.

100. Tretsven, V. E.: Incidence of cleft lip and palate in Montana Indians. J. Speech Hear. Dis., 28:52, 1963.

101. Tünte, W.: Is there a secular increase in the incidence of cleft lip and cleft palate? Cleft Palate J., 6:430, Oct., 1969.

102. Van der Woude, A.: Fistula labii inferioris congenita and its association with cleft lip and palate. Am. J. Hum. Gen., 6:244, 1954.

103. Warkany, J.: Congenital Malformations. Chicago, Year Book Medical Publishers, Inc., 1971.

104. Warkany, J., R. C. Nelson, and E. Schraffenberger: Congenital malformations induced in rats by maternal nutritional deficiency. IV. Cleft palate. Am. J. Dis. Child., 65:882, 1943.

105. Wehrung, D. A., and S. Hay: A study of seasonal incidence of congenital malformations in the United States. Br. J. Prev. Soc. Med., 24:24, 1970.

106. Woolf, C. M.: Congenital cleft lip: A genetic study of 496 propositi. J. Med. Gen., 8:65, March, 1971.

107. Woolf, C. M. and J. A. Turner: Incidence of congenital malformations among live births in Salt Lake City, Utah, 1951–1961. Soc. Bio., 16:270, Dec., 1969.

108. Woolf, C. M., R. M. Woolf, and T. R. Broadbent: Genetic and nongenetic variables related to cleft lip and palate. Plast. Reconstr. Surg., 32:65, July, 1963.

109. Yerushalmy, J. and Melkovick, L.: The evaluation of the teratogenic effect of meclizine in man. Am. J. Obstet. Gynec., 93:553, 1965.

110. Zawoiski, E. J.: Prevention of caffeine-induced cleft palate by L-glutamic acid. Toxicol. Appl. Pharmacol., 35(1):123, 1976.

Suggested Readings

Burdette, W. J. (ed.): Methodology in Human Genetics. San Francisco, Holden Day Inc., 1962. (A collection of papers by leaders in their respective fields contributing to the understanding of the many diverse areas in human genetics. Not a treatise for beginners. It is especially informative concerning the extrapolation of genetic information from epidemiological data.)

McKusick, V. A., and R. Claiborne (eds.): Medical Genetics. New York, Hospital Practice Publishing Co., Inc., 1973. (A well illustrated work by prominent authors on genetic diseases encountered in medical practice. It graphically presents the current knowledge on the transmission of genetic defects. The chapter on Multifactorial Genetic Disease is enlightening.)

Mather, K., and J. L. Jinks: Biometrical Genetics. Ithaca, N.Y., Cornell University Press, 1971. (A compendium on the genetic analysis of continuous variation. Aimed primarily at geneticists, it is nevertheless a good source for understanding the development of the basic assumption underlying the methodology in the study of multifactorial inheritance.)

Nora, J. J., and F. C. Fraser: Medical Genetics: Principles and Practice. Philadelphia, Lea and Febiger, 1974. (An introductory volume covering basic genetic information applied to clinical problems. The multifactorial nature of cleft lip and palate is clearly presented.)

Reesman, L., and A. Matheny: Genetics and Counseling in Medical Practice. St. Louis, The C. V. Mosby Co., 1969. (A good introduction to genetic counseling for clinicians.)

Ross, R. B., and M. C. Johnston: Cleft Lip and Palate. Baltimore, The Williams and Wilkins Co., 1972. (A broad-based and general text that concisely integrates populational, experimental, and clinical data on human orofacial clefts.)

Saxen, L., and J. Rapola: Congenital Defects. New York, Holt, Rinehart and Winston, Inc., 1969. (A comprehensive and readable introduction on the etiology and pathogenesis of congenital defects. Experimental teratology of cleft lip and palate is well documented.)

Stevenson, A. C., B. C. C. Davison, and M. W. Oakes: Genetic Counseling. Philadelphia, J. B. Lippincott Co., 1970. (A helpful book on basic genetics applied to different genetic diseases. Derivation of risk estimates for monogenic traits is clearly presented.)

Stewart, R. E., and G. H. Prescott (eds.): Oral Facial Genetics. St. Louis, The C. V. Mosby Co., 1976. (A comprehensive accumulation of current knowledge from various authors on the genetic aspects of craniofacial maldevelopment.)

Warkany, J.: Congenital Malformation: Notes and Comments. Chicago, Year Book Medical Publishers, Inc., 1971. (A monumental compendium covering all known factors of congenital malformations. Historical aspects of teratology are thoroughly covered, as well as current trends. Malformations are presented by systems affected.)

Chapter Four _____

In the early 1930s H. K. Cooper, Sr., the founder of the Lancaster Cleft Palate Clinic, made what we regard as a landmark observation. He said, in effect, that the clinical care of the child with a cleft lip or palate must be in the hands of a *team* of specialists who will coordinate their diagnoses and treatment, as well as their interpretations of the child's status and progress with the passage of time. Rehabilitation is progressive, not static; each age-period has its unique problems of adjustment.

Dr. Cooper's observation is a recognition of the fact that if we are going to habilitate the whole child with a cleft, we must have a corps of specialists representing many segments of the biological and behavioral spectrum. In a very real sense, a congenital failure such as a cleft palate with or without a cleft lip is a traumatic insult not only to the structures and functions of the child's mouth, but to the entire psychosocial condition of the afflicted child and family.

The specialists involved must consciously function as a team, integrating efforts and viewpoints and working together in total harmony. The use of the word "team" connotes togetherness and orientation to a single goal, with the child and family as the focus. The word also carries the idea of a leader or central participant, for example, the pitcher in baseball or the quarterback in football. For a time the sports analogy holds true in a way for the cleft palate team, because in the first two years after the child's birth, the plastic surgeon is a central participant in his or her care. As Dr. Cooper emphasized in a preceding chapter, however, other members of the team should not be regarded as ancillary to the surgeon, but all should work as coequals in determining the best treatment programs for the patient.

We would like to expand the theme of teamwork by means of the organizational "flow-chart" presented as Table 4–1. This chart was developed on a smaller scale at the Philadelphia Center for Research in Child Growth, founded and directed from 1947 to 1971 by W. M. Krogman. At the Growth Center the central concern was the development of standards of physical growth for normal, healthy, Philadelphia children. The Growth Center staff was small, but it was represented by the disciplines of pediatrics, orthodontics, pedodontics, radiology, and anatomy and physical anthropology. The team, even though it was small, worked together for the developmental and clinical well-being of children classified in many different series: school, orthodontic, cleft palate, endocrinic, male and female, and white and Negro. There were two growth series, birth to seven years and six to 18 years, both followed longitudinally beginning at birth and six years, respectively.

Toward this end the Growth Center created a structural chart of in-

THE CLEFT PALATE TEAM IN ACTION

WILTON M. KROGMAN

terorganizational relationships. We present an expansion of this chart here.* In principle the Growth Center followed the theme of teamwork enunciated by Dr. Cooper many years earlier. It embraced relatively few disciplines in the study of the normal development of the child, but the Cooper Institute, as seen in our chart, embraces many disciplines in a cooperative endeavor. The result is the same: a total effort on behalf of the total child and family.

The team approach is a logical answer to the problem of the child and parents—indeed, it is the only one. Total habilitation of the child with a cleft is so complex that many different aspects must be brought into unison by as many different specialists. Not all team personnel, however, spring into action at the same time; there are, in practice, what may be termed functional subgroups (subteams) acting concertedly.

First of all, services must be provided in what may be termed a series of *developmental stages*, geared to the dynamics of change through time. There are changes owing to physical growth per se, and changes relating to reparative and restorative surgery and dentistry. There are those relating to the progressive unfolding of function, which are categorized under pediatrics, growth and development, speech, and hearing, and those relating to unfolding behavioral patterns, which are studied by psychology and sociology. Changes relating to progressive child and family interactions and to the child's self-concept as it encounters emergent maternal, paternal, sibling, and peer reactions are given consideration by social service. The habilitative pattern is an exquisite—and quite individual—combination of the physical and the behavioral. The cleft palate team must supply the loom upon which this pattern is designed and woven. For each child with a cleft, guidance and understanding must be based upon experience (clinical) and knowledge (research); *these two major themes are inextricably related to one another*. The phrase "clinical research" is one with deep and far-reaching connotations!

In recognition of the foregoing, our chart is based upon sequential change. We have set up eight major stages: prenatal, birth, birth to one year, one year to two years, two years to six years, six years to 12 years, 12 years to 18 years, and 18 years and over (adult). These stages are not arbitrary; nor are they always clear-cut. They are established for two major reasons: (1) they represent the dynamism of change in and of itself; and (2) they represent times at which special skills must be grouped to achieve maximum efficiency in the overall habilitative process. These eight stages are vertically oriented in our chart.

---

*A similar chart, though in less detail, was drawn up by Weatherley-White in 1968.[6]

145

Text continued on page 150

TABLE 4-1   The Team Approach

Age in Years	Obstetrics, Pediatrics	Plastic Surgery	Dentistry: Prosthodontics, Orthodontics	Genetics
Prenatal	Gestation and delivery. Maternal health history and examination upon delivery.	No role	No role	If family history is (FH+), secure pedigree. Counsel prospective parents.
Birth	Pediatrician examines infant; first awareness of cleft or other orofacial anomalies. First talk to parent may be by pediatrician or nurse; discussion should be coordinated with counseling by geneticist and social worker.	Examination of cleft type; appraisal of involvement of lip and palate. Advise parents of operative procedures, extent, and time. Surgeon and dental specialist work together and discuss tooth-arch-bone relationships. First evaluation of soft palate in terms of future competency (?).	No precise role, but acts as consultant to surgeon. Observe for anomalies associated with cleft. Dental specialist and surgeon work together and discuss tooth-arch-bone relationships.	Counsel parents regarding type and severity of cleft. With surgeon discuss prognosis as to repair, speech, appearance, etc. Work with social service worker and both discuss case with pediatrician, surgeon, and dental specialist. Cooperation with cytogeneticist if indicated (HMC).
B-1:0	Pediatrician is health advisor to child and mother; feeding problems discussed and dietary regime set up. Height and weight progress watched to advise regarding health risk in surgery. Feedback from mother made available to social worker.	Upon approval from pediatrician, surgeon operates on lip c. 0:3. Prescribes postoperative care. With dental specialist follows progress of palatal cleft. With growth and development specialist evaluates craniofacial growth pattern at birth (prenatal growth) and during first year.	With surgeon evaluate palate in terms of closure or prosthesis. Take photographs, arch casts, and x-ray head films at 0:3, 0:6, and 1:0. Work with growth progress and possible catch-up growth. Note teeth in crypts (deciduous and permanent). Record associated dental anomalies.	From pedigree geneticist evaluates risk probabilities; counsels in terms of reoccurrence risk. Works with social worker, family, and community.
1:0-2:0	Continues role as health and feeding advisor. Evaluation of improvement in feeding after palatal repair.	Evaluation of lip function and cosmesis and their relation to cleft and anterior deciduous teeth. Closure of palate in possible stages (hard at c. 1:2, soft at c. 1:6). Evaluation of VP competence in structure and function.	Work with surgeon on possible prosthetic aid. Work with growth researcher on arch growth in size, symmetry, and upper to lower arch relations; x-ray head films and casts at 1:0, 1:6, and 2:0. Watch eruption of deciduous teeth in this period.	Continue role as counselor.
2:0-6:0	Continues role in health and nutrition. Height and weight observation continued.	Follow-up care on cosmesis and function of lip. Soft palate studied to check if pharyngoplasty is later necessary. Speech specialist and surgeon work together.	Possible need for prosthesis and speech bulb; oral hygiene followed; crossbite situation checked. Arches studied for malocclusion. Child seen each year on birthday: casts, x-rays, etc. taken. Role of orthodontist considered here.	Family contacts maintained. If siblings are born, pedigree adapted; counseling as necessary.

TABLE 4–1 The Team Approach *(Continued)*

AGE IN YEARS	OBSTETRICS, PEDIATRICS	PLASTIC SURGERY	DENTISTRY: PROSTHODONTICS, ORTHODONTICS	GENETICS
6:0–12:0	Role continues as in 2:0–6:0. Prepubertal growth acceleration evaluated. H-W data continued.	Patient checked for need of secondary surgery of lip, palate, or nose. Cooperation with dental specialist, speech specialist, audiologist, and researcher in growth and development; latter works with orthodontist in tooth to arch relationships.	Role continues as in 2:0–6:0. Close association with orthodontist, speech specialist, surgeon, and growth researcher for timing of growth. Participates in Residency Program.	Role continues with consultation as necessary. Counseling directed more toward patient.
12:0– 18:0	Health care placed in hands of general practitioner.	Possible cosmetic (esthetic) follow-up for lip and nose, especially basic in adolescent self-concept.	Problems are basically orthodontic. If cleft is not closed surgically, must be follow-up with prostheses.	Counseling role moves on to premarital risk statements in late adolescence.
18:0 + (Adult)	Continuation of 12:0–18:0.	Doubtful if role of surgeon extends beyond 18:0.	Dental care in adult life mainly in hands of general practitioner.	Counseling role increases in adult marriage patterns.

AGE IN YEARS	OVERALL SUMMARY
Prenatal	History of gestation and maternal health; close supervision first trimester. If FH+, counseling of parents, especially by geneticist and social worker. This is time of great developmental speed. Cleft may or may not be part of syndrome involving many structures developing at time cleft occurs. Embryonic period (3 l.m.) = differentiation; fetal period (7 l.m.) = growth.
Birth	Pediatrician discusses cleft condition with parents, with cooperation of geneticist and social worker. Surgeon discusses cleft type and advises of operative procedures. Dental specialist appraises arch relationships, especially in bilateral cleft palates; checks for associated oro-dental anomalies. Growth researcher obtains data on prenatal history, including maternal health; confers with geneticist regarding family pedigree; evaluates degree adjacent structures (on time-linked basis) are involved in the dysplastic effects of the cleft.
B–1:0	Pediatrician advises on feeding (problem) and dietary regime; watches child's health and early development. Surgeon closes lip ("rule of 10") at c. 0:3. Dental specialist secures models, x-ray head films, and height and weight at 0:3, 0:6, and 1:0. Genetic pedigree secured, evaluated. Social worker counsels on family situation. Pediatrician, surgeon, dental specialist, geneticist, and social worker coordinate family counseling. Growth researcher evaluates craniofacial status at birth; follows growth progress first year. ENT specialist continues ear observations. Audiologist begins hearing tests via "noise" response at 0:6; gets family hearing history. Earliest speech = "babbling." Speech pathologist and surgeon discuss possible VP insufficiency and incompetence. Child progresses through several early stages of speech and language development in preparation for use of the first true words, which appear about first birthday.
1:0–2:0	Pediatrician continues role in health and nutrition. Surgeon evaluates effect of lip repair. Hard palate closed 1:2, soft palate 1:6, in conference with dental specialist. Speech pathologist evaluates VP structure and function; confers with dental specialist on possible prosthesis. Dentist and growth researcher work together on craniofacial arch relationship, etc., and follow growth pattern. Geneticist and social worker counsel as before. ENT watches ear condition. Audiologic hearing tests. Speech specialist, surgeon, and dentist work together in VP evaluation, and with growth researcher evaluate x-ray films of oropharyngeal development. Child's vocabulary goes from c. 10 to c. 270 words by 2:0.

Table continued on the following page

TABLE 4–1 The Team Approach (*Continued*)

SOCIAL SERVICE	GROWTH AND DEVELOPMENT	AUDIOLOGY	SPEECH: PATHOLOGY AND THERAPY
Participation in prenatal counseling.	Embryogenesis of orofacial defects	No role	No role
Secure complete family history in terms of total socioeconomic background and sociocultural milieu. Work with geneticist and both discuss case with pediatrician, surgeon, and dental specialist. Orientation of family to Institute's services, programs, policies.	Conference with surgeon and dental specialist to consider time-linked growth and development. From obstetrician and pediatrician get information on gestation history and delivery. From geneticist get data on family history. Evaluate child in terms of data on growth risk from files of geneticist.	Alert parents to overt signs of possible hearing loss (audiologist).	Counsel parents concerning possible speech problems (degree and extent). Advise how to guide beginning speech in terms of instilling proper habits (first visit).
Work with geneticist in counseling; they aid and substantiate one another. With surgeon's cooperation, counsel regarding prognosis.	Initial assessment at birth of degree to which orofacial anomaly has affected growth pattern. Work with serial x-ray records and dental casts; follow general growth via H/W. Use standards; get familial x-rays.	Complete otologic examination to rule out middle ear disease. Test hearing via sound field stimuli, first at 0:6; test same each time child has appointment. Counsel parents on possible hearing problems. Impedance tests begin at 0:6.	Earliest vocalization: "babbling." Analysis of socialization role of baby's "talk." Consult with surgeon on the functioning of the VP port mechanism during speech. Counsel parents regarding child's speech development. Observe child's vocalization.
Continue role as counselor. Study family attitudes toward problem of child with a cleft; also cleft child's attitude toward siblings and attitude of parents toward noncleft siblings.	Continue growth assessment 1:0, 1:6, and 2:0. Evaluate, if possible, postoperative growth and if surgery is a traumatic factor; continue height weight data. Note growth of bones and soft tissue of oropharynx.	Continue otoscopic observation and corrective measures when indicated. Continue testing hearing in terms of response level to sound field stimuli and assess middle ear function by impedance tests.	Continue counseling. Provide home (play) exercises, using sounds and words child can produce morphologically and maturationally. Consult with surgery, prosthodontics and growth on function of velopharyngeal port during speech.
Counseling continued. Study of preschool child for evaluation of attitude formation of child and family as patient begins school.	Continued study of height weight. In craniofacial growth, x-rays casts, etc., assessed for age changes. Growth trends evaluated and prognosis of "catch-up" growth given.	Patient checked regularly for ear pathology. Pure tone thresholds and middle ear function regularly assessed. Speech reception threshold and discrimination tests may be administered.	Formal testing of speech and language development on a regular and progressive basis. Consult with all disciplines in monitoring child's physical and social maturation. Speech therapy as needed. Special studies, e.g., cine speech studies, as necessary.

TABLE 4–1   The Team Approach *(Continued)*

SOCIAL SERVICE	GROWTH AND DEVELOPMENT	AUDIOLOGY	SPEECH: PATHOLOGY AND THERAPY
Changes in peer relationships in school situation are focus of study; impact of psychosocial change in patient upon family. Participates in Residency Program.	Study of craniofacial growth intensified with heightened velocity of circumpubertal "spurt." Close association with orthodontist and dental specialist. Study form and function of oropharyngeal soft tissue. Height and weight data continue.	Ears checked for pathology. Audiometric data collected on schedule. Work closely with speech. Teachers notified of hearing loss.	Continue longitudinal monitoring of speech and language development. Consult with all other specialties. Provide concentrated speech training in selected cases. Cine records as pertinent. Participate in Residency Program.
Focus on male/male, female/female, and male/female peer problems; counseling.	Craniofacial growth c. 90% complete at end of pubertal "spurt"; growth studies focus on possible relation to malocclusion.	Continued attention to aural health and hearing sensitivity.	Continuation of role in 6:0–12:0.
Follow-up studies in life situations on rehabilitation of adults with clefts that have been operated on.	Little or no further craniofacial growth. May be residual orthodontic follow-up care.	Periodic checks on hearing.	Continuation of role in 6:0–12:0.

AGE IN YEARS	OVERALL SUMMARY
2:0–6:0	Pediatrician's role is the same. Surgeon has follow-up role; works with speech pathologist on effect of surgery on VP function. Dental specialist notes oral segmental relations, with reference to crossbite and malocclusion (with orthodontist); casts and x-rays taken annually. Genetic role slight. Social worker notes preschool child's development of attitudes toward self and peer relations; continues role as counselor. Growth researcher follows craniofacial growth for progress in postoperative "catch-up" trend; growth pattern analyzed. ENT specialist continues services. Audiologist begins audiometric and impedance tests at 2:6; hearing evaluated in terms of cleft type. Speech data are recorded for articulation, voice quality, etc. Speech specialists, surgeon, dentist, and growth researcher work closely together. Period of rapid speech and language growth.
6:0–12:0	Pediatrician's role as in 2:0–6:0. Surgical follow-up for possible need of secondary repair of lip, palate, or nose. Residency Program begins: dentistry, speech, social work closely interrelated. Dental specialist and orthodontist teamed closely with growth researcher. Role of geneticist not significantly changed. Growth focuses on more rapid craniofacial growth of "prepubertal" acceleration. ENT specialist continues. Audiologist and speech specialist work together; progress in speech and hearing noted. Speech therapy as required. Cineradiography taken for oropharyngeal form and function. Speech matures to adult levels at 7–8 years. Grammar is refined and vocabulary expanded.
12:0–18:0	Surgical follow-up on lip and nose; focus on orthodontic care. Geneticist may give premarital counseling. Social worker begins intensive study of attitude development in adolescence and in child to parent relationship. Growth researcher works with dentistry, speech, orthodontics. ENT and audiology continue as in 6:0–12:0. Speech therapy and counseling as indicated.
18.0+ (Adult)	Health in hands of general practitioner. Surgical role moot. Dental care probably by general dentist. Geneticist and social worker counsel mostly in premarital and marital terms, mainly regarding risk and parent to child relationships. Hearing and speech as needed. Speech is mature; vocabulary continues to expand.

The chart then presents the specialties that are represented in the cleft palate team, either primarily or secondarily: obstetrics; pediatrics; plastic surgery; dentistry; orthodontics; genetics; social service; growth and development; otolaryngology and audiology; and speech. These specific services are horizontally oriented in our chart.

PRENATAL PERIOD AND BIRTH

In the prenatal period and at birth the obstetrician is reponsible for the maternal health and nutritional record, the circumstances of delivery, and the examination of the child at delivery, in which the pediatrician joins. During this time the plastic surgeon and the dentist are not specifically involved. If the family history, either maternal or paternal, is positive for clefts (FH+), the geneticist has a role: obtaining the family line pedigree, and as a genetic counselor discussing with the prospective parents the possibilities of a cleft occurring in the unborn child. If there is an FH+ history, then there should be feedback to the obstetrician, whose duty it will be to monitor the possibility of teratogenic factors in the first trimester. He is involved in a reciprocal relationship between obstetrician and geneticist. Counseling is not only genetic, for the social worker may complement the risk data provided by the geneticist by discussing with the parents-to-be the socioeconomic and psychosocial problems that may be encountered.

The prenatal period, comprising that of the embryo (the first three lunar months)* and that of the fetus (the last seven lunar months), is of great potential importance to the surgeon, the dentist, and the researcher in growth and development. At birth the type and the extent of the cleft must be analyzed in terms of how greatly it has insulted — inhibited or deviated — normal nasal, labial, oral, or pharyngeal embryogenesis. In other words, the growth researcher must evaluate just how and where the cleft has disturbed the normal craniofacial pattern. At this stage the concern is largely one of structural disturbance of both hard (skeletal) and soft tissues. The embryogenic (congenital) failure will give the researcher in growth a picture of the extent of the cleft and its possible repercussions upon future structural and functional changes in growth. The total situation has a sort of "as the twig is bent so is the tree inclined" potential. The otolaryngologist, audiologist, and speech therapist are not actively involved in the prenatal period.

The presence of a cleft is revealed at birth. Here the pediatrician's role begins, for it is usually his initial examination that reveals the orofacial anomaly (a cleft lip is at first obvious, a cleft palate may not be). Most frequently it is the pediatrician who breaks the news of the cleft to the mother; sometimes it is a nurse. Whatever the circumstances, this is the time for unified counseling by the pediatrician, geneticist, and social service worker: they are a biobehavioral subgroup of the total cleft palate team. This observation is a recognition of the fact that the pediatrician is in contact far more

---

*The human gestation period lasts for 10 lunar months (l.m.) of 28 days each for a total of 280 days; this is roughly nine calendar months.

frequently with the mother than is any other team member. There is another factor to consider here: the pediatrician carries the prestige of health care and will be listened to most closely by the mother, thus becoming an effective spokesman for the subgroup filling the counseling role.

At birth the plastic surgeon and dental specialist unite in appraisal, evaluation, planning, and prognosis. At this time they constitute a powerful clinical subgroup in terms of the morphological and functional implications of the cleft. The surgeon has a major counseling role in discussing what can be done and what must be done to repair the congenital defect. The assurance of favorable prognosis by the surgeon is the most vital, the most comforting counseling that the parents may receive. Surgeon, geneticist, and social service worker reinforce one another here, in the same manner as do pediatrician, geneticist, and social service worker. At this time the surgeon and dental specialist also come together to survey the bone, dental arch, and tooth involvement in terms of the entire dentofacial structure.

A cleft lip and a cleft palate—most notably the latter—are basically problems of dentofacial (maxillofacial) tissue and bony adjustments. Involved is a deep-seated disturbance of midfacial form and function, a disturbance so fundamental that it is almost automatically a matter of orthodontic concern. This may seem to be involving orthodontics a bit too early in the life of the child, but it is really a recognition that every severe congenital failure in the palate carries with it the genesis of a malalignment of tooth and bone, leading to a malocclusion.

Geneticist and social service worker extend the rapport they have earlier established between themselves and the affected family. In the special instance in which a craniofacial syndrome may be involved, the geneticist may call for karyotyping to be performed by the Hershey (PA) Medical Center, of which the Institute is an affiliate. The social service worker now has three major contributions: (1) securing the total socioeconomic background of the child's family, advising of estimated costs, and telling of possible state, federal, and insurance aids; (2) informing the parents of the child enrolled at the Institute of the complete range of services available here and the nature and intent of each of the services; and (3) explaining that if the child is enrolled in our Research Series, these services will be continuing at a semiannual rate until two years of age and annually thereafter.*

At birth research in growth and development has its real beginning. Surgical, dental, genetic, and pediatric data are made available to the researcher as a background for each patient, including information for case histories, classifications of details of the cleft and of the palatal arch and dental arch relationships, lateral and posteroanterior x-ray head films, and dental models. Based upon these birth data the growth researcher makes his first appraisal: (1) What are the structural interrelationships of the skeletal elements involved? (2) What is the extent to which the skeletal craniofacial pattern is affected, i.e., deviated, inhibited, or distorted? and (3) How do the lateral and posteroanterior x-ray head film tracings relate to non-cleft (normal) lateral and posteroanterior x-ray head film standards? In sum, what is the craniofacial construct at birth, and what degree of skeletal harmony is to be

---

*Frequency may be greater than semiannual and annual in individual cases, depending upon clinical needs.

achieved? At birth the growth researcher evaluates status and may advance an opinion as to the correction of that status and the direction of restorative change. For example, a malrelationship between the upper and lower jaws may be noted. The lower jaw may be absolutely or relatively retruded compared with the upper jaw, and this condition, if it continues during growth, may lead to a Class II, Division 1 malocclusion (lower teeth back relative to the upper). As previously noted, birth is very early to anticipate this sort of orthodontic problem, yet if the degree of the malrelationship is severe enough, there may be reason at this point to warn of incipient (and later) occlusal complications.

Some time after birth (or during the first year) the otolaryngologist may examine the child with a cleft palate for the possibility of fluid in the middle ear. At the time of surgery to close the cleft lip, the otolaryngologist may perform a myringotomy.

BIRTH TO ONE YEAR

The first year is one of the most important years of the entire course of postnatal growth. Apart from the initial adjustment to the traumatic circumstances of "living on its own," the child will experience a terrific velocity in growth that it will never again know. For example, weight at birth will increase 200 per cent in this year, and length at birth 50 per cent. Most of the craniofacial dimensions will share in the latter percentage increase, though they will do so differentially, i.e., some will grow faster than others. Most important, it is in this first year that the child with a cleft must develop integrative patterns of function, especially eating and breathing, the two functions directly involving the nasal and oropharyngeal cavities.

During the first year the role of the pediatrician will be an important one, especially if there are feeding problems. A feeding procedure will be set up involving, if necessary, the sheer mechanics of getting food down the throat, i.e., the possibility of slow manual feeding, the use of special nipples on formula bottles, and other methods. An intake formula, balanced in amount and calorie and vitamin content, will be worked out. The pediatrician will, of course, work in concert with the surgeon, the otolaryngologist, and the dentist. There is another realm of cooperative endeavor: in this first year the mother will impart to the pediatrician her anxieties, her fears, her frustrations, and even her feelings of inadequacy. The pediatrician, if not too pressed for time to establish a relatively complete rapport with the mother, must certainly utilize the skills and advice of the social service worker. The medical-behavioral duo can do much to affirm one another's understanding of the mother-child problems, the one mediating health problems, the other incipient behavioral problems.

When the "rule of ten"* has been acceptably observed (at about three months), the pediatrician will give the go-ahead to the plastic surgeon for lip repair. It goes without saying that the plastic surgeon, before and after lip

---

*Ten pounds weight, 10 g. hemoglobin, white blood count not over 10,000 per cu. mm.

surgery, will relate to parent and to pediatrician with reassuring counsel. The cleft lip, an external manifestation of a birth defect, will arouse parental concern in terms of later cosmetic appearance, particularly if the child is a girl. "Will it show?" is the concern of the parent. "Can I restore good function?" is the concern of the surgeon. Form (appearance) and function (effective repair) thus become joint concerns of clinician and parent. In a longer view, adequately established lip function may play an important role in facilitating the processes of palatal union by narrowing the palatal cleft if lip and palate are both cleft. Mazaheri, Harding and Nanda have shown that lip repair may be a factor in reducing the width of the palatal cleft before palatal surgery.[1] Apparently, lip closure sets in motion a series of functional reactions that leads to a (compressive?) medialward movement of the palatal shelves.

Concurrently, the dental specialist is very much in the picture and with the surgeon appraises the relationships of the palatal complex (premaxilla, maxilla, nasal septum). The relationship of the premaxilla and maxilla must involve considerations of both mesiodistal and mediolateral alignment of palatal segments and dental arch configuration. The dental specialist in this first year initiates the basic morphological research that will longitudinally follow the clinical and developmental progress of the child with a cleft. Certain data, both clinical and morphological, will be gathered: (1) bilateral (right, left) segmental relationships will be assessed via a Panorex x-ray film; (2) a face mask will be secured at three months; (3) dental models will be done at three and six months and at one year; (4) roentgenographic cephalometry will be done, also at three and six months and at one year (lateral and posteroanterior oriented x-ray head films); and (5) dental histories will be secured and may be compared with, or related to, medical histories. The dental history will include dental anomalies (if they exist) associated with the cleft. Developing teeth, deciduous and permanent, are observed in their crypts, and possible eruptive complications (spatial and occlusal) may be anticipated.

During the first year the specialists in speech and hearing also have an important role in counseling. During the patient's first visit the parents should be advised of the type (and degree, if possible) of communication problems that may develop as a result of a VPI involvement and an accompanying loss in hearing sensitivity (either fairly constant or fluctuant). At this time the speech pathologist may give the parents instruction and material for verbal-play games designed to stimulate correct labio-oral movements during the patient's early speech attempts. The audiologist should advise and alert parents to possible signs of middle ear problems, e.g., fluid stains on the pillow or pulling and scratching of the ears. Furthermore, over the next several years parental alertness to signals of hearing loss should be emphasized, i.e., inattention to normal sounds and conversation-level speech, frequent quizzical looks suggesting incomplete comprehension, and, after speech has begun, frequent requests to repeat a statement, a question, or an admonition.

In this first year the counseling of the geneticist and social service worker must be done at maximum efficiency, geared to the degree of parental need and concern. It is at this time that the parent poses the big questions: "Why?" "Who?" "Will it happen again?" The first two queries may reflect a sense of guilt and recrimination ("it never happened in *my* family before!"). In such circumstances, the social service worker must virtually serve as a marriage counselor, ameliorating possible tensions between husband and wife. If there are siblings (usually unaffected), advice as to how to handle the child with a cleft with respect to them must be shared in order that overprotection or rejection can be avoided. The social service worker must also deal with a family situation in which the socioeconomic facts of life have suddenly become very real; the total medical and dental care of the infant with a cleft imposes a strain upon the average income. The parents may need financial aid, which can be derived from various agencies and other sources. Fees for pediatric care, surgery, dental care, and other services are explained as they are scheduled; methods and times of payment are also explained and established (see chapter on the social worker).

The geneticist continues in the first year the data gathering that began at birth or shortly thereafter. During this time, initially gathered family histories (pedigrees) are completed and carefully appraised. Questions centering on the likelihood of reoccurrence can be answered and assurance given. Genetic interpretation is thus linked with social service in a buttressing of family morale.

By the end of the first year, the combined efforts and advice of pediatrician, plastic surgeon, dental specialist, geneticist, and social service worker will have led the family to understanding, hope, and, most of all, have given confidence in the habilitative process.

Also within this first year the child has developed his or her first true word. Communication has developed through the stages of reflexive crying, babbling, and jargon, all in preparation for use of the first true words. The speech pathologist is able to counsel the parents regarding the type of speech problems that the child may present as a result of the nature of the cleft. Instruction of the parents of a child with a cleft palate as to sounds and words that the child will be physiologically capable of producing prior to closure of the palate will also be provided. Conferences with the parents and observations of the child's vocalizations enable the speech pathologist to advise the surgeon as to the functioning of the velopharyngeal valve during speech.

The data made available by surgeon and dental specialist are the basic materials of the growth researchers; here, the clinician (medical, dental) and basic scientist (growth researcher) join forces. The growth researcher has determined the degree to which the defect has affected the total craniofacial complex and is confronted with the fact that status gives way to motion, to the dynamic movement of differential increments of growth in the bones and tissues of the head, face, and jaws. Via the serial data collected by the prosthodontist, the growth researcher becomes the referee of the unfolding pattern of growth of the child with a cleft. A number of questions are now asked: Is differential growth affirming or modifying the pattern evaluated at birth? Is the modifying factor worsening or improving the birth condition, i.e., if there is a basic asymmetry of palatal segments, is it being intensified, or is there a compensatory, adjustive "catch-up" toward a more normal faciodental complex?

Questions such as the foregoing are answered—at least in part—by the use of roentgenographic cephalometric standards. At Lancaster we use two such standards (both concern craniofacial growth and development of healthy, non-cleft, American white children): the Broadbent-Bolton Standards of Cleveland, Ohio, and the Krogman Standards of Philadelphia, Pennsylvania.*

In recent years the growth researcher and geneticist have joined in the analysis of a possible familial patterning in craniofacial structure. The question posed is this: Can we discern in the x-ray head films of the parents of a child with a cleft certain morphological traits or trait complexes that foreshadow a tendency to clefting? Consider the following: (1) an experimental group of the mother and father of a child with a cleft; (2) a control group of the mother and father of a child without a cleft. Lateral x-ray head films are secured for groups 1 and 2 and, ideally, for all siblings in each family. In group 1 we will have data on mother, father, and all children. Analysis of data will be oriented to degrees of family and child resemblance in each group: Do parents in group 1 differ significantly from parents in group 2 in craniofacial details (form, size, proportion), and, if so, is the difference such that the parents of group 1 are similar in overall craniofacial "pattern" to an individual with a cleft? The problem can be put (in perhaps oversimplified terms) in the question: Do parents of children with a cleft look as if they have an incipient— but unrealized—cleft faciodental construct, and do parents of children without clefts in faces and jaws look like "normal" non-cleft adults? There is another aspect of the problem: If we accept an overall familial pattern of growth in head and face, is such a familial pattern closer (in group 1) to the child with a cleft than to the siblings without clefts? (These and other group questions are discussed in the chapter on genetics.)

In the first year the otologist and audiologist work closely with each other and with the speech pathologist. Obviously, the otologist continues the clinical care begun early, but observation is also made into the realm of function (hearing), in which the otologist joins hands with the audiologist, who begins testing hearing via sound field stimuli at six months of age. This, in addition to various impedance measures, represents the beginning of serial observation (age-related changes) on hearing.

The audiologist, working with the geneticist, may gather a family history of hearing problems to check upon the possibility of a familial tendency toward conductive hearing loss. Additionally, the audiologist may gather data on the hearing of parents and non-cleft siblings. Counseling of the parent may be initiated in the case of a child who does not "pay attention" because of faulty hearing. Discussion with the parents as to the possible hearing loss of the child with a cleft will aid greatly in parent and child relationships in terms of parental awareness.

The speech pathologist now enters the picture and works with the surgeon, dental specialist, and audiologist. The surgeon and the speech pathologist join in the first appraisal of the soft tissue structures of the mouth and pharynx. The focus will be upon problems of relative velar insufficiency and competence. The surgeon may predict how palatal repair may affect velar function (closure) and, hence, speech. The dental specialist, looking at

---

*The Cleveland Standards are available in both lateral and facial views, the Philadelphia Standards in the lateral view only.

dental models of the palate, may indicate how surgical closure may affect palatal segments, the dental arch, and possibly occlusion, all of which may later be factors in the relationships between the teeth, pharynx, and tongue that affect articulation.

In the early part of the first year, speech, per se, is not a basic factor, but vocalization expressed in babbling may play a socializing role in the mother and child relationship. The importance of the situation at this time is not so much in the sounds as such, but rather in how the mother may give them meaning and react to them. These psychosocial data are of interest to the social service worker in providing maternal counseling.

ONE TO TWO YEARS

In the second year a major event in the postnatal life of the child with a cleft occurs: surgical repair of the palate. The pediatrician will continue to monitor the feeding and health care of the child with a cleft. It is quite likely that much of his function as a counselor will be transferred to the plastic surgeon, who in this year occupies the center of the stage. Effectiveness of lip closure in terms of form (appearance) and function (tissue) can be appraised. The evaluation of the amount of scar tissue in the lip is important: if the amount is excessive, then the lip may act as a constricting band (literally an orthodontic appliance), inclining the upper anterior teeth in a lingual direction and thus providing for a potential anterior crossbite and a retrusive midface. Also, as has been noted, lip closure may have a reciprocal effect on the narrowing of the width of the palatal cleft.

Surgical closure of a cleft of soft and hard palates may proceed in two stages: hard palate at about 14 to 16 months, and soft palate at about 18 to 20 months. If there is nasal involvement, either septal or alar, repair will await further growth at a later age.

The surgeon, dental specialist, growth researcher, and speech pathologist all have a role in this second year. The dental specialist and the surgeon must confer on the possibility of a prosthetic aid in the event that the palatal cleft is so wide or so horseshoe-shaped that surgical repair is contraindicated and an obturator is necessary—in other words, closure is not surgical, but dental. Surgeon and dentist in this year may provide a firm evaluation as to velar sufficiency, i.e., in terms of absolute and relative velar length, and can so advise the speech pathologist accordingly.

The geneticist and social service worker, especially the latter, continue counseling. The patterns of interaction between the family and cleft child, family and non-cleft siblings, and cleft child and non-cleft siblings all begin to form definitive shapes, so that psychosocial counseling takes on a directive and orienting nature in the sense that efforts are made to maximize intrafamily harmony and adjustment.

The growth researcher, utilizing the data and interpretations of the surgeon and dentist, is now moving into a very strategic position. By the age of two years, with growth data collected at six months, one year, 18 months, and two years, there are four endpoints of progressive age-related changes that indicate a *growth trend* in terms of amount, speed, and direction. At this age an initial approximation may be made as to the effect on growth of the trauma of surgery. Has there occurred inhibited growth or a redirected growth of either a compensatory and adjustive or a deviant nature? At this age answers will, of course, not be definitive, but they can be evaluative in the sense of a possible positive (ameliorative) or negative (discrepant) result.

The otolaryngologist and audiologist continue and amplify the roles they established in the first year. The relation between possible ear pathology and hearing loss becomes a matter of increased joint concern. Additionally, clinical ear problems relate to speech in terms of hearing and speech integration; to learn to speak clearly, the child must hear clearly. In effect, inadequacy in the area of hearing may lead to inadequacy in speech and language.

By two years of age a normal child uses approximately 272 words and sentences that are on the average about two words in length. The mechanisms of speech can be evaluated in terms of what surgery, dentistry, and growth and development have to offer. Surgeon and dental specialist can tell the speech researcher about velopharyngeal conditions, and the growth researcher can advise in terms of the gross morphology of skeletal and tissue structures at two years. If clinically indicated, cineradiography may elucidate oropharyngeal function in terms of deglutition (phonation comes later).

We feel that by the age of two years, the framework for biological and behavioral habilitation is pretty well established. A total pattern is discernible in the child; we have a fair idea of what he or she can be expected to achieve and what can be done to facilitate that achievement. The child has grown enough and, in a sense, is "mature" enough to be malleable, moldable, and receptive to various kinds of remedial therapy leading to better all-around adjustment.

TWO TO SIX YEARS

With this in mind, the next stage, two to six years, is one of extension and amplification of the two-year stage. It is the period of early childhood and a fairly rapid but consolidative period of growth. As far as the face and jaws are concerned, it is the time of completion of the eruption of the deciduous dentition and the threshold of the replacement by the permanent dentition. Psychosocially, however, this is a very important period of development for the child with a cleft; it is the time of entrance to kindergarten and school, the time of a "brave new world" of peer reaction in a greatly extended social realm, and the time of psychosocial "weaning" as the child with a cleft leaves but does not lose the home environment for the outside world of contact with others.

The pediatrician continues to support the child and family in an essentially medical (health) capacity. We feel that it is still important that the general growth of the child with a cleft—at least in height and weight—be watched and evaluated. By the age of six years, with a background of height and weight data in the maternal and paternal lines, we can assess the potential of "short," "average," or "tall" stature, and the potential of "slender," "average," or "stocky" body build.

In the period from two to six years, the role of the surgeon is mainly one of support and follow-up care. Lip repair can be judged cosmetically and functionally. Palate repair must be looked at basically in terms of soft tissue function. The surgeon and speech pathologist confer as to the possible need for a velar lengthening operation to achieve successful velopharyngeal closure.

The dental specialist works with the surgeon in this period, as well as with the speech pathologist. Again, the problem of a prosthesis may arise, and a speech bulb may be indicated. Care must be devoted to problems of oral hygiene, circumstances of tooth eruption, development of crossbites, and the possibility of occlusal malrelationships owing to palatal segmental asymmetry or malplacement. In this period the incipience of an orthodontic problem may be envisioned.

The primary role of the geneticist as counselor has been well realized by the age of six years. By this age in the child with a cleft, the parental decision as to having another child has been made, one way or the other.

Now the social service worker takes a very active habilitative role. At Lancaster we have a program directed toward the preschool child. The focus is largely on the genesis of attitudes of the child with a cleft to self, family, and peers. We know from Peter's studies[2, 3, 4, 5] that adult individuals with a cleft differ significantly from those without a cleft in certain psychological, social, and economic respects.* The problem at issue is when and how these differences arose. We feel that the preschool period and the first introduction to school may hold partial answers. This is the first major exposure of the child with a cleft to the possible realization that he or she is "different" in appearance (lip, nose) and different in behavior (clarity of speech, nasality).

Growth research is a carry-over from the two-year stage. All serial data (dental models, x-ray head films) unite in the interpretation of unfolding craniofacial growth. Our research has demonstrated postoperative catch-up growth by the age of six that has taken the faciodental complex to within the lower end of a normal range of variation, as compared with control non-cleft faces. By the age of six the anterior moiety of the dental arches, upper and lower, is finished growing (as measured in front of a line tangent to the posterior margin of the first permanent molars).

The otolaryngologist continues clinical surveillance and evaluation and may initiate medical and surgical procedures. The audiologist now moves full-swing into research, since the child has reached an age when more objective tests may be administered; serial tests of pure tone air and bone conduction begin regularly at two years, six months. Thresholds of air and bone conduction are analyzed in terms of cleft type, ear pathology, and postoperative recovery. Testing of impedance is now initiated at two months. Hearing sensitivity is reported to all disciplines, and speech evaluation programs are set up accordingly.

The child makes the largest gains in speech and language development during this period. This development is monitored by the speech pathologist through the use of formal speech and language tests and tape recordings at regular intervals. The functioning of the velopharyngeal port during speech is closely monitored by the speech pathologist. Cineradiographic studies of the oral speech mechanism, specifically the velopharyngeal port, are secured when deemed necessary by the surgeon, prosthodontist, and speech pathol-

---

*Studies were based on patients who had been treated at the Lancaster Cleft Palate Clinic.

ogist. The films are then analyzed by the speech specialist for oral function and by the growth specialist for oral morphology. As delays in speech development are identified and the causes determined, the team institutes management procedures. These include surgery, prosthodontia, and speech therapy.

SIX TO 12 YEARS

By the age of six years the child with a cleft is launched into the world of peers that will judge him or her. Biologically this child has achieved about 75 per cent of the physical growth and 60 per cent of the maturational progress destined to be completed in the two decades of postnatal growth allotted to everyone. From the ages of six to 12, the child is in a relatively quiescent period of growth.

Mention has been made of the residency program that will begin in the period of six to 12 years. The program will be discussed in greater detail in the chapter on speech, but we feel it merits mention here, too. The program is one of intensive remedial care of a basically dental, speech, and psychosocial nature. The children, organized on the basis of age (early school, later school, adolescence), live in a dormitory and share a common organized experience of speech therapy, dental care, and general socialization. It is good for each child to learn that his or her "problems" are not unique, and that others find a need for adjustive behavior. Moreover, since the classes are small in size, each child is the recipient of speech correction almost individualized for his benefit. Over the years this program, originated in Lancaster, has proved itself, for many of its alumni have gone on to well-adjusted, productive lives. Our preschool study will give us better insight into the handling of the program.

At the time the child reaches the age of 12, there is little or no change in the role of the pediatrician. The surgeon is more or less on a stand-by basis, and if additional surgical repair is needed on nose or lip, achieved growth is such that correction will not be embarrassed by additional growth. In some cases remedial palatal surgery may be undertaken at this age. The dental specialist works increasingly closer with the orthodontist in those cases in which occlusal problems present themselves.

By this age the individual child with a cleft may also be the recipient of genetic counseling, in terms of explaining to him or her the nature of the cleft situation and its probable relation to an inherited predisposition in family lines on the mother's or the father's side.

At twelve years the child is just about ready to move on to the circumpubertal carousel, with its bewilderingly rapid series of structural, functional, and behavioral metamorphoses. More importantly, the grouping of peers is redefined: no longer boy-boy, girl-girl, but boy-girl. The social service worker takes a special interest in the adolescent, once more extending insight into the genesis of self-role concepts. The total impact of the new social structure upon the child and family becomes the focus of intense investigative concern.

Biologically, this is the time of the deciduous to permanent transition in the dentition. Lack of synchrony at this time in dentofacial growth in breadth, height, and depth may lead to transitory "ugly duckling" stages. Hence, the growth researcher, dental specialist, and orthodontist will join hands in the appraisal of normative versus deviant growth in the face, jaws, and teeth.

Otolaryngology and audiology maintain their roles, both clinically and in research. The audiologist again conveys to the school system (the teacher), as he or she did in the early school years, information on those children with clefts who have a hearing loss and should be understood and worked with in this light.

The speech pathologist continues monitoring speech and language development, and speech therapy is recommended as needed. When progress is slow, psychosocial counseling is offered through social service. Special studies, such as cineradiographic speech analyses, are reserved for cases in which observation of the velopharyngeal port is necessary. Concentrated speech therapy is available at the Institute for patients, cleft and non-cleft, who do not have a speech therapy service readily available in their communities.

TWELVE TO 18 YEARS AND ADULTHOOD

At 12 years the child enters into the full blossoming of the complex of age-related changes; biologically, the girl becomes a woman, the boy a man. The period from 12 to 18 years takes the child through adolescence to the threshold of adulthood. At this time the surgeon may have some follow-up correction (usually cosmetic). Dentistry gives way mainly to orthodontic care, with, however, a follow-up by the dental specialist in individual cases.

The geneticist may play a role in late adolescence as the individual with a cleft gives voice to his or her concern over the possibility of genetic (hereditary) transmission of the cleft lip or palate. By 18 years, marriage and a family are in mind and there is logically a need to answer the question, "Will a child of mine face the same problems that I did?" Here the geneticist and social service worker advise together as the behavioral study of the adolescent continues toward its objectives.

Faciodental growth is in its terminal phases: rapid before puberty, slow and approaching adult values after puberty. Here the growth specialist and orthodontist team up. The hearing and speech specialists continue their roles and consult with one another and with the child with a cleft.

The final stage, 18 years and over, is almost anticlimactic. Pediatrician, surgeon, and dental specialist have essentially secondary roles. Medical and dental care are almost always in the hands of the general practitioner. Genetic counseling has now gone full cycle, i.e., the counseling passes on from parent to prospective parent, and the pedigree could well be activated by yet another generation. The counseling of the social service worker may take on a dual role: aiding the adult with a cleft to cope with adjustive problems at the adult level, and counseling him or her regarding possible problems in marrying and starting a family.

The team has done its habilitative job: a generation has been aided and counseled. That aid and counseling must inevitably influence and, hopefully, guide the next generation. The team thus takes its rightful and useful place in the human generational chain of command.

References

1. Mazaheri, M., R. L. Harding, and S. Nanda: The effect of surgery on maxillary growth and cleft width. Plast. Reconstr. Surg., *40*:22, 1967.
2. Peter, J. P., and R. R. Chinsky: Sociological aspects of cleft palate adults: I. Marriage. Cleft Palate J., *11*:295, 1974.
3. Peter, J. P., and R. R. Chinsky: Sociological aspects of cleft palate adults: II. Education. Cleft Palate J., *11*:443, 1974.
4. Peter, J. P., R. R. Chinsky, and M. J. Fisher: Sociological aspects of cleft palate adults: III. Vocational and economic aspects. Cleft Palate J., *12*:193, 1975.
5. Peter, J. P., R. R. Chinsky, and M. J. Fisher: Sociological aspects of cleft palate adults: IV. Social integration. Cleft Palate J., *12*:304, 1975.
6. Weatherley-White, R. C.: The operation of a cleft palate clinic. *In* Stark, R. B. (ed.): Cleft Palate: A-Multi-Discipline Approach, New York, Harper & Row, pp. 70–83, 1968.

Chapter Five

INTRODUCTION

Change is a continuum, and to select a specific year to mark an advance in medicine is somewhat arbitrary. But several events clustered around the beginning of the fifth decade of the twentieth century permit one to suggest that the present era of cleft lip and palate rehabilitation began about the year 1940. Prior to that time medicine had devoted much of its attention to the infectious and nutritional diseases. Then in 1940 Warkany and his associates in Cincinnati reported that they had induced cleft palate in the offspring of laboratory rats that had been fed a diet deficient in riboflavin during pregnancy. In the following year Gregg, an Australian ophthalmologist, reported the finding of congenital cataracts, deafness, cardiac defects, and mental retardation (in various combinations) among infants born to women who had contracted rubella during an epidemic in 1940.

These two discoveries, made on opposite sides of the globe, and subsequent related research created considerable excitement because there was now evidence that congenital malformations could result not only from hereditary factors but from environmental insults as well. The concept evolved that many facial clefts might be caused by teratogenic agents acting upon a labile constitution, and thoughts turned to the possibility of preventing certain congenital defects.

It was in 1940, too, that penicillin, which had been discovered by Alexander Fleming in 1928, was shown to be clinically effective against pathogenic bacteria. The dawning of the antibiotic age soon brought many of the more serious infectious diseases under control, and it then became obvious that many could be cured. At about that same time came the tremendous development in the preservation and "banking" of human blood and the use of blood substitutes.

The historic events just mentioned had far reaching effects upon medicine in general and made possible improvements in the care of cleft lip and palate patients. Although the prevention of congenital disorders would not become a reality for another 30 years, with the adoption of genetic counseling on a wide scale, another innovation beginning shortly before 1940 was of great importance to patients with a facial cleft. This was the advent of the interdisciplinary team dedicated to the total care of patients with cleft lip and/or palate. Persons from different disciplines, working in concert with mutual respect and restraint, began to exert a profound influence upon the management of these patients. Since 1940, many interdisciplinary groups have been organized throughout the United States, and the inter-

ROBERT L. HARDING

related disciplines and groups have joined together in a national organization, the American Cleft Palate Association. More recently, an International Congress on Cleft Palate has been formed.

Among the developments of great importance to the advancement of surgery, including operations for cleft lip and palate, was endotracheal anesthesia, which although suggested in the early 1900s was not employed until years later. The Magill endotracheal tube, introduced by Sir Ivan Magill in 1937, was just gaining acceptance in 1940. It permitted better control of the patient during surgery and enabled the surgeon to work with greater ease. Another forward step was board specialization and its accompanying certification for physicians. This began with the American Board of Ophthalmology in 1917, increased to 14 boards by 1940, and was given considerable impetus by World War II. Medical progress is dynamic and, as we have said, it is undergoing continual change. But the historic events during and around the year 1940 had a profound effect on surgery, and hence we feel that probably that year should be considered the beginning of the present era of cleft lip and palate rehabilitation.

_____ THE CLEFT LIP

Since 1940, several surgical innovations in cleft lip repair have caused surgeons to become more critical of their own results. During the early 1940s, the Blair-Brown modification[8] of the Mirault operation[53] was still quite popular. In this operation, a small triangular flap of tissue was transferred from the base of the lateral side of the cleft to fill a defect in the medial side of the lip. In addition to Mirault, Blair and Brown, Jalaguier, Hagedorn,[26] Koenig,[31] and a few others endorsed the concept of transposing a flap of tissue from one side of a cleft to the other. In 1950, Brown and McDowell[11] reported on their experience with a modification of the Blair-Brown procedure in which a small lateral triangular flap was transferred into the medial side of the base of the cleft.

In 1946, LeMesurier conducted a one-day clinic in Toronto at which time he presented his results of ten years' experience with a modification of the Hagedorn quadrilateral flap lip repair. Then in 1949 he published his results in the *Journal of Plastic and Reconstructive Surgery*, in which he gave full credit to Hagedorn for the quadrilateral flap design.[37] W. H. Steffensen, who had been present at the Toronto meeting, also published his results with the quadrilateral flap procedure in 1949.[74] He demonstrated the application of this flap design to all cleft lip repairs. In this operation, one-half of the cupid's bow is destroyed and a new half is constructed on the lateral side of the cleft. As surgeons came to appreciate the advantage of the quadrilateral flap procedure, emphasized by LeMesurier and Steffensen, the popularity of the straight-line repairs of the Rose-Thompson type diminished, except for repairs of the minimal cleft. But when many of the lips repaired by the quadrilateral flap method later elongated on the operated side, this procedure gave way to still newer and improved operative designs.

One of these was the triangular flap method for cleft lip closure published by Tennison in 1952.[78] It was referred to as the stencil method because he used a bent wire as a stencil in laying out the operative pattern. This simplified maneuver, in which a triangular flap was transferred from the lateral side of the base of the cleft into a defect on the medial side, gained wide acceptance among surgeons. Marcks, Trevaskis, and DaCosta adopted the method, clarified the technique, and discarded the stencil for calipers. Other surgeons, including Hagerty, Cronin, and Brauer, recommended modifications, and then in 1959 Randall published his modification and described the operation in clear mathematical detail.[61]

Millard presented his rotation-advancement operation in 1955[46] and has continually revised the initial plan since that time. In his approach, the medial side of the repair is rotated downward from beneath the columella to its normal horizontal level, and the defect is corrected by advancing a triangular flap from the superior part of the lateral side of the cleft. The resulting scar is essentially a Z-plasty with an eccentric extension along the site of the philtral column. By virtue of improved revisions in the initial operation, developed especially by Millard himself, a Millard I and a Millard II rotation-advancement (R-A) operation for cleft lip have gradually evolved. The primary difference in the two operations is that the flap on the medial side of the cleft is utilized in the nasal sill in the R-A I procedure and in the columella in the R-A II operation. Presently, the triangular flap and the rotation-advancement operations are the most widely accepted methods among surgeons in the United States, and these have contributed greatly to the improved aesthetics of cleft lip surgery. In 1969, the late Tord Skoog published results concerning his utilization of triangular flaps.[72] His operation has been popular in Europe and has gained advocates in this country. For simplicity, the popular operations of the day can all be referred to as triangular flap operations. The Tennison-Randall design has a triangular flap in the lower part of the cleft repair. The Millard rotation-advancement operation and the Wynn procedure have essentially a triangular flap in the upper part of the cleft. Skoog's operation utilizes a triangular flap at both the top and bottom of the cleft. It is surprising that so much of the normal lip anatomy, which is present but distorted in patients with a cleft, was for so many years overlooked and destroyed during surgical operations.

Closure of a cleft lip is performed for both aesthetic and functional reasons. The face is an important anatomical region with several sophisticated functions, one of which is to identify us as human beings. A face with an unoperated cleft is not within the range of normality or social acceptability in our society (Figure 5-1). A carefully detailed repair of a cleft lip will not only restore the face to an aesthetically acceptable norm but, acting

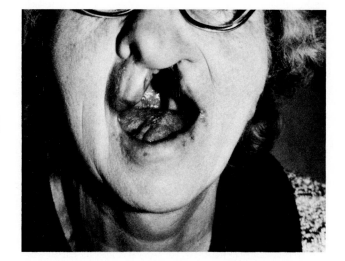

FIGURE 5-1 Normal midface development in a patient with an unoperated unilateral cleft lip and palate.

as a supple soft tissue matrix, it will gently mold the underlying structural elements into a more favorable relationship, which is so important to aesthetics, structural relations, and function.

TIMING OF THE CLEFT LIP REPAIR

Distressed by their infant's appearance, the parents are naturally anxious to know how soon something can be done about it, and this is one of the first questions addressed to the surgeon. It is technically possible to close the lip during the first day or two of life, and some surgeons elect to do this by choice. At that early period, however, the lip is less well developed and the vermilion border and tissues are not as distinct as they will be a few weeks later. Parents rarely resent a delay, provided there is an advantage to be gained. And when they are properly instructed, they do not find feeding a problem during the waiting period. We, like the majority of surgeons, prefer to delay the operation until the criteria for the "rule of tens" are satisfied. At approximately 10 weeks of age, the baby should weigh 10 pounds (4.54 kg.), the hemoglobin should be at least ten grams for adequate oxygenation of vital tissues, and the white blood cell count should not exceed 10,000. By that time the lip will have increased in size and the vermilion tissues and white skin roll will be more distinct, a situation that facilitates more exact realignment during the operation. The baby will have had a start in an external environment, and there will be ample time for a medical review and the collection of timely preoperative data and records by the team. Even though the preoperative care of the baby is the responsibility of the primary care physician, the surgeon must also be certain in his own mind that the baby is ready for the operation. A lip repair is an elective procedure, so in addition to satisfying the rule of tens, the baby should be in as good a state of health as possible and free of infections.

PREOPERATIVE RECORDS

Before embarking on a surgical program, it is important to obtain appropriate records, in addition to those for medical documentation, and to repeat or add to these at scheduled intervals. Records that have been helpful to us prior to repair of the lip include photographs, cephalometric films, face masks, and dental casts. At appropriate times, sound cinefluorographic films and speech and hearing recordings, as well as the opinions of all members of the cleft palate group, are incorporated in the patient's record. Not all of these studies and evaluations are economically practical or necessary in all situations. Photographs; lateral cephalometric films in the rest and functional positions, particularly for velopharyngeal relations; and a good clinical evaluation are the important prerequisites to all reparative cleft lip and palate planning. With that documentation, a competent surgical service can be provided to the patient. Good, complete records are difficult to acquire, but they are essential in longitudinal studies and in retrospective evaluations of the quality of one's own work. Too often we are left with clinical impressions but without documentation.

ANESTHESIA

In order to perform a cheilorrhaphy with a high degree of accuracy and alignment, it is essential for the baby to be quiet. Our preference, therefore, is for oral endotracheal anesthesia with a well-fitting, noncuffed tube resting gently on the midportion of the lower lip and chin. Immediately following the intubation and prior to draping, a catheter is passed into the stomach to evacuate the air bubble and any secretions present in the mouth and throat when the catheter is withdrawn. This permits better expansion of the lungs and a smoother anesthetic. A catheter can easily be passed into the stomach of an infant, and the procedure requires not more than 15 seconds. The endotracheal tube is marked with tape or a dye to determine if it moves in or out during the operative procedure.

The anesthesiologist sees the baby preoperatively and selects the anesthetic agents. Ordinarily we use halothane and oxygen. In addition to the general anesthesia, the operative field is blocked with 0.5 per cent lidocaine containing 1:100,000 parts of epinephrine. This anesthetic agent is injected around the field in such a manner so as not to distort the site of the operative design. A total of 2 ml. or less is usually adequate to aid in hemostasis and provide supplemental regional anesthesia. We have used lidocaine containing epinephrine in conjunction with halothane anesthesia for several years with no ill effect. At the conclusion of the operation, the patient should be breathing well and will probably be crying on leaving the operating table. The baby reacts rapidly and frequently will be given a bottle containing 5 per cent glucose and water within an hour. This will do more to quiet the baby than either restraint or sedation. Some surgeons prefer to repair the lip with sedation and local anesthesia alone. We have repaired some lips by this method, but our preference is for general anesthesia because of the technology and agents available today. Our main objection to the use of sedation and local anesthesia alone is that the baby may be heavily medicated and may require close postoperative supervision for several hours.

TYPES OF CLEFT LIP SURGERY

Clefts of the lip can be grouped under the headings of the prenatal scar, the minimal cleft, the partial or incomplete cleft, and the complete cleft. It is also helpful for descriptive purposes to divide the extent of clefting into minimal, one-third, two-thirds, or three-thirds. The cleft can also be identified as narrow, average, or wide.

We are fortunate in having available more than one good operative design for the repair of a cleft of the lip. Presently, the most commonly used operations are the Tennison-Randall triangular flap, the Millard rotation-advancement operation, the Skoog procedure, and the Rose-Thompson straight-line repair. All of these operations have undergone revisions with time, either by the originator or by other surgeons. The triangular flap procedure, in particular, has been revised by Marcks, Cronin, Brauer, Hagerty, Randall, and others. Occasionally, a revision may be of such magnitude that the procedure will bear a new name, such as the Wynn operation, which in part resembles the Millard rotation-advancement technique. Wynn raises a triangular flap with the apex inferior on the lateral side of the cleft to fill the rotation gap on the medial side. All of these operations, with the exception of the Rose-Thompson procedure, use a broken line closure that frequently resembles a Z-plasty. This reduces the risk of a straight contracture with its associated elevation of the vermilion tissue at the site of repair.

The wise surgeon will be familiar with all of these techniques and their modifications and will select an operative plan that appears to be most appropriate for each individual patient. No two surgeons will execute an operation in exactly the same manner. This is because some degree of visual empiricism is essential in addition to noting the specific skin markings. No two patients are exactly alike and no two lips are identical. It is important to examine the lip carefully before performing the operation. Some details to be noted are the length and breadth of the lip, asymmetry in lip length between one side and the other, the cupid's bow, the vermilion tissue and white skin roll, areas of tissue deficiency, the presence of a muscle bulge lateral to the cleft, the associated nasal deformity, and the level of the attachment of the alar base. In addition to the extent and width of the cleft, the position of the underlying structural elements should be noted. These observations will help the surgeon to select the best operation for each patient. In all of surgery, the first surgeon has the best chance, and this is particularly true in repair of a facial cleft. No surgeon always attains a good result at the first operation. It is more difficult to obtain an optimal result with a secondary repair, but all is not lost if lip tissue has not been needlessly sacrificed during the first operation. Since the operation on the lip is so important to the patient's future, we agree with those surgeons who prefer not to dilute their attention at that time with time-consuming accessory operative procedures.

PREOPERATIVE MAXILLARY ORTHOPEDICS

The purpose of presurgical maxillary orthopedics is not only to improve the alignment of the maxillary segments but to narrow the cleft to facilitate the lip repair. The cleft of the lip cannot be narrowed independently of the underlying arch. Narrowing the cleft of the lip preoperatively will permit a repair with less dependence upon relaxing incisions and the consequent fibrosis with its potential effect upon the anterior drift or growth of the maxilla. Various types of extraoral and intraoral appliances utilizing some form of traction have been recommended. All of these require supervision and parental cooperation. We are of the opinion that presurgical appliances have not significantly enhanced the final result in our hands. For the more difficult and wide cleft of the lip, we will occasionally use the Randall-Graham lip adhesion or surgical Simonart's band. This will mold the underlying segments and enhance the definitive repair within six months (Figure 5–2). To construct this adhesion, a rectangular flap is elevated on either side of the upper pole of the cleft and the two flaps are then sutured together across the cleft. Unfortunately, in the wide cleft it is still necessary to make a relaxing incision in the labial sulcus to permit a secure closure. However, the mobilization of tissues does not have to be as extensive as in the case of a complete repair of a wide cleft of the lip. The main

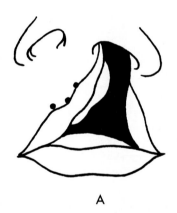

A

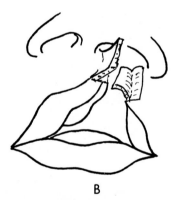

B

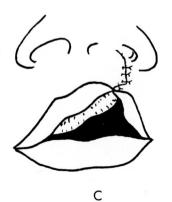

C

FIGURE 5–2 Illustration of the Randall-Graham lip adhesion or surgical Simonart's band.

disadvantage of the lip adhesion is that it may gradually dehisce or create a scar at a site that may interfere with the planned definitive lip repair. Construction of this adhesion does add an operation, but from our study on the effects of hospital experience, we have not found that to be a significant disadvantage. The advantage to be gained needs to be weighed against any disadvantage.

We have gradually abandoned nearly all preoperative maxillary orthopedic appliances designed to alter structural relations. By means of a retrospective study, we learned that the arch and segmental relationships will undergo favorable change owing to the influence of growth and the eruption of the deciduous dentition, provided the lip is supple and maxillary segments are not locked in position by surgical intervention.

UNILATERAL CLEFT LIP

The Rose-Thompson Operation

The Rose-Thompson operation, or the straight-line repair, is practical only for the minimal cleft, the prenatal scar, and the partial median cleft. The minimal cleft has a notch or cleft limited to the vermilion tissue, with the vermilion border usually being elevated and a groove extending on up into the nostril floor. The groove is due to a partial separation of the underlying muscle. There is usually an associated slight asymmetry of the nostril on the cleft side. The Rose-Thompson operation will leave a straight-line scar on the full length of the external surface of the lip that continues on the underlying mucosal surface (Figures 5–3 and 5–4). In a repair of this type, there is an increased risk of postoperative scar contracture with recurrence of a notch in the vermilion and an elevation of the mucocutaneous border at the repair site. In order to obviate this, a Z-plasty may be introduced in the vermilion tissue with interdigitation of the

FIGURE 5–3 The Rose-Thompson repair for a minimal cleft of the lip. There is a notch in the vermilion tissue, the red-white line is slightly elevated, and a groove extends to the nasal sill. Excision of tissue in the nasal floor may create a small nostril. This repair terminated at the base of the columella without complete transection of the lip to the nasal sill.

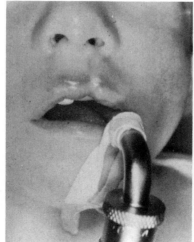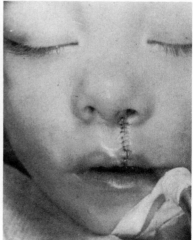

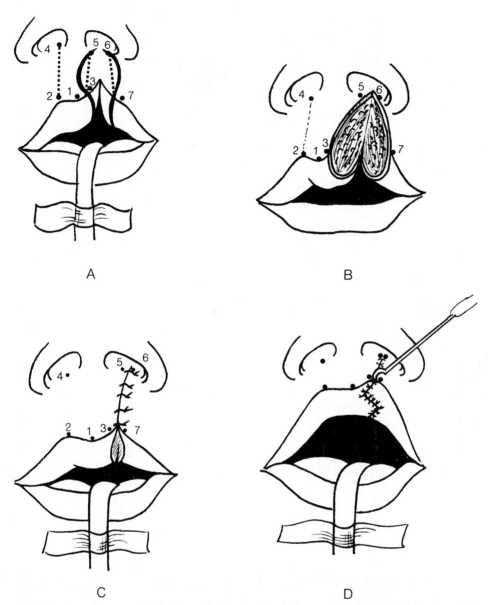

FIGURE 5–4   Illustration of the Rose-Thompson straight line repair. The elliptical excision (*A*) should be conservative to avoid unnecessary sacrifice of lip tissue and the creation of a tight lip. A Z-plasty can be designed on the mucosal surface (*D*) to reduce the risk of a straight line scar contracture.

mucosal flaps to interrupt the straight-line scar. Another method that we frequently use is to insert an offset or a small triangular flap just above the vermilion border (Figure 5–5). It is not wise to elect the Rose-Thompson operation for any other than a minimal cleft, as it tends to create a tight, flat lip when used for a complete cleft lip repair because of the amount of tissue sacrificed within the elliptical excision.

On executing the Rose-Thompson operation (Figure 5-4), methylene blue or another aniline dye is used to mark symmetrical dots on either side of the base of the columella, which represents the top of the philtral crease (4,5). A dot is placed at the apices of the cupid's bow (2,3) and equidistant from a dot located in the center of the bow (1). Another dot is placed at the end of the white skin roll on the lateral side of the cleft (7) and symmetrical to its matching point on the apex of the bow on the medial side of the cleft (3). One can gain some concept of the increase in length needed on the cleft side by locating the points for the inverted V-excision. On the normal side the length is measured down the philtral crease to the red-white junction, and the caliper is set for this normal length of the lip (4,2). Using this normal length as a guide, one point of the caliper is placed on the predetermined point in the cleft nostril floor, and an arch is swung so that it transects the vermilion border both on the columellar side and on the alar side of the cleft (3,7). This locates three points (5,3,7) of which one is in the nostril floor and two are on the vermilion border, which form landmarks for an inverted V-excision. If the points for the V-excision on the vermilion border coincide with that on the cupid's bow on the cleft side and on the end of the white roll on the alar side, a V-excision properly executed will create a lip of normal length on the cleft side. Ordinarily this will not occur; therefore, an ellipse is designed to lower the vermilion border so as to preserve tissue in the lower third of the lip. Using methylene blue, the ellipse is outlined about the groove or inverted V in the lip from the nostril floor to the points selected on vermilion border (3,7). The blue lines then extend straight through the full thickness of the vermilion on either side of the notch. The planned elliptical excision, which is somewhat arbitrary, should be conservative in the initial outline to pre-serve tissue; any correction can be made in the level of the vermilion border after the first excision.

Prior to making an incision, the operative field is blocked with a small amount of 0.5 per cent lidocaine containing 1:100,000 epinephrine, without distorting the tissues. The lip is cut in a positive manner through the skin with a No. 15 blade. If necessary, the excision is then carried through the full thickness of the lip with a No. 11 blade. It is not always necessary or advisable to cut through the full thickness of the lip, especially if the vermilion border does not have to be lowered. After the tissues within the

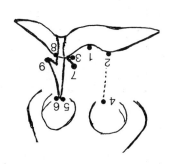

A

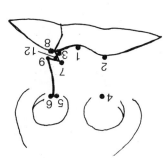

B

FIGURE 5-5 The modified Rose-Thompson repair with a small triangular flap or offset. The design can be planned more accurately and with conserva-tion of lip tissue.

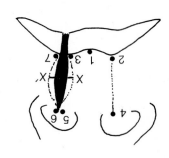

FIGURE 5–6 If the red-white line is still elevated following the Rose-Thompson elliptical excision, the vermilion border can be additionally lowered by small horizontal cuts in the midlip (X,X'). This will determine the depth of the arc of the additional ellipse required for vermilion symmetry.

ellipse are excised, the length of the operated side can be checked against the length of the normal side by approximating the tissues with skin hooks or by aligning the vermilion border with a single suture. The length can be checked visually and with calipers. If the length is still inadequate, a small transverse cut (X–X') can be made into each edge of the freshly cut ellipse at the midlip level (Figure 5–6) while holding the lip down with a skin hook. When the vermilion border is lowered to its normal level, the ellipse can be additionally cut, using the end of the transverse cut to determine the depth of the arc of the ellipse. It is important to remove as little tissue as possible from the floor of the nose because there is a real risk in creating a nostril that will be too small compared with the normal.

After the tissue within the ellipse is removed, the lip is definitively repaired. The muscle layer is accurately approximated with a 4–0 absorbable suture. The skin is then repaired with 6–0 monofilament nylon suture, placing the first suture in the vermilion border and the second between the columella and base of the ala. The remaining skin sutures are then placed. A Z-plasty can then be performed in the vermilion tissue, and the mucosal surfaces are approximated after interpolation of the flaps (Figure 5–4).

A modified Rose-Thompson operation with a small, triangular flap above the vermilion has become our choice for this repair, particularly when it is necessary to lower the vermilion border (Figures 5–5 and 5–7).

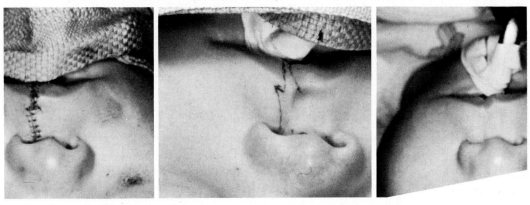

FIGURE 5–7 A minimal cleft of the lip repaired with a modified Rose-Thompson procedure with an offset or small triangular flap.

By using this modified operation, which admittedly creates a small triangular flap, we sacrifice less tissue in the substance of the lip, accentuate the pout, and obtain a better transverse relationship of the cupid's bow. In addition, we can outline this operative plan with a little more precision by following the basic plan for the triangular flap design. Again, the length on the normal side of the lip is determined from the top of the philtral crease · to the red-white line (4,2). The distance is then measured from the base of the columella to the apex of the cupid's bow on the cleft side (5,3) and the difference between this and the normal determines the length of the line (7,3). The operative design is planned as a triangular flap repair. The sides of the triangle 9–12–8 are each equal to the medial triangular defect that opens after a cut is made from 7 to 3. The lip is then cut, and a lesser amount of tissue is sacrificed than with the Rose-Thompson operation. After adjustments are made in the vermilion tissue, the lip is repaired in three layers, starting with an accurate approximation of the muscle layer.

The Triangular Flap Operation

Surgeons who are interested in exact measurements and mathematical design are often attracted to the Tennison-Randall triangular flap operation

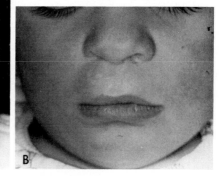

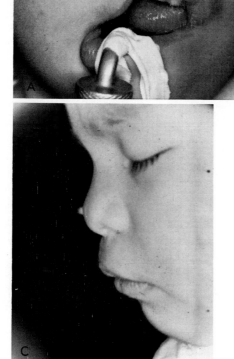

FIGURE 5–8 A wide cleft lip repaired by the Tennison-Randall triangular flap method. It is important to obtain a supple nonrestrictive lip that drapes over the lower lip. This repair was accomplished without any type of preoperative maxillary orthopedics.

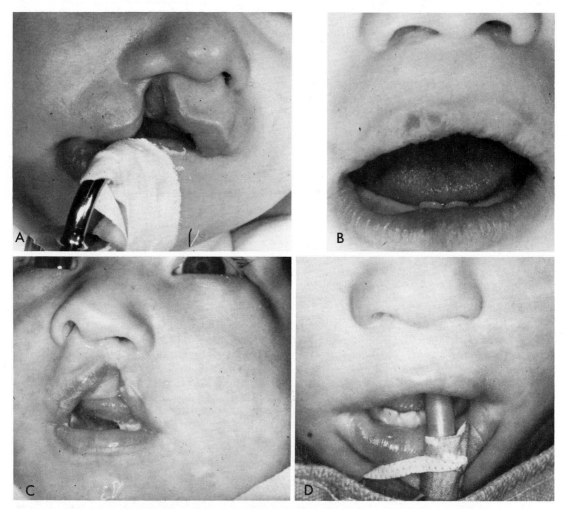

FIGURE 5-9 *A* and *B*, A cleft lip of average width. Note the highlights outlining the accentuated cupid's bow on the preoperative photograph. This lip was repaired by the triangular flap method, but it could have been repaired by Millard's or Wynn's rotation advancement methods. *C* and *D*, A partial cleft lip repaired by the triangular flap method.

for a cleft lip. It is a good procedure in which little tissue is sacrificed, enabling the creation of a full, supple lip with a good pout. We have been able to repair all types of lateral lip clefts by this method, and it is our preference for the wide cleft in which the cupid's bow is drawn well up toward the nostril (Figures 5-8 and 5-9). Regardless of the design selected for a lip repair, it is important to obtain a supple lip that will drape over the lower lip and gently mold the underlying structural elements into a more favorable relationship. A tight, flat lip is not only aesthetically poor but constricts the underlying bony arch and limits the forward drift or growth of the maxilla (Figure 5-10). The orthodontist will be unable to make structural corrections against a restrictive lip matrix.

The wire stencil proposed by Tennison was discarded years ago.

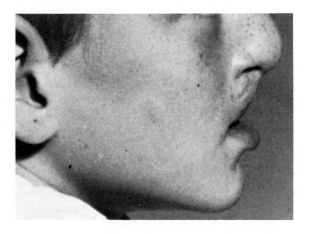

FIGURE 5–10 A restrictive postoperative cleft lip that will constrict the maxillary arch and limit the forward drift of the maxilla. A cross-lip or Abbe flap will be required to restore symmetry.

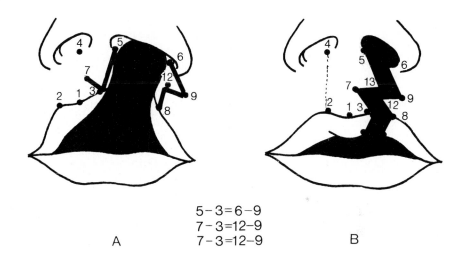

5 – 3 = 6 – 9
7 – 3 = 12 – 9
7 – 3 = 12 – 9

A   B

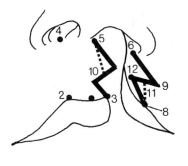

C

5 – 10 + 11 – 8 = 4 – 2

FIGURE 5–11 Randall's description and clarification of Tennison's (1952) triangular flap repair of a cleft lip published in 1959. There is less risk of acquiring a long lip postoperatively on the cleft side with this detailed repair than was true with the Hagedorn-Le Mesurier quadrilateral flap. (See Figure 5–8.)

Instead, the surgeon follows the location of the points in the operative plan as first described in detail by Randall[61] (Figure 5–11). A methylene blue dot (4) is placed at the base of the columella and another on the summit of the cupid's bow (2) on the normal side. A dot is then placed at the midpoint of the depth of the cupid's bow and another at the apex of the bow on the cleft side (3). Distance 2–1 and 1–3 should be equal. A symmetrical point (5) is then placed at the base of the columella on the cleft side, and this is best determined by pushing the distorted columella into a more normal midline position. Another point (6) is placed near the inner base of the ala on a transverse plane symmetrical with point 5. Point 7 is placed in the philtral dimple so that the line 7–3 is approximately at right angles to the mucocutaneous ridge. The distance 5–3 plus 7–3 is equal to the normal length of the lip 4–2. The point 9 is arbitrarily selected at first so that the distance 6–9 is equal to 5–13 and the distance 12–9 is equal to 12–8 is equal to 7–3. Point 12 was picked so that 9–12 equals 8–12. Point 11 is at the midpoint of the transverse line 12–9, and point 10 is at the midpoint of the transverse line 7–13. The distances 6–11–8 and 5–10–3 are both equal to the normal length of the lip 4–2 (Figure 5–12). Point 9 can be varied so that the distance 8–11 is the proper minor vertical length. When the distance 8–11 needs to be shortened, the equilateral triangle 9–12–8 becomes an isosceles triangle.

After all measurements are checked and the lines are drawn, the lip is blocked with 0.5 per cent lidocaine with 1:100,000 epinephrine in a manner that will not distort the tissues. The lip is then cut with determined strokes, using a No. 15 knife blade held at right angles to the skin. The medial side of the cleft is always cut first. If necessary, a relaxing incision can be carried along the reflection of the sulcus but not beyond the canine area on the non-cleft side. Relaxation of the tissues is obtained without elevating or disturbing the maxillary periosteum. A very small bit of tissue is sacrificed on the medial side of the cleft at the nostril floor. The cupid's bow is dropped to its horizontal position and is held down with a skin hook.

While the medial side of the cleft is in its horizontal position, the measurements on the medial side are again checked, particularly those in the triangular defect. It will frequently be found that the distance 7–3 from the vermilion border into the philtral dimple will have lengthened after cutting the lip. If that is so, correction must be made in the matching distance 12–8 before cutting the lateral side. Otherwise the triangular flap will not fit into the defect, and there will be a discrepancy in the vermilion border that will present a difficult correction at a subsequent operation. The cut from point 3 and point 8 may be made straight into the vermilion. The skin on the lateral side of the cleft is cut and then extended through the full thickness of the lip, usually saving much of the vermilion tissue. It is always better to be safe, as once the vermilion is cut off, it is too late if a need for this tissue is found. When there is any evidence of a deficiency with need for additional vermilion tissue, the mucosal flaps turned down from the margin of the cleft, particularly the lateral side, can be turned under the lip and used to augment the vermilion.

A relaxing incision may be necessary on the lateral side, and if so, the soft tissues are mobilized above the level of the periosteum to reduce

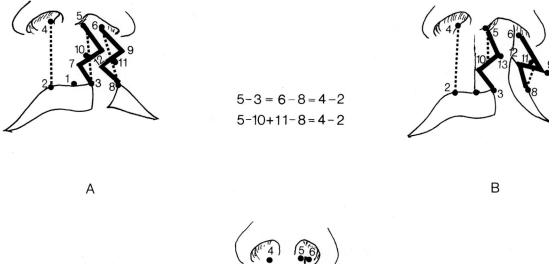

$$5 - 3 = 6 - 8 = 4 - 2$$
$$5 - 10 + 11 - 8 = 4 - 2$$

A

B

C

FIGURE 5–12 Illustration of measurements to determine proper lip length with the triangular flap method of repair.

tension on the suture line. Relaxation of tissues is usually necessary in the complete cleft but not in the partial cleft lip. The lip is then closed accurately, approximating the muscle layer with fine absorbable suture material. The first buried suture is placed at the level of points 5 and 6. This is a critical suture that brings the base of the ala into a normal relationship with the columella. The skin is closed with 6–0 nylon, after placing the first skin suture at 5,6 and the second at the mucocutaneous white roll. The triangular flap helps in the alignment of tissues. Finally, the vermilion and mucosal surfaces are approximated after making any adjustments in the vermilion.

Muscle reorientation, as initially recommended by Fara[20–22] and later by Randall,[64] often complements the lip repair from an aesthetic and functional point of view. Reorientation of the orbicularis oris muscle does not appear to be an essential step in all complete unilateral cleft lip repairs. It extends the area of surgical intervention from the cleft margin to a vertical line passing through the outer attachment of the alar base, which means additional edema and fibrosis. In the first few postoperative days, the lip demonstrates the appearance of added surgical trauma. For those patients who have evidence of a deficiency of tissue on the medial side of the cleft or a noticeable muscle bulge on the lateral side, the muscle reorientation enhances the quality of the repair and in such instances is a step that has long been overlooked. It is a technique that also enhances the quality of some secondary repairs. Muscle reorientation is especially helpful to patients with a conspicuous lateral muscle bulge, an accentuated deformity on whistling, or an area of thin vermilion in the midlip. Accurate approximation of the muscle layer is important in all types of repair with or without reorientation. Following dissection of the muscle from the skin and mucosa, its attachment near the nasal sill and base of the ala is cut and dropped to a horizontal level. It should be pointed out that muscle fibers do not extend up to the base of the ala in every patient. The muscle flap is securely fixed to muscle on the medial side at least to the midline. Then the rest of the lip is repaired, as already described.

The Rotation-Advancement Operation

The rotation-advancement (R-A) principle by Millard has undergone revisions and extensions in an attempt to correct some of the shortcomings inherent in the initial operative design. This operation, which is widely endorsed by the younger surgeons, can be executed with a free, artistic hand utilizing a visual cut-as-you-do principle with less of the exactness demanded by the triangular flap type repair. However, the surgeon should resort to a few caliper checks. Millard has tailored the operation for use in the incomplete, the complete, and the wide cleft lip and has presented some pleasing results in all situations. The cleft lip surgeon should be a perfectionist and, as such, will find shortcomings in all operative plans. The need for secondary revisions in cleft lip surgery is common. Many of these corrections are easier to perform following the R-A method than the triangular flap procedure. This operation is ideally suited for the partial cleft and the complete cleft of average width. It is not used for the minimal cleft, and our preference for the wide cleft, in which the cupid's bow is drawn well up toward the nostril, is the Tennison-Randall triangular flap method.

For the wide cleft, it, is usually necessary to make a back-cut at the extremity of the rotation incision on the normal side, permitting the cupid's bow to drop down to its normal horizontal position. The scar then falls below the base of the columella and may even extend obliquely across the philtral dimple. The scar may not follow the philtral line, which is one of the good qualities of the R-A operation. In developing an adequate lateral advancement flap to fill the rotation gap in a wide cleft repair, there is a risk of carrying the incision along the mucocutaneous ridge beyond the beginning point of the full thickness of the vermilion. This additional sacrifice of vermilion tissue shortens the distance from the summit of the bow on the cleft side to the commissure, as compared with the normal side. The tip of the advancement flap obtained from the region of the floor of the cleft nostril is usually thin and lacking in adequate subcutaneous tissue to fill the defect at the end of the rotation incision. The triangular flap procedure also violates the dimple, but in all fairness it should be noted that most lip wounds heal well with minimal scarring during infancy. The greatest tension following an R-A repair is in the upper third of the lip, and following the triangular flap procedure, such tension is in the midthird of the lip.

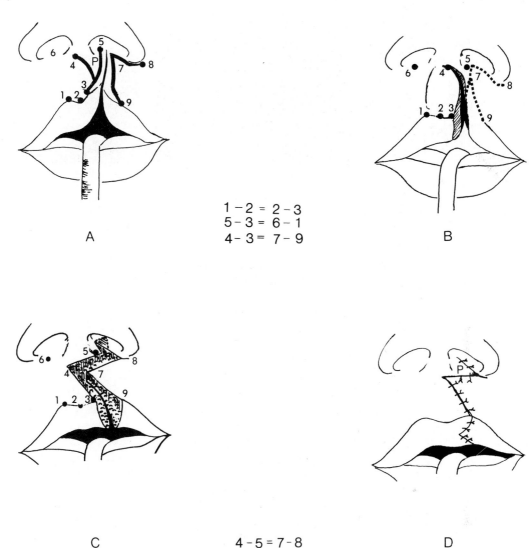

$$1-2 = 2-3$$
$$5-3 = 6-1$$
$$4-3 = 7-9$$

A   B

C $$4-5 = 7-8$$ D

FIGURE 5-13   Millard's initial rotation-advancement repair of a cleft lip reported in 1955. In this operation, a small skin flap (P) on the medial side of the cleft is used to build up the nasal sill.

Millard's first operation was simpler than the later ones in which he has incorporated extensions and revisions (Figures 5-13 and 5-14). A methylene blue dot is placed at the summit of the cupid's bow on the normal side, another at the depth of the bow, and a third at the summit on the cleft side so that 1-2 is equal to 2-3. A dot (6) is placed at the base of the columella on the normal side and another on the opposite side of the columella (5), and a symmetrical dot (7) is placed inside the base of the ala on the cleft side. Then a dot (9) is placed at the end of the white roll on the lateral side of the cleft, which is usually the site of the beginning of the normal fullness of the vermilion. A line is then drawn from the peak of the bow on the cleft side along the margin of the cleft and then curving horizontally across the base of the columella to its midpoint. The upper

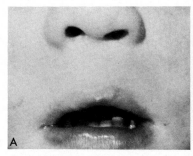
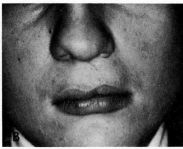
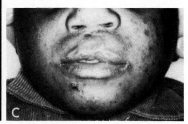

FIGURE 5–14 The clefts in both *A* and *B* were repaired by Millard's initial rotation-advancement plan. The cleft in *C* was repaired by Wynn's method in which a triangular flap was raised on the medial aspect of the lateral lip element and rotated up to fill the gap below the columella. There is a similarity in the scars following the philtral columns.

line for the advancement flap on the lateral side extends around the base of the ala to the edge of the cleft. Another line is drawn just inside the mucocutaneous junction to the end of the white roll. The vertical height of the normal side of the lip is determined from point 1 to point 6. The same routine of blocking the lip with 0.5 per cent lidocaine containing 1:100,000 parts of epinephrine without distorting the tissues is followed in all cleft procedures prior to cutting the lip.

The rotation incision on the medial side of the cleft is cut first. Slight traction is placed on the lip with a skin hook while the rotation cut is made until the cupid's bow is in its normal transverse position. The vertical height on the cleft side (5–3) can then be checked with the calipers against the distance 6–1. If the rotation incision does not need to extend beyond the midpoint of the columella, the scar will be well camouflaged and the operation will be ideally suited to the repair. As the incision is extended to obtain more relaxation, the scar tends to drop away from its ideal location. The small triangular skin flap (P) at the base of the columella on the cleft side is freed and utilized in the nasal sill. The lateral flap is then cut. An incision (8–7) is made about the base of the ala and then across the nasal floor to the edge of the cleft. Another incision (7–9) is made in a determined fashion along the mucocutaneous junction to the end of the white roll. Relaxing incisions are made along the underlying sulcus on either side of the cleft, if needed, to reduce tension. The lateral flap is then advanced into the rotation gap. The key suture fixes the end of the flap into the extremity of the rotation incision. A check should then be made to determine symmetry and the vertical length of the lip. The wound is closed in layers with accurate approximation of the muscle layer first. The base of the ala is aligned with the columella. Then the vermilion border is aligned. The skin is then closed with interrupted 6–0 monofilament nylon sutures. The vermilion tissue may have to be adjusted, and all normal vermilion tissue can be salvaged in this operation. The mucosal surface is then closed with nylon or silk sutures, and the site of the relaxing incisions is loosely closed with an absorbable suture. This simpler R-A principle, referred to as R-A I, is still a good operation in properly selected cases and will give the patient a supple lip that will gently mold the underlying structural elements.

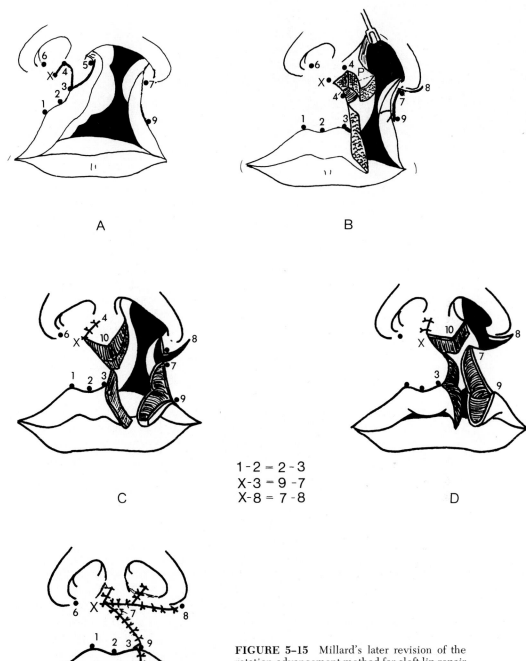

$$1-2 = 2-3$$
$$X-3 = 9-7$$
$$X-8 = 7-8$$

A

B

C

D

E

FIGURE 5-15 Millard's later revision of the rotation-advancement method for cleft lip repair in which a small flap (P) is used to provide some length to the columella on the cleft side.

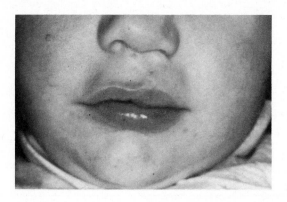

FIGURE 5–16 The rotation gap extended to the philtral column on the normal side in this rotation-advancement repair. There is some fullness of the lateral vermilion, which, when present, is corrected during another scheduled operation, such as a pharyngeal flap or palatal repair.

In the more recent R-A repair, which has been modified for the wider clefts and known as the R-A II, the same points and operative design are laid out (Figures 5–15 and 5–16). The rotation or relaxing incision on the medial side of the cleft will have to extend beyond the columella but should not violate the philtrum on the normal side. Instead, a back-cut (4–X) is made downward and medial to the philtral column as far as necessary to permit the cupid's bow to drop to its normal transverse position. The small triangular skin flap (P) attached to the base of the columella is mobilized and used to provide some length to the columella on the cleft side rather than in the nasal sill. As estimate of the vertical length on the cleft side should be compared with that on the normal side, 6–1. When the lateral flap is cut, the distance 7–9 must be equal to the length of the rotation incision. The upper incision of the advancement flap curves around the alar inset and crosses the nasal floor to the cleft (8–7). An adequate relaxing incision in the sublabial sulcus will be necessary to reduce tension at the site of repair. The key suture again attaches the end of the advancement flap into the extremity of the "back-cut" of the rotation gap defect. It may be necessary to extend the lower incision on the lateral side beyond point 9 to establish vertical length. If so, this shortens the distance between the summit of the cupid's bow on the cleft side and the oral commissure and may result in the sacrifice of usable vermilion tissue. A small interdigitating flap at the mucocutaneous border is fashioned to break up the scar line and to help accentuate the white roll. The lip is then definitively closed, accurately approximating the muscle layer first, then the skin and mucosal tissues, and finally the site of the relaxing incisions.

Millard and some other surgeons do varying amounts of nasal tip revision at the time of the primary lip repair. The nasal tip surgery is performed when there is buckling of the vestibular skin with blockage of the nasal airway. This optional procedure improves nostril symmetry at the primary operation. How much nasal surgery should be done with the initial lip repair is still both an issue that is debated and a procedure that is practiced. We cannot recall a patient with an underdeveloped nasal tip resulting from early surgery. Most surgeons would agree that it is inadvisable to cut and traumatize nasal tip cartilages at an early age. In most instances, we have elected to do a nasal tip adjustment and correct vestibular buckling as a secondary procedure, frequently along with another stage or revision.

A muscle dissection and reorientation is not essential in every patient, even one with a complete cleft, and the design of the R-A procedure tends to place the muscle fibers in a more normal position. When there is a lateral muscle bulge or evidence of tissue deficiency on the medial side, a reorientation of the muscle can easily be carried out with the rotation-advancement operation, and this will enhance the result in some patients. Accurate approximation of the muscle layer with or without reorientation is essential for a good result in all repairs.

Both the R-A principle and the triangular flap repair can give consistently good results in a high percentage of patients when executed properly. Even though the rotation-advancement operation is performed with a free hand, it must be carried out with a high degree of accuracy and supported with a few caliper checks. It is possible to create a lip that is vertically too long or too short on the cleft side with either the R-A or the triangular flap repair. However, there is a greater tendency for a vertical length that is too long with the triangular flap repair and one that is too short with the rotation-advancement procedure. In the very wide cleft with the cupid's bow drawn well up toward the nostril, it has been our observation that the risk of sacrificing too much usable vermilion is greater with the R-A procedure than with the triangular flap. This too is an issue that is debated.

The Skoog Repair

The technique for Tord Skoog's lip repair was first published in 1958, and revisions and optional procedures have been added since. These are incorporated in the description of his lip repair published in 1974.[72] The basic Skoog repair utilizes a triangular flap at the base of the cleft, a "mini-triangular" flap at the vermilion border, and a third triangular flap in the region of the nasal sill. The nasal floor is restored with nasal mucoperiosteal and mucoperichondrial flaps. In recent years, Skoog incorporated certain optional procedures, such as nasal tip surgery with readjustment of the alar cartilage, the transfer of a maxillary periosteal flap into the maxillary cleft, and an orbicularis oris muscle reorientation. The illustrations that Skoog presented, using his method, were not excelled by any other procedure. His follow-up illustrations a few years after repair revealed a persistently good lip with apparently normal nasal development. None of these patients, however, appeared to be adolescents, and unfortunately it does take a number of years to follow patients through puberty to determine the full impact of an operation upon growth and structural relations. It is unlikely, however, that the presence of good structural relations and development at six to eight years of age will change drastically in the teens.

There are potential risks in Skoog's extended repair. Vestibular stenosis may develop if the medial mucoperiosteal and mucoperichondrial flaps are dissected up on the nasal septum. Extensive nasal tip surgery at the time of the primary lip repair is not uniformly practiced. Some surgeons prefer to correct the nasal deformity as a secondary procedure, perhaps in conjunction with another stage or revision. If the nasal tip surgery is well executed without injury to the cartilage, normal development is unlikely to be impaired. There is a real risk to normal facial growth in the anteroposterior or sagittal dimension if one closes the maxillary cleft at an early age with a periosteal flap. This is because of the associated wide dissection over the maxilla and the consequent scar tissue. In procuring the periosteal flap, the dissection is carried over the anterior and lateral surface of the maxilla as high as the infraorbital foramen. This evidently does not interfere as much with the forward growth of the maxilla as Skoog had previously noted among his patients following early primary bone grafting, but the hazard is real. Growth and segmental changes take place in a favorable manner under the influence of a restored, supple lip and during the eruption of the deciduous dentition. Additional width in the maxillary ridge occurs about 11 years of age or even later. For that reason, many individuals are of the opinion that it is better to delay closure of a cleft involving the alveolar process and thus to interfere as little as possible with normal biological growth processes and their effect upon structural change. We have adopted a philosophy of delaying some of the optional procedures, such as bone grafting and periosteal flaps, that might impair growth and development when carried out at an early age. We prefer to delay bone grafts and periosteal flaps until 12 years of age. It is true that dental supervision and dental orthopedic appliances might help to reduce the impact of surgical intervention on morphological change. However, a substantial economy can be realized if a surgical protocol is developed that will require minimal dependence on corrective appliances.

As is apparently true with the other operative plans, the reorientation of the orbicularis oris muscle does not seem to be warranted in all cases. It will enhance the quality of repair when a deficiency is obvious on the medial side or a muscle bulge occurs on the lateral side. The lateral muscle mass is dissected free from the overlying skin and underlying mucosa but not beyond the alar base, and the superior fibers are then detached. The muscle fibers are rotated to a horizontal position and advanced into the medial side of the cleft behind the skin and muscle of the prolabial section. The muscle is sutured to the muscle of the opposite side at the midline, and the key suture attaches the lateral muscle to the tissues at the base of the nasal spine. A muscle reorientation can be performed as a secondary procedure through a mucosal approach underneath the lip or in conjunction with a lip revision.

In planning Skoog's repair, the length of the lip is first determined on the normal side, as with other repairs (Figure 5–17). Different surgeons use different numbers or letters to designate specific landmarks. One should become familiar with the landmarks themselves because the numbers are unimportant. A point is placed at the summit of the cupid's bow on the normal side (2), another at the depth of the bow in the midline (1), and another at the apex of the bow on the cleft side (3). The summit of the bow on either side should be equidistant from the midpoint. A line is drawn from the midpoint of the base of the columella to the midpoint of the cupid's bow (1) in a slightly curved fashion to conform with the normal curvature of the philtral dimple. Point 5 is selected on the small ridge extending out from the base of the columella. Point 7 is on the midline of the philtral dimple and at right angles from point *a* on the summit of the cupid's bow on the cleft side. A small line is carried transversely from

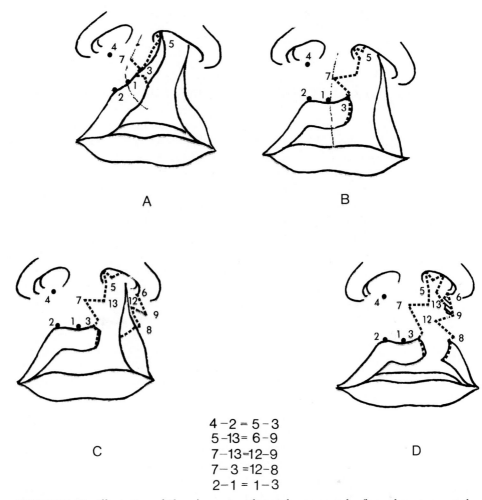

$$4 - 2 = 5 - 3$$
$$5 - 13 = 6 - 9$$
$$7 - 13 = 12 - 9$$
$$7 - 3 = 12 - 8$$
$$2 - 1 = 1 - 3$$

FIGURE 5–17 Illustration of Skoog's repair utilizing three triangular flaps; there is one at the base of the columella, one at the base of the lip, and a third mini-flap at the vermilion border. Optional procedures including a nasal tip revision, an orbicularis oris muscle reorientation and a maxillary periosteal flap transfer to the alveolar cleft were incorporated with the lip repair. It would be unwise to attempt to use Skoog's plan with the three triangles until one has had considerable experience in cleft lip surgery.

point 5 to the base of the columella, which will be the site of the upper triangular defect. The design on the lateral side of the lip can be made at this time, although Skoog defers that step until the labial frenum has been released, the medial side of the cleft has been cut, the nasal tip revision has been carried out, and the periosteal flap has been transferred to the maxillary cleft. A line is drawn from 5 to 3 and from 7 to 3 with methylene blue.

Before cutting the lip, the operative field is blocked by an infiltration of 0.5 per cent lidocaine containing 1:100,000 parts of epinephrine. The lip is then cut with a No. 15 knife blade in a positive manner from point 3 to 5 and then 7 to 3. At point 3, a small 1-mm. defect is created in the vermilion border, and the incision then extends on through the vermilion. The skin-vermilion incision is then extended through the full thickness of the lip with a No. 11 scalpel blade. This releases the lip tissues and permits them to drop down to their normal vertical length. The cupid's bow falls into its proper horizontal position. If it appears that the apex of the bow on the cleft side is still above that of the normal, it can be dropped further by extending the line 7–3, but under no circumstances should the line 7–3 extend beyond the philtrum on the normal side.

A mucoperiosteal flap is then elevated on the medial side of the cleft in the nasal floor and on the premaxilla, and a lateral mucoperiosteal flap is elevated low on the lateral wall. The two flaps are sutured together to bridge the cleft and close the nasal floor. The maxillary periosteal flap is turned in underneath these mucoperiosteal flaps. The operative design is then drawn on the lateral side of the cleft. A point (8) is placed at the end of the white roll or at the beginning of the full red lip. Another point (6) is placed medial to the alar base and symmetrical with 5. Points 5 and 6 should be located so that when they are approximated in the final repair, the width of the nasal floor will be equal to that of the normal side.

The operative plan is similar to that for the standard triangular flap repair. The line 5–13 should equal 6–9. The triangle 9–12–8 should match the defect 13–7–3. Before the lateral lip is cut, the dimensions should be checked with a caliper against the defect on the medial side of the cleft while that side of the lip is held down in its normal horizontal position. The lateral lip is then cut, leaving a small offset at the vermilion border to fit in the small triangular defect on the medial side. This small offset is designed to accentuate the white roll and vermilion border. The rectangular flap of tissue 6–9–12 is mobilized after the lip is cut and turned into the nasal sill and the defect in the base of the columella. This restores tissue in an area of a common deficiency. The muscle reorientation is then carried out, and the muscle layer is accurately approximated. Then 5 and 6 are approximated, which will elevate the alar attachment on the cleft side. The next suture is placed in the vermilion border. The rest of the skin is then closed with interrupted 6-0 nylon sutures. The mucosal tissues are then closed, as well as any remaining incisions in the sublabial sulcus.

Skoog's modifications and options are related primarily to the complete cleft lip. For the partial cleft lip, the standard triangular flap repair would apply, although the small offset at the vermilion border could be included, as recommended in Skoog's complete lip repair and as carried out in Millard's R-A procedure.

Summary

A pleasing lip can be accomplished with any of the methods described. Each method has its shortcomings, and there are complications associated with all methods. The plastic surgeon must be a perfectionist in a lip repair, executing the operation with exactness and pausing for a critical look as the procedure progresses. The wise surgeon who wishes to practice above the level of mediocrity should become familiar with all operative designs, and an indication can be found for each operation.

BILATERAL CLEFT LIP

The repair of the lip is an exceedingly important first step in a patient's total plan of habilitation. Important as it is, it is only the first step in a total interdisciplinary habilitation program that goes on into maturity. We like to see these patients in a group conference every six months during the early years when maturation and growth changes are rapid and there is need for professional advice and assistance. The plan is somewhat flexible because a patient with a bilateral cleft lip and palate needs far more service than does a patient with only a partial cleft of the lip. When the need for service decreases, recall is on an annual basis and in some instances may be required only every two years (see Figure 5–9B).

The bilateral cleft of the lip can be symmetrical or asymmetrical, with the extent of the involvement being the same or different on each side (Figure 5–18). The malformation on either side can vary from a minimal cleft to a complete and wide cleft. As the extent of the cleft increases, so do the deficiencies and distortions. In a complete cleft, the premaxilla may protrude for varying degrees along an arc, being attached only to the tip of the nose and the nasal septum. The columella may be deficient or almost totally absent. The prolabium, which forms the vertical height of the midlip, is devoid of muscle. It may vary in size from a well-developed lip segment to a small dome-shaped mass of tissue. The prolabial vermilion is deficient and may vary in color and texture from that of the normal lateral vermilion. As the malformation becomes more extensive, the cupid's bow, lip dimple, and philtral columns disappear. A complete bilateral cleft of the lip and palate, with its deficiencies, distortions, and shortness of midline tissues, is a major surgical challenge in which the best results often leave much to be desired. J. B. Brown once stated that a bilateral cleft lip is twice as difficult to repair as a unilateral cleft and the results are only half as good. The deficiencies and distortions associated with a bilateral cleft are more than double those of a unilateral cleft. The physical alterations associated with a bilateral cleft lip and palate need to be carefully observed and recorded. A successful

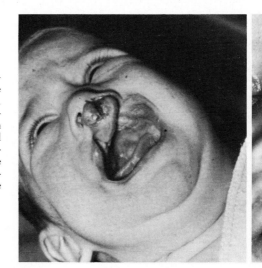

FIGURE 5–18 An asymmetrical bilateral cleft of the lip, being complete on the left and incomplete on the right. The side with the most extensive involvement is always repaired first. In this situation, the restored lip will mold the premaxilla into a more normal position within a few weeks. The partial cleft on the right side can be repaired in 6 to 8 weeks following the first stage repair.

habilitation program will require the maximum effort of a concerted interdisciplinary team.

The bilateral cleft lip can be repaired in one or two stages. When the repair is staged, the first operation is usually performed when the baby weighs 10 to 12 pounds and the second stage 6 weeks later, although some surgeons prefer a longer delay. Several good operative plans are available for repair of the bilateral lip, and the surgeon should be familiar with the acceptable methods in order to provide a sophisticated service and to make one's practice more gratifying. The surgical philosophy for the straight-line repair, the triangular or zig-zag flap, the rotation-advancement principle, the Skoog operation, and other repairs has been applied to the bilateral cleft. There are situations in which one operation may be more suited to a particular case than any other. There may be exceptions, but it is always safer to select a two-staged repair when the operative design requires cutting deeply into the prolabium, such as the rotation-advancement principle. To cut deeply into the prolabium from both sides may embarrass the circulation. We have never lost a prolabium doing this, but we have seen some that were a worrisome dusky color for a day or two. When there is marked protrusion of the premaxilla, a repair on one side will gradually mold the premaxillary segment toward that side. The second side then becomes more difficult to close because the cleft becomes wider and the prolabium becomes thinner as these structures are rotated and drawn toward the repaired side (see Figure 5–25A). When a two-stage repair is done, the measurements used for the operative design on the first side are recorded and made available at the time that the second side is closed. If one chooses, a few key points can be tattooed on the delayed side when the initial repair is being carried out.

All operations designed to turn down a flap of skin, muscle, and vermilion from the lateral side of the cleft to the lower border of the prolabium should be avoided. The reasons are generally understood. These procedures are designed to increase the length of the prolabium, but in so doing they create a restrictive lip that is frequently too long and too narrow. The resulting tight lip destroys the normal profile, restricts and constricts the underlying structures, and limits the capabilities of the orthodontist. The prolabium, regardless of its apparent size, should be used to obtain the vertical height of

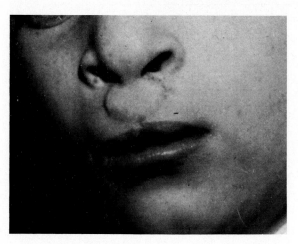

FIGURE 5–19 A ring scar in the lip caused by turning lateral skin-vermilion flaps below the prolabium. The unsightly ring scar needs to be interrupted to improve the aesthetics. Frequently the lip is too long and narrow following this type of repair.

the midlip. However, the prolabial vermilion can be augmented with mucosal flaps from the lateral margins of the clefts. The lateral skin-vermilion flaps create a ring scar on the lip, within which the skin tends to rise and form an unsightly dome-shaped mass and which attracts attention (Figure 5–19). These patients are referred to as "ring-nose" by their peers, and it becomes necessary to flatten the prolabial tissue and interrupt the ring scar, possibly with a Z-plasty on either side.

The Premaxilla

The size of the prolabium and the protrusion of the premaxilla are problems that can complicate a bilateral cleft lip repair. Occasionally a small Simonart's band will hold a premaxilla in a relatively normal position when the bilateral cleft is otherwise complete (Figure 5–20). If the premaxilla is in fairly good position or the protrusion is only moderate, the lip can be repaired in one or two stages without undue tension on the suture line. When the protrusion is extensive, a lip repair may be a technical impossibility without first recessing the premaxilla enough to relieve tension on the suture line (Figure 5–21). A premaxilla should never be recessed to its apparent normal position in the maxillary arch. This overcorrection will lead to a retrusion of the maxilla and an abnormal profile. In a complete bilateral cleft, the premaxila will have to rest anterior to the maxillary segments to provide a normal profile. Time, especially the period through the eruption of the deciduous dentition, will improve the structural relations.

Both external and intraoral traction methods have been suggested and used by different surgeons to recess the premaxilla. These usually require time, supervision, and parental cooperation and are not without complications. Some of these technologies for recessing a premaxilla can also cause compression of the maxillary segments unless the segments are stabilized with a hold prosthesis. This is a matter for interdisciplinary discussion. A lip

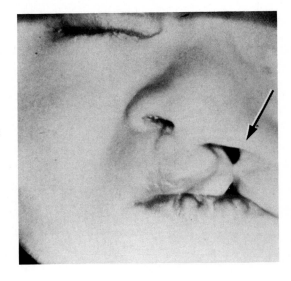

FIGURE 5–20 A Simonart's band capable of retaining a premaxilla in a normal position.

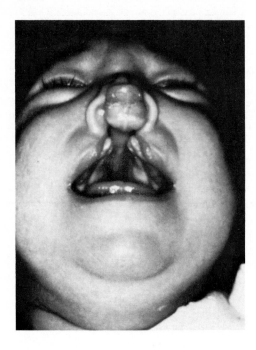

FIGURE 5–21 Marked ventroflexion of the premaxilla. This premaxilla must be recessed enough to permit repair of the lip. It should not be recessed into the maxillary arch. The prolabium is well developed.

FIGURE 5–22 The premaxilla will dorsiflex under the influence of a restored lip, although a limited surgical recession or maxillary orthopedics may be required to enhance closure of the lip. The premaxilla should rest anterior to the maxillary segments and not in the arch. The segmental relations will improve through the period of eruption of the deciduous dentition.

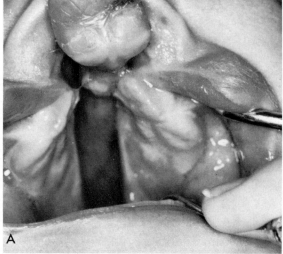

A

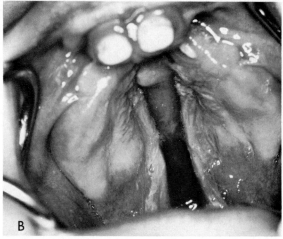

B

adhesion, as proposed by Randall and Graham[63] will gradually mold a premaxilla (see Figure 5–2). If there is marked protrusion of the premaxilla, it will be necessary to place a relaxing incision in the sulcus adjacent to the cleft to gain enough relaxation to create the adhesion. There is still a risk of dehiscence or inducing scar tissue that might interfere with the later definitive repair.

A surgical recession of the premaxilla will not cause maxillary retrusion if it is a limited recession that will permit closure of the lip without undue tension, but without its being compressed back into the arch (Figure 5–22). In order to recess the premaxilla, we usually make a small incision in the base of the midseptal or vomer region posterior to the bulge representing the prevomerine-vomer suture. The mucosal flaps are elevated on either side of the vomer, and a section of cartilage about 5 mm. wide is removed with a single bite of a small rongeur or with an osteotome. That procedure alone may cause enough dorsiflexion of the premaxilla to permit a repair. If the retropositioning is inadequate, the septal cartilage can be cut with a septal knife from the point of resection anteriorly to allow the premaxilla to slide back a little. Rather than cutting the septal cartilage, it can be freed from the groove in the underlying crest of vomerine bone to permit the premaxilla to slide posteriorly a limited amount. Some surgeons prefer to stabilize the premaxilla with a small Kirschner wire. We usually do not and instead depend upon the repaired lip to provide some stability. The small mucosal wound on the base of the vomer is then repaired with an absorbable suture material.

The Rose-Thompson Repair

The Rose-Thompson straight-line repair described for a unilateral cleft lip can also be used to repair a bilateral minimal cleft of the lip. Both sides can be repaired at the same time, and a Z-plasty can be added in the vermilion tissue to interrupt the straight-line scar. If the vermilion is tented up at the cleft site, a small triangular flap just above the mucocutaneous ridge will lower the peak of the vermilion tissue to its horizontal position. The breadth of the nasal floor may be increased with a minimal cleft, but the columella and premaxilla do not usually present a problem. The technique for a straight-line closure of a minimal cleft was described in more detail in the section on the unilateral cleft.

The Veau III Operation

A bilateral lip repair can be carried out in a single operative stage by the Veau III straight-line repair or by one of its modifications. We seldom use this operation anymore and never when the prolabium is small. If there is significant protrusion of the premaxilla, a recession must be accomplished first. We have had some pleasing results with the Veau III repair, and this procedure should be considered when both sides of the cleft are to be repaired during the same operation. Our preference is usually for one of the other methods described in the section on the unilateral cleft (Figures 5–23 and 5–24).

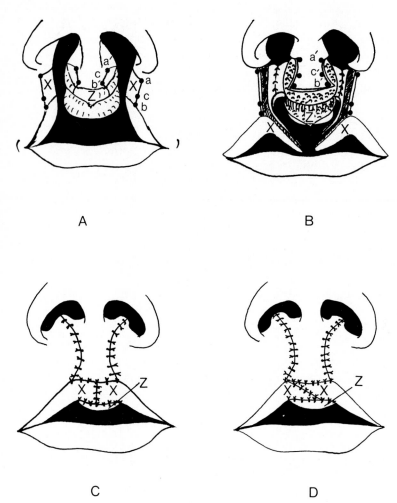

A

B

C

D

FIGURE 5–23 Illustration of the Veau III technique. The line a'c'b' should follow the philtral line. The flap is turned down laterally to serve as inner lip lining, and the skin edge is cut off. The lateral flap a,c,b is turned down inferiorly, and the skin is cut off, saving only vermilion tissue to help build up a tubercle. The vermilion flaps can overlap to form a **Z** or meet as a butt-joint. Or the flap-**X** can be placed under the prolabial vermilion without disturbing the mucocutaneous ridge.

FIGURE 5–24 A postoperative one-staged Veau III bilateral lip repair.

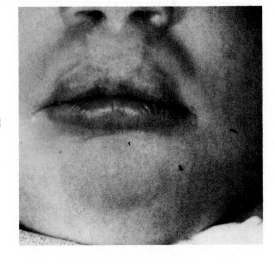

The Triangular Flap Repair

A straight-line repair does not routinely produce an adequate pout or fullness in the lower part of the lip. A multi-directional scar is usually less conspicuous than the straight-line scar. The triangular flap procedure provides more tissue in the lower lip, where it is needed to create fullness and eversion of the lip. This method also eliminates the sharp vermilion peaks that are commonly associated with a straight-line closure.

In all bilateral lip repairs, conservation of tissue is essential. There is a place for nearly all lip tissue, and preservation of the prolabial vermilion is important in the repair of a bilateral cleft. It is better to execute the triangular flap procedure and all other multi-directional designs one side at a time, especially when there is a protruding premaxilla. This causes less chance of circulatory embarrassment of the prolabium, and the magnitude of the procedure is reduced. Closure of one side at a time seems to conserve tissue, and it gradually molds the underlying structural elements. The side of the initial repair heals well in the absence of tension, and the scar is often barely visible. Repair of the second side is more difficult because the premaxilla has swung over to the side of the initial repair, making the cleft on the delayed side wider (Figure 5–25). The prolabium is also thin and drawn toward the

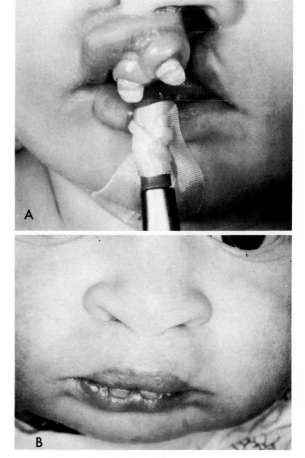

FIGURE 5–25 *A*, Following the first stage of the lip repair, the premaxilla swings toward the repaired side and the edge on the unrepaired side protrudes out into the cleft. The skin and vermilion on the unrepaired side are thin and drawn toward the repaired side, making the second stage lip repair more difficult. *B*, After repair of the second side, the premaxilla is gradually molded back to a midline position. The columella lengthening is a delayed procedure.

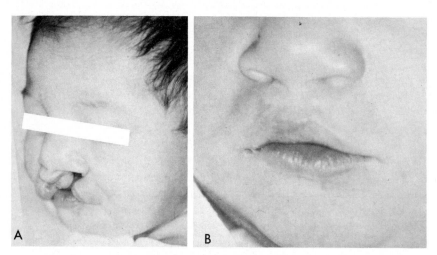

FIGURE 5–26 *A,* Preoperative complete bilateral cleft lip and palate. *B,* Postoperative two-staged bilateral lip repair by the triangular flap method. Note some hypertrophy of the scar on the patient's right, which is the side of the second stage of the repair.

repaired side, and the edge of the premaxilla on the unrepaired side protrudes out into the cleft. Occasionally, it is difficult to determine the exact measurements of the triangle on the repaired side after healing has taken place. Because of this, accurate measurements made during the initial repair are available for use at the second lip operation. This has been very helpful in laying out the design on the second side because the tissues have been distorted by being pulled toward the repaired side. Following repair of the second side, the premaxilla will gradually move back to a midline position. Because of greater tension on the repair of the delayed side, there is an increased risk of developing a hypertrophied scar. This will usually soften and flatten within six to twelve months (Figure 5–26).

The plan for marking the triangular flap procedure is similar to that described for the unilateral cleft. However, the philtral dimple and cupid's bow are absent, so that some of the landmarks used in the repair of a unilateral cleft are not present in the complete bilateral cleft. If there is asymmetry of the bilateral cleft lip, the side with the greater involvement is repaired first (Figure 5–27). Point 1 is placed at the midpoint of the mucocutaneous border of the prolabium. Points 2 and 3 lie equidistant on either side of the midline point 1 and at a location at which one would estimate the apices of the cupid's bow to lie. This will simply be an estimate and will vary somewhat with the size of the prolabium. Point 5 is at the mucocutaneous junction on a level with the base of the columella. Point 6 is inside the alar attachment. Point 6 is often a little lower than point 5 so that the alar attachment is elevated to a normal columnar relationship when the cleft is closed. One needs to use self-restraint and not plan to excise too much nasal floor tissue or the nostril will be too small. Point 7 is selected so that a line 3–7 will be at right angles to the vermilion border. A line is drawn from 5 to 3 and from 7 to 3. The length of 3–7 is approximately half the length of 3–5. The upper edge of the triangular gap 7–3 should not extend to the midline or it will contact the cut from the

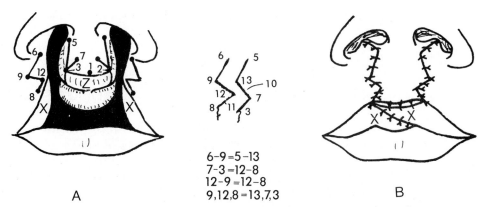

FIGURE 5-27   Illustration of the bilateral triangular flap repair. This is carried out as a two-staged operation with the second half of the lip closed after an interval of 6 weeks.

opposite side following the second stage repair and leave a ring or oval scar. Some surgeons prefer to outline the operative plan and cut the lateral segment of a bilateral cleft first and then make adjustments in the prolabial segment. Point 8 is placed at the end of the white roll or at the beginning of the normal full thickness of the vermilion. Point 12 is placed above point 8 on the vermilion border at a distance representing approximately one-third the height of the lip. Line 3–7 should equal line 8–12. A line is drawn at right angles to point 12. Point 9, which is negotiable, is placed on this line so that the distance 12–9 is about equal to 12–8. The distance 6–9 should equal 5–13. The sides of the triangle 12–9 and 12–8 should be equal, and the triangular flap should fit properly into the triangular gap in the prolabium.

Our preference has been to cut the prolabial side first. The prolabium often sits on the premaxilla as a round, dome-shaped mass of soft tissue similar to skin surrounded by a circular scar. To facilitate cutting the prolabium, it is flattened out by exerting pressure on it with the tip of one index finger. The lip is then cut while the prolabium is compressed by the finger, and this will control bleeding when the first skin incisions are made. The initial cuts are then deepened while the surgeon is still compressing the prolabium. A mucosal flap medial to the line 5–3 is turned down and left attached to the premaxilla to serve as a lining on the undersurface of the lip. A relaxing incision is then carried along the prolabial sulcus from point 3. The prolabium is partially raised from the premaxilla, and the elevation should not extend beyond the midline. With a skin hook holding the medial side of the cleft down, the vertical height is viewed to determine if the mucocutaneous ridge has dropped to a normal horizontal position. If additional lowering is needed, this can be accomplished by a slight extension of the line 7–3. At that time the measurements and the size of the triangular gap are determined and compared with the diagram on the lateral side. An adjustment is made, and the lateral side is then cut. An incision is made from points 8 to 12, then from 9 to 12, and from 9 to 6. At point 8 the cut turns at right angles and passes just through the mucocutaneous junction and then follows superiorly near the vermilion border. This will preserve a flap of vermilion tissue that can be used to augment the prolabial vermilion.

After the initial cut is made, the incisions are carried through the full thickness of the lateral lip. A relaxing incision is usually necessary and extends from the upper pole of the cleft laterally along the sublabial sulcus. The lip tissue is mobilized above the periosteum to relieve tension at the site of the repair. The prolabium is deprived of muscle, but a muscle flap is usually not advanced into the prolabium during the initial repair. The subcutaneous tissues on the prolabial side lack strength to hold a muscle flap, except near the base of the columella. The lip is then closed, and the prolabial subcutaneous tissues are approximated to the subcutaneous tissues on the lateral side using a 4–0 or 5–0 absorbable suture. The skin flap inside 6–9–12 can be mobilized and turned up for use in the nasal sill, similar to a modification in the R-A principle. When this is done, a triangular gap must be created in the base of the columella. Points 6 and 5 and points 8 and 3 are then approximated. Then the rest of the skin is closed with 6–0 monofilament nylon. The mucosal or vermilion flap left attached to the lateral lip segment is then notched on the superior edge near the vermilion border, placed in a wound underneath the prolabial vermilion, and sutured to the mucosal edges. This provides additional fullness to the prolabial vermilion. The mucosal flap is sutured in place with an absorbable suture material.

Some surgeons prefer to insert the lateral vermilion flaps along the mucocutaneous border of the prolabium and turn down a prolabial flap to serve as an inner mucosal lining. The lateral vermilion flap extends beyond the midline of the prolabium, and the surplus tip of the flap can be discarded. A corresponding area of prolabial vermilion is turned down for lining on the underside of the lip. When the delayed side of the bilateral cleft is repaired, the opposite vermilion flap will form an end-to-end relationship with the first vermilion flap, or the two vermilion flaps may overlap to form a Z closure. When a bilateral cleft lip is repaired in a single operation, both vermilion flaps are joined simultaneously at the midline, either as an end-to-end or an overlapping Z closure. Adjustments of the vermilion are easier during a single-staged repair. Our preference has been to place the lateral vermilion flaps underneath the prolabial vermilion just above the sulcus rather than to open the mucocutaneous junction. The triangular flap repair is accomplished with the sacrifice of very little tissue. At the conclusion of the procedure, points 1, 2, 4, 6, 8, 9 and 12 or any lesser number of critical points can be tattooed on the opposite cleft side to make it easier to lay out the plan of repair on the second cleft. We imprint all the initial points and measurements 5–3, 7–3, 6–9, 9–12, and 12–8 on a tongue blade with the points of the calipers. The tongue blade is sterilized and saved for use as a guide during the repair of the second side of the lip.

Some surgeons like to incorporate a nasal tip adjustment at the time of the primary repair. Bauer, Trusler, and Tondra[4] freed the skin widely over the lower nasal cartilage through both the lateral wound and the wound at the base of the columella to permit some readjustment. Millard, Skoog, and others have been more aggressive in early nasal tip correction. Furthermore, there are others who prefer to delay surgery on the nasal tip.

If nasal tip surgery is done at the first stage, it will also have to be done on the opposite side during the second operation. The second side of the lip can be repaired after a six weeks' delay. Softening of the tissues seems to take place rather rapidly in infants. The design for the second stage is the same as that for the first operation, and it is made easier by having available a record of the measurements from the initial repair or a few critical dots tattooed during the first stage. It is also well to check the vertical height of the repaired lip as a guideline. The operation is then carried out on the second side but with greater difficulty than the first because of the rotation of the premaxilla toward the repaired side. More extensive relaxation of the lateral lip segment may be required on the second side. The mucosal flap that is turned down from the edge of the cleft on the lateral side is placed in the prolabial sulcus between the premaxilla and the previous mucosal flap. A flap of mucosa from the medial side of the cleft is also preserved to help line the inner surface of the repair on the second side.

Even with augmentation, the prolabial vermilion may still be inadequate to form a normal tubercle, and the middle third of the vermilion may be thinner than the lateral lip segments. The prolabial skin will flatten out and develop following the lip repair. The eventual vertical height of the prolabial segment will vary from patient to patient, as it does in the normal population. If there is a persistent lack of fullness and vermilion tubercle in the midthird of the lip, the overall aesthetic result can be enhanced by a combined V–Y plasty and orbicularis oris muscle reorientation. This is carried out as a secondary operation. A V incision is made in the lip vermilion and mucosa, with its apex in the region of the labial frenum and the open portion of the V near the vermilion border at the junction of the prolabium and lateral lip segments. The V-shaped mucosal flap is elevated, and the muscle in each lateral segment is then dissected free from its overlying skin and underlying mucosa. The muscle fibers are detached at the nasal sill and alar base and rotated down to a horizontal position. It is frequently possible to overlap the muscle from each side at the midline, which strengthens the repair and provides adequate bulk in the region of the tubercle. After completing the muscle transfer, the V-shaped wound is repaired as a Y, which helps to build up the tubercle (Figure 5–28). This provides enough advancement to cover the muscle and brings in some lateral lip tissue toward the midline.

The triangular flap operation has provided many patients with a satisfactory lip repair. It does encourage tissue conservation, since a minimum

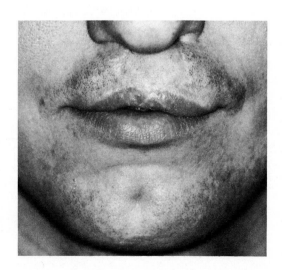

FIGURE 5–28 A postoperative bilateral cleft lip that initially had a conspicuous deficiency of vermilion tissue in the midlip region. This was corrected with a V–Y mucosal advancement and orbicularis muscle reorientation from an approach on the mucosal side of the lip.

amount of tissue is sacrificed. The procedure also provides tissue in the lower part of the lip where it is needed.

The Rotation-Advancement Operation

The rotation-advancement (R-A) principle has been presented by Millard for repair of a bilateral cleft of the lip, both incomplete and complete, symmetrical or asymmetrical, and as a single or two-staged procedure. The plan is the same as for the unilateral lip repair with some modifications to accommodate for bilateral cleft lip deficiencies and distortions (Figure 5–29). On occasion, we have witnessed circulatory embarrassment in the island of prolabial skin following a one-staged bilateral lip repair that occurred when the rotation incisions met at the midline (Figure 5–30). This occurred even though the prolabium was not elevated from the premaxilla. There was no loss of tissue, but a dusky discoloration can lead to a restless night for the surgeon. In the initial R-A plan, the end of the rotation incisions met at the midline beneath the columella, but in a later revision Millard left a bridge of skin between the ends of those incisions. This was a progressive step because, unlike the initial operation that created an objectionable ring scar in the lip, the later revision permitted the scar to follow a more normal philtral line. The separation of the advancement flaps at the midline also lessens the tendency for increased vertical length of the lip. The small bridge of tissue at the base of the columella may also improve circulation following a one-staged repair.

A cleft of the lip is basically a triangular defect with the apex of the triangle in the floor of the nostril and the base of the triangle at the free lip margin. In the absence of a significant protrusion of the premaxilla and with a well-developed prolabium, Millard suggested that primary forked flaps can be raised on each side of the prolabium lateral to the normal line of the philtral ridge. These flaps are then advanced into the columella to increase its length and to raise the depressed nasal tip. Following that, the bilateral rotation-advancement procedure is carried out to completion.

In a complete bilateral cleft lip, the prolabium is deprived of muscle. Because of this, Schultz[70] separated the prolabium from the premaxilla and united lateral mucosal-muscle flaps behind the prolabium. This will provide more body to the lip repair. In the wider clefts, union of mucosal-muscle flaps

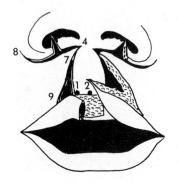
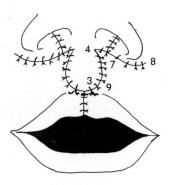

FIGURE 5–29 Rotation-advancement operation for bilateral incomplete cleft lip. If the rotation gaps do not meet at the midline below the columella, the lip scar will follow the path of the philtral columns and the operation can be performed in a single stage.

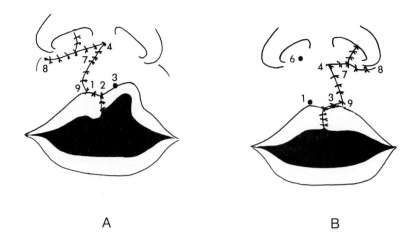

FIGURE 5–30 A two-staged rotation-advancement illustration. When the rotation incision extends beyond the midline, it is better to repair one side at a time.

at the midline may create a tight lip and reduce the breadth of the lip, which is a dimension that should not be compromised. If the prolabium is completely elevated from the premaxilla, the R-A procedure must be carried out in two stages to avoid circulatory embarrassment.

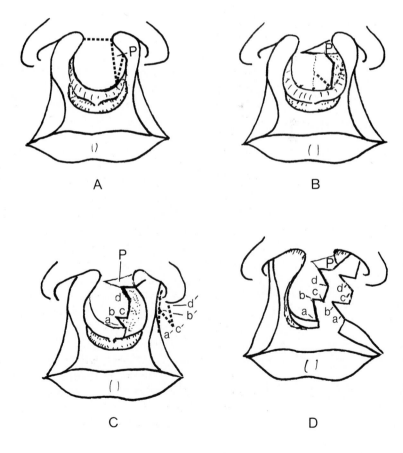

FIGURE 5–31 Skoog's two-staged bilateral cleft lip repair. The P-flap is used to provide some length to the columella. This should only be considered when the prolabium is large. A small flap is of little value. This method, with its multiple triangles, leaves little room for error and probably should not be attempted until one has considerable experience in cleft lip surgery.

The Skoog Repair

Skoog's repair of a bilateral cleft lip is essentially the same as his unilateral repair and is carried out as a two-staged operation (Figure 5–31). Following the initial stage, the premaxilla rotates toward the repaired side and the prolabium becomes thin on the side of the remaining cleft, just as it does in other two-staged repairs. Skoog raised a triangular flap on the lateral side of the prolabium and rotated this into the base of the columella to provide length. This is essentially one-half of Marcks' method for lengthening the columella. During the second stage of the lip repair, a triangular flap is raised on the other side of the prolabium and this flap is also placed in the base of the columella below the first flap. That completes the Marcks type of columellar lengthening operation in conjunction with the lip repair.

When the prolabium is a small mass, it is inadvisable to use tissue for lengthening the columella at the expense of the lip repair. Small flaps do not provide adequate release of the columella and nasal tip. It is only in the presence of a large prolabium, when there may be a tendency to sacrifice some prolabial tissue, that consideration should be given to incorporating a columellar lengthening procedure along with the lip repair. In our experience, we have generally preferred to consider the lengthening of the columella as a secondary procedure.

THE CLEFT PALATE

The aim in cleft palate surgery is to restore a functioning, anatomical structure that will improve speech, oronasopharyngeal physiology, and aesthetics without interfering with the form and function of all related parts. Presently, there seems to be an increasing interest in conservatism in cleft palate surgery with less emphasis on the more radical operations. There is greater attention to a balance between growth, structural relations and function and the type and timing of operations. Much of this came about from longitudinal studies on patients with a cleft lip and palate and from retrospective observations of long-term results. Laboratory studies on primates have given support to some clinical impressions. Improved interdisciplinary communication has helped to bring new knowledge and experiences together for us in a more effective manner and time sequence. The cleft of the palate is the hub of the wheel of the interdisciplinary services to patients with a facial cleft.

The normal anatomy and physiology of the palate and oronasal pharynx will not be reviewed, since this is available in appropriate manuscripts and texts. Some fundamental knowledge of anatomy and craniofacial biology is particularly important in a surgical program. There are some students of anatomy who believe that the levator veli palatini are the sole muscles utilized in normal velopharyngeal closure, while others are not entirely in agreement. The proponents hold that the levator veli palatini muscles are responsible for the elevation and traction of the soft palate and the posteromedial movement of the lateral walls on a level with the torus tubarius. The normal intact muscle forms a sling that extends across the palate from the posterior palatine aponeurosis anteriorly to the uvula posteriorly. In the cleft palate patient the levator palatini muscles are reduced in volume and tend to fatigue more easily. Muscle fibers extend anteriorly to the posterior border of the hard palate in those individuals. The salpingopharyngeus muscles are now known to be absent on one or both sides of the pharynx in about half of those with a cleft. The theory upon which the Hynes' pharyngoplasty is based then loses much of its validity. The tensor veli palatini muscles contain a superficial and deep portion. The superficial portion ends in a tendinous structure that passes around the hamular process of the sphenoid bone to spread out in the palatine aponeurosis in the anterior third of a normal palate, where it functions as its name applies. The deep portion arises from the lateral wall of the auditory tube. There is, therefore, no reason why a fracture of the hamular process would affect eustachian tube function, and this impression is supported by clinical investigation.

Important information to support surgical judgment is available in the field of craniofacial biology. It is now generally recognized that the form and function of the craniofacial structures are dependent upon the integrity of all related structures and systems, and the distortion or dysfunction of any structure may affect all related structures and systems. A mandible may be genetically normal, for example, but may develop an abnormal form and function because of its relations with an abnormal maxilla and an altered tongue position. Some of these problems are best studied in animal models. There are well-documented studies and observations in primate models and in man of the effects of surgery on growth and development and on the form and function of the structural elements. Craniofacial growth, which is not

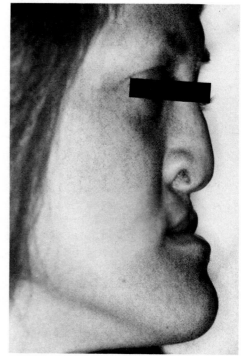

FIGURE 5–32 Maxillary and midface retrusion secondary to bilateral cleft lip and palate surgery. There was no evidence of a genetic predisposition to retromaxillism.

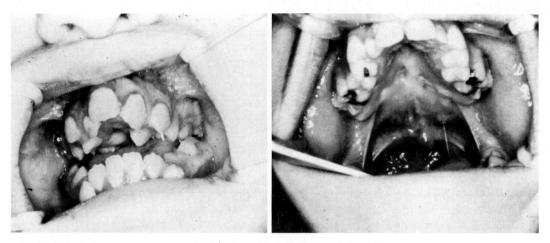

FIGURE 5–33   Two patients with marked dentoalveolar deformity secondary to scar contracture. The patient on the left has a heavily scarred palate with no vault. The one on the right has an "hour-glass" deformity.

clearly understood, is probably the result of several interacting systems. All of the structures have a morphogenetic ability to grow and a capacity to react. Restrictive scar or fibrous tissue is probably the common factor affecting midface growth following surgical intervention (Figure 5–32). A maxilla may be genetically deficient at birth, and poorly planned surgery may make the situation worse. It now appears possible to predict the pattern of facial growth and to plan a surgical program that will not complicate future development.

Prior to orthodontic intervention, most patients with a repaired cleft lip and palate will demonstrate some degree of arch asymmetry and deformity, varying from a crossbite limited to the canine on the cleft side to the extremes of retromaxillism or midface retrusion and the "hour-glass" deformity (Figures 5–32 and 5–33). We have been able to demonstrate a growth lag for as long as six months following a procedure as simple as a vomer flap. This lag is followed by a period of increased rate of growth or "catch-up" growth, so that recovery takes place within one year. An extensive and traumatic surgical episode may limit this recovery because of fibrosis and a false ankylosis.

In primate models, Kremenak[32-34] demonstrated that the removal of a strip of mucous membrane 4 mm. wide from the crest of the ridge will produce a growth disturbance. Later he removed a strip of mucosa from one palatal shelf, and this resulted in a narrowing or growth interference of approximately 12 per cent as compared with the normal side. Although one cannot always extrapolate from animals, nevertheless these experiments do give cause for concern about the location of palatal relaxing incisions and the denudation of bone at an early age. The surgeon facing the demands of society must be concerned about form and function, both of which are essential to aesthetics.

Retrospective studies by several surgeons (Rehrmann,[65] Dingman, and others) and animal models by Kremenak,[32-34] Atherton,[2] and other investigators have demonstrated that oral mucoperiosteum is related to bone growth and the direction of bone modeling. The dislocation of the mucoperiosteum and the contractural capabilities of fibrous tissue following an operation on

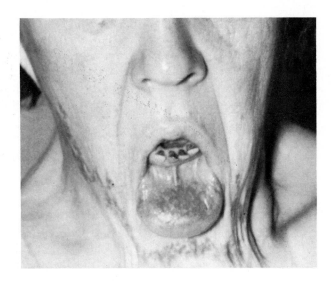

FIGURE 5–34 A burn scar contracture on the anterior neck has caused a deformity in the body of the mandible so that the lower incisor teeth are horizontal. Scar contracture on the palate can also cause structural deformities, which in turn can affect function and aesthetics.

the bony palate at an early age can lead to structural malrelations. Scar contracture on the anterior neck can deform or bend a developing mandible, and this serves as a conspicuous example of the powerful contractural capabilities of scar tissue (Figure 5–34).

Knowledge based on research and clinical experience now seems to us to provide firm support for a conservative surgical program during the periods of the child's active growth. Emphasis is on gentle technique and respect for complex biological growth processes, neurovascular supply, and the adverse effects of scar tissue. Enough time has passed so that we now realize that we have not had our best results in cleft palate surgery following the extensive mobilization of flaps over bony structures, such as in lengthening operations, the vonLangenbeck repair, or any method that might create scar tissue capable of restricting normal midface development. It is possible, of course, in reviewing the treatment of malformations as complicated and diversified as orofacial clefts, to learn that some patients turn out well by any of these methods, but there are others who develop complicated structural malformations. Respect for young growing parts cannot be overemphasized.

Following repair of a bilateral cleft lip and palate, there is constant favorable change in the segmental relationship of the premaxilla and the lateral maxillary segments, provided the alveolar clefts are not closed at the time of the primary lip and palate surgery and biological processes are not altered by scar tissue. Spatial relations will improve through the period of eruption of the deciduous dentition under the influence of a restored lip matrix and dentoalveolar adaptation, provided the lip is supple, the alveolar segments are not locked in, the tongue is normal, and the genetic background is favorable. There is a tissue deficiency in the anterior aspect of an affected maxillary alveolar segment. By the sixth year, the alveolar length approaches normal if it is not inhibited by surgical intervention and scar tissue. During periods of cleft palate surgery, temporary growth lags occur and may persist for six months. These are followed by a period of accelerated growth that will approach the normal within a year, again provided the operative design and resultant fibrosis are not restrictive. Hence, with all the knowledge now available from both research and clinical experience, a strong case can be made for a careful and conservative surgical philosophy on the part of the interdisciplinary group responsible for the care of cleft lip and palate patients. Such a conservative philosophy relating to facial cleft surgery should not imply use of only a single surgical protocol, but rather a constant awareness of the complexities of craniofacial growth and the adverse effects of scar tissue. Young, growing maxillary segments should be treated with the same surgical respect that one gives to a nerve or tendon repair. Scar tissue can impair normal relations and function in each situation.

TIME FOR CLEFT PALATE REPAIR

There has not been unanimity of opinion concerning the best time to repair a cleft of the palate, such as has prevailed with respect to the lip repair. Probably one should not fix on a single point in chronological time to repair clefts because of the wide variations in this malformation. In the past, growth morphologists have warned of the risks associated with early operative surgery on the palate, but they did so without much consideration for the various types of cleft. Many speech pathologists, on the other hand, have taken the position that early surgical correction leads to better speech with a need for less therapy. A healthy infant can tolerate cleft palate surgery very well at an early age. Narrow clefts with adequate tissue available can be repaired at six months of age if the surgeon so chooses. Some surgeons elect to repair the hard palate with a vomer flap at the same time that the lip is repaired. Probably the most popular period among surgeons has been 18 to 24 months, which is prior to the development of speech habits. A smaller group of surgeons would defer a primary repair until five to seven years of age, at which time considerable growth of the craniofacial complex has already taken place. The mean age at which we initiate most of our cleft palate repairs is about 12 months, usually shortly after the yearly examination by the team. We have not found this early period to be a disadvantage in our hands, so long as a conservative surgical program is adopted.

TECHNIQUE OF REPAIR OF CLEFT PALATE

Because there is no single procedure uniformly acceptable for the repair of all types of cleft palate, the literature contains descriptions of many different operations. Like other surgeons, we have used many of them at one time or another and have then abandoned those that were associated with a higher incidence of undesirable results. We have continued to alter our surgical protocol based on retrospective examinations of our longitudinal data. And we have finally selected only those operations that created the fewest structural malrelations for the patients in our longitudinal series.

The cleft palate operations that have been most helpful in our hands will be described and illustrated. Preoperative care and general anesthesia are essentially the same as that for the cleft lip patient. Since this is an elective procedure, it should not be undertaken until the hemoglobin level is adequate for the age and is not less than 10 grams. The child should also be free of infection, respiratory and ear infections being the most prevalent. Some patients with a cleft will also have cardiac and other anomalies, but the majority of them will tolerate the operation very well. Those patients with cardiac anomalies usually do well under general anesthesia because they are at rest with an increased oxygen tension.

The operations that we have utilized in our longitudinal series included the following:

A. Cleft of the soft palate only:
   1. Three layer closure—nasal mucosa, muscle layer, and oral mucosa—was performed.
   2. Some repairs were combined with the Veau-Wardill-Kilner two-flap pushback procedure.
   3. A primary pharyngeal flap was occasionally done when there was need for additional tissue to close the cleft.

B. Complete cleft palate:
   1. The vonLangenbeck repair was used in a comparatively few instances.
   2. The hard palate was closed with sliding mucoperiosteal flaps as part of a two-staged repair in some patients.
   3. When technically feasible, the hard palate was closed with bilateral vomer flaps in some patients. The soft palate was then closed four months later.
   4. Some patients had a two-flap lengthening procedure along with the closure of the soft palate.
   5. A primary veloplasty was done in some, with a delay of the repair of the hard palate.

C. Cleft lip and palate:
   1. When feasible, the hard palate was closed with a vomer flap that extended anteriorly only to the incisive foramen.
   2. The hard palate was closed with sliding mucoperiosteal flaps in another group of patients.
   3. The soft palate was closed four months after the repair of the hard palate in the two-staged repair.
   4. Some patients had a combined two-flap lengthening operation along with the closure of the soft palate.
   5. A vomer flap, soft palate closure, and two-flap lengthening procedure was done in one stage in a few patients.
   6. A primary veloplasty was done in still other patients, with a delay of the hard palate repair.
   7. A reorientation of the levator muscles was done in a comparatively few patients.

Cleft of the Soft Palate Only

Clefts of the soft palate, like the lip, can be divided into thirds for descriptive purposes, namely one-third, two-thirds, or three-thirds, depending upon the anterior extent of the cleft in the soft palate. A category of minimal cleft can also be added. Clefts of the palate also vary in width from narrow to wide. It is desirable to record the width at the widest point. The soft

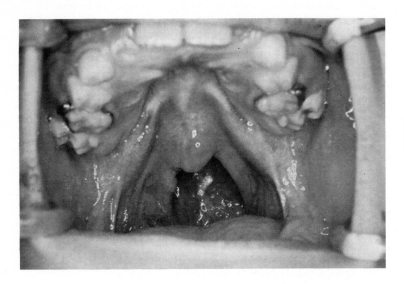

FIGURE 5–35 A congenitally deficient soft palate in which the uvula is at the posterior aspect of the hard palate.

palate will also have varying amounts of deficiency from slight to extreme, in which the uvula may be near the posterior border of the hard palate (Figure 5–35). Other factors should also be noted, such as any evidence of a neurological deficit with limited movement of the soft palate, asymmetry between the halves of the palate, and the size of adenoid and tonsil masses. Before the cleft is closed, one may be able to view the depth or expanse of the nasopharynx. If the surgeon wishes to make a dental cast recording of the cleft of the palate, this can be done after the patient is anesthetized. In an interdisciplinary team, face masks and dental casts are made by the dental specialists.

The Repair of the Soft Palate

The surgeon sits comfortably at the head of the table, and the palate is exposed with a mouth prop of the Dingman or Dott type. A small amount of 0.5 per cent lidocaine (Xylocaine) with epinephrine 1:100,000 is infiltrated into the soft palate and at the site of the lateral relaxing incisions without ballooning and distorting the tissues. It is important to handle the soft palate tissues gently with skin hooks in preference to crushing forceps. Even trauma from a suction tip can cause considerable edema of the uvula.

An incision is made from the anterior pole of the cleft entirely along one margin of the cleft. This allows the oral and nasal mucosa to retract and separate. The raw surface can be expanded by slight undermining of the mucosa with a fine pointed scissors or a scalpel. No tissue is sacrificed, except possibly a small amount of marginal mucosa on each half of the uvula. The same procedure is then performed on the opposite side. For convenience, it is well to learn to do one side with the right hand and the other with the left. The margins of the cleft are prepared before the palatal flaps are mobilized.

The relaxing incisions can then be made. A modified S-shaped incision is carried along the pterygomandibular raphe to the posterolateral aspect of the tuberosity and is then curved medially around the tuberosity to the posterior border of the hard palate. It then extends anteriorly along the line demarcating the alveolar process and palatal shelf, just far enough to permit closure of the soft palate flaps. Frequently, the incision can be terminated after curving medially around the tuberosity without extending it anteriorly on the hard palate. A cleft that extends into the posterior edge of the hard palate can be closed by elevating the adjacent mucoperiosteum through the lateral relaxing incision without extending the lateral cuts onto the hard palate. If the lateral incision extends onto the buccal mucosa, the buccal fat pad may be released into the field. This is a nuisance but causes no problem, provided it is buried in the cheek.

The index finger is then slipped into the wound behind the tuberosity along the pterygomandibular raphe. The area of separation is just lateral to the hamular process and the inner wall of the pharynx. The hamular process can be fractured with the finger during this maneuver, although it should not be fractured needlessly. As the finger moves inward to separate the palatal flap from the dense, glistening pterygomandibular raphe, the pressure of the finger should be against the firm lateral wall or raphe to avoid tearing the flap. It will be necessary to separate the attachments at the posterior aspect of the hard palate for clefts involving more than two-thirds of the soft palate. The posterior neurovascular bundle should be preserved in all palate repairs, although it will not be visualized in most partial clefts of the soft palate. After completing the opposite side, it should be possible to approximate the flaps with ease. There is a risk of dehiscence if the flaps are closed under tension. When the surgeon is convinced that the palate can be closed without tension, no further relaxation or dissection is needed unless there is an apparent advantage in the realignment of the levator veli palatini muscles.

The palatal flaps are then ready for closure. The nasal mucosa is closed first, using a 4–0 absorbable suture material. The muscle layer should then be accurately approximated without leaving suture knots between the approximated muscles. One technique that has worked well is to pass a 3–0 chromic suture from one lateral relaxation incision through the muscle layer of both palatal flaps and out the opposite relaxing incision. The suture is then passed

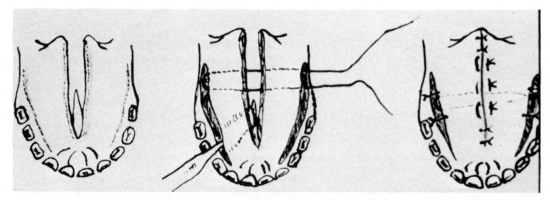

FIGURE 5–36 Illustration of transfixion suture in the muscle layer of the soft palate. The suture is passed through the muscle layer of both halves of the palate and then back to the relaxation incision, similar to a horizontal mattress suture. Ordinarily three sutures are used; one in the anterior third, one in the middle third and another at the base of the uvula. We have had extremely few postsurgical fistulae and no necrosis of tissue.

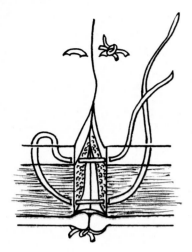

FIGURE 5–37 A vertical mattress-type suture to approximate the muscle and oral mucosal layers. The nasal mucosa is sutured separately.

back on the same level to form a horizontal mattress-type suture. Three such sutures are adequate, with one in the anterior third, one in the middle third, and one at the base of the uvula. These hold the flaps together effectively with no knots buried in the repair site and without strangulation of tissues. The oral mucosa is then closed, making sure it is everted at the repair site. We have had extremely few palatal fistulae develop with this method (Figure 5–36).

Another method that we have used and one that avoids knots in the repair site is to pass a suture through the oral mucosa and muscle to the nasal mucosa, then across the cleft beneath the nasal mucosa, and out through the oral surface. This suture, essentially a vertical mattress type, then picks up the edges of the oral mucosa and is tied (Figure 5–37). It closes muscle and oral mucosa and everts the mucosal edges with no buried knots. The lateral relaxing wounds are loosely closed with absorbable sutures, using 4–0 chromic catgut. A Z-plasty is frequently done between the tuberosity and the retromolar area to minimize the bowstring contracture often seen at that site in the relaxing incision (Figure 5–38).

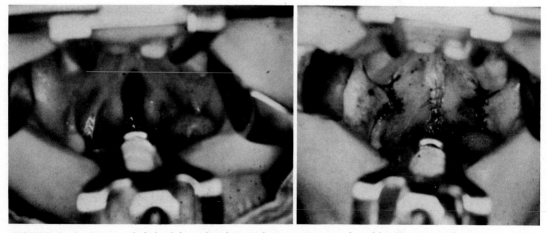

FIGURE 5–38 Repair of cleft of the soft palate without an associated pushback. Frequently a Z-plasty is done to reduce bow-stringing at the site of the lateral relaxation incision, as demonstrated on the patient's right side.

Following this operative procedure, most of the palates have exhibited elevation and traction of the velum, provided there was no preoperative neurological deficit. If the surgeon prefers, the levator veli palatini muscle on either side can be dissected out and realigned to restore a sling in a manner similar to realignment of the orbicularis oris muscle. The reconstruction of the levator sling is an important advancement for some patients in whom the cleft of the soft palate is complete (Figure 5–38). The muscle is detached from the posterior border of the hard palate in all cleft repairs involving more than two-thirds of the soft palate. Elevation of the palate has been good regardless of whether the muscle was realigned, provided the muscle layer was well approximated.

Complete Cleft Palate

Any cleft that does not extend forward to the incisive foramen is a partial cleft or an incomplete cleft. Clefts of the hard palate, like clefts of the lip and the soft palate, can be divided into thirds—one-third, two-thirds, and three-thirds. A cleft palate is frequently referred to as a partial cleft or a complete cleft, but it is probably more accurate to state that it is a cleft involving three-thirds of the soft palate and three-thirds of the hard palate if the cleft extends anteriorly to the incisive foramen. The risk of creating a structural malformation is greater when the cleft extends into the hard palate because the repair may violate the integrity of the oral mucoperiosteum and lead to scar contracture in some patients (Figure 5–39). The bone flap technique of Dieffenbach[16] was designed to repair the hard palate cleft by

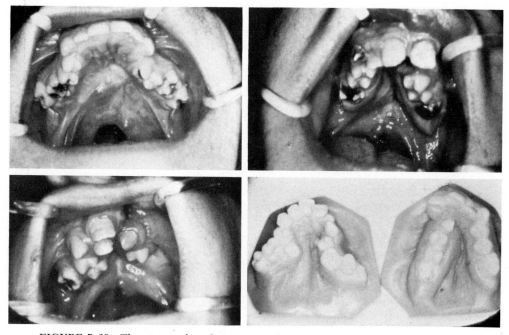

FIGURE 5–39   Three examples of patients we have seen with contractural deformities of the palate and maxillary dental arches.

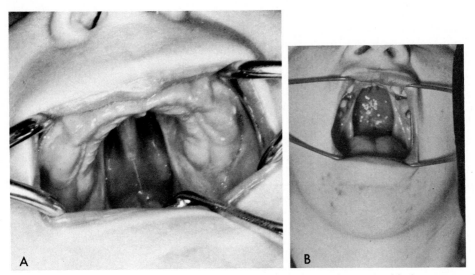

FIGURE 5–40   Two patients with wide complete clefts of the palate not suitable for a repair of the hard palate by either bilateral vomer flaps or sliding mucoperiosteal flaps. Clefts as extensive as these are best treated with a prosthesis.

moving the palatal shelves medially and leaving the overlying mucoperiosteum intact. Most clefts of the hard palate that are not associated with a cleft involving the lip and alveolar process are not suitable for a repair by a vomer flap (Figure 5–40). This is because the cleft is too wide, or the septum is too high above the palatal shelves, or the hard palate is only partially clefted.

In order to reduce the incidence of surgically acquired structural malrelations, we decided to treat some of the patients who had a complete cleft of the palate with a primary veloplasty and to delay the repair of the hard palate. The length of delay for closure of the hard palate depends upon growth and structural changes and frequently may extend to the age of six years or older. As soon as the patient is cooperative, the cleft of the hard palate can be covered with a temporary dental prosthesis, and this is determined in our group conference. We try to design a surgical plan that takes advantage of biological growth processes with little dependence upon prostheses to resist structural change. There are situations in which the infants are too young to cooperate in the wearing of a prosthesis, or have problems with retention due to shedding of teeth, or have poor oral hygiene so that a prosthesis is inadvisable.

We formerly closed all clefts involving the hard palate at about one year of age with either a vomer flap or sliding mucoperiosteal flaps. We now delay the closure of the hard palate and consider a primary veloplasty when a bilateral vomer flap is not feasible. Admittedly, a primary veloplasty is not suitable for all patients, particularly those with a wide cleft of the soft palate, unless the surgeon acquires additional tissue by means of a pharyngeal flap. Closure of a wide cleft of the soft palate by a primary veloplasty will shorten a soft palate that is already deficient and will contribute to poor speech. There are some patients in whom it is better to delay all surgery on the palate until about six years of age, and many of these children can wear a temporary prosthesis.

The operations that we formerly used for repair of a complete cleft of the

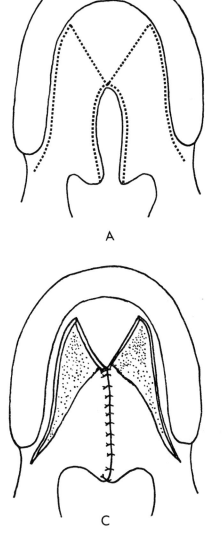

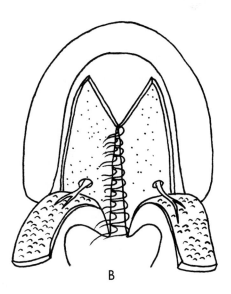

FIGURE 5-41   The W/V-Y lengthening procedure performed in some patients along with closure of the cleft of the soft palate. In a two-staged procedure, the W/V-Y was part of the second stage.

palate were predominantly of three types. If the vomer extended well down between the palatal shelves in a complete cleft of the palate, the hard palate would be repaired at one year of age with a bilateral vomer flap, and the soft palate would be repaired four months later. A Veau-Wardill-Kilner two–flap type pushback operation was carried out in conjunction with the soft palate repair in about half of the patients (Figure 5–41). In another group of patients, the hard palate was closed with sliding mucoperiosteal flaps of the vonLangenbeck type, provided the vomer flaps could not be used. This repair was also staged, with repair of the soft palate carried out four months later in the manner previously described. This two-stage repair was essentially a two-staged vonLangenbeck procedure, in which it was possible to obtain a better palatal vault and less postoperative shortening of the soft palate than

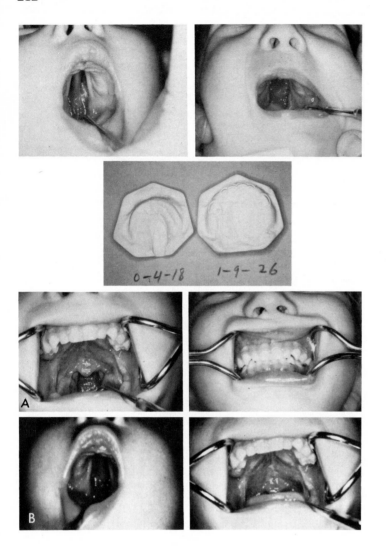

FIGURE 5–42 Two patients with complete clefts of the palate that were closed in two stages to preserve a better vault and length.

with a one-stage repair (Figure 5–42). Closing the hard palate with sliding mucoperiosteal flaps and delaying the soft palate closure made it possible to retain attachments at the posterior border of the hard palate at the first operation. It was reasoned that this might tend to resist postoperative shortening of the soft palate from any scar contracture in the hard palate. Scar contracture is three-dimensional, and we did create some narrowing of the maxillary arch by cicatricial orthodontia in some patients treated by this method. We were unable to predict with accuracy in which patients this would occur. A W/V–Y two-flap lengthening procedure was also carried out in conjunction with the soft palate repair in some of the patients.

A third group of patients, particularly those in whom the cleft of the palate extended only through the posterior one-third or two-thirds of the hard palate, was treated in a single operative procedure with sliding vonLangenbeck flaps or with sliding flaps associated with a Veau-Wardill-Kilner lengthening operation (Figure 5–43). We did not create structural malrelations with a bilateral vomer flap repair, but we did produce narrowing and dental

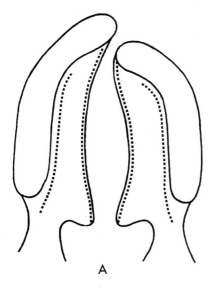

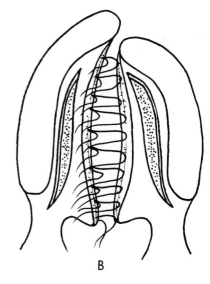

FIGURE 5-43 Illustration of vonLangenbeck's sliding flaps. Because of the development of structural malrelations in some patients, we have curtailed this method of palatal closure.

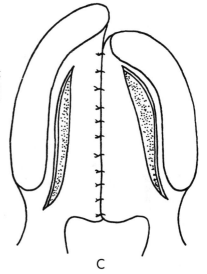

malrelations in the posterior arch in some, but not all, of the patients in whom the oral mucoperiosteum was widely elevated. Consequently, we have gradually altered our philosophy and have curtailed those procedures that require wide mobilization of the oral mucoperiosteum at an early age. We now prefer to do a primary veloplasty for some patients when the hard palate cannot be closed with vomer flaps or to defer the palate repair entirely if the cleft is wide. A dental prosthesis is then used until such time as the repair is associated with less risk of structural impairment.

Occasionally, when the cleft of the soft palate is wide, a superior-based pharyngeal flap is used to supply additional tissue. This will lessen the risk of a tight closure with increased shortening of the soft palate and will reduce the size of the velopharyngeal gap.

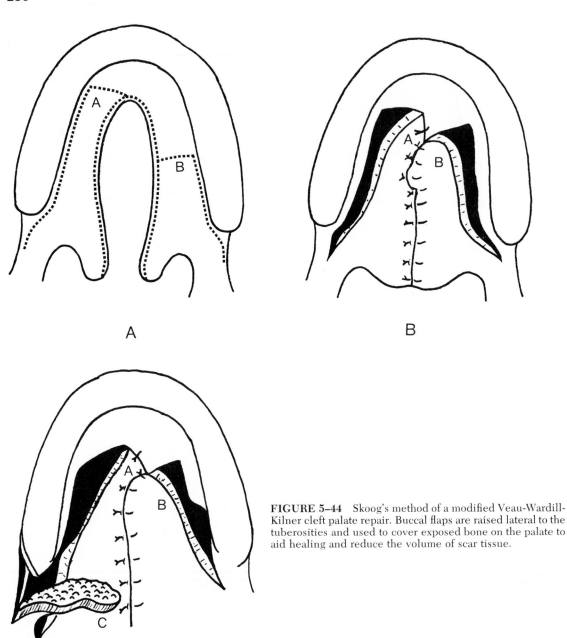

A

B

C

FIGURE 5-44 Skoog's method of a modified Veau-Wardill-Kilner cleft palate repair. Buccal flaps are raised lateral to the tuberosities and used to cover exposed bone on the palate to aid healing and reduce the volume of scar tissue.

Skoog's Method of Palate Repair

In Skoog's method (Figure 5–44) bilateral asymmetrical oral mucoperiosteal flaps are elevated to close the hard palate. On one side, a flap is raised beyond the anterior pole of the cleft, and this is rotated medially to cover the full length of the cleft. A shorter flap is raised on the opposite side. The nasal mucoperiosteum is then mobilized and repaired in the midline throughout the full length of the cleft. The posterior neurovascular bundles are preserved, and the muscle is detached from the posterior border of the hard palate. The long flap is rotated over the cleft and sutured to a wedge of intact oral mucoperiosteum anterior to the short flap. The short flap is rotated medially across the cleft and sutured to the oral mucoperiosteum of the opposite side. The surgeon then closes the soft palate, making certain that the muscle layer is well approximated. A flap of buccal mucosa is raised lateral to the tuberosity and rotated to the palate to partially cover the denuded bone at the donor areas of the mucoperiosteal flaps. Skoog believed that these buccal flaps closed most of the wound, promoted healing, and reduced the amount of scar formation, which is a decided advantage. The operation is essentially a modification of the V–Y principle, and there is some gain in the length of the palate.

Perhaps in the future medical control of scar tissue and contracture will open the door to new surgical concepts.

Complete Unilateral Cleft of the Lip and Palate

A complete cleft of the palate in association with a cleft of the lip is now usually managed surgically in one of two ways. If structural relations make a vomer flap feasible, the hard palate is closed at one year of age with a vomer flap that extends anteriorly only to the incisive foramen. A vomer flap is not always technically suitable for a repair of the hard palate. One alternative is a primary repair of the velum or Schweckendiek veloplasty, carried out as the initial procedure with a delayed closure of the hard palate. Some surgeons elect to do a vomer flap at the time that the lip is repaired. Many surgeons close the cleft in the alveolar process along with the vomer flap, and we used to do this type of complete closure. For several years now our preference has been to repair the hard palate with a vomer flap at one year of age, leaving the alveolar ridge open so that the segments would be free to undergo molding and dentoalveolar adaptation under the influence of normal biological growth processes. We have observed that under these circumstances arch relations begin to change about the third year and improve through the period of eruption of the deciduous dentition. The patients will frequently develop an end-to-end or butt-joint approximation between the maxillary alveolar segments without the aid of dental orthopedic appliances. There have been very few complaints relative to the leakage of food or fluids through the alveolar cleft, particularly after the segmental relations have improved (Figures 5–45 to 5–48). The alveolar clefts are usually closed at about 12 years of age. There is an increase of about 2.5 mm in the width of the anterior maxillary ridge at about 11 years of age. For that reason, the alveolar cleft repair is delayed until after that growth spurt. The alveolar clefts are closed with mucoperiosteal flaps and sometimes with bone grafts.

All surgery has an effect upon growth when carried out over the bony parts at an early age. Following a procedure as simple as a vomer flap, there is a lag in the growth curve compared with normals that lasts approximately six months. Following the lag, a period of accelerated or "catch-up" growth occurs, so that within a year the growth curve approaches normal. After some

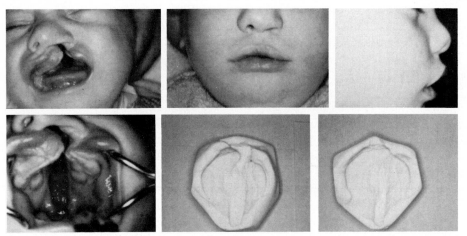

FIGURE 5–45   Following closure of the cleft lip, there is reduction in width of the hard palate cleft as illustrated in the casts.

of the more extensive operations, the recovery may not be complete. This is one of the reasons why we have some concern about operations that extensively violate the oral mucoperiosteum at an early age.

To raise a vomer flap, an incision is made along the base of the vomerine bone at the junction of the oral and nasal mucosa and is extended anteriorly to

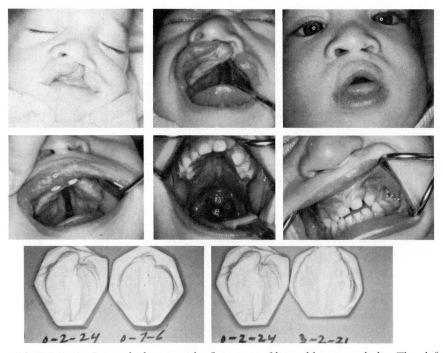

FIGURE 5–46   Patient had a triangular flap repair of lip and has a supple lip. The cleft of the hard palate then becomes narrower. The hard palate was closed at 1 year with a vomer flap that extended anteriorly to the incisive foramen. The soft palate was closed without a W/V-Y push-back 4 months later. The arch relations are good. The patient has a buccal crossbite on the left side, which is easily corrected by orthodontia.

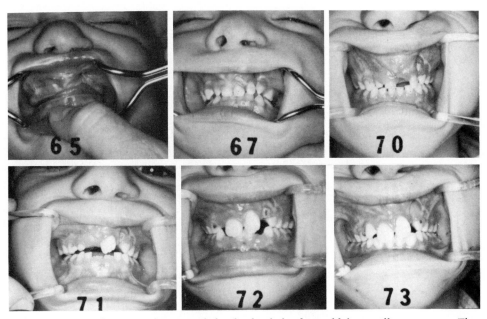

FIGURE 5–47 This patient has a supple lip that has helped to mold the maxillary segments. The patient also had a two-staged palate repair without a pushback. The dentoalveolar relations have improved and remained satisfactory through the period of eruption of the deciduous dentition.

the region of the incisive foramen. The vomer flap is elevated and turned over in order to be sutured underneath the raised edge of the oral mucoperiosteum on the opposite side. There is minimal violation of the oral mucoperiosteum. The open wound will heal by second intention, closing the cleft of the hard

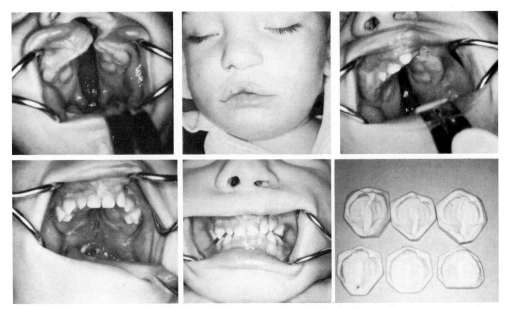

FIGURE 5–48 This patient had a lip repair and a two-staged palatal procedure without a pushback. The dental-arch relations are good without the use of orthopedic measures. Normal dental arch relations are important in both function and aesthetics.

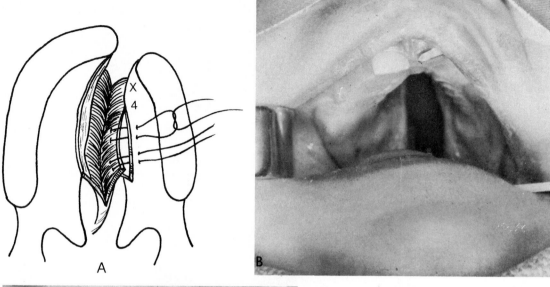

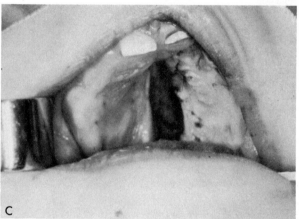

FIGURE 5–49   Illustration of vomer flap that extends anteriorly only to the incisive foramen. The alveolar cleft is left open to encourage molding of segments and dentoalveolar adaptation. There is minimal violation of the oral mucoperiosteum.

palate. This leaves a cleft of the soft palate posteriorly and of the alveolar ridge anteriorly (Figure 5–49).

Following closure of the hard palate with the vomer flap, the soft palate is repaired about four months later, in some cases with and in some without an associated two-flap W/V–Y type lengthening procedure for evaluation purposes. In a few instances, we have closed the cleft of the hard palate with a vomer flap and have repaired the cleft of the soft palate in conjunction with a lengthening operation in a single stage.

For those patients for whom a vomer flap repair is not feasible, we have now adopted the primary veloplasty in many instances. The primary veloplasty is best suited for the patient with a complete cleft lip and palate.

Primary restoration of the soft palate matrix is followed by a narrowing of the cleft of the hard palate. The cleft becomes narrow from molding of the segments, similar to that which occurs following repair of the cleft of the lip. In addition, there is growth of the palatal shelves; the shelf on the cleft side grows more slowly than that on the normal side. Should any lowering of the

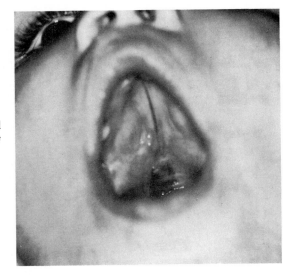

FIGURE 5–50   Following a primary veloplasty, the hard palate cleft narrowed to a slit. The baby had a complete unilateral cleft lip and palate.

palatal shelves occur, it would help to narrow the cleft further. In some instances the cleft may gradually narrow to a slit or a point of contact between the palatal shelves so that air pressure can be built up and there is less interference with speech development (Figure 5–50). The hard palate can then be closed by simply elevating the margins of the cleft and suturing them together without extensive violation of the oral mucoperiosteum and the associated risk of scar contracture. If the cleft of the hard palate remains relatively wide, we may close the hard palate with a temporary dental prosthesis whenever the patient is cooperative and defer surgical closure of the hard palate until six years or older, depending upon the circumstances.

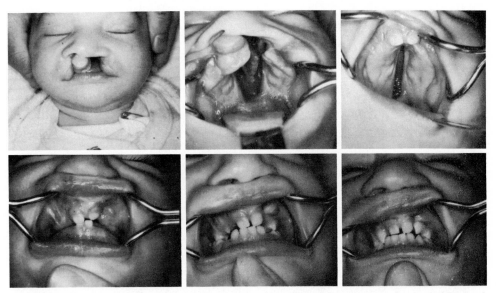

FIGURE 5–51   An asymmetrical bilateral cleft of the lip and palate with narrowing of the hard palate cleft following the lip repair. The palate was closed in two stages without a pushback. The dental and arch relations improve through the period of eruption of the deciduous dentition under the influence of normal biological growth processes, provided the segments are not restricted by scar tissue and the alveolar clefts are not "locked in."

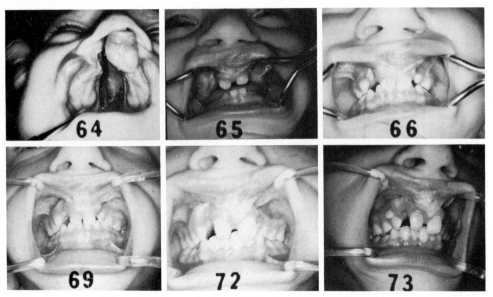

FIGURE 5–52 A bilateral cleft lip and palate with the development of satisfactory arch relations.

Bilateral Cleft Lip and Palate

The bilateral cleft palate is managed in a manner similar to that described for the unilateral cleft lip and palate. The cleft of the palate varies in width, depending in part upon the relationship of the maxillary segments. The cleft

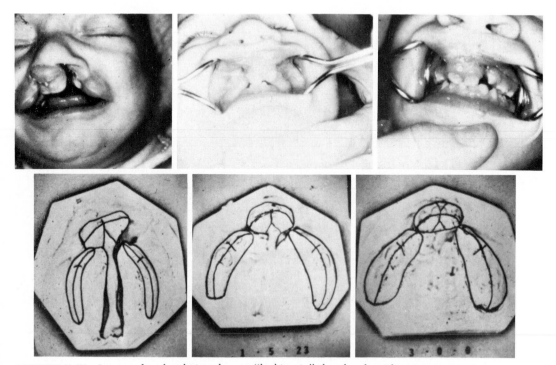

FIGURE 5–53 Improved arch relations by not "locking in" the alveolar ridges to encourage dentoalveolar adaptation.

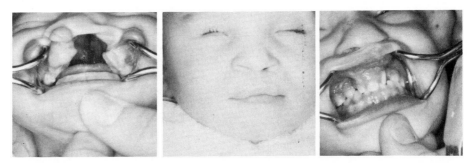

FIGURE 5-54 A postoperative bilateral cleft lip and palate. The lip is supple, the palate is not restrictive, and the alveolar clefts are left open. The patient developed satisfactory arch relations through the period of eruption of the deciduous dentition.

may be wide and the septum may appear to be deficient and high above the palatal shelves. If the nasal septum is suspended between the palatal shelves and the cleft is not wide, we would elect to close the cleft of the hard palate with bilateral vomer flaps, again extending anteriorly only to the level of the incisive foramen (Figures 5–51, 5–52, 5–53, and 5–54). The clefts in the alveolar ridge are left open to enhance molding and dentoalveolar adaptation. The soft palate is repaired four months later, and we have combined the repair with a two-flap lengthening operation in some patients but not in others. If the structural relations are not conducive to a vomer flap palatoplasty, the repair of the hard palate is delayed and a primary veloplasty may be carried out at one year of age (Figure 5–55).

The Primary Veloplasty

Based on a review of our longitudinal data, we have curtailed operations that extensively challenge the oral mucoperiosteum at an early age, such as the lengthening operations, the island flaps, and the vonLangenbeck

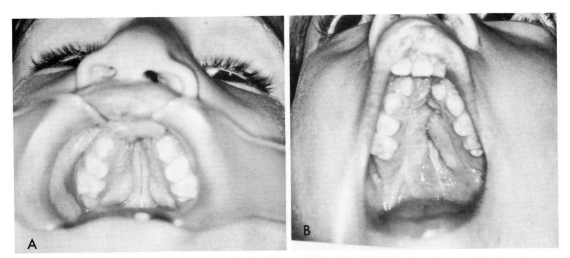

FIGURE 5-55 A, This baby had a bilateral cleft of the lip and palate. In properly selected cases involving the lip and palate, the hard palate cleft may narrow considerably. B, A bilateral cleft apparently closed by the vonLangenbeck method with constriction of the maxillary arch. With good case selection, many structural deformities can be avoided.

palatoplasty. We have elected to do a larger number of primary veloplasties and to study our results with this procedure. Closure of at least two-thirds of the soft palate restores the posterior matrix but also tends to shorten the soft palate. When performing a primary veloplasty, the lateral relaxing incisions are usually made first. These extend along the pterygomandibular raphe to the tuberosity and then around the tuberosity to the posterior border of the hard palate. The relaxing incision does not need to extend anteriorly on the hard palate. After the flaps are mobilized, one can determine the extent to which the margins of the cleft will need to be opened for the repair. Ordinarily we like to close as much of the soft palate as possible and attempt to close at least two-thirds in the wider clefts. We usually do not use a primary pharyngeal flap (P-flap) with a palate repair, but this does provide additional tissue when one is attempting to close a wide cleft of the soft palate as previously mentioned. In addition, the P-flap reduces the size of the velopharyngeal gap and

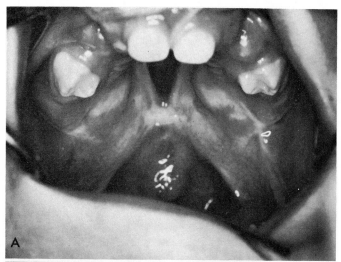

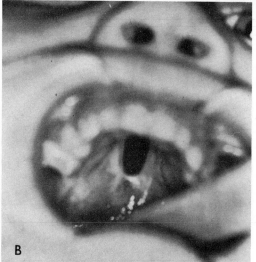

FIGURE 5–56 *A,* A primary veloplasty that encourages poor speech. The anterior cleft or fistula is wide, and the soft palate is short, with the uvula at the posterior border of the hard palate. Proper selection of cases for this procedure is important. *B,* A persistent wide cleft of the hard palate following a primary repair of the velum. The patient had a complete cleft of the palate. This hard palate opening will need to be closed temporarily with a prosthesis and surgically at the proper time.

enhances the chance of velopharyngeal competence when the cleft is wide and the palate is shortened by the repair.

The quality of speech is one measure of function that helps to evaluate the quality of palatal surgery. A speech evaluation was carried out on a group of patients who had had a two-staged palatal repair without an associated lengthening operation and excluding those who had had a primary veloplasty. It was determined that 73 to 76 per cent of these patients had a good quality of speech without hypernasality. After evaluating them, the examining therapists arrived at a range rather than a single number. In evaluating the speech of a large group of patients, it was found that some do not perform equally well on each visit, which suggests that some may have a borderline velopharyngeal competence. This range is approximately that of the national average for palates repaired by other methods.

The primary veloplasty is not a routinely satisfactory operation, but it is a technique that should be considered in a cleft palate program. It is best suited for patients who have a complete cleft lip and palate because there is a greater chance of significant narrowing of the hard palate with no major speech maladjustment. In those with cleft palate only and those with wider clefts, there will be less narrowing of the hard palate cleft but increased shortening of the soft palate with a larger velopharyngeal gap (Figure 5–56). Hence, a poorer quality speech with compensatory maladjustments will result. If a primary veloplasty is part of the plan of management of a complete or a wide cleft palate, a temporary prosthesis will be essential to help the patient build up oral pressure until the final surgical measures are carried out.

Congenital Velopharyngeal Incompetence and Submucous Cleft Palate

These are two entities that now occupy more attention in a cleft palate program. Patients with a congenital velopharyngeal incompetence (VPI) do not have a submucous cleft palate but rather a disparity between the length or function of the soft palate and the size of the oronasal pharynx. The diagnosis is often made following removal of the tonsils and adenoids because of a persistent oronasal imbalance (Figure 5–57).

A patient with a submucous cleft palate will exhibit a soft palate that is short compared with the normal. There is a submucous separation of the soft palate musculature, a palpable notch in the posterior border of the hard palate, and frequently a notching or clefting of the uvula. The presence of a submucous cleft is not an indication for an operation, and when indicated, the restoration of muscle continuity alone is inadequate (Figure 5–58).

Patients with congenital VPI or a submucous cleft palate with VPI should first have an adequate speech evaluation and perhaps a trial on therapy. If there is evidence of a neurological deficit or fatigability, we frequently recommend a trial with a palatal lift prosthesis for a few months. This may help to improve muscle function so that an operation is unnecessary, or it may enhance the level of velopharyngeal competence. If VPI with speech impairment persists, definitive therapy is carried out, usually with a pharyngeal flap.

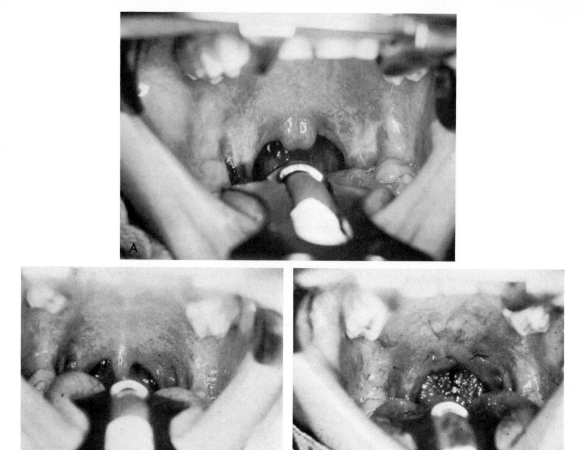

FIGURE 5–57 *A*, Congenital velpharyngeal incompetence. The levator veli palatini muscles are intact and united at the midline, and there is no notch in the posterior border of the hard palate. The patient does have a shallow groove in the uvula. *B*, Congenital velopharyngeal incompetence treated with a superior based pharyngeal flap because of persistent hypernasality.

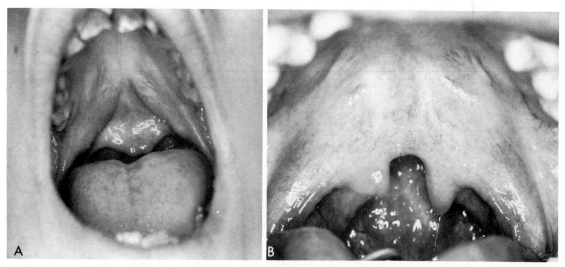

FIGURE 5–58 *A*, Patient with submucous cleft palate saying "ah" to demonstrate notch at posterior border of hard palate. *B*, This patient has a submucous cleft palate with thin mucosa at the site of separation of the levator veli palatini muscles, a cleft of the uvula, and a notch in the posterior border of the hard palate. Repair of the muscle and cleft uvula is inadequate to correct velopharyngeal incompetence.

The care of a patient with a cleft palate is best managed by an interdisciplinary group in which there is mutual respect and restraint. The question that needs to be answered is what to do and when to do it. The type and timing of surgical and other services are most important, and these decisions are best provided by the concerted effort of the cleft palate team. It is important to restore a cleft palate, but it is equally important to be aware of the results of surgical intervention and its effect upon structural relations, aesthetics, and function. There is probably no situation in which an awareness of the effects of surgery on growth and development is more essential than in cleft palate surgery on an infant. A surgical protocol should not rely too heavily upon dental services to prevent or correct malformations resulting from operative intervention. There is enough need for the service of dental specialists in the normal care of a patient with a cleft palate.

If a retrospective review of the results of surgery reveals too many structural malrelations, perhaps the surgical program needs to be revised. Cleft of the palate is not a simple problem, although we do have many options and surgical procedures. It is unlikely that there will ever be a single surgical procedure applicable to all cleft palate cases. We are fortunate in having enough options to provide a sophisticated surgical service. A familiarity with biological growth processes, altered pathophysiology, and the results of related research projects will provide a basis for judgment if our surgical approaches must be modified. We believe that we have improved our overall results in cleft palate management since our surgical protocol has been revised to avoid extensive surgical intervention over the bony parts at an early age. We now have greater respect for the integrity of the oral mucoperiosteum and the capabilities of the fibroblast and scar contracture. We still are faced with structural malformations following surgical intervention, but they are fewer in number and more easily correctable, without the need to rely upon major secondary procedures. The cost in time, money, and disappointment of some surgically induced malformations is very high. We are particularly anxious to avoid the major malformations, such as a midface retrusion. The common crossbites, such as those involving the canines, are a minor orthodontic problem.

VELOPHARYNGEAL INCOMPETENCE

Velopharyngeal incompetence is a condition in which there is inadequate functional valving or balance between the oral and nasal cavities. A hypernasal quality to the speech or rhinolalia aperta is frequently an early indication of incompetence. Other signs may develop, such as nasal air escape or emission, compensatory maladjustments including facial grimaces, glottal stops, and articulatory problems with distortion of sibilant sounds. Velopharyngeal incompetence may be camouflaged by an active superior pharyngeal constrictor muscle, a large adenoid pad, or nasal impedance.

The velopharyngeal mechanism may vary in its degree of competency or incompetency from a functional closure to a very large gap. The quality of speech may vary from one that is intelligible with good articulation to one that is totally unintelligible. Speech is a complicated and highly sophisticated human function, and it is one criterion upon which the success of cleft palate surgery is based.

The anatomical variations commonly associated with VPI are:

1. A congenital short palate in association with a normal pharynx. The door is too small for the frame.

2. A congenital large pharynx with an apparently normal soft palate. The frame is too large for the door.

3. A submucous cleft palate in which there is a submucosal separation of the soft palate muscle mass, a palpable notch in the posterior border of the hard palate, and a short soft palate.

4. A palate with a cleft. All clefted palates are short compared with normals, and this may persist postoperatively.

5. A neuromuscular deficit with partial or complete paresis of the soft palate.

6. A deficiency of the soft palate due to trauma, disease, or excisional surgery.

At some point every clinician who sees a large cleft palate population will find a patient with an unoperated cleft and intelligible speech. And there will be other patients (usually young adults) who, based on clinical inspection of the oral cavity, should be talking poorly but do not. They are in oronasal balance in spite of what appears to be a very short palate.

DIAGNOSIS

The diagnosis of velopharyngeal incompetence is usually made from a speech sample. But a speech sample alone is not enough to support a complete and accurate diagnosis and the recommendation for surgical intervention. If the surgeon undertakes a pharyngeal flap without further assessment of the patient, it may turn out to be simply a surgical exercise. An adequate medical and social history is fundamental in the management. Family cooperation is most important in assisting the patient to develop intelligible speech.

It is also helpful to have some concept of the patient's level of intelligence. Every effort should be made to provide those who have great potential with a quality of speech that is as good as possible. Then there are individuals at the opposite extreme, such as those destined to be institutionalized, who will need a palate repair but will gain little with a pharyngeal flap and velopharyngeal competence. There are also physical findings of importance. These include dental health, hearing status as revealed by audiometric studies, structional relations and palatal vault, the position and function of the tongue, palatopharyngeal muscle function, the size and health of the tonsils and adenoids, and evidence of a neurological deficit with decreased muscle activity. It is also essential to inspect the soft palate for perforations, excessive fibrous tissue, midline separation of the levator veli palatini muscles, and the thickness of the palate. The patency of the nasal airway should be determined. An estimate of the size and shape of the velopharyngeal port is quite significant in relation to prognosis. In short, one should make a broad assessment of the problem and not simply determine the presence of hypernasal speech.

Sophisticated instruments and examination methods are available for studying velopharyngeal competence. These include cephalometric films with a lateral, frontal, basal or Towne's view in a functional and rest position; sound cinefluorography; multiview videofluoroscopy; laminagraphy; fiberoptic nasendoscopy (an invasive technique); ultrasonography; sonograms;

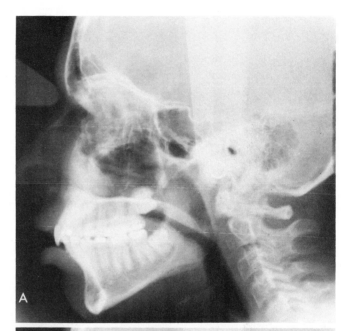

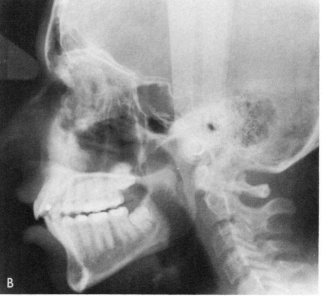

FIGURE 5–59 *A*, Lateral cephalometric film in rest position. *B*, Lateral cephalometric film in functional position. This is a static view, but it does provide valuable information to the clinician.

electromyography; TONAR or oronasal acoustic ratios; aerodynamics; and others. There are also helpful clinical tests such as flowing devices, fogging mirrors, listening devices, and so forth, but these are of little value for investigative purposes.

It is both possible and practical to conduct a clinical practice with a high degree of competence without the advantages of all the sophisticated technology essential to research. If one has obtained a good history and a thorough clinical evaluation, including an adequate speech assessment, velopharyngeal incompetence can be diagnosed and treated adequately. Probably the single most important technical aid is a good lateral cephalometric film in a position of rest and function (Figure 5–59). These x-ray films provide a static view of velar elevation, velar stretch, depth of the nasopharynx, an anteroposterior diameter of the velopharyngeal port at rest and during function, the size of the adenoid pad, and the elevation of Passavant's ridge. Cephalometric films also present a sagittal contour of the cranial base and the position of a pharyngeal flap, if one is present. Investigative projects with the aid of expensive and sophisticated technology should lead to new knowledge and principles that will enable clinicians to provide a competent service without the necessity of relying on expensive instrumentation. In this way, adequate patient services can be provided at a more reasonable cost.

Velopharyngeal competency depends upon the size and shape of the velopharyngeal orifice, lung output, vocal cords, tongue, lips and nasal impedance. Warren found that velopharyngeal insufficiency begins when the area of the velopharyngeal orifice is within the 10 to 20 sq. mm. range. Competency is also dependent upon the shape of the orifice, and hypernasality can be present when the area is less than 10 sq. mm., depending largely upon the shape. When the velopharyngeal mechanism is incompetent, the patient develops hypernasality, nasal air escape, reduced pressure or volume, and compensatory maladjustments such as facial grimaces, glottal stops, altered tongue position, and so forth. There is no substitute for a good speech evaluation in determining velopharyngeal competence.

TREATMENT

The diagnosis and best management of velopharyngeal incompetence require the cooperative effort of the interdisciplinary cleft palate group. A number of proposals have been made for the improvement of the velopharyngeal mechanism. This is primarily because of the variations in the nature of the problem and because the treatment is not always successful. Many factors have a bearing on the results of treatment. Whether or not the patient has a hearing loss and what the patient hears are important. A parent with hypernasal speech and defective articulation will be a poor home teacher. Intelligence and cooperation of the patient and family are important. These are but a few of the factors that should be considered when contemplating construction of a pharyngeal flap.

The following are some of the proposals for improving velopharyngeal competency.

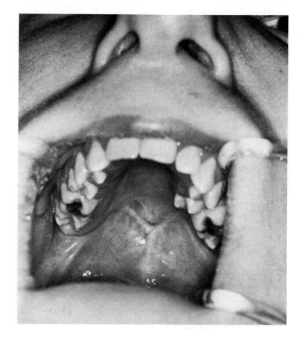

FIGURE 5–60 A hypertrophied scar outlining the two flaps of the W/V-Y repair. One band of scar leads directly to the medially malposed bicuspid.

Palate Lengthening

Palate lengthening operations as an independent procedure are generally unsatisfactory. Substantial palatal lengthening is associated with the risk of maxillary growth impairment of structural malrelations. This is because of the denudation of large areas of bone and the limitations resulting from fibrous tissue. This risk diminishes with increasing age. There is also the surgical risk of acquiring a neurological deficit of the soft palate musculature. The accidental disruption of the posterior palatine neurovascular bundles can also occur, but this does not appear to impair structural growth or survival of the palatal flaps. Usually there is some postoperative shortening of the palate following lengthening operations that is due to wound healing, scar formation, and contracture.

The postoperative contracture may occur with or without a lining on the nasal palatine surface. So far as speech is concerned, we have found little significant difference between patients who have had a two-flap lengthening operation of the Veau-Wardill-Kilner type and those whose palate was not lengthened. However, the two-flap or W/V–Y lengthening procedure does facilitate closure of clefts of the soft palate that tend to be a little wider than the average. Its use must be balanced against the risk associated with denuding bone in a growing infant (Figure 5–60).

Posterior Wall Implants

Posterior wall implants have been used for many years. The most acceptable materials have been Teflon, soft silicone prostheses, and cartilage. Insertion of materials in the retropharyngeal space probably should be limited to those patients with a palatopharyngeal gap of less than 1 cm. and with a functional palatopharyngeal musculature. There has been a high risk of loss of these materials, as they are often extruded or drift caudally in the retropharyngeal space. They have also been used to reduce the size of an incompetent lateral port following a pharyngeal flap. Their popularity has dwindled considerably, and presently we do not use this technique.

Temporal Muscle–Fascial Sling

This operation serves primarily as a palatal lift. The temporal muscle is an elevator that assists in raising the mandible and as such cannot function as an effective rapidly moving muscle in speech, other than to lift the soft palate into a more functional position.

Pharyngoplasties

Several types of pharyngoplasty have been recommended, some of which are becoming of historic interest. The Hynes pharyngoplasty that had its greatest popularity in England has fallen into disrepute. In this operation, bilateral myocutaneous flaps utilizing the salpingopharyngeus muscle were transferred from the lateral to the posterior pharyngeal wall. This muscle is absent in about half the cleft palate patients. Moore and Sullivan transferred lateral myocutaneous flaps with palatopharyngeus muscle to increase length. Orticochea used similar flaps but sutured them to an inferior-based pharyngeal flap. More recently, Jackson and Silverton sutured lateral myocutaneous flaps with palatopharyngeus muscle to a superior-based pharyngeal flap. They considered the palatopharyngeal flaps to contain functional muscle units that would provide some sphincteric action.

Thompson transplanted a free autogenous muscle graft for VPI, but no one has been able to reproduce his results. Song and Bromberg reported on an intravelar veloplasty in which they used a palmaris longus tendon with a purse-string effect to reduce the area of the palatopharyngeal port. Thompson performed the same operation but used an extensor tendon from the foot. The use of tendons for this purpose is somewhat controversial.

Prostheses

The speech-aid prosthesis has been employed by choice for selected cases, such as the horseshoe-shaped cleft palate, or as a temporary or permanent restoration when there is reason to defer a surgical repair either temporarily or permanently (Figure 5–61). We have also found it to be helpful as a physical therapy modality. By gradually reducing the size of the pharyngeal section or bulb, it is possible to improve palatopharyngeal muscle function prior to transposing a pharyngeal flap. If the gap on either side of the pharyngeal flap gradually enlarges and hypernasality recurs, a speech-aid prosthesis with a split or Y-shaped pharyngeal section may serve as an obturator or training device.

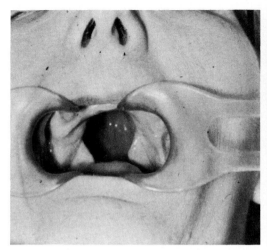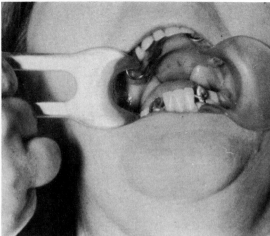

FIGURE 5–61   Prosthesis used to close a "horse-shoe" cleft to the palate.

In geographical areas in which sinus disease with a postnasal drip is common, a prosthesis might be considered for those individuals with troublesome disease. When there is a persistent, heavy postnasal drip, mucus is usually suspended over the pharyngeal flap, creating an unhygienic situation. The prosthesis is an advantage here because it can be removed for cleaning. It can, in addition, be designed to restore missing teeth.

A speech-aid prosthesis should also be considered if the patient has a paresis of the palate, for when there is a neurological deficit of the soft palate, surgery alone cannot be depended upon to provide oronasal balance with acceptable speech. The ports on either side of the pharyngeal flap must be functionally occluded by the musculature to acquire good quality speech. If occlusion is inadequate, no more than limited postoperative improvement can be anticipated. The nasal airway should never be occluded with a P-flap to correct hypernasality. Rather than sacrifice nasal breathing, it would be preferable to prescribe a prosthesis with an adequate pharyngeal section.

A palatal lift prosthesis is occasionally used as a crutch to elevate a sluggish palate. This device will often lead to improved muscle function prior to transfer of a pharyngeal flap. Here again, these decisions are best made by the interdisciplinary cleft palate group.

Posterior Wall Pharyngeal Flaps

Schoenborn introduced the pharyngeal flap operation in 1876.[69] Since that time the operation has passed through periods of rising and falling popularity. The procedure was technically more difficult and failures were common earlier in the twentieth century, which was the reason for the decline in popularity. The posterior pharyngeal wall flaps, whether superior or inferior-based, are an adynamic, mucosal-covered fibromuscular tube that tethers the soft palate to the posterior pharyngeal wall. They reduce the size of the palatopharyngeal gap to a point at which the lateral ports can be obstructed by a surrounding functional musculature.

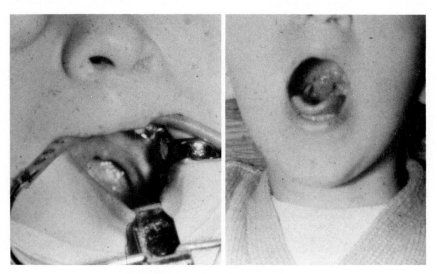

FIGURE 5–62   An inferior-based pharyngeal flap.

More recently, lateral-based flaps have been proposed to retain the nerve supply and create a dynamic structure with activated muscle. The lateral-based flaps, whether a bipedicled flap or two opposing flaps, should be placed as near the level of normal palatopharyngeal wall contact as possible. A functional unit that is located too low will tend to drag the soft palate inferiorly. Our preference has been almost exclusively for the superior-based flap. It can be inserted at an optimal level of function, which is usually at the level of the torus tubarius or eustachian cushions. In large velopharyngeal gaps, the inferior-based flap is too low and drags the palate downward (Figure 5–62).

It is probably wise to have the tonsils and adenoid mass removed at least three months before transposing a superior-based pharyngeal flap. There will be no access to the adenoids following the operation. If the tonsils are hypertrophied, they will interfere with the technical aspect of the operation. They may also occlude the airway postoperatively as they move closer together when the donor site of the pharyngeal flap is closed.

The superior-based pharyngeal flap is lined with a rectangular flap raised on the nasal surface of the soft palate and based posteriorly. This flap is similar to Passavant's palatine flap used to correct velopharyngeal incompetence.[59] With the two flaps opposing each other and with closure of the donor site in the posterior pharyngeal wall, the operative field is converted into essentially a closed wound. This enhances wound healing and reduces the risk of complications such as postoperative hemorrhage.

Pharyngeal Flap Technique

The pharyngeal flap technique is illustrated in Figures 5–63 to 5–65.

The anesthesia for the pharyngeal flap operation is a general oroendotracheal anesthetic in which the endotracheal tube is held in position and the mouth is propped open by a Dingman mouth-gag. The surgeon sits comfortably at the head of the table. The posterior pharyngeal wall is

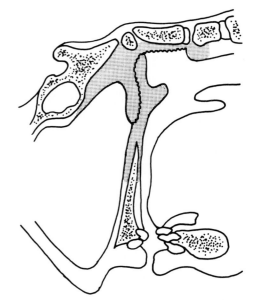

FIGURE 5–63 Line drawing illustrating the P-flap and the opposing nasal palatine flap.

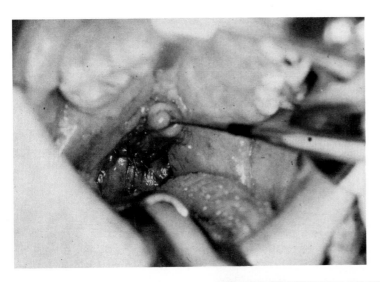

FIGURE 5–64 View showing nasal palatine flap lining the caudal surface of the P-flap and sutured into the posterior pharyngeal wall at the base of the pharyngeal flap.

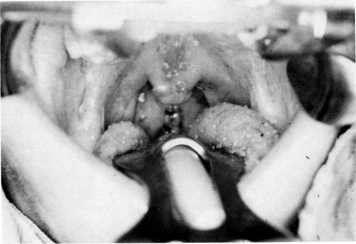

FIGURE 5–65 The superior based flap is often above the level of vision. The donor site in the posterior pharyngeal wall is closed.

inspected for pulsating vessels and any posterior wall bulge. Lidocaine (Xylocaine), 0.5 per cent with epinephrine, is infiltrated into the posterior pharyngeal wall and the soft palate. About 2 or 3 ml. is used.

An incision is made from the oropharynx along, but not within, the lateral gutter on each side up to the nasopharynx at a level near the base of the dens of the second cervical vertebra. The two lateral mucosal incisions are then connected far enough caudally to permit the flap to cover at least two-thirds of the nasal surface of the soft palate. With pointed scissors, one lateral wound is deepened to the whitish prevertebral fascia. Then with long curved or angled scissors of the type designed for nasal tip surgery, the flap is undermined at the level of the fascia. The mucosal wounds are completed to the proper depth and the flap is raised superiorly, frequently without the need to ligate any vessels. Should small vessels be encountered, they can be electrocoagulated. A suture is placed through the tip of the flap and held forward by attaching it to the spring on the mouth-gag. The donor site of the flap is then closed with interrupted 3–0 slowly absorbable suture material. Closing the donor site helps to keep the flap in its superior position. The pharyngeal flap is then released to temporarily hang loose.

Using a skin hook, the velum is everted to expose the nasal surface. Parallel incisions are made through the mucosa on either side of the nasal surface far enough apart to accommodate the pharyngeal flap. With pointed scissors, the soft palate is split midway between the oral and nasal mucosa from one lateral wound to the other. A cut is made with scissors between the anterior ends of the wounds on the nasal surface to create a bed over two-thirds of the posterior aspect of the soft palate. The flap is raised and based posteriorly, and it will survive as a viable flap if the incisions are no deeper than half the thickness of the palate. As the palatal flap is being raised, the surgeon can feel the release of the midline scar contracture in postoperative cleft palates. We do not section the soft palate in the midline to raise nasal palatine flaps or to create a bed to receive the P-flap.

A 4–0 nylon suture is passed through the soft palate near the midline just posterior to the hard palate. It passes through the raw nasal bed, through the tip of the pharyngeal flap, and then back through the pharyngeal flap and soft palate as a mattress-type suture. It is tied on the oral surface so as to approximate the raw surface of the pharyngeal flap to the raw surface on the nasal surface of the soft palate. Two other mattress-type sutures are placed laterally, one on either side, so that the three sutures will fix the end of the pharyngeal flap anteriorly in the bed. Usually all three sutures are placed before they are tied down. Each suture must engage the mucosa of the pharyngeal flap or it will not hold. The tip of the rectangular nasal palatine flap is then sutured into the posterior pharyngeal wall at the base of the pharyngeal flap. The sides of the two flaps are then sutured together (Figure 5–66). As this is done the size of the lateral ports is determined by using a 4 mm. (14 French) sterile flexible suction catheter, available on the anesthesia table. The size of the ports can be adjusted as the sides are sutured together. This then creates a lined pharyngeal flap that will maintain a better caliber and one that is well stabilized and unlikely to separate. One cannot always quantitate 20 sq. mm. surgically, but conceptually it is important to try to obtain a functional port. Some surgeons prefer to split the soft palate in the

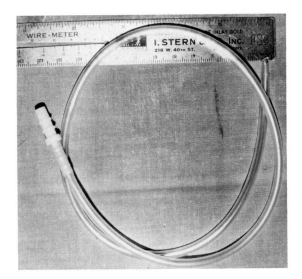

FIGURE 5–66 The sterile suction catheter (4 mm.) used to determine size of the velopharyngeal ports.

midline to facilitate placement of the superior-based flap. We have rarely found that to be necessary in our present technical plan.

The inferior-based flap is easier to execute because it is seated on the oral surface of the soft palate. It can also be lined by fixing an oral palatal flap on its superior surface. The flap is elevated in the same fashion as the superior-based flap except that the lateral wounds are joined above and the flap is based caudally.

Postoperative Care

Following a pharyngeal flap operation, patients have a sore throat and often some stiffness or limitation of neck movement for about two days. Other than medication for their comfort, there are no specific orders. The patients are given general care and a regular soft pediatric diet. They are discharged on the third or fourth postoperative day and advised to avoid exertional activities and the playing of wind instruments for about two weeks. Speech therapy can be started after one month.

THE CLEFT LIP NOSE

A typical cleft lip nose is often more conspicuous in the teenager than is the repaired lip. Restoration of nasal balance will frequently divert attention away from the midface. The unilateral cleft lip nasal deformity is the result of opposing forces acting on a fairly normal structure. The continued tension on the lower lateral cartilage on the cleft side creates an alar cartilage that is distorted, displaced, usually thin, and of poor structural quality compared with the normal side. The attenuated cartilage may not be capable of providing adequate support to the nasal tip (Figure 5–67). Even though similarities exist among all cleft lip noses, there are infinite variations in the

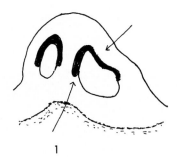

1

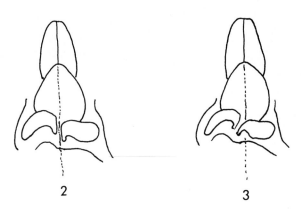

2

3

FIGURE 5–67 Distorted, displaced attenuated alar cartilage on the cleft side. The nasal tip may have an apparent twist (2) or a real twist (3).

deformity and the extent of the involvement. There may be little nasal deformity associated with a minimal or incomplete cleft of the lip. In a complete cleft of the lip and palate, the nasal floor is open because of clefting of the soft tissues and bony shelves, and the nasal tip on the affected side is a low, flat bridge of tissue spanning the cleft. The typical unilateral cleft lip nose presents the following physical findings:

1. The columella is oblique, and its base is directed away from the cleft.

2. The maxillary segment on the medial side is rotated outward, carrying the nasal spine, the lower septum, and the base of the columella away from the cleft as a result of an unopposed muscle force.

3. The entire nasal tip and even the upper lateral cartilages appear to be drawn toward the non-cleft side.

4. The flaring alar base is displaced laterally and is often below its normal horizontal position. This again is the result of an unopposed muscle force.

5. The deviated nasal septum may elevate the dome of the tip on the non-cleft side above its normal height.

6. The nasal floor, sill, and bony shelf are absent.

7. The entire ala and the lower lateral cartilage are flattened. The medial crux of the lower cartilage on the cleft side is lower than that of the normal side. The free margin of the ala lacks a normal curve and is caudal or below that of its mate on the normal side.

8. The lower lateral cartilage, when viewed during open surgery, appears to be a thin, weak structure.

The goal in cleft lip nasal surgery is to restore nasal balance and facial harmony with an adequate nasal airway. The question is how much surgery and when? There is no agreement among surgeons on an answer. Some favor a rather extensive nasal tip repair during the primary lip closure with realignment and stabilization of the distorted parts. The proponents of this procedure argue that access is easier at that time and that the infant nose is soft and pliable and easier to work on. The opponents of early primary repair and equally competent surgeons recommend minimal surgical intervention on the nose before adult life. Regardless of how much primary correction is made, secondary nasal repairs will invariably be necessary because changes take place through the period of growth and development. A good nasal correction can be obtained when the deformity is minimal, such as that associated with a minimal cleft of the lip (Fgure 5–68). Perfection is rarely, if ever, obtained with a nasal deformity associated with a complete cleft of the lip and palate. The main point of disagreement among surgeons is how much primary surgery can be performed without interfering with the growth of the nasal tip. This point has not been scientifically answered. It now appears that cartilaginous structures can be repositioned without significantly interfering with growth of the tip, provided there is not undue injury to the cartilage and perichondrium. Skilled surgeons should be able to handle these delicate structures competently. At one period in our cleft lip and nasal experience, we elevated the skin rather widely over the nasal tip and repositioned the displaced lower cartilage and fixed it to either the overlying skin or the opposite lower cartilage. Too often the improvement was short-lived, particularly when the cartilage was only attached in a new position to the overlying skin. In many cases it appeared that the result did not justify the

FIGURE 5–68 The symmetry of the nares can be easily improved when a minimal cleft lip is repaired by the Rose-Thompson method. One needs to be careful not to make the involved naris too small.

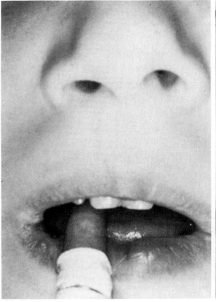
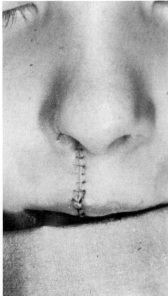

effort. However, in none of these patients did we observe any interference with growth of the nasal tip. The nose is also injured in many growing children; yet there are not many adults with underdeveloped noses as a result of trauma.

Many papers have been written and suggestions made for the repair of a cleft lip nose. The volume of papers and the surgical options are an admission of the inadequacy of all proposals and the continuing struggle for perfection. We usually have to settle for less so far as the cleft lip nose is concerned.

The nasal tip revision can be carried out in conjunction with the triangular flap, the rotation-advancement principle, the Skoog repair, and other operative cleft lip designs. In Millard's latest R-A plan, a small triangular flap is turned into the base of the columella to add some length to the short side. Operative procedures either during a primary lip repair or as a secondary stage have included any or all of the following points:

1. Repair nasal floor and sill.
2. Place nasal septal cartilage in the midline.
3. Reposition displaced tip cartilages and stabilize the lower lateral cartilage on the cleft side to one of the neighboring fixed structures.
4. Trim the excess cartilage and skin lining from the lower edge of the depressed alar cartilage and repair the alar web.
5. Trim all four major nasal tip cartilages unequally to provide symmetry and stabilize the weak alar cartilage.
6. Establish a normal-sized nostril and alar base-columella relationship.
7. Reduce the dome on the normal side and use the upper portion of the normal alar cartilage as a free cartilage onlay graft on the depressed side.
8. Place a cartilage strut in the columella to provide thrust to the tip and support to the ala on the cleft side.

We do not use silicone implants to restore contour or support to the nasal tip. These are placed immediately beneath the skin in an area exposed to frequent trauma and are often extruded, presenting through the skin.

SURGICAL PLAN

We have tried a number of surgical procedures, especially in the adult nose, and too often the results have been less than satisfactory in our opinion. The plan that seems to work best for us can be divided into stages of nasal reconstruction.

The Primary Repair

Important surgical requirements during the primary lip repair are as follows: (1) repair the nasal floor, (2) establish a normal-sized nostril, and (3) establish normal relations between the base of the ala and the columella. A subcutaneous suture between the base of the ala and the columella is a critical stitch as the lip is being repaired (Figure 5–69; see also Figures 5–8 and 5–9).

For the majority of patients in our longitudinal group, we have been limiting the nasal tip surgery in conjunction with the primary lip repair to the requirements just cited. For some of the patients, we made a rim incision in

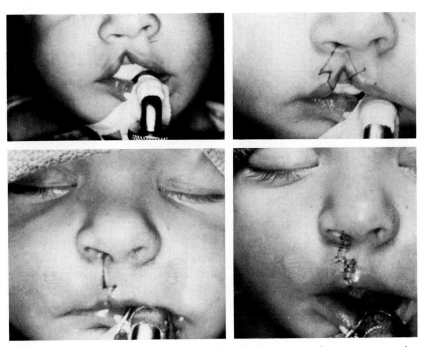

FIGURE 5–69 Improvement of nasal sill and anterior naris during a primary lip repair.

the ala on the cleft side and freed the lower lateral cartilage and its skin lining from the overlying skin. The excess cartilage and lining skin are then trimmed to create a normal alar curve and to correct the alar web. The scar is hidden inside the nostril. We do not do any extensive or additional undermining at that time. A well-repaired lip will mold the underlying maxillary structural elements and bring the columella back to the midline.

Intermediate Nasal Surgery

At about five years of age and before entering the first grade, patients undergo a limited nasal tip correction to make them more presentable before their peers. This is a period when children are inquisitive and unrestrained in their remarks. The operation at this time is designed to provide enough improvement to carry the patient over until a final correction is made on the adult nose. An intermediate stage is often carried out in conjunction with another service, such as a columella lengthening procedure, a lip revision, or perhaps a pharyngeal flap operation. If the columella is being lengthened, the nasal tip cartilages can be exposed, repositioned, and stabilized at the same time. The nasal tip deformity is usually one of flattening of the tip on the cleft side, absence of a normal curve of the free alar margin, and a buckling of the inner vestibular wall. If the nasal tip deformity had been corrected during the initial lip repair, this intermediate stage may be unnecessary. If no tip correction had been made at the primary lip operation, it is done at about five years of age. The plan that

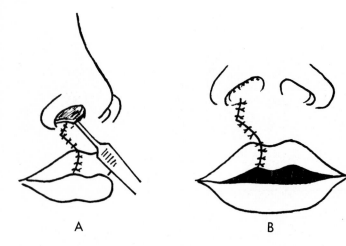

FIGURE 5–70 Illustration of undermining the lower lateral cartilage through a rim incision for exposure and trimming of the rim or lower margin of skin-cartilage to develop a normal alar curve.

has provided a nice improvement in our hands at that point in time has been to improve the curve of the free margin of the ala and correct any alar web and vestibular buckling (Figures 5–70 to 5–72).

A rim incision is made from near the inner side of the alar base to the apex of the nostril and then down the side of the columella for a short distance. The skin is elevated over the lower lateral cartilage, and the undermining is carried down to the base of the ala. The excess vestibular skin and rim cartilage are trimmed to create a curve to match that of the free margin of the normal ala. One or two sutures can be placed to close the rim wound to check the symmetry. The incision at the base of the ala is then carried back inside the alar base, and when undermining is complete, this will allow the vestibular lining to spread out. The excess can then be trimmed and the entire wound closed. The scar is hidden within the nostril beneath the alar rim. This will relieve the vestibular buckling and create a symmetrical alar curve, but some flattening of the nasal tip will often persist on the cleft side. If the nostrils and the alar margins are symmetrical, a little flattening of the nasal tip can be acceptable for the next several

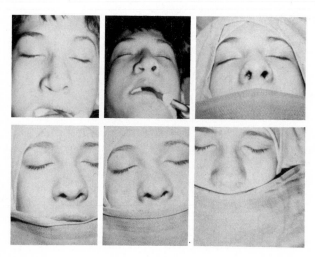

FIGURE 5–71 Improvement of nasal tip and nares symmetry by freeing and trimming the lower edge of the alar cartilage. This is usually done just before the child enters first grade.

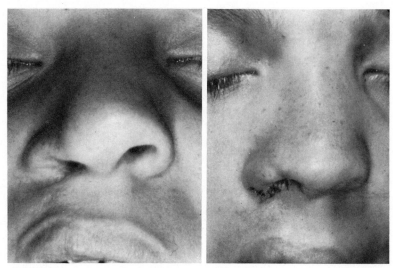

FIGURE 5–72   Improvement of tip symmetry by (1) making a rim incision to the base of the ala and then back-cut along the inner wall of the base, (2) trimming the lower edge of the alar cartilage to create a normal curve, (3) spreading out and trimming the excess of the buckled lining, and (4) improving columellar-alar relations. This provides a satisfactory improvement until a final rhinoplasty is done in the teens.

years. We have not been satisfied with the A-plasty or V–Y plasty for correction of vestibular buckling.

We have, on occasion, raised the superior edge of the lower lateral cartilage through an intercartilaginous incision and stabilized it to the upper lateral cartilage. However, in most instances we have still found it advantageous to trim the rim margin. Occasionally, a patient will have a marked septal dislocation and derangement, so that the nasal airway is occluded on the cleft side and there is continual drainage of nasal secretions onto the lip with excoriation of the skin. In this situation, we do a limited submucous resection to create an airway and enough space to permit nasal drainage to flow posteriorly. We may also fracture the base of the septum and move it toward the midline. This will provide for an adequate airway and proper drainage until a final or more extensive correction can be done in the adult nose.

The Adult Cleft Lip Nose

The adult with a cleft lip nose will present not only with the derangements commonly seen in association with a cleft of the lip but also with the structural deformities common to the general run of the rhinoplasty patients. Dr. J. B. Brown once stated that when treating a cleft lip nose, the surgeon should do a standard rhinoplasty with added attention to the nasal tip. That states very simply our plan for the adult cleft lip nose. The nasal tip procedure can be complicated, and the final result usually falls short of the ideal. We do not tell a patient with a cleft lip nose that one operation is all that is needed. We find it best to tell the individual that a second-stage adjustment of the nasal tip may be necessary in about six months or thereafter. If the patient needs other services, such as a major lip revision, we will plan to do the rhinoplasty first and a secondary tip revision when the lip is repaired.

When treating a cleft lip nose, it is important to study the nasal deformity carefully and make an accurate diagnosis because there are infinite variations, even though the general contour is similar in many patients. The operation is then carried out step by step, just as in a routine rhinoplasty. The nasal tip will, however, require additional attention. The upper and lower lateral cartilages are all trimmed as much as is required, but the extent and location of the trimming may vary somewhat in each cartilage to encourage eventual symmetry. The superior portion of the lower cartilage on the normal side is skeletonized and removed, as in a standard rhinoplasty, leaving the lower rim of cartilage intact. On the cleft side, the same amount of trimming may be done, or it may be necessary to remove less or none of the superior portion of the cartilage. The septum can be shortened to improve the columellar labial angle, and usually a submucous resection and septoplasty are necessary in the cleft lip nose. The approach to the septal cartilage is through the incision in the membranous columella. Following the submucous resection, the retained septal struts may need to be straightened. We have on occasion removed a septal cartilage, straightened it, and then replaced it between its lining flaps.

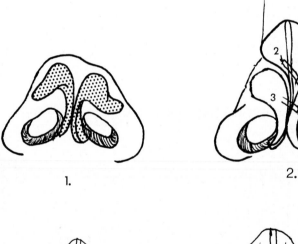

1.

2.

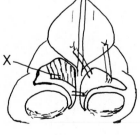

3.

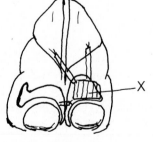

4.

A

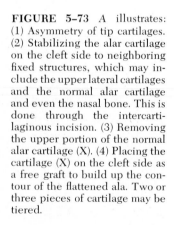

FIGURE 5–73 A illustrates: (1) Asymmetry of tip cartilages. (2) Stabilizing the alar cartilage on the cleft side to neighboring fixed structures, which may include the upper lateral cartilages and the normal alar cartilage and even the nasal bone. This is done through the intercartilaginous incision. (3) Removing the upper portion of the normal alar cartilage (X). (4) Placing the cartilage (X) on the cleft side as a free graft to build up the contour of the flattened ala. Two or three pieces of cartilage may be tiered.

(Illustration continued on opposite page)

The best time to carry out the septal surgery is in conjunction with the rhinoplasty, when access is good. All tissue removed during the course of a reduction rhinoplasty and septal surgery is set aside for later use. After the septum or septal struts are placed in the midline, some additional trimming of the cartilages may be necessary. The dome on the normal side may still be high and have to be lowered. This is done by removing 1 or 2 mm. of cartilage from the lower extremity of the lateral wing of the intact rim of alar cartilage. The lower cartilage on the cleft side may have to be stabilized to the upper lateral cartilage on one or both sides and the rim trimmed through a rim incision.

After the operation is complete, the wound in the membranous septum is closed. The nose is now inspected for asymmetry. The cartilaginous material that had been removed is now fashioned and used as an onlay graft wherever it is needed. The superior portion of the lower cartilage that was taken from the normal side is often employed as an onlay graft over the lower cartilage on the cleft side. The septal cartilage can also be fashioned and used for additional contour. Two or three pieces of cartilage may be tiered to build up the sagging cleft side. A small button of cartilage may be advantageous in rounding out the nasal tip. The problem that we have had is that the nasal tip in the region of the lower lateral cartilages may be too bulbous following replantation of cartilage, even though symmetry may be obtained. If this occurs, the tip can be secondarily trimmed after several months. The intranasal wounds on the cleft side are sutured when an onlay graft is inserted, but otherwise not (Figures 5–73 to 5–78).

There is nothing new about this method of management of the adult cleft lip nose. It is a combination of a standard rhinoplasty and septal

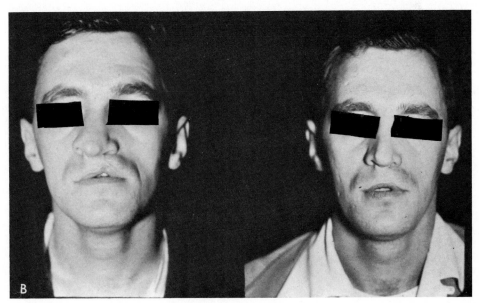

FIGURE 5–73 Continued. B, Cleft lip rhinoplasty and secondary cheiloplasty.

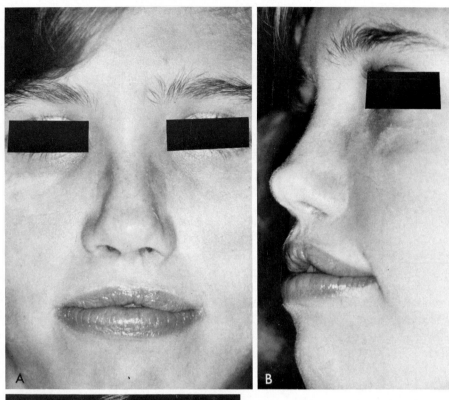

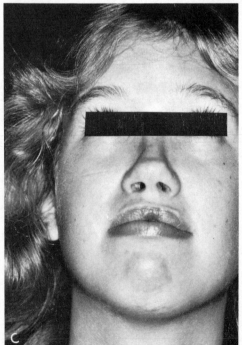

FIGURE 5–74 Following a rhinoplasty as described in the text, this
patient's nose is symmetrical. However, occasionally the tip will be broad
following the cartilage transplant and
will require a secondary trim after 6 to
12 months to improve the definition.
This patient also needs a V-Y and
muscle reorientation to build up the
lip tubercle.

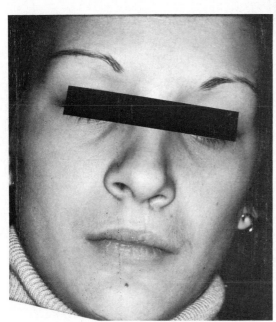
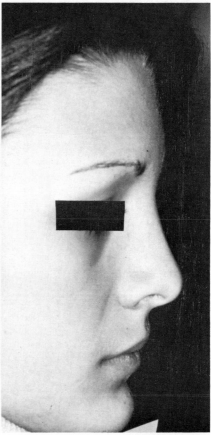

FIGURE 5–75   Postoperative cleft lip nose by the method described in the text.

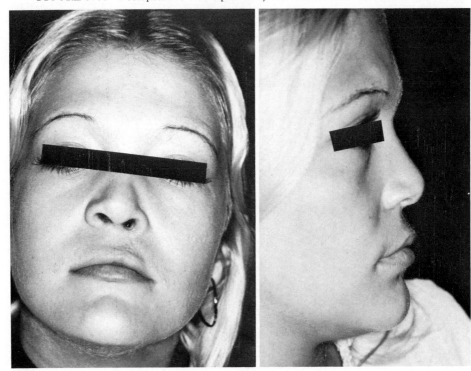

FIGURE 5–76   Postoperative cleft lip nose. This is not perfect, but it does improve midface balance.

245

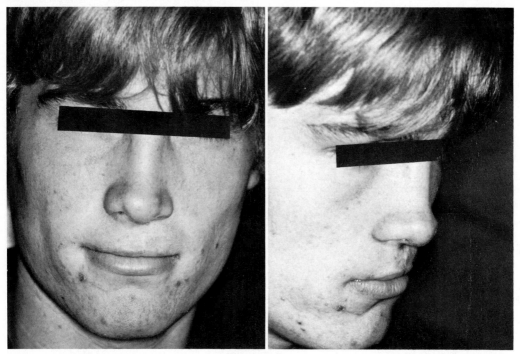

FIGURE 5–77   Postoperative cleft lip nose and long-term cleft lip follow-up.

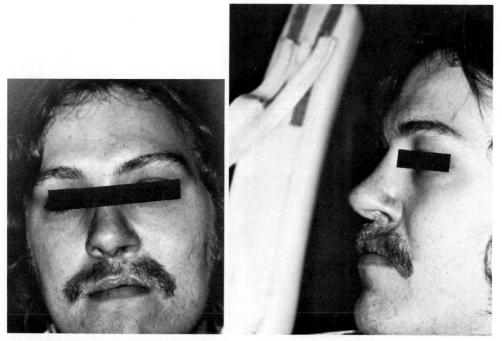

FIGURE 5–78   Postoperative cleft lip nose. This still shows some alar-naris asymmetry.

surgery, together with a combination of options available for the management of the nasal tip. These surgical recommendations have been put together in a plan that seems to be most suitable in our hands.

The Bilateral Cleft Lip Nose

The bilateral cleft lip nose is essentially two single cleft lip nasal deformities with a marked deficiency of the columella. The tip and columella may be broad with separation of the medial crura of the lower cartilages. The deformity is somewhat similar to that of the unilateral cleft except that it involves both sides. Whatever primary nasal tip realignment is planned, it can only be carried out on one side at a time if the lip repair is a two-staged operation. Very nearly all of our bilateral cleft lips are repaired one side at a time, and we try to restore a nasal floor, a normal relationship between the alar base and columella, and a normal-sized nostril. We do not do a nasal tip revision in conjunction with the primary bilateral lip repair. When the columella is lengthened at about four or five years of age, the nasal tip cartilages can be exposed and realigned to elevate and narrow the nasal tip. This procedure is still considered to be an interim nasal operation, and a final repair will be planned on the adult nose, using the principles described for the unilateral cleft lip nose.

SECONDARY SURGICAL PROCEDURES

Secondary deformities and their corrective operative procedures are varied and many. The diversity of repairs necessary to provide a sophisticated primary and secondary cleft lip and palate surgical service is one reason why this field of surgery is so fascinating. There are secondary surgical repairs that vary from a rather simple procedure to a complicated plan that may be more difficult than an initial repair. Before a surgeon undertakes to correct a secondary deformity, it is necessary to determine what has been done and what can be done to restore facial balance. By clinical inspection, it is usually easy to determine what surgical procedures have been carried out. The determination of what to do about this is not always easy.

Secondary operations are designed to improve deformities that occur following surgical intervention. Or they are purposely planned to correct residual deformities that were not incorporated in the primary operative plan. Some surgeons will carry out a rather extensive readjustment of the nasal tip in conjunction with the primary lip repair, while others prefer to treat the nasal tip as a secondary procedure. In carrying out a secondary revision, it may be necessary to utilize either a technique similar to a primary repair or a plastic surgery principle for realignment of tissue, or a combination of the two. Discussion of all possible types of deformities would not be practical, if indeed possible. In this section, only primary bone grafting, orbicularis oris muscle reorientation in the bilateral cleft, the columella raise, and the Abbe flap will be considered.

PRIMARY BONE GRAFTING

We do not use or recommend early primary bone grafting in the cleft lip and palate patient. An autogenous bone graft has been very helpful as a delayed procedure in the stabilization of maxillary segments and the closure of hard palatal fistulae and in providing contour. Bone grafts should be covered on both the nasal and oral surfaces by utilizing a vomer flap, vestibular-gingival flaps, and sliding mucoperiosteal flaps. Since extensive dissection of the lining of the nasal septum and violation of the oral mucoperiosteum during periods of active growth may have adverse effects on midfacial development, we do not use bone grafts until 12 years of age, provided the maxillary segments are in proper alignment. Retrospective studies by several surgeons on the long-term effects of early primary bone grafting support this concept (Figure 5–79).

When the maxillary segments are in their proper relations, a dental holding prosthesis is constructed to maintain stability until a bony union is accomplished. Our preference is for autogenous iliac bone, both as a fashioned solid block and as chips or cancellous bone obtained by curettage. The bone is used to fill the gap in the alveolar process and to support the alar base. Although it is important to cover the bone graft on both the nasal and oral surfaces, it is not essential that this be a watertight seal.

In our present protocol for repair of a cleft of the palate, the alveolar cleft is initially left open and its repair is delayed until about 12 years of age, as previously stated. If the maxillary segments are stable and in good alignment, the cleft can be closed with adjacent vestibular and mucoperiosteal flaps without a bone graft. Bone may grow across small alveolar gaps, but the volume of new bone formed is not enough to fill out the defect completely and restore normal contour. When the alveolar gap is wide or when there is lack of stability, an autogenous iliac bone graft will complement the repair.

Small hard palate fistulae can usually be repaired with a soft tissue closure. For the larger fistulae we like to develop a shelf of iliac bone to provide a solid base for the repair. With our present cleft palate surgical protocol, fistulae of the hard palate are an uncommon occurrence. To repeat, the hard palate is closed with a vomer flap that extends anteriorly only to the incisive foramen when feasible. Otherwise, a primary repair of the velum is considered, and the repair of the hard palate may be deferred until the cleft has narrowed or until such time that a major portion of the maxillary growth has taken place.

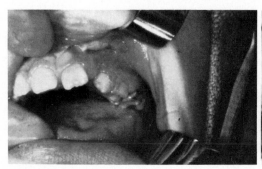 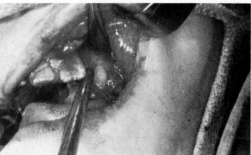

FIGURE 5–79   Direct exposure of cleft stabilized with a healed autogenous bone graft.

MUSCLE REORIENTATION IN THE BILATERAL CLEFT LIP

We have not found it necessary to realign the orbicularis oris muscle routinely in all unilateral cleft lip repairs. When indicated, it is easier to realign the muscle in conjunction with the primary unilateral repair, rather than as a secondary procedure (Figure 5–80). We have also felt that a muscle reorientation is not essential in all bilateral cleft lip repairs, but it is an important final step in the reconstruction of many of the complete bilateral clefts. When bilateral cleft lips are repaired in two stages, a muscle repair in the absence of muscle in the prolabium is essentially impossible. A primary muscle realignment may be carried out with a one-staged bilateral lip repair. However, a muscle realignment at that time tends to sacrifice breadth of the lip, which is an important dimension. There is lack of a tubercle and a deficiency of vermilion tissue in the prolabial section of a lip following many bilateral cleft repairs, even though lateral vermilion flaps may have been used to augment the central vermilion.

Our final stage of a bilateral cleft lip repair for many of our patients

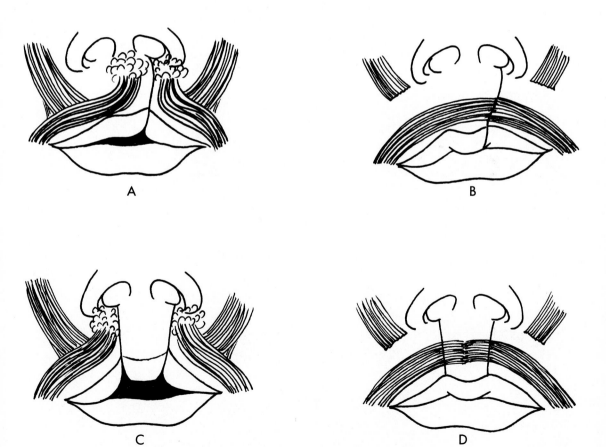

FIGURE 5–80 Direction of orbicularis oris muscle fibers before and after reorientation. The muscle fibers do not always extend to the base of the columella and ala.

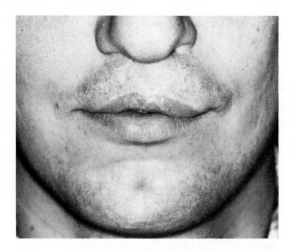

FIGURE 5–81   A deficiency of vermilion in the prolabial portion of the lip has been built up with a V-Y plasty and orbicularis oris muscle reorientation through a mucosal approach.

consists of a V–Y plasty and muscle realignment (Figure 5–81). The V-incision has its apex in the sulcus underneath the lip at the reflection of the labial frenum, and the base is the vermilion border of the prolabium. After the V-shaped flap is elevated, the muscle in the lateral lip segments is dissected free from the covering skin and mucosa and then detached from the nasal sill and base of the ala. The muscle is freed laterally to a vertical line extending down from the outer attachment of the alar base. The muscle is then united behind the prolabium with its fellow from the opposite side with 4–0

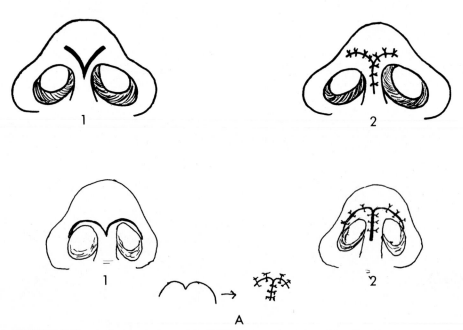

FIGURE 5–82   A, Two variations of the V-Y lengthening of the columella. The V-Y principle has been popularized by Brauer.

(*Illustration continued on opposite page*)

absorbable sutures. In many instances it is possible to overlap the muscle repair. The muscle fibers are placed in a horizontal position in the lower third of the lip to help build up the vermilion and the tubercle. The V-shaped flap is then closed as a Y in order to create a tubercle and fullness in the lower lip where it is needed. This secondary muscle reorientation can be carried out at any age, but preferably should be done between four and five years. Some other secondary procedures, such as possibly a pharyngeal flap, can be carried out at the same time to consolidate operations.

COLUMELLA LENGTHENING

Lengthening of the columella may be carried out as a primary or a secondary procedure. In a complete bilateral cleft lip and palate, the columella may be markedly deficient or totally absent. Millard has utilized bilateral forked flaps from the prolabium and advanced these into the columella to gain length at the time of an initial one-staged bilateral lip repair. In Skoog's two-staged bilateral lip repair, a triangular flap is raised on the lateral aspect of the prolabium and transferred into the base of the columella. This is essentially one-half of Marcks' plan for lengthening the columella. When there is a well-developed prolabial cap on the premaxilla, it is better to utilize any excess skin in the columella, rather than to sacrifice it. All too frequently the prolabial cap is a small, dome-shaped mass, in which case it is better to utilize all of the prolabial skin in the lip repair.

In general, our preference has been to treat the deficient columella as a

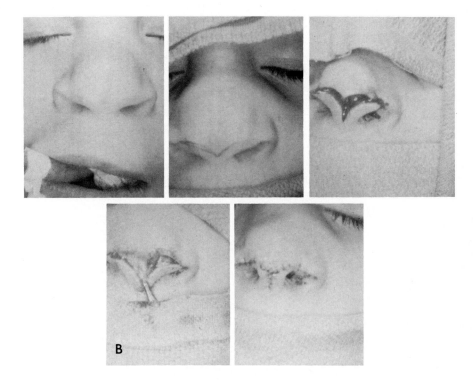

FIGURE 5–82 *Continued.* *B,* V-Y advancement of the columella in a patient.

secondary procedure. Here again, this lengthening operation can be carried out at any age but preferably before the patient enters elementary school and frequently in conjunction with another procedure. There are several operative proposals for lengthening the columella, and no procedure is ideally suited to all cases. The operative plan selected will depend upon the clinical findings. If the patient has a well-repaired lip, one may be hesitant to invade it to raise forked or triangular flaps to lengthen the columella. If the nasal floor is not broad and the alar bases are not displaced laterally, there may not be sufficient tissue to do a Carter or Cronin repair. A composite graft could be used to lengthen the columella, but this is generally unsatisfactory because the risk of loss is high, particularly in an uncooperative young patient. The columella can also be lengthened by a V-Y type procedure performed on the nasal tip. This does place a scar on the nasal tip and tends to create a columella that has a hanging appearance with an obtuse columella-labial angle unless an appropriate correction is made (Figure 5–82). The Straith procedure gives the appearance of an increased columellar length but does not elevate the nasal tip.

The Carter procedure[12] described in 1914 advances tissue from the nasal floor into the columella (Figure 5–83). It has been recommended by a number of surgeons and was extended and refined by Cronin to include the base of the ala. When the anterior nasal floor is broad, the alar base is invariably displaced laterally. A strap of tissue is elevated from the nasal floor, including the alar base, and it must be thick enough to maintain an adequate blood supply. A V-shaped cut is made on the base of the columella where the two nasal floor flaps of soft tissue meet at the midline. The membranous columella is freed from the cartilaginous septum, and the skin is undermined over the nasal tip. The nostrils are rotated, and the flaps are advanced into the columella, creating a V-Y type lengthening. The alar bases can then be freed and advanced into a more normal relationship with the base of the columella. The advancement of the alar bases will create a dog ear on the upper part of the lip, and this is corrected by removing a wedge of tissue from the upper part of the lip repair on either side. The columellar wounds are closed first, and then the

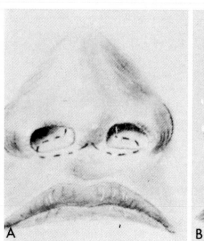 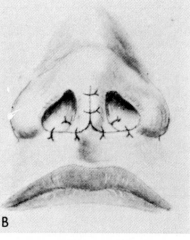

FIGURE 5–83 Carter method for advancing tissue from the nasal floor into the columella.

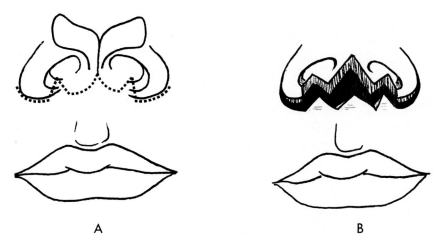

A   B

FIGURE 5–84   A variation of Cronin's method for columella lengthening.

ala is fixed to its new relationship with the columella. This operative plan is a
nice way to correct a broad nasal floor and a laterally displaced alar base when
lengthening a columella. In many instances, the final length of the columella
will be inadequate, so that the tip will still be slightly depressed. However,
this may be camouflaged by reducing the nasal dorsum when doing a final
rhinoplasty in the teens.

The Cronin procedure can be modified by making a single incision along
the edge of the nasal floor and into the base of the columella (Figure 5–84).
The floor of the nose and the septal skin mucosa are raised without creating a
pedicle or strap of nasal floor skin. After adequate relaxation is obtained, the
nostrils are rotated, the columella is lengthened, and the alar bases are
brought in toward the columella. This rotation and advancement procedure is
similar to the Cronin operation. The alar base will need to be secured to its
new position, and a cartilage strut may be helpful in the columella to project
the tip. A separate cartilage graft in the tip may provide a better contour.

In 1833 Gensoul[25] was the first to advance tissue from the prolabium into
the columella as a V-Y advancement. In 1941 Brown and McDowell[11] also

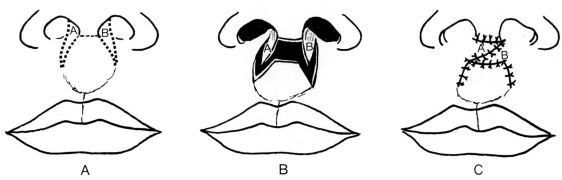

A   B   C

FIGURE 5–85   Illustration of Marcks' method for lengthening the columella.

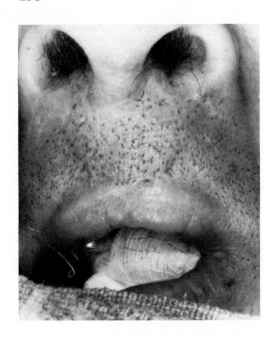

FIGURE 5–86 Columella lengthened by Marcks' method. Length attained is denoted in the patient by a color change. This patient had very little hair in the prolabium, so it was tattooed to resemble beard stubble.

performed a V–Y advancement of prolabial tissue but incorporated a small triangle of skin from the floor of the nose, and these were inserted on either side of the septum to help support the nasal tip. Marcks raised a triangular flap at the site of the lip repair on either side of the prolabium with its apex inferior (Figure 5–85). Each of these triangles can extend all the way to the vermilion border to include a revision of the lip scars. Each flap only needs to be long enough to extend across the base of the columella. An incision is made across the base of the columella to connect the two triangles of lip skin. The columella is then released with an incision in the membranous septum, and the nasal tip can be undermined to permit adequate elevation. The two flaps are then crossed, one above the other, in the base of the columella, and the wounds are repaired. We have been able to obtain some very nice results with this method (Figure 5–86).

When the prolabium is well developed, Skoog utilized Marcks' method of columella lengthening, one side at a time, during the primary bilateral lip

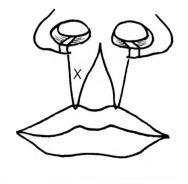

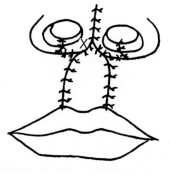

FIGURE 5–87 Illustration of bilateral forked flaps.

A

B

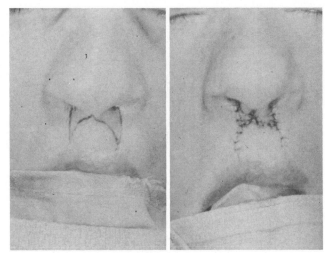

FIGURE 5–88 Bilateral forked flaps advanced into columella.

repair. Millard[47, 52] proposed bilateral forked flaps for a secondary repair, as well as for certain primary repairs (Figure 5–87 and 5–88). The technique is the same for either a primary or secondary lengthening of the columella. The forked flaps incorporate the site of the lip scar on either side of the prolabium and extend down to or just beyond the vermilion border. The medial limbs of the flaps end in an inverted V at the base of the columella. An incision is made in the membranous columella and the flaps are elevated. By this method, it is possible to expose the lower tip cartilages and symmetrically align the medial crura and dome of the two cartilages. A satisfactory lengthening can be accomplished with this plan. It may even be possible to sacrifice the tip of each flap. It is also possible to narrow the anterior nasal floor and realign the alar bases when a forked or triangular flap is raised from the lip.

Occasionally a patient with a bilateral cleft will have a separation of the nasal tip cartilages, creating a broad tip and columella. It is important when lengthening a columella to take into consideration the width of that structure as well as the natural flare of its base. If there is a separation of the tip cartilages and the medial crura, these can be approximated once they are exposed when the columella is raised up.

CROSS-LIP OR ABBE FLAP

Robert Abbe in 1898 was the first surgeon to turn a pedicle flap from the lower lip into a tight upper lip to correct a disparity between the lips following a cleft lip repair. Stein (1848), Buck (1860), and Estlander (1865) all preceded Abbe in turning a flap from one lip to the other but for different reasons. Over the years, there has been little change in the operation as originally described by Abbe.

A tight upper lip may occur when too much tissue has been discarded at the time of the primary repair or when lateral skin and vermilion flaps are turned down beneath the prolabium in a bilateral cleft repair. A tight lip is more frequently seen following a bilateral cleft lip repair. It is more common

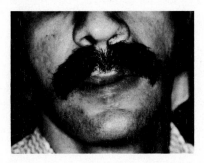

FIGURE 5–89   Hair growing upward on Abbe flap.

in the unilateral cleft following a Rose type of operation than with the present-day offset procedures that make use of various triangles. The cross-lip tissue transfer has been carried out successfully as a free composite graft when its width did not exceed 1 cm. Dufourmentel[18] reported 100 per cent success with free grafts. We have had no experience with this method reported by Dufourmentel, Walker, and others. The procedure requires a cooperative patient, and it would be somewhat disastrous if the graft were lost. The pedicle of the cross-lip flap can be sectioned in 10 to 16 days. It is better not to go by the calendar but rather by a clinical evaluation of the circulation of the flap and the amount of scar tissue present in the upper lip bed. Generally we wait the two full weeks because a great deal is at stake. The flap becomes a functional portion of the upper lip and is completely re-enervated in two years or less. The flap will grow hair but the hairs will turn up, rather than down, as they will on the lateral lip element (Figure 5–89).

We routinely place the flap in the midline of the upper lip, even though the primary operation may have been a unilateral lip repair. The flap can simulate the philtrum and the unilateral scar can be repaired at a later time (Figures 5–90 and 5–91). If there are plans to place the flap at the site of the unilateral lip scar, the cross-lip flap should be taken from the same lateral side of the lower lip, rather than from the midline. Many of the patients in whom we placed the flap at the site of the unilateral lip scar developed a lip asymmetry that was very difficult to correct (Figure 5–92).

The cross-lip pedicle flap operation is performed under local anesthesia in the adult and under oral endotracheal anesthesia in children. Subsequent section of the pedicle and closure of the defect are performed under sedation

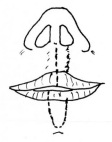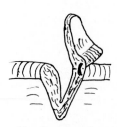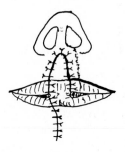

FIGURE 5–90   Abbe flap placed in midline of upper lip.

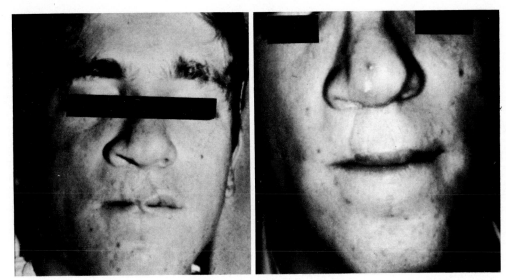

FIGURE 5–91   Abbe flap in midline of upper lip even though the patient had a unilateral cleft.

and local anesthesia in both children and adults. It is useful to measure the breadth of the upper and lower lips and to estimate the width of the flap as being a little over half the difference. A measurement is made from the base of the columella down the midline of the lip to the vermilion border. This measurement will determine the skin length of the lower lip flap. The Abbe flap is usually wedge-shaped with a rounded apex, although occasionally the skin of the tip of the flap may be split in the midline to form a **W** so that each half can extend up around the columellar base. After the flap is designed, the lower lip can be moved back and forth from right to left to estimate the tightness of the lower lip following the removal of the flap. If there is a shortness of tissue in the midline of the upper lip, some length can be gained

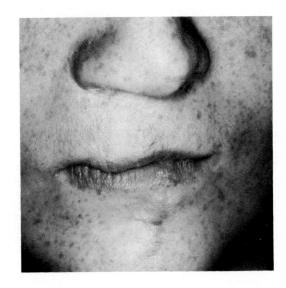

FIGURE 5–92   Asymmetry of lip due to off-center Abbe flap taken from midline of lower lip.

by extending the midline incision around the base of the columella or by removing an ellipse of tissue in the midline similar to a Rose-Thompson procedure. The flap is then cut by completely transecting the lip along one side of the flap and then back up on the other side, terminating about 1 to 2 mm. in the vermilion just beyond the mucocutaneous ridge. One can determine the level of the major vessels on the transected side before completing the cut on the pedicle side. Frequently there are two major vessels on the same level, the posterior vessel being smaller than the anterior one. Bleeding in the lower lip is controlled, and the donor site in the lip is repaired by a three-layer closure. The upper lip is then split in the midline to the base of the columella. Next, the lower lip flap is rotated into position, and a small tongue of muscle at the apex of the flap is securely fixed into the base of the columella to prevent a depression between the flap and the columellar base. The flap is then closed in three layers with alignment of the vermilion borders.

The endotracheal tube is removed after the patient reacts. When the tube is removed, a piece of tubing about the size of a nasopharyngeal tube is placed between the lips on one side of the flap. This will avoid any difficulty with inspiration because of the lips being held together, particularly if the patient has been accustomed to breathing through the mouth. After becoming fully oriented, the patient can remove this tube or replace it between the lips, especially during the first day or two until one becomes accustomed to the

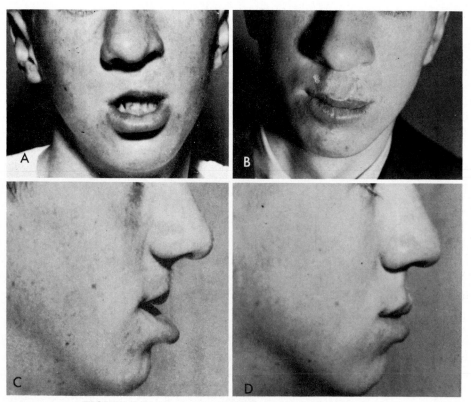

FIGURE 5–93 Pre- and postoperative cross-lip or Abbe flap.

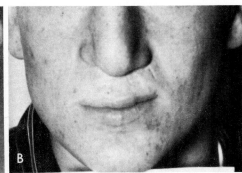

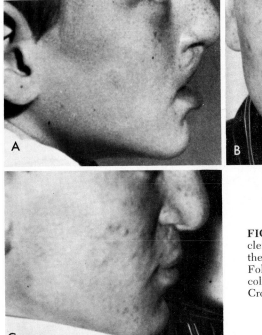

FIGURE 5-94 *A*, Postoperative bilateral cleft lip with tight upper lip, asymmetry of the lips, and a deficient columella. *B* and *C*, Follow-up several years after Abbe flap and columella raise by a variation of the Carter-Cronin method.

change in the airway. The patient is discharged from the hospital, and the food intake is no problem. After the pedicle is sectioned, the donor site in the lower lip is closed and the pedicle stump is inserted into the upper lip. The patient should now have a supple upper lip that drapes over the lower lip in a more normal fashion. If there was previously a malalignment of the upper lip, a revision may be necessary after several months, allowing adequate time for revascularization of the flap and softening of the tissues. A cross-lip pedicle flap is a nice way to restore symmetry between the lips and fulfills one of the basic principles of plastic surgery by replacing lost or deficient tissue with like tissue. It is an operation, however, that should rarely be necessary (Figures 5–93 and 5–94).

Summary

Primary cleft lip and palate repairs are important operations, performed in the early phase of a total program of cleft lip and palate habilitation and rehabilitation that goes on into maturity. During the patient's period of growth and development, the surgeon will find need for a great variety of revisions and secondary operative procedures that will need to be incorporated into a rational time sequence in conjunction with other services rendered by members of a cleft palate team. Osteotomies for malrelations of the jaws and the adult rhinoplasty are but two examples of procedures that must be delayed until the patient's growth is nearly complete. It is not possible to describe all the operative techniques that may be required throughout the history of the individual. Some of these can be grouped together to reduce the total number of operations. Based on an investigative study, we found no ill effects following several hospital admissions compared with a single admission, but the cost factor cannot be ignored. The best way to be prepared for these challenges and to visualize the requirements for correcting a defect or deformity is to have a good foundation in surgery and a firm grasp of the principles of plastic surgery as well as an ability to abstract the patient's needs. The volume of available knowledge has become so massive that the habilitation of a patient born with a cleft of the lip and palate requires the cooperative effort of an interdisciplinary team in which mutual respect and restraint prevail. The need for a concerted effort among specialists has become more and more evident in many patient services as well as for those with a facial cleft.

References

1. Abbe, R.: A new plastic operation for the relief of deformity due to double harelip. Med. Rec., 53:477, 1898.
2. Atherton, J. D., Lovius, B. B. J., and Maisels, D. O.: Growth of bony palate of pig consequent to transpositioning oral and nasal mucoperiosteum. Plast. Reconstr. Surg., 56:110, 1975.
3. Aufricht, G.: Symposium on corrective rhinoplasty (Discussion). Meeting of ASPRS, Los Angeles, Cal., Oct., 1960.
4. Bauer, T. B., Trusler, H. M., and Tondra, J. M.: Changing concepts in the management of bilateral cleft lip deformities. Plast. Reconstr. Surg., 24:321, 1959.
5. Bauer, T. B., Trusler, H. M., and Tondra, J. M.: Bauer, Trusler's and Tondra's method of cheilorrhaphy in bilateral lip. In Grabb, W. C., Rosenstein, S. W., and Bzoch, K. R. (Eds.): Cleft Lip and Palate. Boston, Little, Brown and Co., 1971.
6. Berkeley, W. T.: The cleft-lip nose. Plast. Reconstr. Surg., 23:567, 1959.
7. Blair, V. P.: Nasal deformities associated with congenital cleft of the lip. J.A.M.A., 84:185, 1925.
8. Blair, V. P., and Brown, J. B.: Mirault operation for single harelip. Surg. Gynecol. Obstet., 51:81, July, 1930.
9. Blood banks 1940.
10. Brauer, R. O.: A comparison of the Tennison and LeMesurier lip repairs. Plast. Reconstr. Surg., 23:249, 1959.
11. Brown, J. B., and McDowell, F.: Small triangular flap operation for the primary repair of single cleft lips. Plast. Reconstr. Surg., 5:392, 1950.
12. Carter, W. W.: Cited by Davis, J. S.: Plastic Surgery: Its Principles and Practice. Philadelphia, P. Blakiston's and Co., 1919, p. 492.
13. Cronin, T. D.: Method of preventing raw area on the nasal surface of the soft palate in push-back surgery. Plast. Reconstr. Surg., 20:474, 1957.
14. Cronin, T. D.: A modification of the Tennison-type lip repair. Cleft Palate J., 3:376, 1966.
15. Dieffenbach, J. F.: Bertrage Zur Gaumenmath. Litt. Ann d ges Heilk, 4:145, 1826.
16. Dieffenbach, J. F.: Early description of the bone-flap operation. In Die Operative Chirurgie, Vol. 1. Leipzig, F. A. Brackhaus, 1845.
17. Dorrance, G. M.: Congenital insufficiency of the palate. Arch. Surg., 21:185, 1930.
18. Dufourmentel, C., Mouly, R., Preaux, J., and Marchas, D.: La greffe composee libre de lèure a lèure. Ann. Chir. Plast., 12:119, 1967.
19. Estlander, J. A.: Eine methods aus der einen lippe substanznerluste der anderen zu ersetzen. Arch. fur Klinische Chir., 14:622, 1872.
20. Fara, M.: The importance of folding down muscle stumps in the operation of unilateral clefts of the lip. Acta Chir. Plast. (Praha), 13:162, 1971.
21. Fara, M., and Smahel, J.: Postoperative follow-up of restitution, procedures in the orbicularis oris muscle after operation for complete bilateral cleft of the lip. Plast. Reconstr. Surg., 40:13, 1967.
22. Fara, M., Hrivnakova, J., and Sedlackova, E.: Submucous cleft palates. Acta Chir. Plast. (Praha), 13:221, 1971.
23. Fleming, A.: 1940.

24. Friede, H., and Johanson, B.: A follow-up study of cleft children treated with primary bone grafting. Scan. J. Plast. Reconstr. Surg., 8:88, 1974.
25. Gensoul, M.: J. Hebd. Med. Chir. Pratique 1933. Cited by Davis, J. S.: Plastic Surgery: Its Principles and Practice. Philadelphia, P. Blakiston's and Co., 1919, pp. 491, 494.
26. Hagedorn, W.: Operation der Hasenscharte mit Zickzacknaht. Zentralbl. Chir., 19:281, 1892.
27. Hagerty, R.: Unilateral cleft lip repair. Surg. Gynecol. Obstet., 106:119, 1958.
28. Harding, R. L., and Mazaheri, M.: Growth and spatial changes in the arch form in bilateral cleft lip and palate patients. Plast. Reconstr. Surg., 50:591, 1972.
29. Hynes, W.: Pharyngoplasty by muscle transplantation. Br. J. Plast. Surg., 3:128, 1950.
30. Kilner, T. P.: Cleft lip and palate technique: St. Thomas Hosp. Rep., 2:127, 1937.
31. Koenig, F.: Chirurgie. Lehrbuch der Speziellen Chirurgie fur Aerzte und Studierende, Vol. 1, 4th Ed. Berlin, August Hirschwald, 1898, p. 315.
32. Kremenak, C. R., Huffman, W. C., and Olin, W. H.: I. Growth of the maxillae in dogs after palatal surgery. Cleft Palate J., 4:6, 1967.
33. Kremenak, C. R., Huffman, W. C., and Olin, W. H.: II. Growth of the maxillae in dogs after palatal surgery. Cleft Palate J., 7:719, 1970.
34. Kremenak, C. R., Huffman, W. C., and Olin, W. H.: Maxillary growth inhibition by mucoperiosteal denudation of palatal shelf bone in non-cleft beagles. Cleft Palate J., 7:817, 1970.
35. Krogman, W. M.: Tabulae Biologicae. The Hague, Netherlands, Junk, 1941.
36. Krogman, W. M., Mazaheri, M., Harding, R. L., Ishiguro, K., Bariana, G., Meier, J., Canter, H., and Ross, P.: A longitudinal study of the craniofacial growth pattern in children with clefts as compared to normal, birth to six years. Cleft Palate J., 12:59, 1975.
37. LeMesurier, A. B.: A method of cutting and suturing the lip in the treatment of unilateral clefts. Plast. Reconstr. Surg., 4:1, 1949.
38. Limberg, A.: Nerve wege in der radikolen uranoplastik bei angeborenen spaltendeformationen: Osteotomia interlaminaria und pterygomaxillaris, resectio marginis foraminis palatini und neve plattchennaht, fissura ossea occulta und ihre behandlung. Zentralbl. Chir., 54:1745, 1927.
39. McIndoe, A. H.: Correction of alar deformity in cleft lip. Lancet, 1:607, 1938.
40. McIndoe, A. H., and Rees, T. D.: Synchronous repair of secondary deformities in cleft lip and nose. Plast. Reconstr. Surg., 24:150, 1959.
41. Magill, Sir Ivan: 1937.
42. Mapes, A. H., Mazaheri, M., Harding, R. L., Meier, J. A., and Canter, H. E.: A longitudinal analysis of the maxillary growth increments of cleft lip and palate patients. Cleft Palate J., 11:450, 1974.
43. Marcks, K. M., Trevaskis, A. E., and daCosta, A.: Further observations in cleft lip repair. Plast. Reconstr. Surg., 12:392, 1953.
44. Marcks, K. M., Trevaskis, A. E., and Payne, M. J.: Elongation of the columella by flap transfer and Z-plasty. Plast. Reconstr. Surg., 20:467, 1957.
45. Mazaheri, M., Harding, R. L., and Nanda, S.: The effect of surgery on maxillary growth and cleft width. Plast. Reconstr. Surg., 40:22, 1967.
46. Millard, D. R.: A primary camouflage of the unilateral harelip. In Transactions of the International Society of Plastic Surgeons, First Congress (1955). Baltimore, The Williams and Wilkins Co., 1957, p. 160.
47. Millard, D. R.: Columella lengthening by a forked flap. Plast. Reconstr. Surg., 22:454, 1958.
48. Millard, D. R.: Complete unilateral clefts of the lip. Plast. Reconstr. Surg., 25:595, 1960.
49. Millard, D. R.: Wide and/or short cleft palate: Plast. Reconstr. Surg., 29:40, 1962.
50. Millard, D. R., Jr.: A new use of the island flap in wide palate clefts. Plast. Reconstr. Surg., 38:330, 1966.
51. Millard, D. R.: Bilateral cleft lip and a primary forked flap. Plast. Reconstr. Surg., 39:59, 1967.
52. Millard, D. R.: Extensions of the rotation-advancement principle for wide unilateral cleft lips. Plast. Reconstr. Surg., 43:535, 1968.
53. Mirault, G.: Lettre sur l'operation du hec-de-lievre. J. de Chir., par M. Malgaigne, 2:257, 1844.
54. Musgrave, R. H., and Dupertius, S. M.: Revision of the unilateral cleft lip nostril. Plast. Reconstr. Surg., 25:223, 1960.
55. Musgrave, R. H.: Surgery of nasal deformities associated with cleft lip. Plast. Reconstr. Surg., 28:261, 1961.
56. Ortiz-Monasterio, F., Serrano, A., Valderama, M., and Cruz, R.: Cephalometric measurements on adult patients with non-operated clefts. Plast. Reconstr. Surg., 24:53, 1959.
57. Ortiz-Monasterio, F., Serrano, A. R., Barrera, G. P., Rodriguez-Hossman, H., and Vinegeras, E.: A study of untreated adult cleft palate patients. Plast. Reconstr. Surg., 38:36, 1966.

58. Passavant, G.: Zweiter artikel über die operation der angeborenen spalten des harten gaumens und der domit complicirten hasenscharten. Arch. Heilk., 3:305, 1862.
59. Passavant, G.: Über die beseitigung der Naselden sprache bei angeborenen spalten des harten und weichen gaumens (Gaumensegel Schlundnaht und Rucklagerung des Gaumensegels). Arch. Klin. Chir., 6:333, 1865.
60. Pruzansky, S.: Factors determining arch form in clefts of the lip and palate. Am. J. Orthod., 41:827, 1955.
61. Randall, P.: A triangular flap operation for the primary repair of unilateral clefts of the lip. Plast. Reconstr. Surg., 23:331, 1959.
62. Randall, P.: A lip adhesion operation in cleft lip surgery. Plast. Reconstr. Surg., 35:371, 1965.
63. Randall, P., and Graham, W. P.: Lip adhesion in the repair of bilateral cleft lip. *In* Grabb, W. C., Rosenstein, S. W., and Bzoch, K. R. (Eds.): Cleft Lip and Palate. Boston, Little, Brown and Co., 1971.
64. Randall, P., Whitaker, L. A., and LaRossa, D.: The importance of muscle reconstruction in primary and secondary cleft lip repair. Plast. Reconstr. Surg., 54:316, 1974.
65. Rehrmann, A. H.: Effect of early bone grafting on the growth of upper jaw in cleft lip and palate children. A computer evaluation. Minerva Chir., 26:874, 1971.
66. Reynolds, J. R., and Horton, C. E.: An alar lift procedure in cleft lip rhinoplasty. Plast. Reconstr. Surg., 35:376, 1965.
67. Rose, W.: Harelip and Cleft Palate. London, H. K. Lewis and Co., 1891.
68. Sabattini: Cross-lip flaps. Cited by McDowell, F.: The Source Book of Plastic Surgery. Baltimore, Waverly Press, 1977, p. 331.
69. Schoenhorn, K.: On a method of staphlorrhaphy. Arch. Klin. Chir., 19:527, 1876.
70. Schultz, L. W.: Bilateral cleft lips. Plast. Reconstr. Surg., 1:338, 1946.
71. Schweckendiek, W.: Die Ergebnisse der Kieferbildung und die Sprache nach der primaen Veloplastik, Arch. en Hals. Ohr-Nas-Hehlk-Hk, 180:541, 1962.
72. Skoog, T.: Plastic Surgery. Philadelphia, W. B. Saunders Co., 1975.
73. Slaughter, W. B., and Pruzansky, S.: The rationale for velar closure as a primary procedure in the repair of cleft palate defects. Plast. Reconstr. Surg., 13:341, 1954.
74. Steffensen, W. H.: A method for repair of the unilateral cleft lip. Plast. Reconstr. Surg., 4:144, 1949.
75. Stein, S. A. V.: Lip repair (cheiloplasty) performed by a new method. Hospital-Meddelalser, 1:212, 1848.
76. Straith, C. L.: Reconstructions about the nasal tip. Surg. Gynecol. Obstet., 62:73, 1936.
77. Sullivan, D. E.: Bilateral pharyngoplasty as an aid to velopharyngeal closure. Plast. Reconstr. Surg., 27:31, 1961.
78. Tennison, C. W.: The repair of the unilateral cleft lip by the stencil method. Plast. Reconstr. Surg., 9:115, 1952.
79. Thompson, J. E.: An artistic and mathematically accurate method of repairing the defect in cases of harelip. Surg. Gynecol. Obstet., 14:498, 1912.
80. Veau, V.: Division Palatine. Anatomie, Chirurgie, Phonetigue. Paris, Masson et cie, 1931.
81. Veau, V.: Division Palatine, Paris, Masson et cie, 1931.
82. vonLangenbeck, B.: Weitere erfahrungen im Gebiete der Uranoplastik mittels ablösung des Mukos−periostalen Gaumenüberzuges. Arch. Klin. Chir., 5:1, 1864.
83. Walker, J. C., Callito, M. B., Mancusi-Ungaro, A., and Meijer, R.: Physiologic considerations in cleft lip closure: The C-W technique. Plast. Reconstr. Surg., 37:552, 1966.
84. Wardill, W. E. M.: Discussion on the treatment of cleft palate by operation. Proc. R. Soc. Med., 5:178, 1926/27.
85. Wardill, W. E. M.: Cleft palate. Br. J. Surg., 16:127, 1928.
86. Warkany, J.: 1940.

The Plastic Surgery of Clefts

WILLIAM P. GRAHAM, III

*It is a misfortune of the over celebrated that they cannot
measure up to the excessive expectations of them afterwards;
never can the actual attain the imagined; for to think perfection is easy, and to materialize it, difficult; the imagination
weds the wish and together they always conjure up more than
reality can furnish.[3]*

INTRODUCTION

Surgery and concerns about it often dominate the early life of the child
with cleft lip and palate. Once the initial shock of the child's deformity has
been accepted, or at least the parental guilt and distress have diminished, a
reasonable plan for the surgical treatment can evolve. This must mesh with
the sister disciplines involved in the child's care. Absolute timing is not as
crucial as appropriate integration of the surgical efforts with the need of the
child for care by the other specialists. Guidance, reinforcement, and support
must be given the parents, who will be besieged by well-meaning friends and
family who have heard or have known of similar cases "treated in such and
such a way." The parents must realize that there are many satisfactory ways to
treat the problem surgically and that modifications in the planning may
change with the further growth and development of the child. They must
know that perfection and absolute normality cannot be achieved and that all of
the surgical efforts are directed toward improving function, providing
cosmesis, and enabling the individual to approach sufficiently close to
normality that an enjoyable, productive life can be attained. Such attainment
is *not* achieved by the isolated skill of the surgeon, but through the joint
efforts of the entire team concerned with the child's care.

The initial contact of the surgeon with the child and parents may be in the
perinatal period. This is the time to instill confidence in the parents and to
provide a reasonably brief outline of the potential procedures that the child
will likely encounter. Suggestions with respect to feeding should augment
those already recommended by the pediatrician.

SURGICAL TREATMENT

CLEFT LIP

The sequential surgical treatment of patients with cleft lips is outlined in
Table 5–1.

At an early age, with the use of sedation and local anesthesia, a lip
adhesion operation might be done if the child has an unusually wide
unilateral or bilateral cleft. If myringotomies are required, general anesthesia
is chosen and the two procedures are combined. As a preliminary step, this
operation converts the complete cleft into an incomplete one and initiates
molding of the premaxillary and lateral maxillary segments physiologically
into normal relationships without the use of external traction. The specific

TABLE 5-1 Sequential Surgical Treatment of Cleft Lip

PROCEDURE	AGE OF CHILD				
	1 month°	3 months	6-8 months	10-16 months	6-8 years
Unilateral lip	Adhesion a. Randall b. Walker-Collito	Definitive repair a. Millard b. Tennison			Scar revision
Unilateral lip and unilateral palate	Adhesion°	Definitive vomer flap°		Definitive closure of associated soft palatal cleft	Anterior fistula
Bilateral lip	Adhesion°	Adhesion°	Individual double lip repair (6 months)	Remaining lip (9 months)	
Bilateral lip (alternative)		Definitive unilateral lip	Definitive second lip		
Bilateral lip (alternative)		Double lip repair			
Nasal tip rhinoplasty		Combined with surgery			9-16 years, independent procedure
Scar revisions lip-nose					Usually after puberty unless very unsightly
Rhinoplasty and septoplasty					Usually after age 12 years

°Optional

technique has been described earlier in this chapter. When a lip adhesion is used, the definitive lip repair may be delayed. Alternatively, the performance of bilateral lip adhesions may facilitate early lengthening of the foreshortened columella prior to, or during, definitive lip repair.

Usually, definitive repair of the cleft lip is undertaken at age three months. When myringotomies will be an adjunctive procedure, general anesthesia is used, and the examination of the ears and the insertion of the artificial eustachian tubes are done either at the beginning or the close of the operative procedure.

The surgeon selects the appropriate lip repair procedure based on the width of the cleft, the adequacy of tissues, and the length of the lip that must be attained. Generally, a rotation-advancement procedure, such as that of Millard, or a modification of the Tennison triangular flap procedure is used. Most frequently when dealing with bilateral clefts, the rotation-advancement procedure is preferred, and the definitive repairs are staged several months apart. This diminishes the tension on each repair, minimizes the risk of dehiscence, and lessens the tension on the wound that leads to scar separation or thickening. In conjunction with the definitive correction of the lip itself, repositioning of the alar base is carried out. When this is done, attention must be given to avoid buckling of the upper portion of the alar cartilage within the nostril and obstructing of the vestibule.

The specific techniques of lip repair have previously been discussed.

For the child who has a bilateral cleft of the lip, the second definitive lip repair will generally be done about six months of age. The procedure will be identical to that performed on the first side. Therefore, at the time of the initial procedure, it is helpful to have made specific measurements of the width of the cupid's bow and the height of the lip that are intended.

Columellar lengthening can be facilitated by sliding the excess tissue from the side of the prolabium up into the columella. This can be done as an independent procedure or separately with each definitive lip repair. The use of this technique conserves prolabial tissue and diminishes the chance of needing a columellar lengthening at a later age.

Definitive bilateral lip repairs can be done as a single procedure if the clefts are not wide, with too small a prolabium and marked separation of the premaxilla and lateral maxillary segments. In this instance, the preferred repair is that described by Millard, involving rotation-advancement of the segments and reconstruction of the cupid's bow by the use of lateral vermilion flaps. With any of the lip repairs, a vomer flap can be used to achieve anterior

TABLE 5–2   Sequential Surgical Treatment of Cleft Palate

	AGE OF CHILD				
PROCEDURE	*1 month*	*3 months*	*6 months*	*10–16 months*	*3–6 years*
Submucosal palatal cleft				Closure and lengthening, possible posterior pharyngeal flap	May delay until certain about velopharyngeal incompetence
Bilateral palate				Either posterior palate or complete	Anterior palate, if necessary
Bilateral lip and palate	Adhesion°	Adhesion°	Definitive one side	Definitive other side and soft palate	Anterior palate
(Alternative)		Unilateral lip	Unilateral lip	Soft palate	Anterior palate
Velopharyngeal incompetence					Posterior pharyngeal flap, superior based or inferior based

°Optional

closure of the hard palate along with the closure of the defect in the alveolus. This cannot be done if the cleft is extremely narrow. Closure of the alveolar cleft is facilitated by the use of a buccal mucosal flap.

CLEFT PALATE

In the extremely robust, healthy child, closure of the soft palate can be done as early as nine months, although most often it is carried out between 10 and 16 months of age (Table 5–2). If the second definitive lip repair has not been done, it is carried out at this age, with or without closure of the soft palate. By combining these two procedures, the need for additional hospitalization and anesthesia for the child is eliminated. Throughout the course of cleft lip and palate surgery in the child with a cleft palate, one must bear in mind the need for close observation of the ears and the use of myringotomies and artificial eustachian tubes as indicated. Combining this evaluation with the other necessary operative procedures eliminates unnecessary anesthetics for the child.

Most children by the age of one year are sufficiently large and healthy to permit repair of the soft palate. Here, the choice of the surgeon is dictated by the availability of soft tissue, the width of the cleft, its unilaterality or bilaterality, and what surgery has already been performed with respect to the anterior palate. Three conditions must be satisfied by any surgical procedure: (1) minimize subsequent disturbance of maxillary growth, (2) achieve anatomical closure of the gross defect, and (3) permit physiological closure of the velopharyngeal space.

Generally, the soft palate is lengthened at the time of its closure and an intravelar veloplasty may be performed.

Restoration of the normal levator sling (intravelar veloplasty) is achieved by freeing the muscle from its anterior attachments and interdigitating the two ends across the midline. This releases the abnormal anterior attachment of the levator, facilitates lengthening the palate, and recreates the normal line of pull and attachment of these two muscles to one another at the midline of the soft palate. Criticism of this facet of palatal repair lies in the fact that the necessary dissection is considerably greater than in other methods and may result in greater scarring, precluding good velar function. Routine fracturing of the hamular process is not done unless the closure seems unusually tight.

Combining initial palatal closure with a superiorly based posterior pharyngeal flap is at the election of the surgeon and usually is chosen when the nasopharyngeal vault is extremely spacious or when the soft tissue available for palatal closure appears deficient. For those children whose soft palate is markedly underdeveloped and in whom minimal musculature exists for closure, the use of a speech bulb attached to an anterior prosthesis is often more feasible than multiple operative procedures in the face of deficient soft tissue.

Opinions differ with respect to the early use of the posterior pharyngeal flap at the time of the definitive palate repair and its selection at the earliest sign of velopharyngeal incompetence in the child who has had a cleft repaired. When performed as an isolated operative procedure, the inferiorly based posterior pharyngeal flap is a more simple operation, while the superiorly based flap is usually selected when closing the soft palate and particularly when lengthening it. The specific techniques of palatal repair and posterior pharyngeal flap operative procedures have previously been discussed.

The anterior palate may be closed in conjunction with the lip surgery but is often left open until the child is older to avoid unnecessary scarring. When anterior closure is effected at the time of lip repair, a vomer flap is usually employed. If the anterior defect is closed during the immediate preschool period, growth has often diminished the relative size of the defect and enhances the success of the repair.

Bone grafting of the maxilla is rarely employed. When grafting is done, it is utilized in the older individual (older than 12 years) who has an unstable premaxilla. There is considerable controversy regarding the efficacy of early bone grafting, but our experience has shown that it may prove more of a detriment than an asset when used routinely.

Throughout the period of surgical treatment, the surgeon has to communicate with the other members of the treatment team to be sure that dental extractions, dental banding, impressions, myringotomies, and so forth are not needed also. In addition, the surgeon must be cognizant of the emotional reactions of the child to repeated hospitalizations and surgery. Often, it is well to put off an operative procedure when the child is unduly distressed about the prospect.

In the teens, correction of nasal deviation, palatal fistula, nasal deformity, and the revision of lip and nasal scars can be done at times convenient for the child. Many of these lesser procedures can be done with local anesthesia without the need to admit the individual to the hospital.

References

1. Berkeley, W. T.: Correction of secondary cleft lip nasal deformities. Plast. Reconstr. Surg., 44:234, 1969.
2. Dunn, F. S.: Results of the vomer flap technique used in surgery of the cleft palate during the last eleven years. Am. J. Surg., 92:825, 1956.
3. Gracian, B.: A Truth-Telling Manual and the Art of Worldly Wisdom. Translated by Martin Fischer. Springfield, Ill., Charles C Thomas, Publisher, 1934, p. 31.
4. Kriens, O. B.: Fundamental anatomical findings for an intravelar veloplasty. Cleft Palate J. 7:27, 1970.
5. Mazaheri, M., Harding, R. L., and Nanda, S.: The effects of surgery on maxillary growth and cleft width. Plast. Reconstr. Surg. 40:22, 1967.
6. Millard, D. R., Jr.: Refinements in rotation-advancement cleft lip technique. Plast. Reconstr. Surg., 33:26, 1964.
7. Millard, D. R., Jr.: The unilateral cleft lip nose. Plast. Reconstr. Surg., 34:169, 1964.
8. Millard, D. R., Jr.: Cleft lip. In Grabb, W. C., and Smith, James W. (Eds.): Plastic Surgery. Boston, Little, Brown, and Co., 1973, p. 159.
9. Randall, P.: A triangular flap operation for the primary repair of unilateral clefts of the lip. Plast. Reconstr. Surg., 23:331, 1959.
10. Randall, P. and Graham, W. P.: Lip adhesion in the repair of bilateral cleft lip. In Grabb, W. C., Rosenstein, S. W., and Bzoch, K. R. (Eds.): Cleft Lip and Palate. Boston, Little, Brown, and C., 1971, p. 282.
11. Rehrmann, A. H., Koberg, W. R., and Kock, H.: Long term postoperative results of primary and secondary bone grafting in complete cleft of the lip and palate. Cleft Palate J. 7:207, 1970.
12. Ruding, R.: Cleft palate: Anatomic and surgical considerations. Plast. Reconstr. Surg., 33:132, 1964.
13. Walker, J. C., Jr., Collito, M. B., Mancusi-Unagro, A., and Meijer, R. Physiologic considerations in cleft lip closure: The C-W technique. Plast. Reconstr. Surg., 37:552, 1966.

DIAGNOSIS AND _____
TREATMENT PLANNING

The oral cavity and its complement of teeth play an important role in the growth, development, and appearance of the human face. They are also essential parts of the speech mechanism. In the individual with an orofacial or speech handicap whose dental arch is distorted by a congenital condition, or by disease or accident, the teeth can be of critical importance, for their presence is necessary as an aid in treatment with a prosthetic restoration or an orthodontic appliance. Therefore, every technique for the preservation of the teeth and surrounding structures should be employed by the dentists involved in the care of these patients.

Many people fail to realize that the teeth and periodontal tissues have a direct relationship to their health and their future well-being and appearance, a relationship particularly vital in those with oral deformities. For this reason, our first step in treatment should be to establish the mouth in good hygienic condition and to impress upon the patient that good oral hygiene habits and methods practiced at home can help prevent many dental problems. Not only must the teeth be kept clean and cared for, but the soft tissues surrounding them, which are equally important, must be protected. In fact, in persons past the age of 35, periodontal conditions can become a greater cause of tooth loss than dental caries.

DENTAL CARE

Routine dental care is important in children. The condition of the deciduous teeth, their malposition or their absence, can affect the success of the child's total cleft lip and palate treatment.

A full set of deciduous teeth is normally present by age three, and a dentist should see the child at that time or before. If there is a cleft of the al-

PROSTHODONTIC CARE

MOHAMMAD MAZAHERI

veolar bone, changes generally occur in the structures of the teeth next to the cleft. In some instances extra teeth are present. Any of these teeth may be malformed or may grow outside of their normal position. They may also interfere with feeding to the extent that extraction is required, but it is usually important that all deciduous teeth be kept until they are replaced naturally by the developing permanent teeth.

The dentist takes x-rays as early as possible to help detect carious lesions and supernumerary, malformed, or missing teeth. General inspection alone will not suffice to establish the presence of abnormal dental and periodontal conditions. Parents must be fully aware of how to provide good mouth care. In areas where fluorine is missing from the drinking water, the dentist may recommend the topical application of fluoride to reduce tooth decay.

In persons depending on an appliance for proper mastication, appearance, and good speech, it is absolutely essential that every measure be taken *to insure a good clean mouth and throat. Consequently, we insist that patients learn methods of brushing with a proper tooth brush, flossing, and applying fluoride.* They should also be taught the importance of keeping their appliances clean. Far too often the bands and clasps are blamed for causing carious lesions, while in reality, it was carelessness on the part of the patient in allowing the accumulation of food debris.

DIAGNOSTIC AND EXAMINATION PROCEDURES

Every patient with an oral cleft should be examined by surgical, medical, dental, speech, and hearing specialists. The following procedures will facilitate the proper diagnosis and aid in treatment: (1) case history and recording of defect; (2) study casts and photographs; (3) various radiographic procedures; and (4) medical, surgical, speech, and psychosocial record-taking.

The study casts and photographs, along with various radiographic procedures, help the dentist to appraise the growth and development patterns of orofacial and cranial structures and to observe the effects of surgical and orthopedic intervention upon the physiology and anatomy of the structures involved.

Before the patient is brought to the examination room or dental operatory, however, an interview is conducted at the Clinic, during which an intake caseworker explains the roles that the specialists will play in the rehabilitation program. If the patient is a child, the parents, of course, are principals in the interview. (This subject is discussed in the chapter on social work.)

Case History

A well-designed case history will provide all members of the team with the information they need. This form should not be limited to information about the cleft and the history of its treatment, but should cover details about the patient's general medical background, past illnesses and operations (other than for the cleft), and any treatments undergone or currently taking place for any condition whatsoever. It should also touch upon the family's social and economic background, and it is essential that the information be arranged in concise form for rapid recording and retrieval (Fig 6–1).

Dental History

Special attention should be devoted to the shape of the dental arch (anteriorly, posteriorly, and laterally), the palatal vault height, and the status of the velopharyngeal relationship (the length and the mobility of the soft palate). These morphological details should be charted. All dental anomalies, such as those involving number, shape, and formation of the teeth, the arch and tooth relationship, and the state of the occlusion (type of malocclusion, if present), should be recorded. Other details to be covered in the dental history are dental caries, missing teeth, the condition of gingival and periodontal tissue, periapical lesions, and any other information of dental significance.

Of interest in connection with the recording of the dental history is the following record of the incidence of calcification anomalies and numerical anomalies in the Lancaster Cleft Palate Clinic population. The data were obtained from clinical and radiographic observations and from dental casts.

A. Calcification Anomalies
1. A significant number (56.3 per cent) of the population (131 male, 112 female) presented calcification anomalies.
2. In cases involving the maxillary alveolar ridge there was a slightly higher number of maxillary than mandibular anomalies (116 to 92), but when the alveolar ridge was not involved the incidence of maxillary to mandibular anomalies was about the same (79 to 82).
3. The great majority of the calcification anomalies involved the anterior rather than the posterior teeth.
4. Many more anomalies were found in the deciduous and mixed dentitions than in the permanent dentition.
5. A slight but significantly greater incidence of calcification anomalies was noted in those with clefts involving the alveolar ridge and lip compared with those having only a palatal cleft. In patients with a bilateral cleft of the alveolar process there is a greater number of calcification anomalies than in those with a unilateral cleft of the alveolar process.

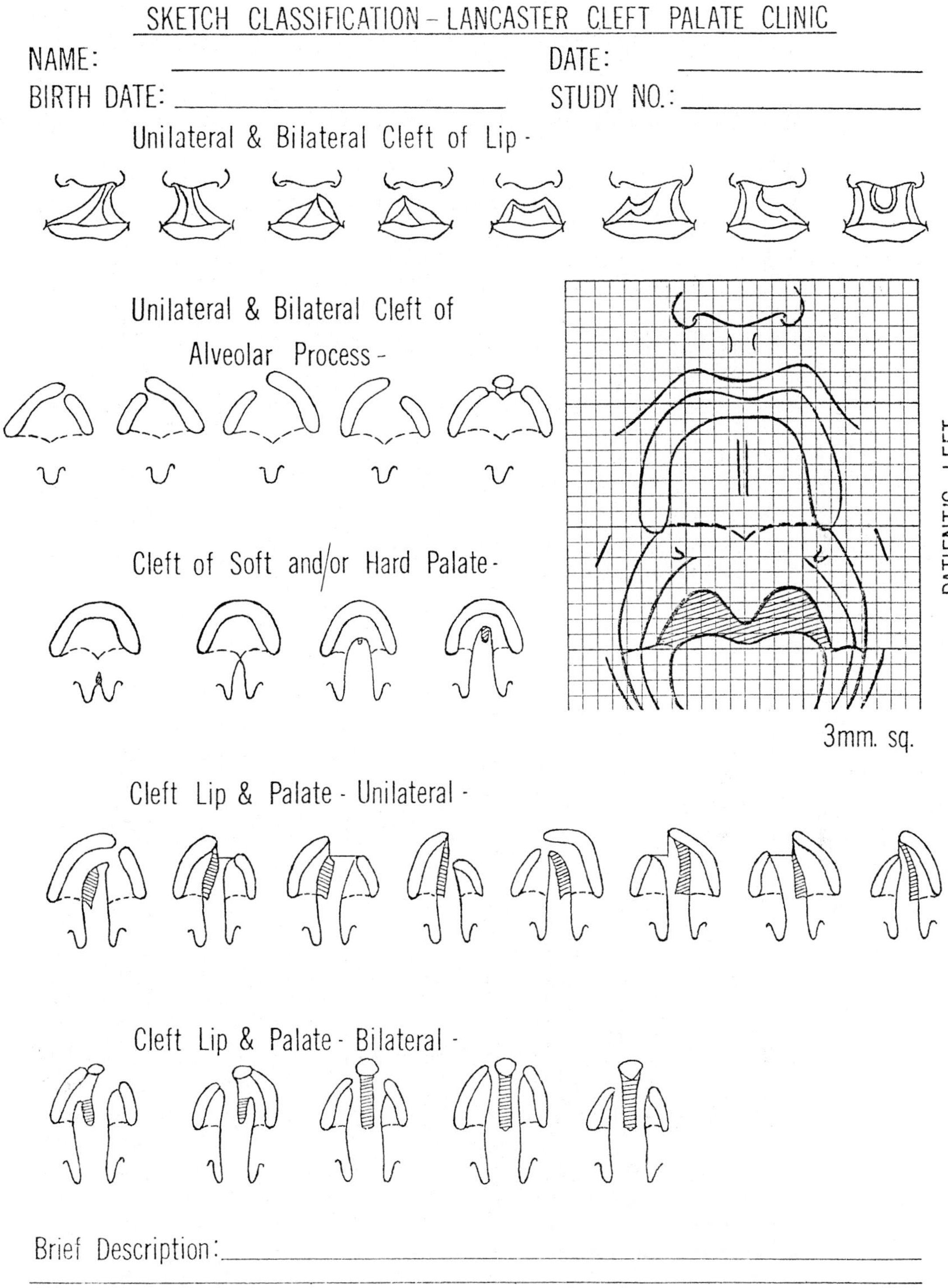

FIGURE 6–1 Cleft classification chart used for each patient at the Lancaster Cleft Palate Clinic. Exact measurement of cleft size is made on dental cast and facial mask and recorded on grid drawing.

B. Numerical Dental Anomalies (Congenitally Missing or Supernumerary Teeth)
 1. A significant number (30.4 per cent) of the population had numerical dental anomalies. This figure includes 21.5 per cent with congenitally missing teeth and 8.9 per cent with supernumerary teeth.
 2. A high incidence (114 out of the total 249) of maxillary lateral incisor anomalies was noticed. Secondary peaks occurred at the location of *both* maxillary and mandibular second bicuspids.
 3. A significant number of dental anomalies were found in the primary dentition at the sites of the maxillary lateral incisors only.
 4. Supernumerary teeth were more common in the primary dentition, whereas missing teeth were more common in the secondary dentition.
 5. A bilateral cleft of the alveolar process was accompanied by almost twice as many numerical anomalies as were found with a unilateral cleft of the alveolar process.
 6. A significantly increased incidence of numerical anomalies was seen in children with a cleft of the alveolar process. Thirty-four to 56.5 per cent of them had missing or supernumerary teeth as compared with a rate of 10 per cent in the subjects with an unaffected alveolar process.
 7. When numerical anomalies were analyzed with respect to their relation to the "unilateral cleft of the lip, alveolar process and palate," it was found that twice as many of these anomalies of the maxillary arch were present on the side of the cleft as on the normal side.

Examination of Infants

As part of the examination of the young patient, Panorex, bite wing, and two lateral cephalometrics are taken (one at rest and one during enunciation of the sound "E"). A posteroanterior radiographic film is also taken, and a cineradiograph is recorded while the patient repeats the following words and sounds:
 1. PAH TAH LAH KAH SAH
 2. Bessie stayed one summer.
 3. AH/A (bat)/EE/OO (boot).
 4. BEAT BAT BOUGHT BOOT.
The patient is then asked to blow in a tube as hard as possible and is instructed to swallow water from a cup.

The dentist's responsibility starts shortly after the birth of a child with a cleft. At this time, and semiannually until the child is two years old, the dentist makes impressions of the infant's maxillary and mandibular regions and also makes cephalometric and photographic records. On the child's second birthday and annually thereafter, the impressions and the radiographic and photographic records are repeated.

Maxillary and mandibular impression trays for infants are not manufactured commercially and must, therefore, be constructed by the dentist. The first step is to shape a piece of baseplate wax against the maxillary or mandibular ridge. The wax is held with one finger and molded against the tissue with the other fingers. The wax pattern obtained is then invested and processed in acrylic resin. The procedure is repeated on different types of clefts until a sufficient number of trays is obtained. Additional trays also can be constructed on the casts collected in the series (Figure 6–2).

Holes are drilled in the tray to provide mechanical retention and means of escape for excess impression material. Additional retention is achieved by painting the internal surface of the tray with an impression adhesive.

An irreversible hydrocolloid material is used for maxillary and mandibular impressions. The amount of water used for these impressions is five sixths of that recommended by the manufacturer, and the water temperature should be 110 degrees F. in order to speed the setting of the material.

The maxillary impression is made with the infant's head tilted at a downward angle of 15 degrees. The head is tilted slightly upward for the mandibular impression. This position makes it possible to maintain a direct view of the oral cavity at all times and directs the flow of the material toward the oropharyngeal space (Figures 6–3 and 6–4).

While the impression is being made, at least four assistants should be available to (1) hold the infant's head, (2) depress the tongue and hold the suction, (3) hold the infant's body and feet, and (4) mix the impression material. The infant is restrained in a receiving blanket.

Proper instruments should be available on the bracket table for gaining access to material should it be displaced or lodged in the nasal and oral pharynx. The tray should not be overloaded with the impression material, nor should too much force be applied in placing the tray in position. The part of the tray that will be directly over the undercut should contain less of the impression material. The procedure for removing the impression from the mouth must be modified according to the location of the undercut.

Flat records of the salient features and dimensions of the impression cast, for filing and for periodic comparisons as the child grows, may be made by the technique illustrated in Figures 6–5 and 6–6, which show how a cast holder assures precise orientation during Xerox reproduction. In Figure 6–7

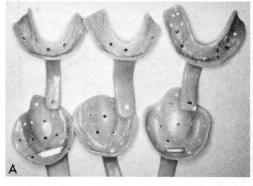
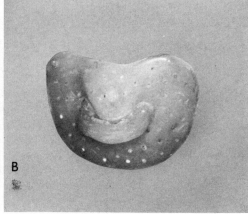

FIGURE 6–2 Custom-made trays for infants (A, intraoral; B, facial) of acrylic resin. Specially constructed trays are needed for the ages of one month, six months, one year, and one and a half years. Stock trays are available for children from age two and thereafter.

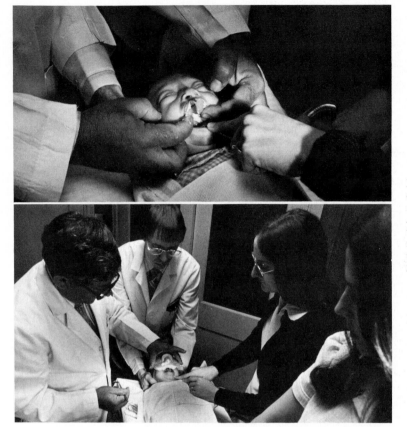

FIGURE 6–3 The infant is properly placed and restrained for intraoral and facial impressions. Adequate suction, direct view of the oral cavity, and assistance and maintenance of airway must be available at all times.

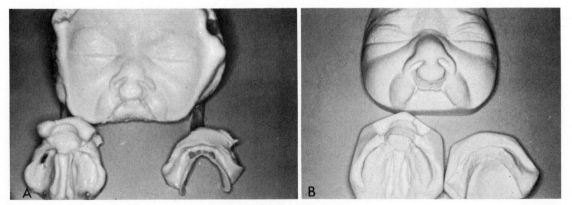

FIGURE 6–4 The maxillary, mandibular, and facial impressions are made in irreversible hydrocolloid, *A*, and then poured in artificial stone, *B*.

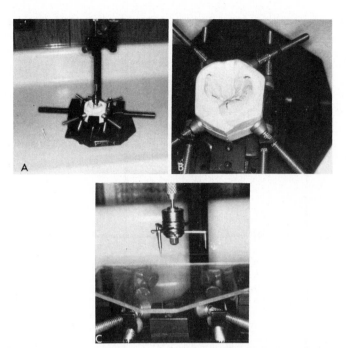

FIGURE 6–5 Techniques used for horizontal orientation of the maxillary and mandibular casts prior to Xeroxing of the cast. *A,* Three orientation points connected to spindle of surveyor rest on landmarks I, T, and T′ (see Figure 6–6), thus orienting cast in desired position. *B,* Model held in a specially designed cast holder with adjustable and flexible screws. *C,* When glass plate is slid over top of holder, it will touch three highest points of cast.

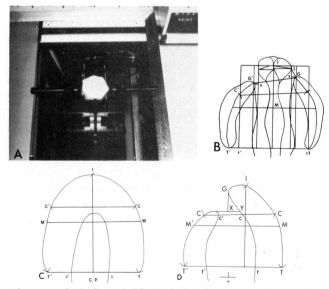

FIGURE 6–6 The cast is locked in a holder and placed in center of Xerox photocopy window *(A).* The three outlines present the graphic view of the photostat of maxillary casts for a patient with a bilateral cleft lip and palate *(B),* cleft of the palate *(C),* and unilateral cleft lip and palate *(D),* demonstrating points from which lines are drawn and measurements are made.

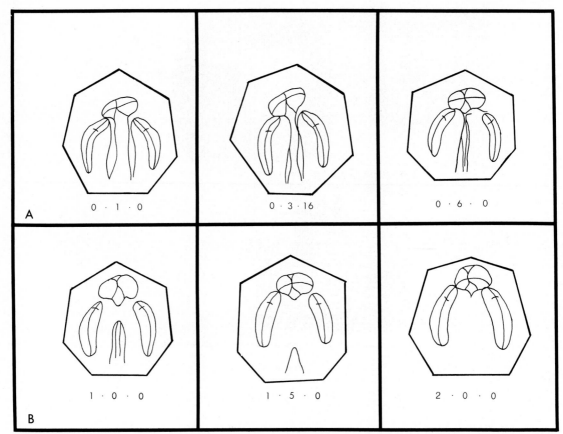

FIGURE 6-7 Photocopy of casts of patient with bilateral cleft lip and palate. Note changes in premaxillary positioning in relation to the lateral maxillary segments before and after lip and palate surgery and at various ages.

are photocopies depicting changes in premaxillary positioning after surgery, at various ages.

Older Children and Adults

A stock tray of adequate dimensions is selected. If a registration of the entire cleft is desirable, the stock tray is modified with modeling compound extending posteriorly to the posterior pharyngeal wall (Figure 6-8). This added section of the tray is under-extended about 4 to 5 mm. in all directions, leaving an adequate space for impression material. The fast-setting irreversible hydrocolloid is used for registering the preliminary impression (Figure 6-9). The following suggestions should be kept in mind when the impression is made:

1. The young patient should be given the opportunity to examine the tray and, in some cases, to try the tray in his or her mouth. The child should be told that cooperation is needed; otherwise, it will

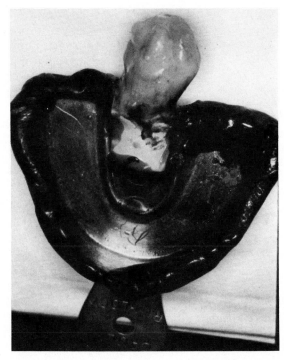

FIGURE 6-8 A stock tray, border trimmed with modeling compound and extended posteriorly with compound and Adaptol, is modified to be used for making the preliminary impression.

be necessary to make several impressions. It is advisable to keep children's minds occupied by talking to them.

2. The patient should have an early morning appointment.
3. The patient should have an empty stomach.
4. A topical anesthetic should be used on a child who has a severe gagging reflex.
5. The tray should not be overloaded with impression material.

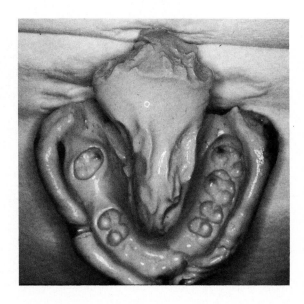

FIGURE 6-9 An irreversible hydrocolloid preliminary impression using the tray in Figure 6-8. Note the registration of hard and soft palatal clefts by the impressions.

Excess material in the nasopharynx will increase the difficulty of removing the impression without a fracture.

6. All oral perforations should be packed with gauze that has been saturated with petroleum jelly.

Roentgenographic Cephalometry

As with the dental impressions, cephalometric data are recorded periodically. A cineradiographic study with synchronized sound, made by the oropharyngeal structures during speech, can help the dentist to evaluate velopharyngeal action and tongue position in postoperative and velopharyngeally incompetent individuals. A series of cephalometric radiographs can also be of great assistance. Sound spectrograms of speech are used for comparative studies of speech changes. A device that measures pressure and flow permits the study of the relationship between nasal emission and speech quality. Forms or charts for collecting data from the various examinations are designed for use with modern computers.

The roentgenographic cephalometer is an accurate, scientific instrument for evaluating craniofacial size, proportion, and growth. Recently many investigators have used it in studying velopharyngeal relationships during various functional activities and in measuring dimensions and observing positions of the lip, tongue, and velum.

Infant Cephalometry

The technique employed in obtaining child and adult roentgenographic cephalometric data was described by Broadbent in 1931.[3] Since that time many others have elaborated and added to this technique. In 1957 Krogman and Sassoni published an extensive discussion. Pruzansky and Lis[31] and Mazaheri and Sahni[28] have described a method for infant cephalometry (Figures 6–10 and 6–11).

Numerous head-holding devices have been introduced (see Figure 6–

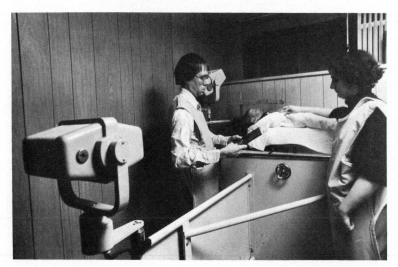

FIGURE 6–10 Infant cephalometric unit with multiple x-ray ports for different exposure planes. Port for anteroposterior plane is mounted beneath stretcher holding infant, who has been sedated. Operator and mother wear lead aprons.

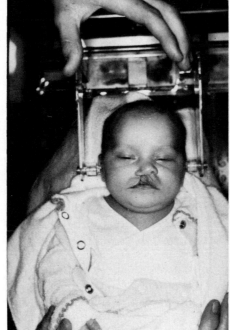
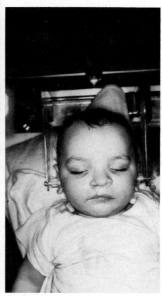

FIGURE 6–11 The ear rod tips are placed in the external meatuses, and the infant's head is oriented in the Frankfort horizontal plane.

12), but immobility is a prerequisite for a precise radiographic examination of the infant and, therefore, we advocate sedation of the child before the procedure is begun. The health of the patient is the chief factor considered in the administration of the sedative. All patients are given a medical examination beforehand. The sedative should have a quick and brief action with minimal side effects. We have found sodium pentobarbital (Nembutal) to be

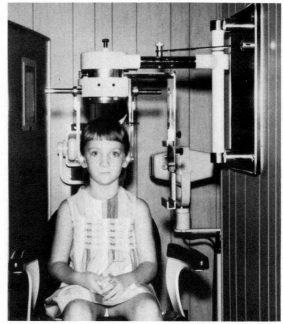

FIGURE 6–12 A B. F. Wehmer cephalometric unit for older children and adults.

the most satisfactory. Since the required dosage is only about half that of most other barbiturates, the aftereffects are fewer and of shorter duration, and there is a wider margin of safety. The dosage is adjusted for the weight and age of the infant and is given orally in the elixir form. The sedated child is placed in a crib in a quiet, darkened room or is held by the parent until asleep. In approximately five per cent of the infants the pentobarbital has no sedative effect, or it may even have a paradoxical stimulating effect. These patients are referred back to the family physician for selection of another type of sedative. We have found chloral hydrate to be effective in some of these children.

It is our experience that children under two months of age require no sedation. These children are scheduled for appointments before their regular sleeping time, and sleep is induced with warm milk prior to the recording procedure. After completion of the cephalometry, the child is gradually awakened, and intraoral impressions are then made. If the child remains drowsy, the parents are told to keep him or her under close observation until fully awake.

The procedure itself is carried out on a special table.* All of the infant's clothing that would obscure points of radiological interest is either removed or adjusted prior to placing the sedated patient on the table in the supine position. The head is centered in a head-holding device that is in fixed relation to the x-ray tube, a unit† mounted on an extension of the table. With a gear and rack apparatus the right and left ear posts are moved simultaneously until they are in line and can be lightly placed within the ear holes. The posts and their supporting arms are made of rigid but radiolucent plastic material, which allows for unobstructed visualization of the anatomic landmarks. The infant's head is kept in the Frankfort horizontal plane and proper postural relations must be maintained between the head, neck, and body. The distance from the anode to the midsagittal plane is 60 inches for the lateral cephalometric radiograms, and the exposure for the average infant is 15 milliamperes at 90 kvp. for $\frac{1}{3}$ second. For the posteroanterior radiogram the distance from anode to transmeatal plane is 36 inches, and the exposure is 15 ma. at 90 kvp. for $\frac{4}{15}$ second. Exposure time will increase proportionately after the child is two years old.

The source of radiation is equipped with a lead grading filter that facilitates proper soft and hard tissue definition in the profile of the face. The film used is 8 by 10 Kodak blue brand.**

Occlusal Radiograms. A General Electric 90 dental unit mounted on a wall is used for making the occlusal radiograms, with a focal film distance of 18 inches. The sedated child remains positioned in the head holder, and a third tray tube, mounted on a wall directly behind the cephalostat, is activated. The tube is adjusted so that the central ray bisects the maxillary line at 90 degrees. The occlusal film is placed inside the mouth and is held in position with a specially designed mounted fork film holder. The exposure used is 15 ma. at 90 kvp. for $\frac{2}{10}$ second (Figure 6–13).

---

*Manufactured by the B. F. Wehmer Company, Franklin Park, Illinois.
†General Electric 90 unit, manufactured by the General Electric Corporation, Philadelphia.
**Manufactured by Eastman Kodak Company, Rochester, N.Y.

Developing and processing of all the radiograms are carried out in the Kodak M5 processing unit, with a processing time of eight minutes for a developing solution at a temperature of 81 degrees F.

Intraoral Radiographs. The intraoral radiograph is used to determine the condition of the teeth and surrounding structures. This type of radiograph includes full mouth x-ray, bite wings, and occlusal x-ray films.

Cineradiography

Although the static radiograph is a valuable asset in determining abnormal conditions and changes in growth in the craniofacial complex, it has limited usefulness in functional analysis of the moving parts. Here cineradiography, with accompanying sound on film, is a most important tool, especially in assessing the results of surgical procedures in the velopharyngeal structures in terms of their functional adequacy. The method can be employed to record on film the action of the mandible, tongue, velum, and surrounding tissues during phonation, blowing, and swallowing. Moreover, the relationship of these velopharyngeal structures in the patient with a

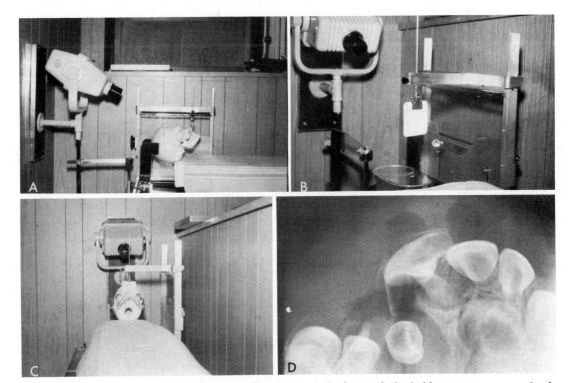

FIGURE 6–13 An x-ray tube mounted on the wall and a specially designed film holder permit a precise fixed-distance radiograph of the anterior maxillary region to be made. For clearer illustration a skull is shown in position with the film holder between the jaws (A). In patients in whom the cleft involves the alveolar process, the bony relationship of the maxillary segments and changes in their movement and position can be accurately measured after surgery of the lip and palate (with and without bone grafting). The occlusal film is placed in line with the x-ray source (B), and C shows, again with a skull, the occlusal film properly positioned. D is an occlusal radiogram showing position of the anterior teeth.

cleft can be compared, on the cineradiographic study film, with the corresponding structures in normal individuals.

Another important application of cineradiography is in isolating the cause of unnecessary displacement of the prosthesis. Direct visual examination has not been satisfactory in this assignment. With the cineradiographic equipment, the relationship of the velar and pharyngeal sections of the prosthesis to the tongue, soft palate, and posterior pharyngeal wall can be observed during swallowing, speaking, and blowing. Both sound and radiographic images can be recorded for careful study. If any movement of the prosthetic speech appliance is revealed, proper adjustments can be made.

The major components of the cineradiographic apparatus are a rotating anode roentgenographic tube with a 0.3 mm. focal spot, a nine-inch image intensifier tube with a light intensification factor of approximately 3600, and an Auricon 16 mm. motion picture camera with its optical system for recording sound-on-film data at 24 frames per second. A specially designed cephalostat consisting of ear rods and plastic forehead positioner calibrated to orient patients to their initial position for subsequent studies can be used.

The distance between the roentgenographic tube and the intensifier tube is fixed, and the tubes are adjusted so that the central rays of the roentgen tube will pass through with no risk to the patient and will strike the center of the receiving screen of the image intensifier. A full-wave generator with an output-smoothing device supplies the power for the rotating roentgen tube. The generator has a stepless control of both kilovolts and milliamperes. The sound-on-film recording apparatus is visually monitored for recording all data presented by the operator or patient. Settings of 65 to 75 kv. and 1.75 ma., with 0.27 mm. copper filter and a 0.5 mm. aluminum filter, are used. The radiation dose received by each subject, for 30 seconds' duration, averages 0.25 R., which is much lower than any standard dental or medical x-ray.

Recording Data

Analysis of skull shape by an electronic method has enabled us to quantify and analyze our cephalometric data with maximal accuracy and minimal professional supervision. The following is a brief description of the technique.

Step 1: Tracings of cephalometric roentgenogram are made with high reliability by trained technicians.

Step 2: To quantify this conventional pattern before using it as a basis for craniofacial analysis, a process known in the computer world as "digitizing" is used. This method converts the cephalometric tracings into a series of coordinates very much as in a mapping program. After a number of experiments and consultations, we adapted 139 coordinated points to represent a description of the basal skull and surrounding soft tissue. The numerical points include all the conventional craniometric landmarks, such as nasion, sella, basion, gonion, and anterior and posterior nasal spines, as well as many intermediate points, geometrically determined, so that there will be enough points to describe adequately the bone and the superimposed soft tissue outline. Figure 6–14 illustrates the 139 points on which our mathematical model of the skull is based.

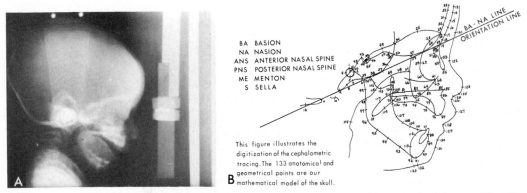

BA BASION
NA NASION
ANS ANTERIOR NASAL SPINE
PNS POSTERIOR NASAL SPINE
ME MENTON
S SELLA

This figure illustrates the digitization of the cephalometric tracing. The 133 anatomical and geometrical points are our mathematical model of the skull.

FIGURE 6–14 *A,* Cephalogram of the infant. *B,* Digitized cephalometric tracing of the same cephalogram. The 139 anatomic and geometrical points map our mathematical model of the skull.

Step 3: The digitizing device used to generate the coordinate points is generally known as OSCAR. Two cross hairs are positioned over the points on the mathematical model, and a recording knob is pressed when the point is to be recorded. A potentiometer generates recording voltages that are then passed through the analogue to the digital converter. This converter then operates an automatic IBM punch card machine, which punches the coordinates on the standard IBM card (Figure 6–15).

Distances, angles, areas, and other dimensions can be computed from the mathematical model very neatly by developing suitable programs to take the measurements of the various coordinates. For instance, each point of the mathematical model is described by two coordinates, the distance along an X axis and the distance along a Y axis. Hence, the distance of any point from the origin becomes the length of the hypotenuse of a right triangle and can be computed from the Pythagorean theorem. Similarly, by employing the same theorem, one can calculate the linear distance between any two points on the mathematical model. The data recorded on either a punch card or magnetic tape are programmed for computer analysis. Frame-by-frame analysis of cineradiographic film using the aforementioned technique is useful in functional analysis of speech organs.

FIGURE 6–15 In the center is an OSCAR model F scanning device, to the right a decimal converter used in conjunction with the OSCAR unit, and to the left an IBM 026 cardpunch. The OSCAR unit records previously designated points from traced cephalometric films as X and Y coordinates. These coordinates are produced at various voltage levels and automatically fed into a decimal converter. The converter then changes the voltage levels into integer numbers and feeds these numbers into a 026 cardpunch, which in turn produces a punched data card. The data obtained by this procedure could be used for multiregression analyses of linear and angular measurements.

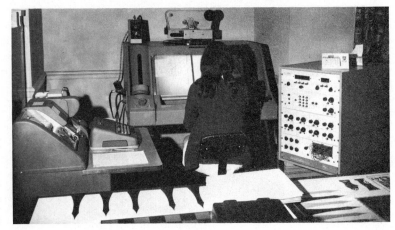

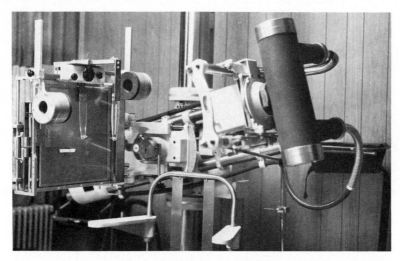

FIGURE 6–16 The Franklin laminographic unit. Note the custom fabricated ear rods attached to the head-holding unit.

Laminagraphy and Pantomography

Laminagraphy has been helpful in the study of craniofacial growth and velopharyngeal orifice size during the sustained sound. Recently, Mazaheri and Biggerstaff[21] introduced a sectional laminagraph for the study of the temporomandibular joint (Figures 6–16 and 6–17).

Panoramic x-rays have been utilized for the clinical diagnosis of the orofacial region and also for growth appraisal of the area.

Photographs

Photographs have been routinely employed in the Cooper Institute in diagnosis, illustration of the patient's situation before and after treatment, and teaching. By precise orientation of the head, it is possible to minimize

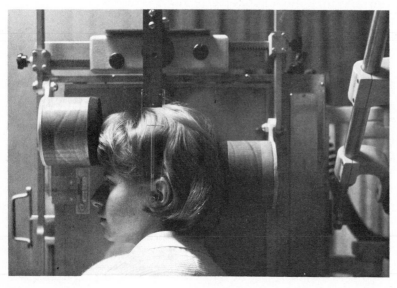

FIGURE 6–17 An anteroposterior view of a patient's head positioned in the Frankfort horizontal plane, with the ear rods and head-holding units in place.

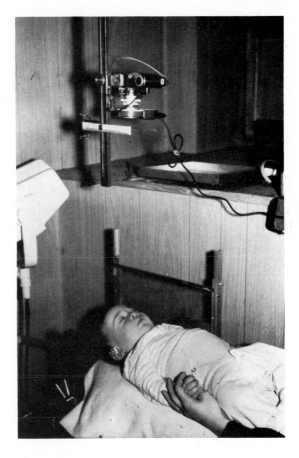

FIGURE 6–18 Infant cephalometric unit is used to photograph the patient with a 35 mm. camera. The ear rods are applied for the positioning and orientation of the head in this procedure.

distortion and magnification, and the photographs can therefore be used for measurement and for analyzing facial type (Figure 6–18). An average of eight photographs is made of each patient, which includes full-face, left and right profile, extraoral, and intraoral views. Photographs of the oral area show teeth in occlusion and the anterior and posterior palate. If the patient is wearing a prosthetic speech appliance, anterior and posterior views of the appliance are also made.

PROSTHODONTICS

Since the early sixteenth century dentists have been making appliances for closing defects in the hard palate (Figures 6–19 and 6–20). Like their predecessors, the prosthodontists of today are also vitally interested in helping the individual with an oral cleft. The prosthetic speech appliances that they make are recommended as a preliminary or secondary treatment for a great many patients with cleft palate. The terms "obturator" and "speech appliance" will both be used in this section. They are frequently used synonymously, but it has become the custom to apply the term "obturator"

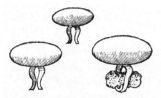

Inftrumentz appellez couuercles, propres pour couurir & eftouper les trouz des os per duz au palais de la bouche, foit de caufe de ve rolle, ou autrement: & fans iceux les patiens ne peuuent proferer leur parolles, mais par lent (comme lon dit vulgairement) regnaut. Ledit Inftrument fera de matiere d'or ou d'ar gent, & de figure courbee, & non plus efpois qu'vn efcu: Auquel fera attachee vne efpon ge, par laquelle eftant appofe ledit Inftrumet dedans le trou, laditte efponge bien toft s'en flera par l'humidite contenue en la bouche, qui fera caufe de le faire tenir ferme : & par tel moyen le patient proferera bien fa pa rolle.

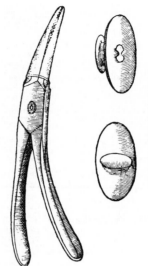

FIGURE 6–19 The first palatal obturators and their sponge or metal retention devices. (From Paré, A.: Dix Livres de la Chirurgie, Paris, Royer, 1564, p. 211. *Reprinted in* Grabb, W. C., S. W. Rosenstein, and K. R. Bzoch [eds.]: Cleft Lip and Palate, Boston, Little, Brown, 1971, p. 147.)

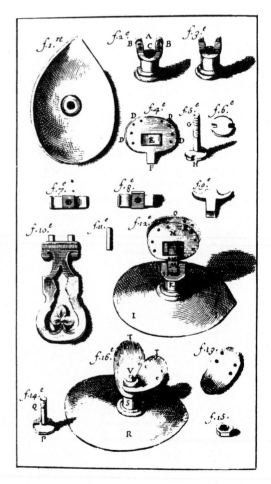

FIGURE 6–20 Designs by Fauchard showing early obturators employed for palatal defects. (From Fauchard, P.: Le Chirurgien Dentiste, ou Traité des Dents, vol. 2, Paris, J. Mariette, 1746, p. 305. *Reprinted in* Grabb, W. C., S. W. Rosenstein, and K. R. Bzoch [eds.]: Cleft Lip and Palate, Boston, Little, Brown, 1971, p. 147.)

to the device used in treating acquired defects and "speech appliance" to that employed in treating congenital clefts.

The design and construction of speech appliances and obturators have changed much in the last 20 years, thanks mainly to improved materials and methods. We have, for example, better wax, acrylics, and impression materials, and superior stone and plaster for the investment process. We have also benefited from improved diagnostic tools for evaluating the results of our prosthetic treatment. Greater coordination of our interdisciplinary team efforts has helped in establishing a more ideal prosthetic concept, one that assures that fixed or removable partial denture prostheses are so managed as to preserve the integrity of all remaining teeth and the surrounding soft and hard oropharyngeal structures.

The decision for prosthetic rehabilitation is based upon the individual's needs, motivation for improvement, and availability for the suggested rehabilitative program. Approximately 70 per cent of all patients with cleft palate will need some type of fixed or removable prosthesis by 30 years of age.

TREATMENT PLANNING

A step-by-step plan and the institution of a program of total health care are essential in the therapeutic management of patients with a cleft. It is especially important to take their general health as well as their dental situation into consideration before any surgical intervention. Fortunately, the interest shown by the dental profession in craniofacial growth and in the behavior of the hard and soft tissues before and after surgery has introduced a new era of closer cooperation between surgeons and their dental colleagues. As a result the dental specialist is now called upon to see the child with a cleft at an early age, before surgery is undertaken.

Analysis of longitudinal maxillary and mandibular casts and of cephalometrics and radiographs has established that there are two major factors causing the growth disturbance of orofacial regions in individuals with a cleft. First is the inherent potential for growth disturbance present among patients with cleft palate, and second is the trauma inflicted by surgical and orthopedic intervention. Since we cannot predict or reduce the first cause, all of our efforts have been directed toward minimizing growth disturbances by performing surgery with the least amount of trauma and scar tissue (see chapter on craniofacial growth). Longitudinal data during the past 10 years concerning surgical closure of the cleft have revealed that conservative surgery, compatible with a knowledge of growth loci, has greatly reduced trauma and scar tissue.

Requirements of a Speech Appliance

1. The prosthesis must be designed to suit the individual patient and situation in relation to oral and facial balance, masticatory function, and speech.

2. All techniques and disciplines involved in removable partial and complete dentures should be kept in mind in designing the maxillary part of

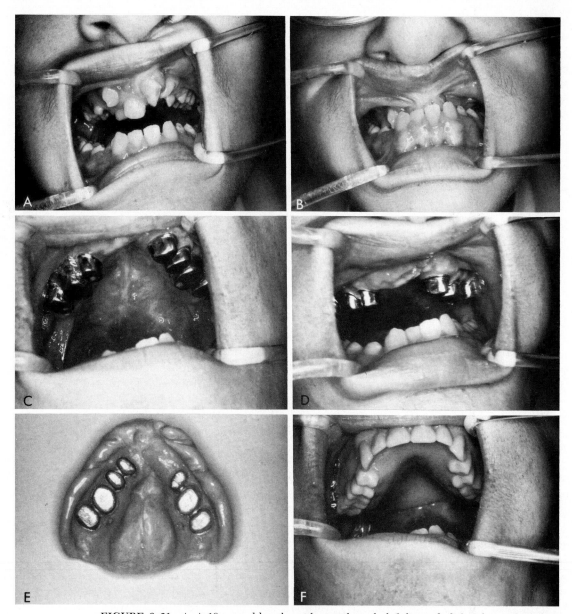

FIGURE 6–21 *A*, A 19-year-old male with a unilateral cleft lip and cleft palate, which have been operated on. The last surgical procedure on the palate was a pharyngeal flap. The remaining maxillary teeth are partially erupted; patient has a generalized gingival hyperplasia; the maxilla is underdeveloped; midfacial deficiency is present. He has both anterior and posterior crossbites, and there is an 11 mm. separation between the maxillary and mandibular teeth when in a position of physiologic rest. *B*, Patient in occlusion. Note the total crossbite and overclosure and reduced vertical dimension. *C*, The prosthodontist and orthodontist decided to have the maxillary incisors removed. The periodontist performed bilateral gingivoplasty and alveoloplasty. The prosthodontist placed copings on the remaining teeth. The copings are parallel and splinted, and the gingival shoulder is placed to prevent overlying denture from impinging on the gingival crest. *D*, The patient after the teeth are crowned and he is in a position of physiologic rest. Note the great distance between the maxillary and mandibular teeth. *E*, The tissue surface of the full denture prosthesis designed to be supported by the remaining maxillary teeth. The cast gold thimbles are held in the resin base by the lateral extension on the casting. *F*, The prosthesis in position.

Legend continued on the opposite page

FIGURE 6–21 *Continued* *G*, Profile of the patient without the prosthesis. *H*, Profile with prosthesis. Plumping out of the lip and correction of facial vertical height have resulted in a more esthetically acceptable appearance.

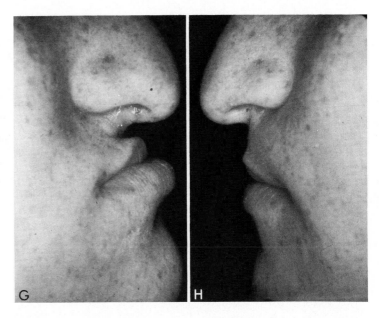

the prosthesis. Preservation of the remaining dentition and surrounding soft and hard tissue in patients with cleft palate is one of the main objectives. So often the proper design of the maxillary part of the prosthesis is neglected. This results in *premature loss* of the hard and soft tissue and further complicates the prosthetic habilitation.

3. The prosthetic speech appliance requires more retention and support than do other devices. This is because of its greater weight and because of displacement pressures produced by the tongue during swallowing. Often patients with clefts, prior to acquiring a prosthesis, attempt to achieve velopharyngeal closure by placing the tongue in that area and by elevating the soft palate by tongue pressure. Therefore, when they begin to use their new prostheses they may persist in this old habit and contine to use the tongue in the same maneuver. This may result in pushing the velo-pharyngeal section of the appliance upward into the nasopharyngeal area, causing anteroposterior leverage that, in seesaw fashion, forces the front portion of the prosthesis downward. The problem can be minimized by firmer retention. In adult patients proper crowning and splinting of the abutment teeth will not only improve retention and support of the prosthesis, but will increase the life of the abutment teeth themselves.

4. Full consideration should be given to the prosthetic treatment of the reduced vertical dimension of occlusion in the patient with cleft palate. Lack of lateral and vertical growth of the maxilla and partial eruption of the deciduous and permanent teeth are often seen as the result of traumatic surgery in patients with congenital cleft lip or palate. Prostheses supported by natural teeth are the ideal treatment for this situation. Gingivectomy is performed to expose enough of the clinical crowns to make them usable. Copings are made for the remaining teeth to prevent decalcification and caries. These teeth are used only for support of the prosthesis and not for retention. (Figures 6–21 and 6–22 illustrate the problems and the procedures in two representative patients.)

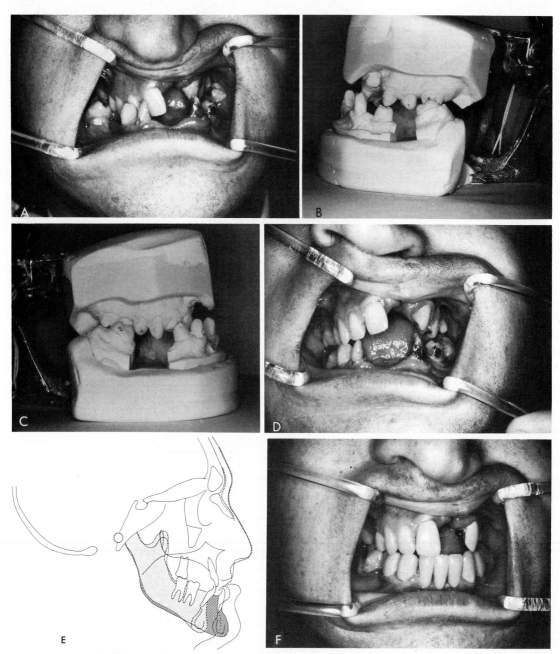

FIGURE 6–22 *A*, Patient with underdeveloped maxilla, anterior and posterior crossbites, protruding mandible, premature loss of several of the permanent teeth, and poor dental restoration. Treatment plan: bilateral ostectomy, mandibular fixed restoration, and crowning of several maxillary teeth. *B*, Study casts are mounted and a section is removed from the left side to indicate site and extent of excision that will give patient proper occlusion. *C*, Larger segment is removed from right side. *D*, Patient after ostectomy is performed as indicated in the study casts. Note dental occlusion. *E*, Cephalometric tracing superimposed before and after ostectomy. Crosshatched area is the profile before the ostectomy. *F*, Patient in occlusion after maxillomandibular fixed restoration and occlusal rehabilitation. (Left upper incisor was later replaced.)

Legend continued on the opposite page

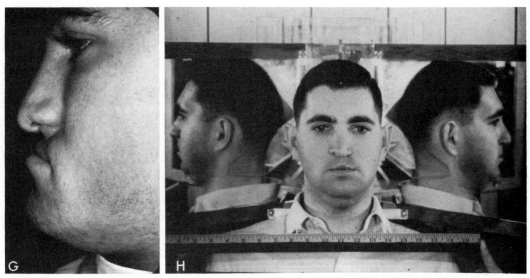

FIGURE 6–22 *Continued*   G, Profile of patient before surgery. H, Patient after surgery.

5. The weight of the prosthetic speech appliance should be kept to a minimum. The materials used should lend themselves easily to repair and modification, usually extension and reduction.

6. Soft tissue displacement in velar and nasopharyngeal areas by the prosthesis should be avoided.

7. The velar and pharyngeal sections of the prosthesis should not at any time be displaced by lateral and posterior pharyngeal wall muscle activities or by tongue movement during swallowing and speech.

8. The nasal surface of the pharyngeal section should be sloped laterally to eliminate the collection of nasal secretions. The oral surface of the bulb section should be slightly concave to allow for freedom of movement for the tongue; no part of the prosthesis should interfere with this movement. The following conclusions summarize the recent investigation of the effect of the location and changes of the speech bulb upon the patient's nasal resonance.

    a. Voice quality was judged best when the speech bulb was positioned in the area in which the posterior and lateral pharyngeal wall activity took place (Passavant's pad) (Figures 6–23 and 6–24).

    b. The inferior to superior dimension of the speech bulb was reduced by three fourths without apparent effect on the nasal resonance. As a consequence the weight of the bulb was reduced considerably (Figure 6–25).

    c. The lateral dimension of the bulb does not have to be changed significantly as the position varies. In the past, we have used the anterior tubercle of the atlas vertebra as a reference point. However, our investigation revealed that the relative position of the tubercle varies in different individuals and that the position of the velopharyngeal structures changes in relation to the tubercle as individuals move their heads. Therefore, we no longer use the atlas bone as the reference point for positioning of the pharyngeal section. In cases in which pos-

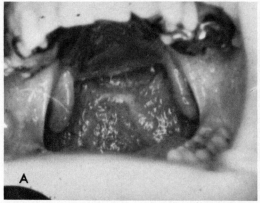

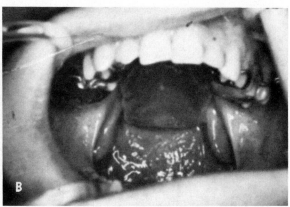

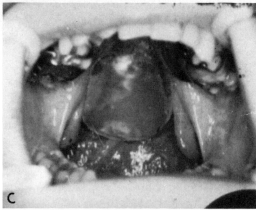

FIGURE 6–23   Three positions of the speech bulb were selected: *A*, superior to posterior pharyngeal wall activity; *B*, over the pharyngeal wall activity; and *C*, inferior to pharyngeal wall activity. We have noted that the best speech quality is achieved if the speech bulb is placed directly over the posterior pharyngeal wall activity as in *B*.[26]

FIGURE 6–24 Superimposed tracing of the original speech bulb and various experimental speech bulbs (*A*, *B*, and *C*) in position in Figure 6–23. The palatal plane was used as a plane of reference along with posterior pharyngeal wall activity, muscle bulge, or Passavant's pad. The posterior nasal spine (PNS), absent in cleft palate subjects, is called posterior palatal point (Ppp) and represents the most posterior point of the remnants of the palatal shelves as shown in the lateral cephalometric film. Median position was judged best.

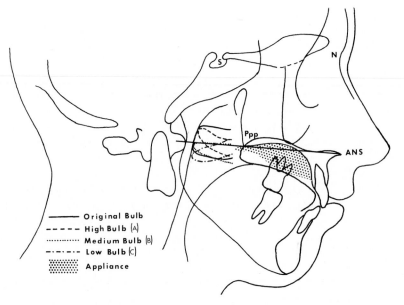

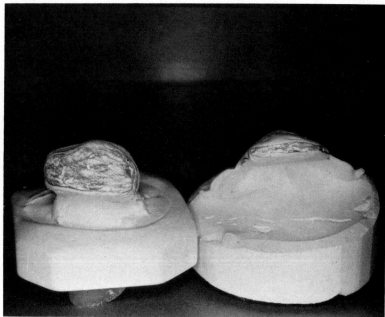

FIGURE 6–25 As a result of our studies[15] we have concluded that the inferior-superior dimensions of the speech bulb do not have a significant effect on speech quality so long as the bulb is properly placed to facilitate good velopharyngeal closure. This dimension was reduced to one quarter of its original size, as shown in cast made during fitting for one patient, without apparent effect on nasal resonance.

terior and lateral pharyngeal wall *activities* cannot be seen because of a long soft palate, the placement of the speech bulb on or above the palatal plane will give satisfactory speech results.

Indications for a Prosthesis in Unoperated Palates

Surgery for cleft palate is not a stereotyped exercise but a service demanding an assessment of all the factors presented by each patient (see chapter on plastic surgery). It follows a reparative surgical plan based on proven principles. The majority of cleft palates can be reconstructed by surgery to enable the patient to develop acceptable velopharyngeal closure. However, there apparently are some situations in which a prosthesis assures the best physical restoration, and the opinion regarding this point should be expressed by the group charged with the habilitation of the patient.

Many clefts of the hard palate can be closed by a vomer flap (Veau, Ivy), and clefts of the soft palate by median suture, with a good anatomical and functional result. The wide cleft and the short palate demand additional attention. Added length may be gained by the Dorrance or V-Y type repositioning operation. The raw nasal surface may be covered with a skin graft (Dorrance), nasal mucosa (Cronin), or with an island flap of palatal mucosa (Millard). The incompetent palatopharyngeal valve can be augmented by a pharyngeal flap either as a primary (Stark) or secondary procedure. The need for additional tissue in a wide cleft can be satisfied by a single or double regional flap.

Although these surgical advantages are now available, some patients with cleft palates also need prostheses. Here trained prosthodontists have methods at their command to assist both the surgeon and the patient. A mutual understanding develops among the specialists in a well-organized team as they consider which procedure will yield the greatest benefit. However, each patient's situation should be carefully assessed in all particulars before a prosthesis is decided upon, for there may be circumstances that argue against this as the best method of treatment.

A prosthesis would not be recommended, for example, if it appears that surgical closure alone would assure a good anatomic and functional result. A mentally retarded individual would not be a good candidate for a prosthesis if it is determined that he or she is not capable of taking reasonably good care of it. Nor should a speech appliance be prescribed if the child and parents are plainly uncooperative.

If caries are rampant, they should be corrected before a prosthesis of any kind is considered. Patients who are edentulous can be fitted if they meet other criteria (Figure 6–26). However, all basic principles governing construction of the full denture prosthesis must be adhered to for such a patient.

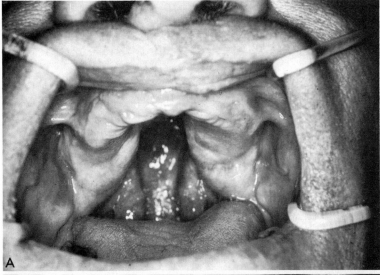

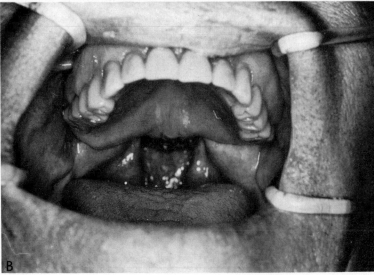

FIGURE 6–26 *A,* An edentulous patient with an unoperated cleft of the soft and hard palate that affects the retention and support of the prosthesis. At no time should a patient with a cleft, especially an unoperated cleft, be rendered edentulous. *B,* The completed prosthetic speech appliance in position.

And because retention and support of the prosthesis are affected by the palatal cleft and can be facilitated by the patient's own teeth, it is important not to render him edentulous if it is at all possible to preserve some of the teeth.

Finally, we should like to emphasize that the construction of a speech device that will really help the wearer achieve satisfactory speech demands a solid understanding of the problem. Prosthodontists engaged in the habilitation of the patient with a cleft palate should be thoroughly familiar with the anatomy and physiology of the structures used in speech. They should also have received adequate training in the principles governing both fixed and removable partial denture prostheses for individuals with cleft palate. If such skill and experience are not locally available, the problem should be discussed frankly with the family and other possibilities explored.

Having made sure there are no contraindications to the prosthetic approach, the cleft palate team will find a number of different situations that do lend themselves to this method of treatment. The principal ones follow:

Wide Cleft with Deficient Soft Palate. Some clefts of this type do not lend themselves to a surgical repair by means of local flaps. Therefore, in these situations a prosthesis is preferable not only to local flaps but to the

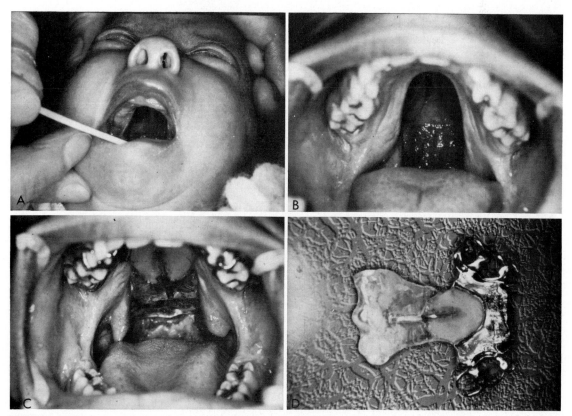

FIGURE 6–27 *A,* An infant with a wide cleft of the soft and hard palate with insufficient local tissue and absence of vomer. *B,* Patient at the age of sixteen years. *C,* Prosthetic speech aid in position. Note that the pharyngeal section of the speech aid is placed directly over the posterior and lateral pharyngeal wall muscle activities. *D,* Oral view of prosthetic speech aid. The utilization of second bicuspids and first and second molars for retention and support will prevent this prosthesis from dislodging into the nasal cavity during swallowing and speaking.

more time-consuming remote flaps. Many of the patients also need the prosthesis to restore missing teeth, whereas the distant tissue would provide only an adynamic mass (Fig. 6–27).

Wide Cleft of Hard Palate. In bilateral clefts the vomer may be high and the cleft of the hard palate wide, so that a surgical repair might produce a low-vaulted palate. It may be possible, however, to close the soft palate with the aid of local flaps and restore the hard palate with a prosthesis. Moreover, a situation similar to that once advocated by Gillies and Fry is created, in which the primary repair of the velum may create a more favorable spatial arrangement for subsequent surgery on the hard palate.

Neuromuscular Deficit of Soft Palate and Pharynx. The repair of the palate does not itself assure the acquisition of good speech. If there is a neural deficiency of the critical muscles involved, as in cerebral palsy or bul-

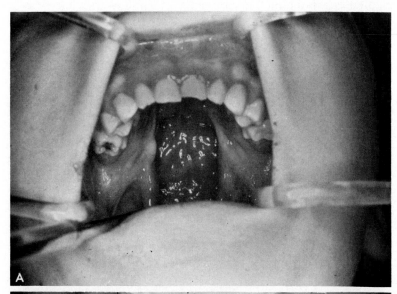

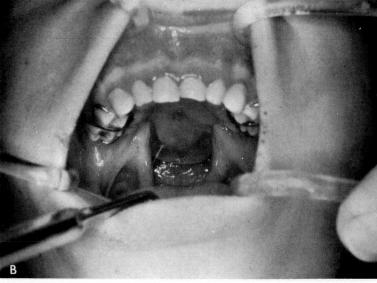

FIGURE 6–28   *A,* A four-and-one-half-year-old girl with a rather wide cleft of the soft and hard palate. We elected to fit her with a prosthesis and to delay the palatal surgery until a later age. *B,* The prosthetic speech aid in position. She tolerated the prosthesis and the speech significantly improved within a six-month period.

bar dysarthria, it is difficult to create and maintain a pharyngeal flap large enough to produce competent palatopharyngeal valving without obstructing the airway. A pharyngeal flap works best if it is surrounded by dynamic musculature. When this situation does not exist, then the pharyngeal section of a speech aid prosthesis should help the valve action and in that way reduce nasality and nasal emission. The prosthesis can also act as a physical therapy modality, providing a resistant mass for the muscles to act against. Should muscle function thereupon improve, definitive surgical measures can be contemplated.

Delayed Surgery.   If surgery is delayed for medical reasons or if the surgeon prefers to repair the palate at a later age, the cleft palate may be temporarily closed with a speech aid prosthesis (Figure 6–28).

Expansion Prosthesis.   We at the Lancaster Cleft Palate Clinic believe that in the period before surgery of the palate, an expansion or repositioning prothesis, with or without bone grafting, should be employed only in selected cases. In the majority of patients with cleft lip and cleft palate, the restoration of the anatomic continuity of the labial muscles, through surgery of the cleft lip, will mold the segments into acceptable relationship with each other and with the mandible. A detailed assessment of the expansion procedure, usually referred to as presurgical orthopedic intervention, appears in the chapter on orthodontics.

Prosthesis and Orthodontic Appliance.   An orthodontic appliance may be combined with a temporary prosthesis to move malposed teeth into a more favorable alignment. A prosthetic speech appliance could be designed such as the one illustrated in Figure 6–29 for a patient receiving full band orthodontic treatment.

Indications for a Prosthesis in Operated Palates

Incompetent Palatopharyngeal Mechanism.   If the clinical cineradiographic analyses suggest that the patient is approaching a functional closure, a prosthesis may serve as a physical therapy modality. The pharyngeal section of the prosthesis is gradually reduced as muscle function improves and the prosthesis can eventually be discarded. If the patient presents a large velopharyngeal gap associated with a neural deficiency, the speech aid prosthesis should be considered as a permanent type of treatment.

Surgical Failure.   A prosthesis should be considered if a patient presents a palate that is low vaulted, heavily scarred, and contracted, or one which has a large perforation or multiple perforations (Figures 6–30 to 6–32). Because of the surgical progress in the last 25 years, plastic surgeons today are not confronted with so many failures in cleft palate surgery. The trained surgeon can now predict with greater accuracy the possible success or failure of an operation and is inclined to avoid a likely failure if an alternative is available.

Contraindications to a Prosthesis

1. Surgical repair is feasible only if surgical closure of the cleft will produce anatomical and functional repair.

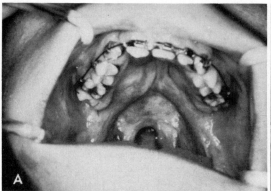
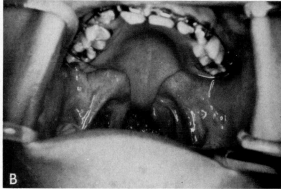

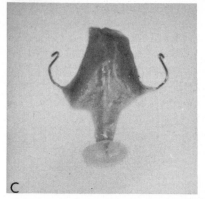

FIGURE 6–29 A temporary prosthetic speech appliance was designed not to interfere with orthodontic treatment while the patient was under active therapy. *A*, View of the palate without prosthesis. *B*, The prosthesis in position. Retention is obtained by placing the retainers above the molar buccal tubes. *C*, View of the prosthesis. After one year of velopharyngeal stimulation by the prosthesis the patient developed adequate posterior and lateral pharyngeal wall activity, resulting in acceptable speech. Prosthesis was then discarded.

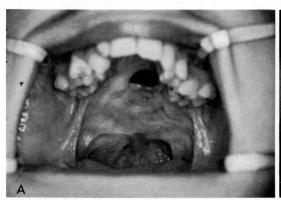
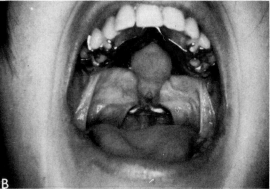

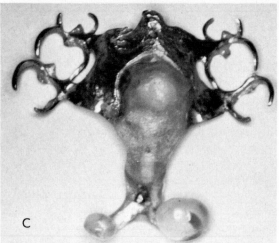

FIGURE 6–30 *A*, Palatal pharyngeal view of a patient with a low-vaulted, heavily scarred and perforated palate. Nonfunctional pharyngeal flap has recently been inserted. *B*, The prosthesis in position. *C*, The prosthesis itself, designed to close palatal defect and seal the orifices on the sides of the flap.

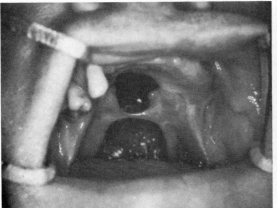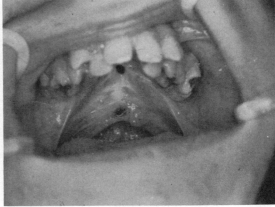

FIGURE 6–31   Two patients with heavily scarred palate and perforation: surgical failures.

2. Mentally retarded patients are not good candidates for a prosthesis, since they are frequently not capable of giving their appliances the care they require.
3. A speech aid is not recommended for an uncooperative patient, or for a child with uncooperative parents.
4. If caries is rampant and not controlled, a prosthesis requires unusual care, and frequent examinations are important.
5. The edentulous condition is *not* a contraindication for a speech aid prosthesis.
6. Since the construction of a functional prosthesis requires the services of a dentist who has had training in cleft palate prosthodontics, it would be better to resort to surgical ingenuity if experienced prosthodontic help is unavailable (examples of poorly constructed prostheses are shown in Figure 6–33 to 6–35).

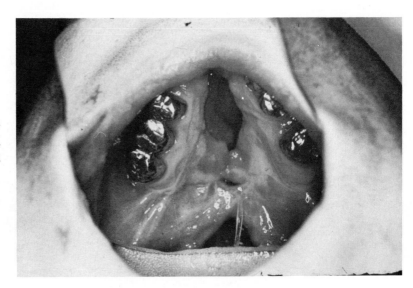

FIGURE 6–32   Patient with large palatal defect and scarring. All the remaining maxillary teeth were crowned and splinted prior to prosthetic habilitation.

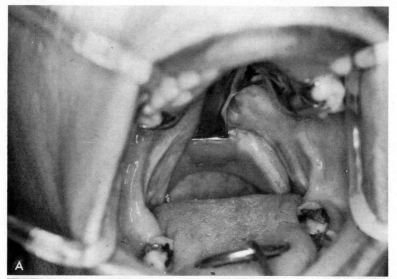

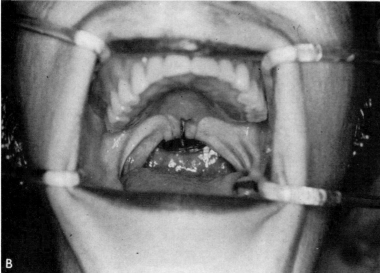

FIGURE 6–33 *A,* A nonfunctional and malpositioned pharyngeal section of a poorly made prosthesis. The prosthesis was easily displaced during swallowing and speaking by muscle pressure on the pharyngeal section. This unstable prosthetic speech appliance caused the two remaining teeth to develop Class III mobility within six months. *B,* The two remaining teeth were removed and a complete denture speech aid was constructed. Note the position of the pharyngeal section in relation to the velopharyngeal musculature.

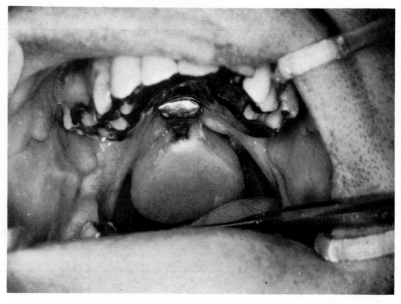

FIGURE 6–34 A poorly designed and nonfunctional pharyngeal section affecting swallowing and tongue position. This prosthesis does not give the patient the desired velopharyngeal obturation.

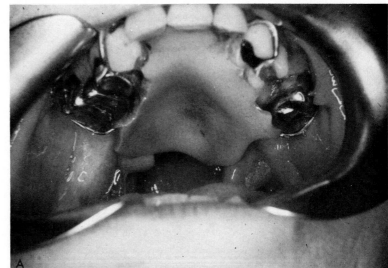
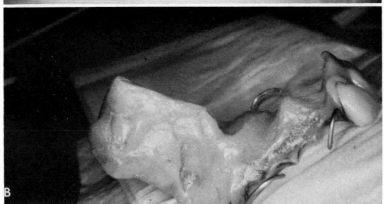

FIGURE 6–35 *A*, A prosthesis with poorly designed direct and indirect retainers and support. *B*, Palatal view of the prosthesis. This is called a meatal prosthesis. It does not give the patient the desired velopharyngeal seal for speech production.

CONSTRUCTION OF PROSTHETIC SPEECH APPLIANCES

All three sections of the prosthetic speech appliance for patients with deciduous, mixed, or incompletely erupted permanent dentitions are made of acrylic resin. Wrought wire retainers without occlusal rest are used (Figure 6–36). In patients in whom the permanent teeth are fully erupted, the anterior section of the prosthetic speech appliance should be made of cast metal or a combination of cast metal and acrylic resin (Figure 6–37).

Preliminary Impressions

These are made by the same techniques used in the initial examination of older children and adults (p. 276).

Preparation for Retention

Most deciduous teeth do not have sufficient undercut for retention; however, a small amount of bilateral undercut can be adequate. The following recommendations will help to produce adequate retention: (1) extend the clasp arms into interproximal areas of the teeth; (2) serrated platinum pins can be inserted into the buccal surface of the deciduous molars to create an artificial undercut for the clasp; (3) bands with a soldered retention lug can be placed on the teeth; and (4) "Rocky Mountain" crowns with a retention lug

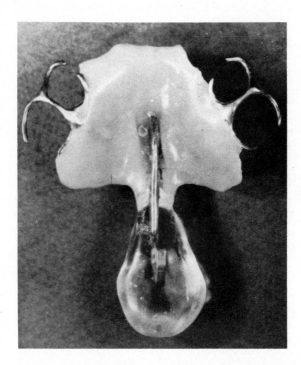

FIGURE 6–36 A temporary acrylic resin speech appliance with wrought wire clasps and full palatal coverage for a child of four years of age.

can be used for teeth with extensive carious lesions or areas of decalcification.

If sufficient space is not available for running the clasps between the teeth, space should be provided for them or the design should be changed. After the clasp design has been determined and the diagnostic casts and the teeth have been prepared for retention, the final impression is made.

If an adequate retention is not available in the permanent dentition, crowning of the molars might be desirable. The crowns are designed for proper retentive areas (Figure 6–38).

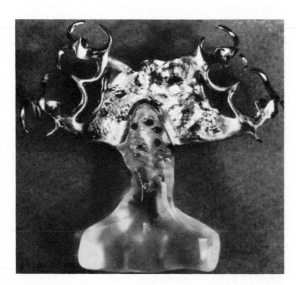

FIGURE 6–37 A permanent cast gold speech appliance with partial palatal coverage for an adult with no missing teeth.

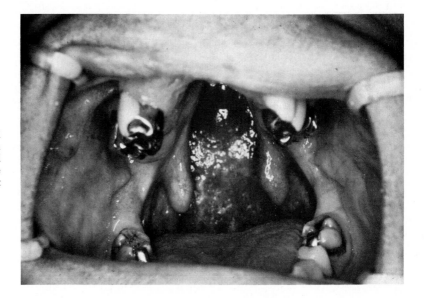

FIGURE 6–38 Crowning and splinting of the abutment teeth will increase the retention and support of the prosthesis and the life expectancy of the abutment teeth.

Final Impression

An acrylic resin tray is constructed over the diagnostic cast (Figure 6–39). The patient is prepared the same as for the preliminary impression and the impression is made in an irreversible hydrocolloid material (Figure 6–40). Then the master cast is poured in stone.

Design of Anterior Framework

Prosthetic design of the anterior portion of the speech aid and obturator apparently is a rather neglected area, as evidenced by the dearth of available information in the literature. To the neophyte there appears to be little guid-

FIGURE 6–39 An acrylic tray is made over the diagnostic cast and the border trimmed with green modeling compound.

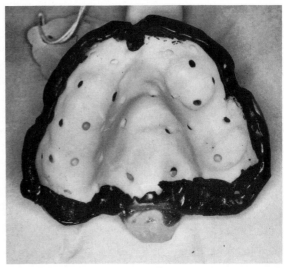

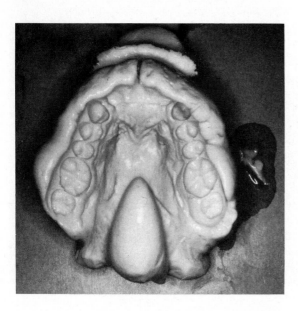

FIGURE 6–40 The final impression is made with alginate material. Note the extent of the registration of the cleft.

ance pertaining directly to actual cast frame design. But certain guidelines must be utilized in order to gain proper support and retention for prostheses.

The design of the anterior section of the obturator and speech aid follows the basic principles for that of the direct and indirect retainers and support for the standard partial and full-denture prostheses. The prosthodontist must be thoroughly familiar with the basic rules governing removable prostheses and knowledgeable in the alterations often required in fabricating appliances for patients with acquired and congenital defects.

It is of great importance to preserve the remaining dentition and supporting structures for the purpose of retaining these prostheses. All efforts should be made to treat and restore the remaining teeth rather than to extract them.[12] Splinting of crowns made for the abutment teeth will increase retention and support for the prosthesis and will aid in the overall life span of these teeth.

Framework design is of primary importance, for it must be balanced to eliminate, as much as possible, harmful torque on the teeth. The palatal coverage with metal or resin or a combination of both should be designed so as not to interfere with tongue positioning. In other words, it should not be too bulky, but one should also keep in mind that rigidity is required for this section. The retainer should be designed to engage the distal undercut on the posterior abutments for support of the pharyngeal section or the speech bulb. Mesial undercuts are engaged for the retention of the anterior replacement. If adequate retention cannot be attained for the prosthesis, then modification of the abutment should be considered. Whenever the abutment needs to be crowned, because of extensive carious lesions or substantial loss of tooth structure, then the crowns should be designed for proper retainer placement and adequate embrasure crossing.

In individuals with collapsed segments or poorly aligned arch form with medially displaced dental units, an overlay denture or veneered appliance may be considered. It is wise to crown all teeth that must lie beneath the appliance in patients who are susceptible to carious lesions.

Generally speaking, the overall aim for the anterior maxillary section of the obturator is to provide as much retention as possible and to distribute the torquing forces over a wide area, in order to include as many teeth as one can. Standard clasp design using primarily cast Akers clasps and interproximal (crib clasps) and T, I, and L bars is the most common approach. Semiprecision and precision attachments are usually not indicated for these appliances. Complex retainers are much more difficult to repair. Simplicity in appliance design allows for more flexibility when taking into consideration the overall requirements of this type of prosthesis (i.e., when the velar and pharyngeal sections require several modifications to reach their final form.) Subjecting precision attachments to repetitive laboratory procedures could ultimately yield an unusable prosthesis.

Vertical and Centric Relations

All the usual steps for recording the vertical dimension of occlusion and centric relations are followed for patients who require a complete or partial denture prosthesis.

The Prosthesis

The master casts are surveyed and the prosthesis is designed by the prosthodontist, but consideration should be given to all the problems involved (Figure 6–41). If the orthodontist feels treatment is not indicated for a patient with a severely constricted maxillary and mandibular arch, the artificial teeth are set up outside the remaining natural teeth to establish the proper occlusion (Figure 6–42).

The prosthetic speech appliance is constructed in three sections. The

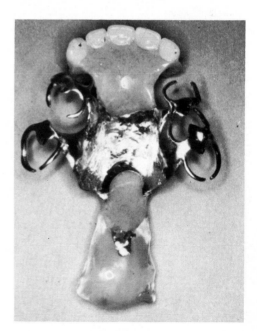

FIGURE 6–41 Cast gold framework. The prosthetic speech appliance requires more retention and support; therefore, all the remaining maxillary teeth of this patient have been used for this purpose. The posterior extension of the framework reinforces the tailpiece and the speech bulb.

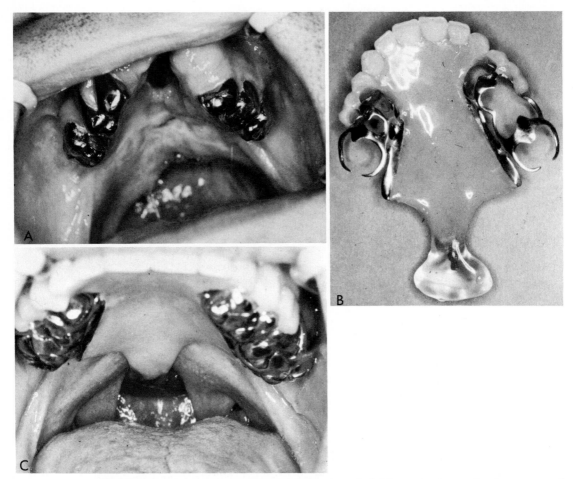

FIGURE 6–42   *A*, A patient with operated unilateral cleft lip and palate. Soft palate is scarred and short and lacks mobility. Maxillary arch constructed, but a large oronasal fistula remains. Prosthetic speech appliance was recommended. All maxillary teeth are crowned and splinted. *B*, Complete prosthetic speech appliance. *C*, Prosthetic speech appliance in position. Note that prosthetic teeth are arranged outside of the remaining natural teeth to give the patient proper occlusion.

design of the anterior portion is similar to that of a partial or complete denture. The number of retainers is increased on partial dentures, if possible. After this section is finished, the patient wears it for at least one week. The length of this adjustment period depends on the patient's ability to adapt to this part of the prosthesis. The construction of the middle part, the tailpiece or velar section, varies for operated and nonoperated clefts.

Velar Section

In nonoperated clefts with the upper prosthesis in position, the extension of the tailpiece over the margin of the cleft is marked on the posterior part of the appliance. The tailpiece extends posteriorly to the anterior margin of the uvula.

In operated palates that are short and require a prosthesis, the position of the tailpiece is marked on the posterior margin of the prosthesis. The tailpiece extends 3 mm. behind the posterior margin of the soft palate. The width of the tailpiece is 5 mm. and its reinforced thickness is approximately 1.5 mm.

A piece of shellac baseplate material of the required width and length is used to act as a tray. It is securely attached to the posterior part of the prosthesis with 2 mm. relief and is brought to the mouth for a check of proper extension. The upper part of the tray is filled with zinc oxide and eugenol impression paste, and the appliance is inserted into the mouth. The patient is instructed to hold his head in a vertical position for one minute to prevent the escape of the impression material into the nasopharynx. After one minute, he is instructed to swallow some water so the muscular movement of the soft palate will be registered in the impression (Figure 6–43). After the material is set, the prosthesis is removed from the mouth and the tailpiece is processed. In order to reduce the number of times the appliance has to be heated, self-curing acrylic resin is used for making the tailpiece. The denture with the finished tailpiece attached is placed in the mouth for testing. Swallowing water stimulates muscle action along the lateral edge of the velar section. If the velar section is overextended laterally, it will cause undue muscle displacement and eventual tissue soreness.

Pharyngeal Section

Two holes are drilled in the posterior part of the tailpiece. A piece of separating wire is drawn through the holes in such a manner that a loop is formed to extend superoposteriorly beyond the superior part of the tailpiece (Figure 6–44). The two ends of the wire are twisted together inferiorly (oral side) and secured to the appliance by sticky wax. The wire loop, which is extended into the nasal pharyngeal area, is bent into an oval form and the appliance inserted into the mouth (Figure 6–45). The patient is asked to swallow, and the wire is adjusted so that it does not contact the pharyngeal walls at any time while the mouth is open. A spray of water with a syringe will stimulate posterior and lateral pharyngeal wall activity. The desired position of the wire is in the area of the maximum posterior and lateral pharyngeal constriction. Green modeling compound is added around the wire loop to reinforce the wire and its attachment to the tailpiece (Figure 6–46). The appliance is inserted into the mouth and the patient is asked to swallow some water. Adaptol,* softened in water at 150 to 160 degrees F. for four to five minutes, is added over the green compound and the appliance is inserted into the mouth. Again the patient is instructed to swallow some water to produce muscle activity that will mold the impression material (Figure 6–47). If gagging occurs, an underextended pharyngeal section is processed, using an autopolymerizer.

The prosthesis is reinserted a number of times, with more Adaptol gradually added to the mass on the wire loop until a functional impression is made of the lateral and posterior pharyngeal walls (Figure 6–48). The impression material is molded by instructing the patient to place his chin against his chest and to move his head from side to side. In the rest position the patient swallows water and speaks, the muscular activity thus further molding the impression material. If the mass is overextended, it will be felt by the patient as he or she swallows and speaks. The overextended bulb im-

---

*J. F. Jelenko and Co., Inc., New York, New York. *Text continued on page 311*

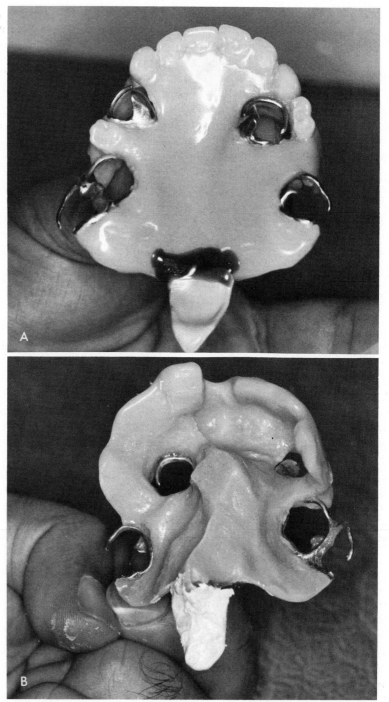

FIGURE 6–43 *A,* Oral view of a prosthesis with attached baseplate tray to carry the material for inpression of the tailpiece or velar section on this operated cleft palate patient. *B,* Palatal view of the zinc oxide-eugenol impression of the soft palate. The upper portion of the tray was filled with zinc oxide and eugenol and an impression of the vascular section was made.

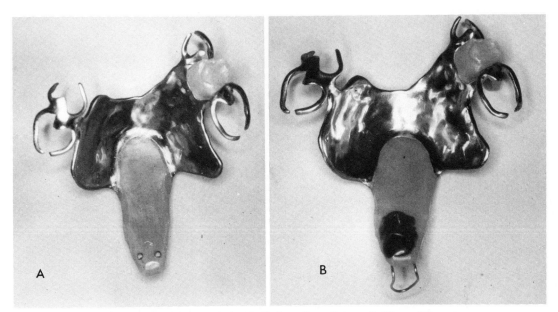

FIGURE 6–44 *A,* The location of the two holes drilled on the tailpiece. *B,* View of the wire formed in a loop, extending supraposteriorly into the nasal pharynx.

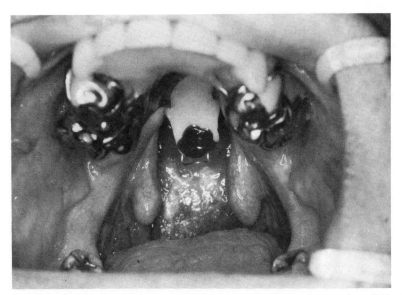

FIGURE 6–45 Wire loop is attached to the tailpiece, inserted into the mouth, and checked to see that it does not contact posterior and lateral pharyngeal walls during swallowing.

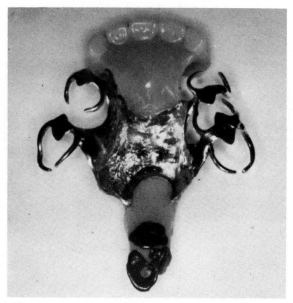

FIGURE 6–46 Modeling compound is added around the wire loop to reinforce the wire and its attachment to the tailpiece.

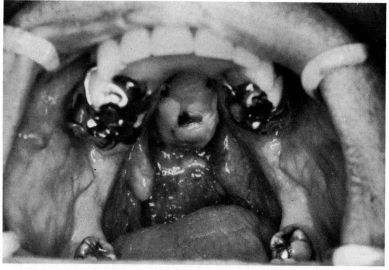

FIGURE 6–47 The Adaptol, softened to 150° to 160° F, is added over the green compound, and appliance is inserted into the mouth. Note the displacement of the material after patient has swallowed some water and rotated the head to each side and down.

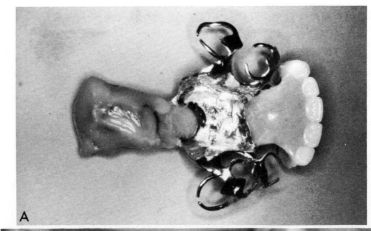

FIGURE 6–48 *A*, Functional registration of the velopharyngeal region using Adaptol. The gradual addition of Adaptol and patient swallowing water and moving the head down and to the sides will give the functional impression of the velopharyngeal region. If any gagging reflex is present, then under-estended pharyngeal section is processed using an autopolymerized. A week or two later the pharyngeal section is modified for addition of the Adaptol. When the speech result is accomplished and patient does not show any gagging reflex, the speech bulb is heat processed. *B*, More Adaptol is gradually added and appliance is inserted until a functional impression of the area has been obtained. In most patients, the speech bulb does not contact the throat wall while the surrounding tissues are at rest.

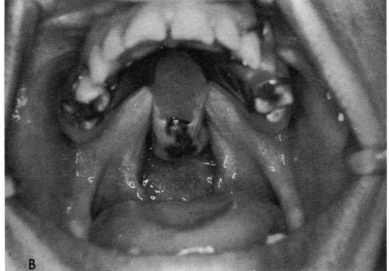

pression is easily modified by simply reheating the bulb on the exterior surface and reinserting it into the mouth while the material is soft. The completed speech bulb impression is then chilled thoroughly in ice water.

To check the position of the bulb, water is injected again. The position of the bulb is checked in relation to the posterior and lateral pharyngeal wall activity. In unoperated clefts, direct visualization of muscle function along the speech bulb during swallowing could be made while the mouth is wide open and water is being injected. If the posterior pharyngeal wall activity is not present or direct visualization is not possible because of the length of the soft palate, a lateral cephalometric radiograph will reveal the position of the bulb in relation to the nasopharyngeal structures. In most instances of this type, the bulb is placed in the area of the palatal plane. When the bulb form has been perfected, the bulb and tailpiece are processed on the denture with heat-cured acrylic resin.

In those patients whose pharyngeal wall tissues, posterior and lateral, are sensitive enough to produce a gag reflex, no attempt is made to obtain a functional impression for the speech bulb on the initial try. Here it is advis-

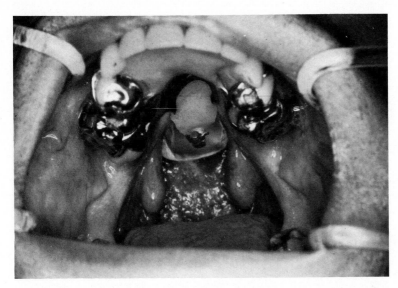

FIGURE 6–49 Processed speech bulb in position.

able to construct an extended bulb, process it in self-curing acrylic resin, and let the patient become adjusted to it for two or three weeks. After the patient is accustomed to the undersized bulb, a final impression is made by adding Adaptol to the bulb, which is then processed by heat-cured acrylic resin (Figure 6–49).

A length of 11-gauge half-round wire is incorporated in the appliance and the bulb. It should extend from the anterior part of the appliance to the speech bulb to prevent swallowing of the bulb in case the tailpiece is fractured. If the anterior part is made of cast metal, the frame should be ex-

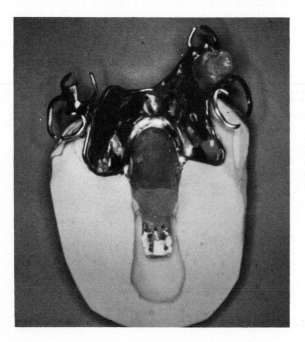

FIGURE 6–50 The nasal and lateral sides of the speech bulb, tailpiece, and a portion of the palatal area of the anterior section are placed in dental stone. These parts of the appliance are made of acrylic resin.

tended as far posteriorly as possible to strengthen the velar and pharyngeal section (Figure 6–50).

The finished speech appliance is inserted into the mouth and checked for (1) muscular adaptation to the speech bulb during swallowing and phonation, (2) excessive pressure against the posterior and lateral walls of the pharynx, (3) stability of the appliance during function, and (4) the improvement of voice quality.

In most patients we found that if the bulb is positioned too low, the pharyngeal section has the following undesirable effects: (1) a tendency to be displaced by the dorsal part of the tongue during tongue movements, (2) a failure to make proper contact at the point where normal velopharyngeal closure takes place, and (3) a detrimental effect upon the quality of the voice. Caution should be exercised not to block or extend the speech bulb into the eustachian tube.

SUMMARY

A patient with a cleft palate who is not a subject for functional surgical repair is a challenging problem for the interdisciplinary treatment approach. Some of the cases for which a prosthetic speech appliance is suggested are as follows:

1. A wide cleft of the palate with a deficiency of the soft palate.
2. A wide cleft of the hard palate with a high vomer.
3. A neuromuscular deficit. A sphincteric velopharyngeal action may not be attained even with a pharyngoplasty if the deficit is marked.
4. A surgical failure.

We strongly object to the use of remote extraoral flaps in cleft palate surgery. A prosthesis seems to be more correct. There have been claims that such a prosthesis may be a cause of cancer, but convincing evidence is lacking, and in my opinion, the relationship is quite unlikely. There has been no evidence of increased hearing loss in our patients wearing a prosthesis. A prosthesis should not be used in a patient not competent to care for it or to maintain proper hygiene.

A prosthodontist engaged in treating orofacial and speech handicapped people should be thoroughly familiar with the anatomical and physiological deviations of the region involved and the basic principles involved in prosthetic dentistry. He should also be willing to acquire further knowledge in this field.

FIXED PROSTHESES

Whenever it is possible to replace missing teeth with a fixed prosthesis, this should be the method of choice. The three basic requirements for a fixed restoration should be kept in mind:

1. Acceptable alveolar bone.
2. Good crown to root ratio.
3. Normal periodontal membrane.

Deficiency of the alveolar support often is present on the side of the root

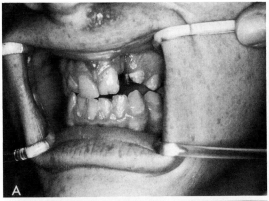
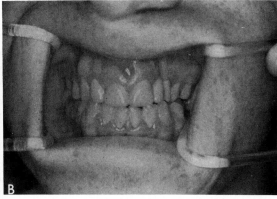
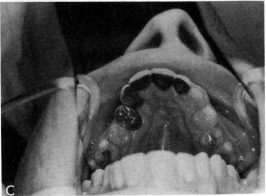

FIGURE 6–54 A, Patient with unilateral cleft lip and palate. The left cuspid and lateral incisor are missing; first bicuspid is partially erupted and has calcification anomalies along with upper left central. Patient has deficiency of alveolar support on the sides of the roots of the teeth adjacent to the cleft. Prescribed treatment: gingivectomy around upper left first bicuspid, crowning of upper right lateral and central and upper left central and upper left first bicuspids. B, Patient in occlusion after cementation of the crown. C, Palatal view of the fixed prosthesis.

VELAR ELEVATION AND VELOPHARYNGEAL STIMULATION

Before getting into methodology, let us briefly outline the symptoms and etiology of the velopharyngeal inadequacy that requires prosthetic stimulation and elevation.

The principal symptoms are hypernasality, or nasal emission, and the accompanying decrease in intelligibility. The situation results from one or more of the following conditions: (1) congenital or acquired cleft of the palate; (2) congenitally short soft palate, palatal paresis, or velopharyngeal insufficiency; (3) velar paralysis or velopharyngeal incompetency; or (4) abnormal nasopharyngeal size.

In addition to these factors, most of which are congenital and therefore prenatal in origin, several conditions may arise postnatally that also affect speech. The removal of tonsils and adenoids may create spatial abnormalities that result in hypernasality. Partial or complete paralysis of the velum may be produced by damage to the central or peripheral nervous system from any one of numerous causes: myasthenia gravis, bulbar poliomyelitis, traumatic brain injuries, cerebral vascular accidents, degenerative diseases of the central nervous system, or amyotrophic lateral sclerosis.

SPEECH PROBLEMS

Hypernasality and decreased intelligibility owing to weak consonant production are probably the commonest speech problems among those with velopharyngeal insufficiency and incompetency, but many patients with VPI develop a glottal stop substitution in compensating for production of pressure consonants. The patient with a neurological disease that has caused complete or partial paralysis of the muscles of the lip, tongue, larynx, or respiratory organs frequently has an abnormal articulatory pattern. A diminution of breath pressure (which in turn causes a reduction of oral pressure and flow) is accompanied by a reduced rate and extent of articulatory movements.

TREATMENT

The closure and obturation of palatal clefts and defects for patients with congenital and acquired clefts have been reported for many years. Doubtless early man used stone, wood, gum, cotton, and other foreign bodies to obturate the palatal opening. In recent years several methods have been advocated, satisfying the main objective of socially acceptable speech for these patients. Among these concepts are:

1. Certain traditional speech treatments, such as lip, tongue, and palatal exercises for the stimulation and physical therapy of musculatures (myofunctional therapy), designed to effect an increase in velar movement.
2. Surgical methods for reducing the velopharyngeal gap or lumen, employing velar lengthening procedures, velopharyngeal flaps, implants (cartilage, bone, silicone, teflon), and combinations of these several methods.
3. Faradization and electrical vibration massage to stimulate palatal function.
4. Prosthetic methods for elevating and stimulating the soft palate in patients with velopharyngeal incompetency, or for elevating, stimulating, and obturating velopharyngeal lumen in patients with velopharyngeal insufficiency.
5. Combination of surgical and prosthetic methods. (Redivision of the soft palate for the purpose of pharyngeal bulb placement should not be considered under any circumstances.)

Lift and Combination Prostheses

With respect to prosthodontic methods there are two prostheses available to us in the treatment of patients with velopharyngeal inadequacies: lift type and combination of lift and bulb.

The lift type of prosthesis is used to elevate the soft palate to the maximal position attained during normal speech and deglutition. Reducing the velopharyngeal gap and lumen will decrease nasal air flow, increase oral pressure for consonant articulation, and improve voice quality. The lift may also assist in repositioning the tongue and act as a physical modality for stimulating velar and pharyngeal musculatures, thus preventing velar *disuse atrophy* (Figures 6–55 to 6–60).

Text continued on page 321

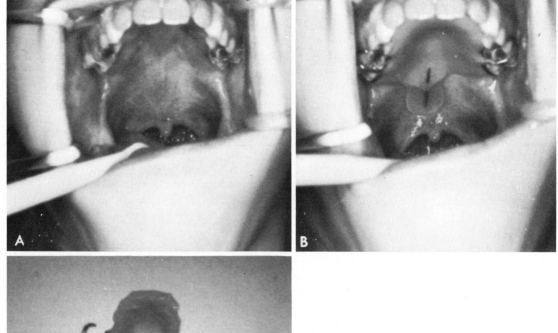

FIGURE 6–55 *A*, Patient with palatopharyngeal insufficiency. The treatment procedure is the stimulation of the soft palate by a palatal lift prosthesis followed by pharyngeal flap surgery; *B*, view of palatal lift prosthesis in position; *C*, palatal view of the lift prosthesis.

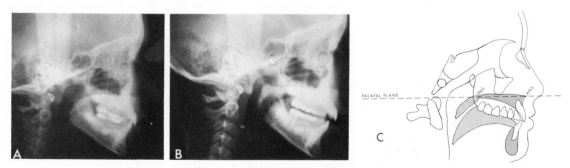

FIGURE 6–56 *A*, Lateral radiograph of patient in Figure 6–55 demonstrates the palatopharyngeal relationship prior to elevation and stimulation; *B*, height of velar elevation during the sound "E"; *C*, tracing of the cephalogram in *A*.

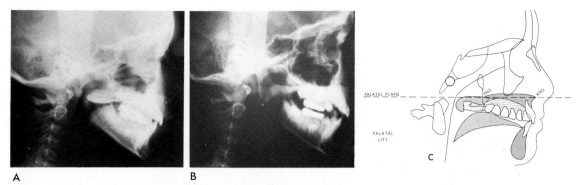

FIGURE 6–57 *A*, Radiographic view of the palatal lift prosthesis of patient in Figure 6–55 in position. Note the degree of palatal elevation. *B*, Increased mobility of the soft palate after one year of prosthetic stimulation. Pharyngeal flap surgery was done after 14 months of soft palatal stimulation, after which the lift prosthesis could be discarded. *C*, Cephalometric tracing of the palatal lift prosthesis and the degree of velar elevation accomplished by the lift.

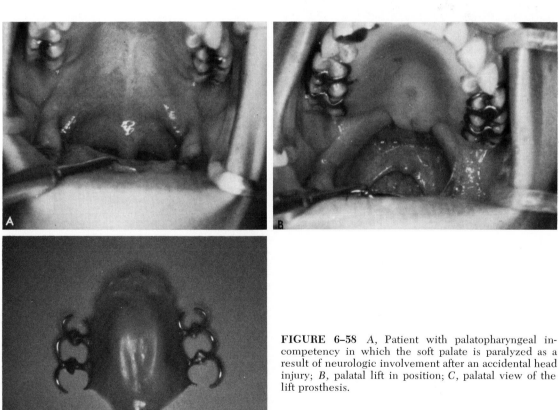

FIGURE 6–58 *A*, Patient with palatopharyngeal incompetency in which the soft palate is paralyzed as a result of neurologic involvement after an accidental head injury; *B*, palatal lift in position; *C*, palatal view of the lift prosthesis.

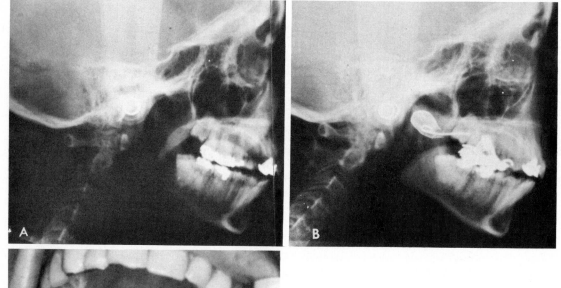

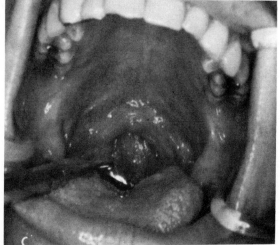

FIGURE 6–59 *A*, Lateral radiograph of the patient in Figure 6–58 prior to stimulation saying "E". *B*, The palatal lift prosthesis in position elevating the soft palate. *C*, Note the increase in the degree of palatal elevation. After 11 months of stimulation and speech therapy patient is saying "E." Note the substantial increase in the velar elevation.

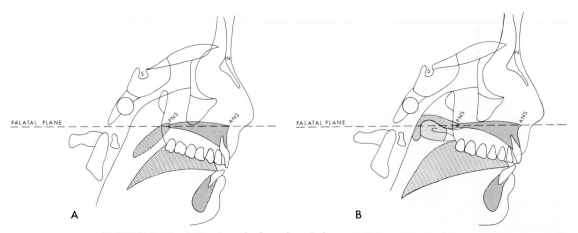

FIGURE 6–60 *A*, Tracing of a lateral cephalogram of the patient in Figure 6–58 prior to soft palate stimulation by a palatal lift prosthesis; *B*, Tracing of the palatal lift prosthesis and elevated soft palate.

When the soft palate is insufficient for the proper velopharyngeal closure, the combined lift and bulb type prosthesis, made by adding a speech bulb to the lift, should be the method of choice. This is used to elevate the soft palate, to obturate the gap, and to stimulate velopharyngeal development and pharyngeal constriction (Figures 6–61 to 6–67).

Requirements

1. The maxillary portion of the prosthesis is designed to achieve optimal retention and stability.
2. The lift portion should be properly placed so that velar elevation occurs in the area in which normal velopharyngeal closure takes place.
3. Elevation of the velum should be gradual so that the velum becomes less resistant to displacement.
4. The pharyngeal section should be placed in the area in which posterior and lateral pharyngeal constriction takes place, so that it increases the chance of further stimulation and muscle activation.
5. The reduction of the pharyngeal section, when indicated, should be gradual.

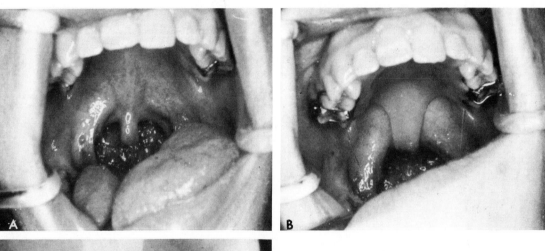

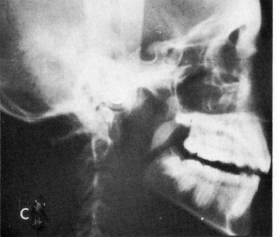

FIGURE 6–61 *A*, Patient with a palatopharyngeal insufficiency in which the soft palate is short and has limited mobility. *B*, Combination palatal lift pharyngeal section in position. The uvula was displaced by the prosthesis without causing any irritation. *C*, Lateral radiograph demonstrates short soft palate and large nasopharynx.

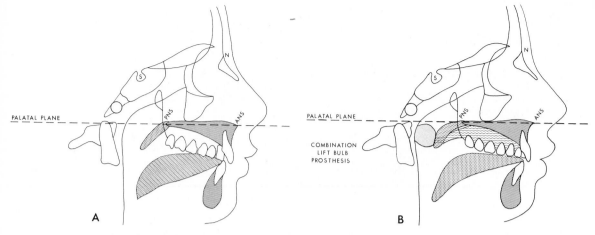

FIGURE 6–62 *A*, Tracing of the lateral cephalogram of the patient in Figure 6–61. *B*, Tracing of the combined palatal lift/pharyngeal section prosthesis in position.

6. Speech therapy, such as lip, tongue, and palatal exercises and placement, should be properly instituted in conjunction with the construction and insertion of the prosthesis.

Results

There are several methods of evaluation for this type of prosthesis:
1. Speech testing procedures.
2. Radiographic evaluation such as cineradiography, cephalometrics, sectional laminagraphy, or tomography.
3. Oral and nasal air pressure and air flow assessing devices.
4. Electronic instrumentation such as tonar and sonograph.

The optimal result will depend upon the type of oropharyngeal involvement. If the neurological disorder is more localized to the velopharyngeal region, and the patient has little or no articulatory impairment, then the

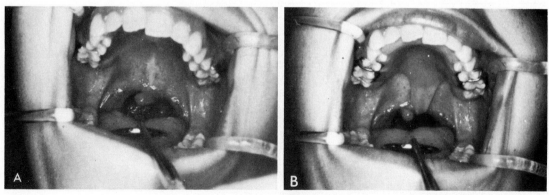

FIGURE 6–63 *A*, Patient with velopharyngeal insufficiency. *B*, Combined lift/pharyngeal section in position. In this patient the uvula, because of its position, did not have to be displaced by the velar section of the prosthesis.

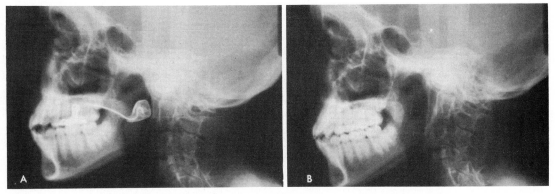

FIGURE 6–64 *A*, Radiographic view of patient in Figure 6–63 with combination lift in position; *B*, note the short soft palate and deep nasopharynx.

prosthetic result will be optimal. Patients with muscular paralysis of the tongue, lips, larynx, and respiratory organs usually respond less favorably to the prosthetic care. Their phonatory and articulatory distortions usually remain after the prosthetic treatment. These patients often require more intensive and coordinated myofunctional therapy.

Tolerance and acceptance of the prosthetic treatment varies. Some patients have less difficulty becoming accustomed to the palatal and velopharyngeal coverage and decreased oropharyngeal space.

We have also noted variations in muscle response to the mechanical stimulation. The velum of some patients, shortly after the placement of the lift, becomes more active, and after six months to one year, prosthetic stimulation and support can be discontinued. Whether the increased velar elevation is the result of prosthetic stimulation or neuromuscular recovery is difficult to assess. However, in our experience with similar patients who receive speech

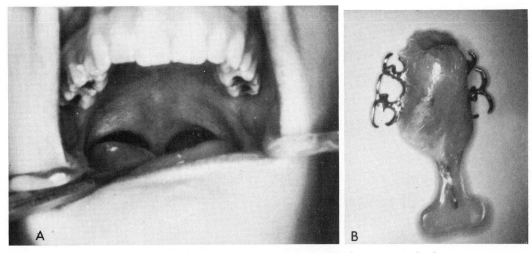

FIGURE 6–65 *A*, Patient with velar disuse atrophy occurring after a cerebral stroke; *B*, palatal view of combination lift designed for this patient.

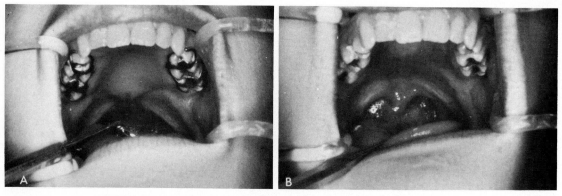

FIGURE 6–66 *A*, Combination lift in position for patient in Figure 6–65; *B*, note the increased velar elevation after eight months of prosthetic stimulation and speech therapy.

therapy as the only mode of velopharyngeal stimulation, their functional recovery was less noticeable over the same period of time than that in patients fitted with prostheses (Figures 6–68 and 6–69).

In our series of patients, we have found that the response of the pharyngeal musculature to prosthetic stimulation was more marked than the velar response. With the velopharyngeal bulb, the patient often develops compensatory muscular constriction requiring frequent reduction in the size of the pharyngeal bulb (Figures 6–70 and 6–71). In some patients, the

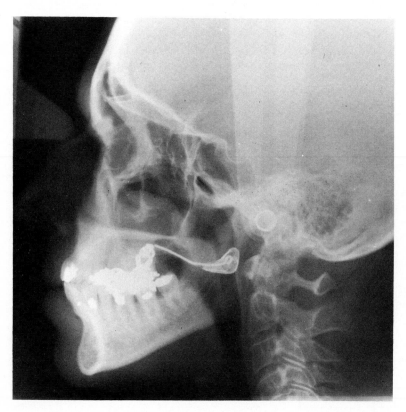

FIGURE 6–67 Radiographic view of patient in Figure 6–65 with combination lift in position.

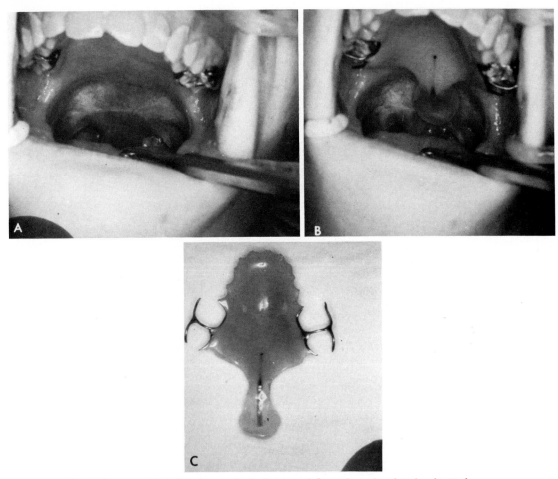

FIGURE 6–68 *A,* Patient with inferiorly attached pharyngeal flap. The soft palate has limited mobility, and there is no palatopharyngeal closure. *B,* The palatal lift prosthesis elevates and stimulates the soft palate and pharyngeal flap. *C,* Oral view of the prosthesis.

complete elimination of the bulb was accomplished. We believe that the reason for the variation in the degree of response in patients with velar incompetency and in those with velopharyngeal insufficiency is that we have two separate phenomena to consider. For one patient, we are trying to stimulate muscular activity by prosthetic physical therapy, and for the other patient, we are attempting to create muscle build-up or constriction as a result of prosthetic placement.

Among the more unusual indications for a prosthetic stimulator was the case of an infant boy we first saw in 1965, whose chief problem was liquid coming through his nose. He was then three months of age. By one year, the difficulty had subsided, but the patient was kept under observation. At the age of two and one half, when he began saying words and making sentences, it was noted that he was hypernasal. Cephalometric and cineradiographic studies were suggested. It was found that the patient had a unilateral paralysis of the soft palate. We continued observing the child. At the age of four,

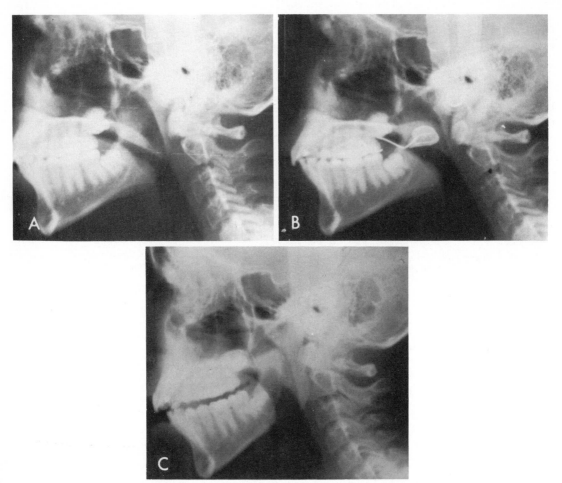

FIGURE 6–69 *A*, Lateral radiograph of patient in Figure 6–68 prior to stimulation; *B*, elevation of the soft palate is accomplished with palatal lift prosthesis; *C*, further soft palate elevation accomplished after ten months of prosthetic stimulation and speech therapy.

intensive speech therapy was initiated at the Clinic, but no substantial improvement was noted for the next two years.

At the age of six, a pharyngeal flap type of surgery was performed. Our annual observation of this child revealed that the soft palate on the affected side continued to be shorter than the nonaffected side. We noted continuation of velar deficiency and shortness after palatal surgery.

At the age of seven, a prosthetic stimulator was recommended to stimulate the posterior and lateral pharyngeal walls surrounding the right orifice of the flap. Stimulation continued for a period of one year, and there was a substantial increase in mobility of the structures in this area. The pharyngeal section of the prosthesis was gradually reduced, and after one and a half years, it was discarded. The speech quality continued to improve and in our last observation, December 1975, the patient's speech quality and articulation were normal by our standards.

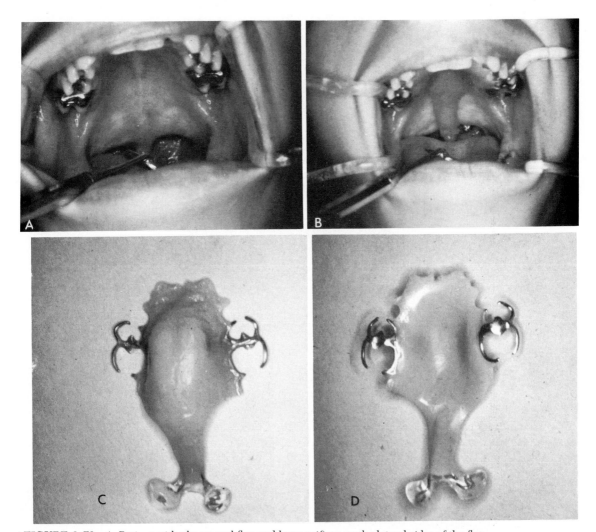

FIGURE 6–70 *A*, Patient with pharyngeal flap and large orifices on the lateral sides of the flap, resulting in inadequate palatopharyngeal closure. This patient also had limited posterior and lateral pharyngeal wall muscle activity. *B*, Split pharyngeal section prosthesis is in position to accomplish stimulation and palatopharyngeal closure. *C*, Palatal view of the prosthesis. *D*, Oral view of the prosthesis.

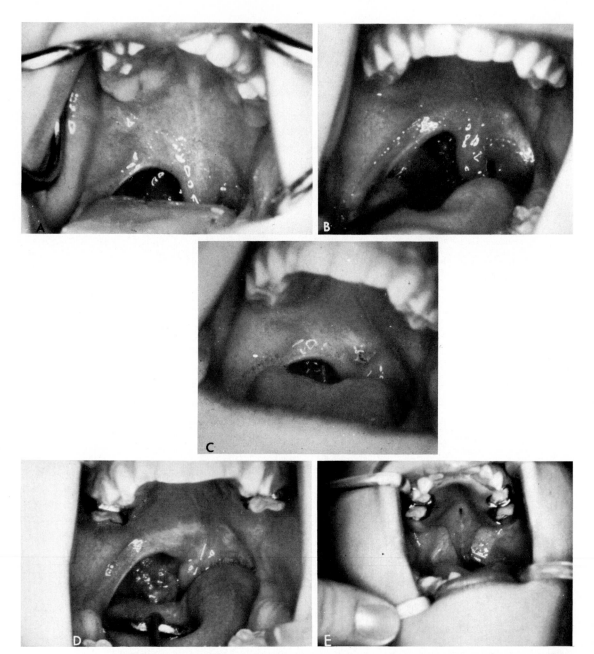

FIGURE 6–71 *A*, Three-year-old patient with unilateral paralysis of the soft palate resulting in hypernasal speech. Note velar hemiatrophy. *B*, Patient at the age of five years; hemiatrophy continues to exist. *C*, At the age of six and one-half years patient had pharyngeal flap surgery performed. *D*, At the age of eight years, velar hemiatrophy continued to exist along with hypernasality. *E*, Prosthetic speech aid to act as a stimulator was constructed for the patient. Patient wore the prosthesis for one year. The increased muscle function of the posterior and lateral pharyngeal wall of the right orifice resulted in a discontinuation of prostheses. At present, patient is 12 years old and has been seen annually. Speech continues to be satisfactory and hypernasality no longer is present.

SUMMARY

1. Velar elevation should be gradual in order to put less pressure upon the teeth retaining the prosthesis and to reduce the possibility of mucosal irritation.
2. Prosthetic stimulation should be initiated as soon as velar paralysis is noted in order to reduce the occurrence of velar disuse atrophy.
3. The palatal lift prosthesis is used as a temporary or permanent measure for the correction of velar incompetency. As soon as adequate elevation occurs, the prosthesis should be discarded. Otherwise, the patient could wear the prosthesis as a permanent supportive device.
4. The construction of the combination lift bulb requires a program of gradual velar elevation and molding of the pharyngeal bulb, so as to reduce the gag reflexes and to increase velopharyngeal adaptation to the prosthesis. After the initial placement, the modification of the velopharyngeal section becomes less troublesome to the patient.
5. Speech and myofunctional therapy should be instituted in conjunction with the prosthetic treatment.
6. Prosthetic lift and combination is more effective for patients with less severe neurological impairment and speech articulatory errors.
7. The prosthetic lift has been more effective for patients with velar incompetency without involvement of other oropharyngeal musculatures, while the combination type has been more effective for patients with velopharyngeal insufficiency without marked articulatory disorders.

There are still several questions that require further investigation:
1. What is the relationship between palatal stimulation and degree of neuromuscular function and recovery?
2. What is the relationship between stimulation and degree of occurrence of disuse atrophy?
3. What is the relationship between pharyngeal stimulation and muscle constriction?
4. What is the degree of stability of velopharyngeal function and constriction after stimulation?

CASE HISTORY: R.E.G.

Adult patients occasionally present themselves at the Cooper Institute and Clinic, either through referral or on their own, seeking improvement in their appearance and speech. Most have had surgery for a cleft lip or palate earlier in life. A few have palatal clefts that have not been repaired. But in nearly all cases the surgical results have not been completely satisfactory to them.

Although the principles of restoration of form and function are basically the same for these individuals as for our child patients, the procedures are usually complicated by the rigidity of the distorted oral structures with which the surgeon and dentist must work and by years of neglect with respect to oral hygiene and dental attention.

We present here a detailed case history of such a patient, who was treated by us over a period of two and one-half years, from March 1966 to November 1968. Many visits were required, but eventually a good result was obtained.

Patient.   R. E. G., male, 31, Caucasian, divorced.

Occupation: Laborer.

One child, a son age 10 at time of patient's admission. Child has no congenital anomalies. Another son died at the age of four from a bowel infection.

Date of Admission.   March 23, 1966. Referred by a cousin, who is a Clinic patient.

CONSULTATION

Chief Complaint.   Unilateral, postoperative cleft lip and unoperated cleft palate (type III). Residual notch in the vermilion tissue. Cleft palate speech. Objectionable oral condition because of lost teeth, with resulting poor esthetics and inability to masticate properly. Patient is dissatisfied with his poor speech, previous lip surgery, difficulty in chewing, and his appearance. "I have been ridiculed continuously," he said, "because of my speech and my looks."

General Appearance.   Upper lip is short and lacks support. A depressed scar remains on left side. Lower lip has a slight forward projection. Nose is slightly elevated to the right.

Medical History.   Examination of his medical record revealed no systemic or neurologic diseases. He is one of two siblings. Both parents are living and in good health, although both are completely edentulous. Condition of the teeth in the family is poor. There are several cases of cleft lip or palate in the father's family, including patient's first cousin, who is receiving treatment at the Lancaster Cleft Palate Clinic.

Patient experienced the usual childhood diseases. Tonsils are present. Cleft of the lip was surgically repaired in infancy. No history of running ears, mastoiditis, or hearing loss.

No early dental care, and oral hygiene was poor by his own admission. First teeth lost were the maxillary first molars and second molars, owing to advanced caries. The other missing teeth had been surgically removed, because of advanced caries, over a period of 12 years, between 1954 and 1966.

Patient has not had any previous experience with prosthetics. Before his admission to our Clinic, a dentist in his home town had removed his maxillary left and right cuspids, the maxillary left and right central incisors, and the mandibular third molar. The dentist had suggested that a removable partial maxillary denture could be constructed, but patient did not return to him for this prosthetic treatment.

He denies the habit of bruxism or clenching of teeth.

Education.   Finished grade school, but because of his poor speech, he did not continue on into high school.

Birth History.   Patient's mother was 24 when he was born. He was born at home, and the mother had not been under medical supervision during pregnancy. Length of pregnancy was normal, and there was no history of illness, bleeding, x-radiation, excessive vomiting, injury, or any other adverse health condition during the first trimester.

Mother had difficulty feeding him; he was fed during infancy with a medicine dropper.

Mental Attitude.   Patient is very anxious to start the treatment program, and he has complete confidence in being rehabilitated.

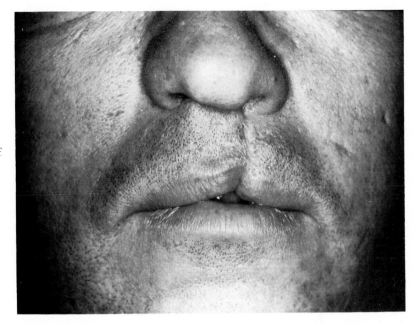

FIGURE 6–72 Front view of the patient before treatment.

PLASTIC SURGERY EXAMINATION

Lip. The patient has a postoperative cleft of the lip on the left side. The scar is depressed; the vermilion border is uneven; and there is a residual notch in the tissue of the vermilion border (Figure 6–72).

Nose. The nose is fairly good, but it appears to deviate to the right slightly, partly owing to flattening of the right ala. He has reduction of the left nasal airway from closure of septum.

Palate. Patient has a cleft of the soft and hard palate (Figure 6–73).

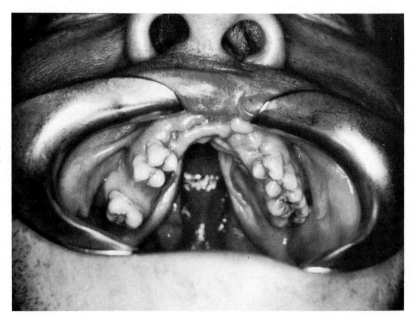

FIGURE 6–73 View of the patient's unoperated cleft of the soft and hard palates.

ORAL EXAMINATION

Preliminary examination revealed a badly crippled masticatory apparatus, with extensively restored teeth and carious lesions. Some of the decayed teeth had been repaired with acrylic resin and amalgam alloys, but the restorations had been poorly done. They had been improperly contoured and had not been polished.

The right second molar and first and second bicuspids, and the left first and second bicuspids and first and second molars were present in the maxilla. Present in the mandible were the left bicuspids, cuspid, lateral incisor, and central incisor, and the right central incisor, lateral incisor, cuspid, and second molar.

Enamel decalcification had taken place on the labial surfaces of all the maxillary and mandibular teeth, and there was evidence of poor oral hygiene habits.

The tongue and the buccal and labial mucosa appeared normal and healthy. There was no mobility of the teeth and all were vital on the vitalometer test. Gingival pocket depth throughout was considered normal.

The character and thickness of the mucoperiosteum in all edentulous areas was determined by digital examination. It appeared uniform in thickness and was only slightly displaceable. All soft tissue attachments had been placed so as to interfere very little with the denture borders. The patient had a thick, ropy saliva.

The shape of the arches was noted. The upper and lower second molars were inclined mesially and also drifted anteriorly. The upper right bicuspids had a considerably mesial drift. Slight forward drift of the maxillary bicuspids and molars was noted.

Vertical dimension at physiological rest and centric occlusal positions were recorded. The path of opening and closing of the mandible was observed and centric relation and centric occlusion determined to be identical. Slight shift of maxillary midline was noted (Fig. 6–74).

The patient did not have a very active gag reflex.

The interalveolar space at centric occlusion in the left posterior region was deficient. Patient had a class II, division I malocclusion.

The palatal cleft originated in the midline of the hard palate at a point par-

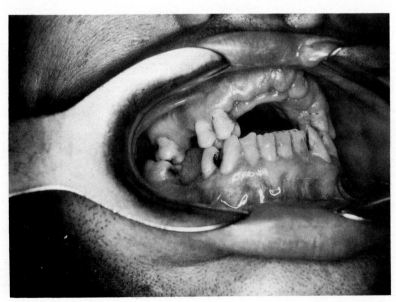

FIGURE 6–74 Patient in centric occlusion before treatment.

allel mesially to the second bicuspids. The cleft started as a point and became wider posteriorly. The width of the cleft at the junction of the soft and hard palate was 14 mm. The width of the nasopharynx was 32 mm. and the anteroposterior length of the cleft was 40 mm. The cleft had not been surgically repaired.

SPEECH AND HEARING EVALUATION

The patient read diagnostic sentences for the evaluation of voice quality and general articulatory pattern. The overall voice was very nasal. The plosive sounds K, T, and P were very weak and produced with nasal emission of air. The fricative sounds F, V, and TH were produced as weak sounds accompanied be nasal emission of air with the substitutions of F for voiceless TH, and V for the voiced TH. The sibilant sounds S and Z were produced in the pharyngeal area (they are commonly called laryngeal fricatives). These sounds should be made within the oral cavity, with the anterior teeth in a biting position. The sounds of K and G, likewise, were produced as guttural or pharyngeal sounds. During the process of phonation, with reference to sibilants particularly, the patient produced a snorting sound with great frequency.

The tongue could move in the general directions necessary for sound placement. The lingual frenum attachment was satisfactory.

Although voice quality was hypernasal, the vital capacity test indicated no loss of air through the nose while blowing. The patient accomplished this by elevating his tongue into the nasal cavity and allowing air to escape laterally. By thus occluding the nose, he was able to produce a breath pressure equal to the intraoral pressure he could develop while holding his nose and blowing into the spirometer.

The patient reported no hearing problems associated with ear aches or ear infection. Puretone audiometric evaluation, using a Beltone 15–A or C clinic audiometer, revealed the following air conduction test data: right ear above 5 db throughout speech range (500 to 4000 cycles per second); left ear in the range of 500 to 2000 cycles per second indicated a similar pattern to the right ear. For the left ear at 4000 cycles per second level, the patient fell off to 20 dB. It was felt that the patient's hearing was within normal limits bilaterally.

The sonogram showed overtones of each vowel to be enhanced, thus producing a nasal pattern. Middle frequency formants were missing, indicating lack of vowel intelligibility.

ROENTGENOGRAPHIC EXAMINATION

A full mouth x-ray study, utilizing 14 periapical films and two bite-wings, revealed 17 vital teeth (Figure 6–75). The restorations were not properly con-

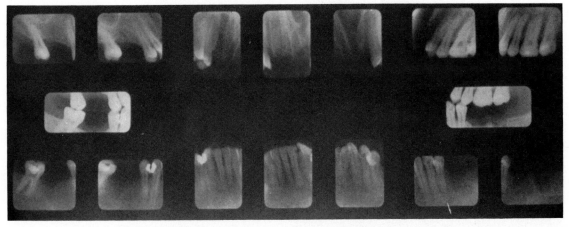

FIGURE 6–75 Roentgenograms before treatment.

toured, and they had overhanging margins. Interproximal and occlusal carious lesions were noted in several of the maxillary and mandibular teeth. Evidence of some alveolar resorption around the existing maxillary and mandibular bicuspids and molars was noted in the x-rays. Mesial inclination of maxillary and mandibular second molars existed. Alveolar resorption around the maxillary molar was related to premature contact in centric and eccentric relationship. Since the mandibular molar was stronger than the maxillary molar, the latter tooth received most of the damage. The trabeculae of the alveolar bone were closely meshed and the healthy appearance of the bony support around the existing teeth, which had been carrying an additional load for some time, gave a favorable prognosis for the rate of resorption of the alveolar bone under a correctly constructed removable prosthesis.

The interproximal bony crests were high and well formed, except in the upper and lower bicuspids and molars, where some resorption had taken place. The pulp chambers appeared normal. There was no evidence of root canal therapy or apical lesions.

The length, shape, and inclination of each root was noted. There was no calculus present.

The edentulous areas were free of cysts, residual roots, or other foreign matter. The floor of the antrum appeared high; no nutrient canals could be identified.

CINERADIOGRAPHIC EVALUATION

A cineradiographic study was completed without a prosthetic device in position. The patient showed no velopharyngeal closure with the remnants of the soft tissue present. During the process of blowing and phonation, no posterior pharyngeal activity was seen.

STUDY CASTS

Maxillary and mandibular alginate impressions were poured in artificial stone and mounted on a Hanau model H articulator with a face-bow transfer (Figure 6–76). An interocclusal wax record in centric occlusion was obtained. An interocclusal wax record in protrusive relation was obtained and condylar inclination guides on the articulator adjusted. The only tooth contacts in protrusive relation were two maxillary and mandibular teeth.

The maxillary right bicuspids and molar drifted mesially and the right lower molar also appeared mesially displaced. Molars were in crossbite relationship.

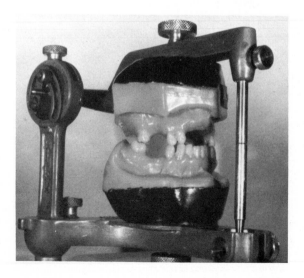

FIGURE 6–76 Mounted study casts in centric occlusion.

The maxillomandibular relationship was class II, division I in character; but the lower posterior extension (edentulous area) was in a favorable relationship. Edentulous areas are classified as mandibular class II–P and maxillary class IV–P (after Kennedy, Applegate).

The position, inclination, parallelism, and shape of all clinical crowns were noted. Duplicate study casts were placed on a surveyor and the lingual inclination of the mandibular bicuspids and molars noted.

The survey of the soft tissues at 0–degree tilt disclosed some undercuts on the lingual side of the mandibular left posterior region, and on the mandibular right buccal and also the maxillary labial portion. A severe undercut was noted in the region of the palatal cleft.

The width, depth, and length of the palatal cleft, the position of the alveolar cleft, the shape and height of the vault, the condition of the rugae, and the position of the labial, buccal, and lingual frena were noted.

The disuse atrophy of the edentulous areas, caused by the elapsed time between extractions and insertion of a prosthesis, which left narrow ridges in some regions, is evident. The left retromolar pad is not well defined.

TREATMENT PLAN

After a careful study of the hard and soft structures in the mouth, the length and width of the cleft and nasopharynx, the speech and psychological evaluation of the patient, the roentgenograms, the cineradiographic studies, and the mounted study casts, the following course of treatment was decided upon by the members of the staff:

1. Full coverage of the abutment teeth with nine acrylic resin veneer crowns and three full cast gold crowns was planned, with splinting of the maxillary left bicuspids and molars, maxillary right bicuspids, mandibular left bicuspids, and mandibular right cuspid and bicuspid.

The replacement of the maxillary central and lateral incisors as a part of the removable prosthesis was indicated because a better esthetic result could be obtained with that method than by replacing them with a fixed prosthesis. The necks of the maxillary central and lateral incisors would therefore be placed labially in a position that would be necessary in a fixed prosthesis to obtain a better lip support.

The splinting of maxillary and mandibular right molars with bicuspids on the same side was considered, but abandoned as unnecessary because the prosthesis would be designed to act as a splint for these teeth.

2. Fabrication of a removable maxillary prosthetic speech aid replacing the missing teeth, restoring the hard palate cleft, and obtaining velopharyngeal closure was decided upon in order to reduce the amount of air flow through the nose and produce better speech.

3. A removable partial mandibular denture replacing the missing posterior teeth was to be fabricated.

The maxillary central and lateral incisors do not contact the mandibular teeth to provide a zero incisal guidance and give the patient a better esthetic result because of a short upper lip.

The protrusion of the alveolar ridge of the maxillary anterior region would give sufficient horizontal overlap of the incisor teeth.

4. Surgical revision of the lip, rhinoplasty, and septoplasty was decided upon.

5. Intensive speech therapy was indicated.

PRETREATMENT DISCUSSION

The cuspal inclination and occlusal horizontal dimension of the clinical crowns will be decreased in the fabricated crowns where possible. Allowance will be made in the crowns for the reception of the partial dentures and the prosthetic speech aid. The crowns will be surveyed, and favorable undercuts built into them at the buccocervical surface wherever possible. The retentive elements of the clasps will rest on the gold of the acrylic resin veneer crowns. The lingual surfaces will be parallel to each other unilaterally and bilaterally. Allowance will be made on the lingual surfaces to accommodate the reciprocating segments of the clasps on the crowns. This will reduce the buccolingual contour of the crowns and make the lingual clasp segments less irritating to the tongue.

Full coverage of the abutment teeth was decided upon because of the high caries index, extensive restoration, decalcified enamel, poor cuspal relationship, and occlusal disharmony. Alteration of pitch, contour, and shape will be accomplished for esthetic improvement as well as for reception of the prosthesis.

Splinting of the abutments will be done to create multi-rooted abutments, aiding in the preservation of the periodontium because of the additional resistance to torque stress.

All crowns will have rest stops in them, prepared so that the vertical forces will be directed toward and parallel to the long axis of the teeth. Minor connectors will be placed flush against the abutment teeth on the proximal side, to decrease the force in a mesiodistal direction and aid the occlusal stops in distributing the vertical stresses in a direction parallel to the long axis of the teeth.

All the clasps will be slightly passive in order to promote a stress-breaking action as the denture base moves slightly on the displaceable tissue.

Torque stresses causing rotational movements around the abutments adjacent to the posterior extension of the denture base will be dissipated by the retentive arms of the clasps. The rigid bracing arm and properly prepared occlusal rests offer resistance to lateral displacement and also superior displacements of the maxillary prosthetic speech aid.

Rigid major connectors will be utilized in the mandibular denture. The full palatal coverage, utilizing gold laterally and gold mesh filled with acrylic resin in the middle, will be employed. Care will be taken in making the maxillary impression to prevent the sagging of the alginate material, so that a seal along the posterior border of the prosthesis will be assured. Caution also will be taken not to extend the impression material too far inside the nasal cavity to prevent the removal of the impression in one piece.

The posterior palatal seal will be placed along the posterior border of the maxillary prosthesis to prevent leakage of air. Clasped teeth will have a clearance of 3 to 4 mm. between the necks of the teeth and the major connectors, wherever possible.

Indirect retention is provided on the lingual side of the cuspid crown and is further aided by an accurate impression and accurately determined borders of the denture bases. Intimate contact of the rest extensions in their prepared seats must be maintained for the indirect retainers to function.

Denture bases in the posterior extension areas will be extended to obtain maximal coverage of tissues. The mandibular base will extend distally to cover the retromolar pad and laterally to the external oblique line, utilizing the entire buccal shelf for support. The lingual and distolingual borders will be determined by the muscle-trimmed impression of this area with the tongue at rest, its tip and lateral borders touching the occlusal surfaces of the teeth.

Care will be exercised in establishing the borders of the denture bases to avoid irritation to the soft tissue and eliminate tension on the borders in certain movements with referred stress to the abutment teeth.

All cuspal inclination will be kept to the minimum to reduce horizontal and torque stresses on the abutment teeth. Rational posterior teeth will be employed.

The maxillary prosthetic speech aid will be fabricated in two or three separate procedures, making an anterior section, velar section, and pharyngeal section. This will give the patient the chance of easy adaptation and a more comfortable adjustment period. The velar section will cover 2 mm. of the lateral border of the cleft. A functional impression of the pharyngeal section with suitable material will be obtained.

Methyl methacrylate resin will be used in the fabrication of the denture bases, velar section, and pharyngeal section. Use of this material instead of gold provides the advantages of lightness in the maxillary prosthesis and ease of rebasing and adding to the pharyngeal section if required.

Upon the completion of the prosthesis, the revision of the lip, rhinoplasty, and septoplasty will be performed. Intensive speech therapy will follow.

TREATMENT RECORD

First Appointment. The medical history of the patient and the parents and the financial status of the patient were taken. A complete visual, digital, and roentgenographic examination of the oral structures and a plastic surgical examination of the lip and nose were done. Speech, hearing, and psychological evaluations, plus cineradiographic studies, were also completed. Alginate impressions were made, into which study casts were poured. Interocclusal records in centric occlusion and protrusive relation were completed and a face-bow registration accomplished. Measurements of the vertical dimension at the centric occlusion and physiological rest positions were recorded. Front, profile, and intraoral Kodachrome exposures were done.

At the staff meeting following the completion of diagnostic procedures, the plan of treatment was discussed by the members of the team and approved.

Second Appointment. Plan, cost, and approximate duration of treatment were discussed with the patient, who expressed his approval of the plan. Since the patient was not able to undertake the complete cost of treatment, it was decided to proceed with treatment and allow the patient to pay minimal fees.

Under local two per cent lidocaine hydrochloride (Xylocaine) anesthesia, the full veneer crown on the maxillary right bicuspid and the mandibular right cuspid and bicuspid were prepared. Maxillary and mandibular molars were prepared for full gold crowns. Full-mouth rubber base impressions were completed. The face-bow registration and wax interocclusal records were made. Temporary crowns of autopolymer acrylic resin were placed on all the prepared teeth. Because of the position of the maxillary right first bicuspid, its preparation was modified to receive a cuspid crown.

Third Appointment. The castings were seated and checked. A procedure similar to that in the second appointment was performed on the maxillary and mandibular bicuspids and molars.

Fourth Appointment. All 12 crowns in which the plane of occlusion, angulation for survey, rest stops, and lingual receptacles had been worked were now tried in the mouth and adjusted. Plaster indices were registered in preparation for soldering of the maxillary right bicuspids, left bicuspids and molars, and mandibular left bicuspids and right cuspid and first bicuspid.

The soldered crowns were tried on the teeth and checked. Full mouth maxillary and mandibular plaster impressions were taken with crowns in position. Face-bow registration and wax interocclusal records were completed.

With all the crowns on the cast mounted on the articulator, centric and eccentric occlusions were thoroughly studied.

Fifth Appointment. The splinted crowns with veneers added were placed on the teeth and checked (Figures 6–77 to 6–82). Maxillary and mandibular alginate impressions of the preparation under local anesthesia were made. Kodachrome exposures were recorded. All the crowns were cemented at this time. Maxillary and mandibular alginate impressions were made in the perforated stock trays.

Sixth Appointment. Maxillary and mandibular alginate impressions were made in autopolymer acrylic resin trays. Casts were poured and surveyed for the most favorable path of insertion. The crowns had been surveyed during their fabrication for the equal infrabulge retentive areas and parallel guiding planes. Attention was given to the tissue undercuts as well.

Seventh Appointment. The cast gold framework was tried in the mouth, checked, and adjusted (Figure 6–83). Wax occlusal rims were attached to the metal framework in the edentulous areas. A face-bow registration was accomplished and interocclusal wax records of the teeth in centric occlusion and protrusion were completed.

Text continued on page 341

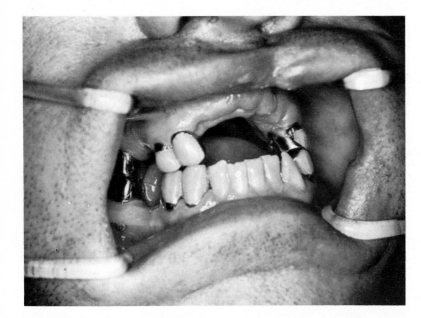

FIGURE 6–77 Patient in centric occlusion after the restoration of the abutments.

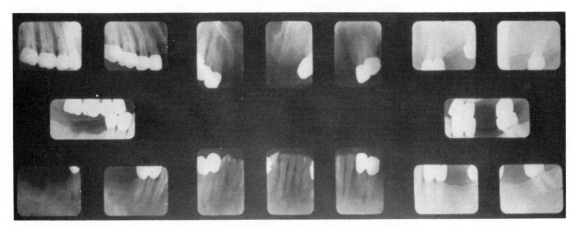

FIGURE 6–78 Roentgenograms after treatment.

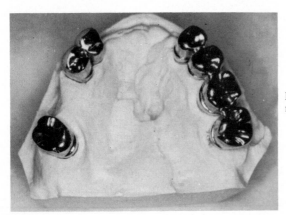

FIGURE 6–79 View of crowns designed to support and retain prosthesis prior to cementation.

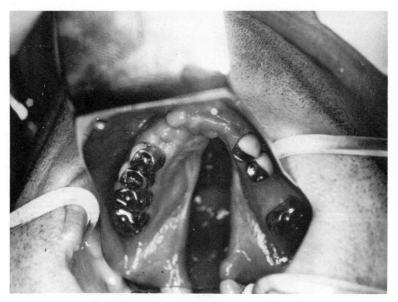

FIGURE 6–80 Splinted crowns cemented.

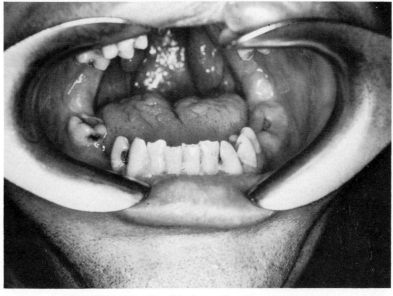

FIGURE 6–81 Mandibular teeth prior to restoration.

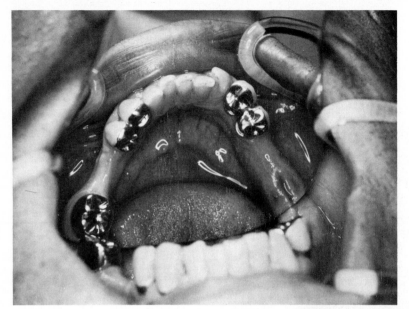

FIGURE 6–82 After restoration of the abutment.

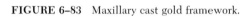

FIGURE 6–83 Maxillary cast gold framework.

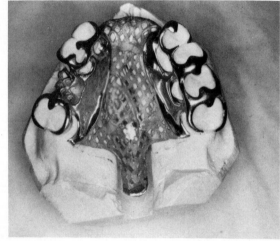

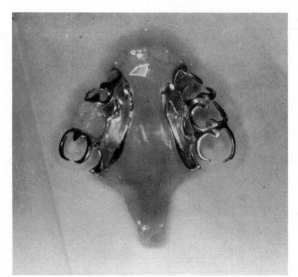

FIGURE 6–84 View of the prosthesis prior to the construction of the speech bulb (pharyngeal section).

Eighth Appointment. The removable partial denture and prosthetic speech aid framework with the teeth attached were tried in the mouth and checked. The trial denture bases in the posterior extension and anterior edentulous areas were of autopolymer resin and attached to the metal framework.

Ninth Appointment. The completed dentures (without the speech bulb) were placed, and occlusion checked. Minor adjustments were required to correct slight occlusal discrepancies (Figure 6–84).

Tenth Appointment. The patient returned with a complaint of gagging several times in a day owing to contact of the velar section of the prosthesis with the soft palate. He was assured that this would eventually subside.

Eleventh Appointment. The Adaptol impression of the pharyngeal section, or speech bulb, was made. Special attention was given to the displaceable nasopharyngeal tissues and to providing comfort for the patient during swallowing, head movements, and speech exercises. A lateral head plate roentgenogram of the speech bulb in position was taken to check the position of the bulb in relation to the anterior tubercle of the atlas bone. Cineradiographic studies reveal that velopharyngeal closure in a normal individual takes place at an area anterior and superior to the anterior tubercle of the atlas bone. We position our speech bulb in this area (Figures 6–85 to 6–88).

During this same visit, a sonogram was made. A sonographic analysis (frequency versus time as related to intensity) indicates the improvement in voice quality following insertion of a prosthetic speech aid. Vowels are easily identified and the voice has improved projection with reduction of nasality and nasal snorting during phonation. With the prosthetic speech aid in position, the sonogram and disc recording of the patient clearly indicate the reduction of nasal voice quality. The goal of the remaining program is to retrain the patient's articulation pattern to increase speech intelligibility. The prognosis, with speech training and good results, is socially acceptable speech.

Cineradiographic studies with the prosthetic speech aid in position reveal that the speech bulb rests against the postpharyngeal wall at a level anterior to the external tubercle of the atlas bone. The appliance does not move during the process of phonation. There appears to be adequate room within the oral cavity for phonation.

Twelfth Appointment. Patient returned without any discomfort. The max-

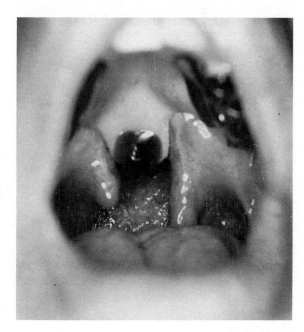

FIGURE 6–85 Two holes are drilled in the posterior part of the tailpiece (velar section). A piece of separating wire is drawn through the holes in such a manner that a loop is formed beyond the superior part of the tailpiece. The two ends of the wires are twisted together inferiorly and secured to the appliance with a sticky wax. With the prosthesis in position, if desired, a lateral cephalometric x-ray is taken to locate the position of the wire in relation to the palatal plane. This wire would also help to hold the speech bulb impression in position.

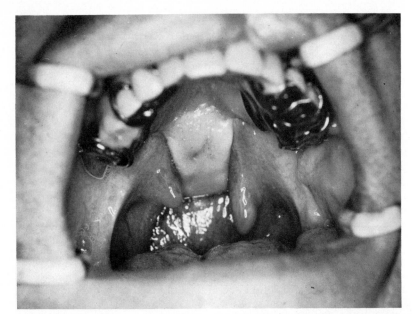

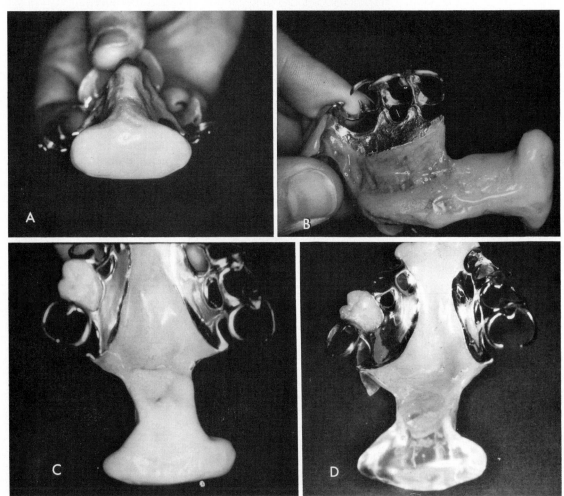

FIGURE 6–87 *A*, Posterior view of the speech bulb where it contacts the posterior pharyngeal wall; *B*, lateral view. *C*, Oral view of the speech bulb prior to processing. *D*, Completed prosthetic speech aid.

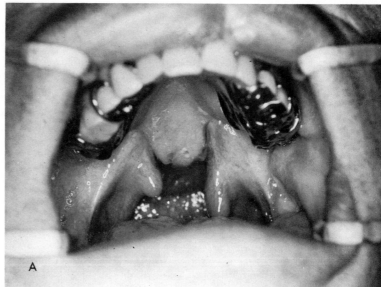

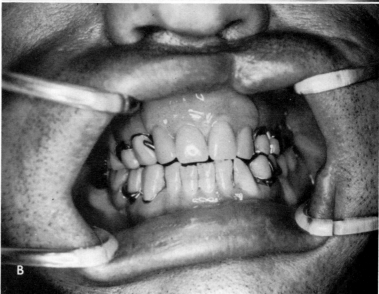

FIGURE 6-88 *A*, Prosthetic speech aid in position. *B*, Patient in centric occlusion with the prosthesis in position.

illary and mandibular alginate impressions, with and without the prosthesis, were obtained. Kodachrome exposures and full mouth x-rays of the patient were made. Patient received speech therapy.

Thirteenth Appointment. The patient had no complaints and continued to receive speech therapy. A disc recording, sonogram, and cineradiographic studies were made with the prosthesis in position.

Fourteenth Appointment. Lip revision was performed.

Fifteenth Appointment. Postsurgical observation and Kodachrome exposures of the lip after surgery were made.

POSTTREATMENT DISCUSSION

Considerable thought has been given to the design of these removable partial dentures and prosthetic speech aids, and to how they would be converted in case one or more abutment teeth were lost. Multiple clasping is one possible solution.

The distal extension side could be dispensed with by making an intra-coronal attachment, but this was decided against in favor of a passive clasp that would permit stress-breaking action to the horizontal, vertical, and torque stresses. The torque and horizontal stresses have been minimized by placing all occlusal contacts on one plane and eliminating inclinations in the occlusal scheme.

Retention clasp segments in all areas are resting on gold rather than acrylic resin veneers of the crowns. This problem could have been eliminated by using porcelain veneer crowns. However, the lack of facilities at the Clinic, much greater expense to the patient, and difficulty in obtaining a suitable shade for this type of porcelain prevented its use.

SUMMARY AND CONCLUSION

Correct diagnosis and treatment planning are essential to successful cleft lip and palate rehabilitation and prosthodontics. When a careful diagnosis is ac-complished by a well-organized team of medical, dental, speech, and other spe-cialists interested in the welfare of the patient, when these specialists work together as a team and utilize all the available diagnostic tools to their best ad-vantage, and when a well-thought-out treatment plan is executed, a favorable prognosis is assured.

Upon completion of this extensive treatment, the patient was extremely grateful and happy. He told me: "For the first time in my life I could chew bet-ter, I look nicer, and the people don't make fun of me because of my speech. The whole thing looks like a dream to me. I don't know how to appreciate what you have done for me. I pray that some day I can repay you for your work."

There is no greater reward than when a patient has good results, especially in the field of cleft palate rehabilitation. I am proud of the fact that our dental profession plays an important role in rehabilitating and habilitating these hand-icapped individuals.

FACIAL CANCER AND _____
PROSTHETICS

Patients who have undergone surgery for an orofacial malignancy are frequently left with defects that seriously impair their speech and mastica-tory functions. In many instances the tumor is so extensive that the resulting postsurgical defect cannot be closed by surgical methods. For these patients we have been able to construct prostheses of plastic materials that can re-store their oral functions, including speech, and greatly improve their ap-pearance (Figure 6–89).

Following are (1) a case history of a man of 65 that details the surgical and prosthetic management of an intraoral tumor (Figures 6–90 to 6–101), and (2) brief notes concerning two other patients who were fitted with prostheses following surgical treatment of facial cancers.

Text continued on page 350

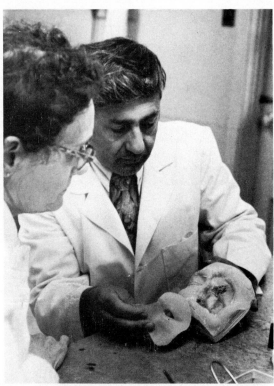

FIGURE 6–89 The Clinic's own laboratory provides the skills and equipment for designing and producing all types of dental appliances and orofacial prostheses. Here, Mazaheri and Dorothy Biesicker, a dental technician, check a moulage and prosthesis for a patient who had undergone extensive surgery for facial cancer.

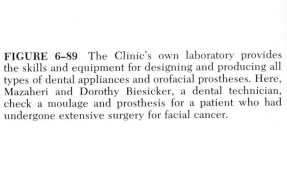

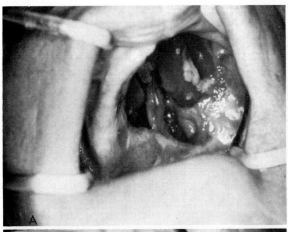

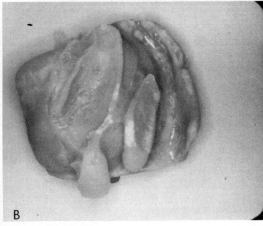

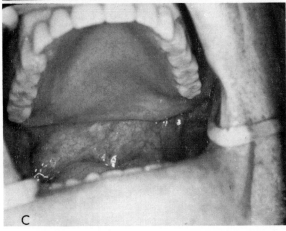

FIGURE 6–90 A, An edentulous patient with a resection of most of the maxilla. B, Nasal view of the obturator. To gain more retention, the utilization of the nasal undercuts by the prosthesis was undertaken. The prosthesis is relined with Silicone 390. This type of soft lining material has to be frequently replaced owing to changes caused by oral environment. C, The prosthetic obturator in position.

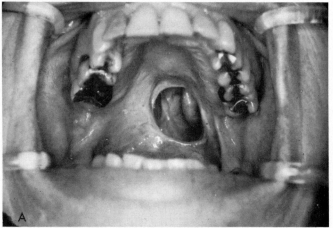

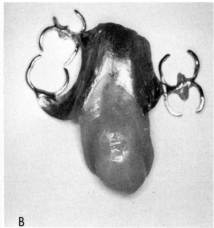

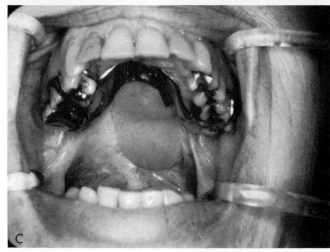

FIGURE 6–91 *A*, Patient after excision of a lesion in the soft and hard palate. *B*, The nasal view of the prosthesis and obturator. *C*, The prosthesis in position.

FIGURE 6–92 Palatal view showing preoperative lesion of the left maxilla and antrum.

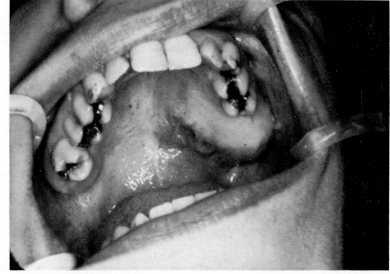

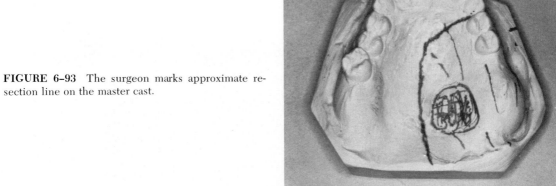

FIGURE 6–93 The surgeon marks approximate resection line on the master cast.

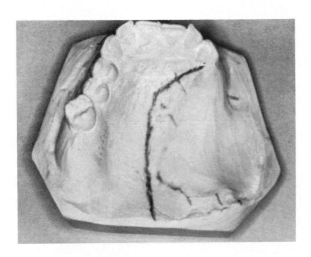

FIGURE 6–94 Trimming of the teeth and jaw on the cast on the resection side.

FIGURE 6–95 Palatal view of an immediate temporary obturator.

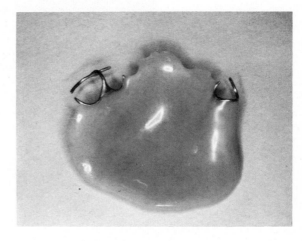

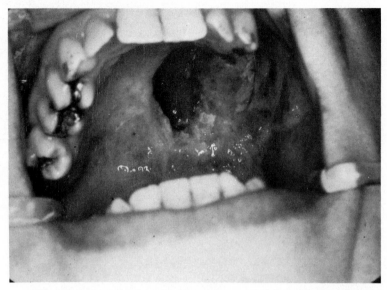

FIGURE 6–96   Palatal view of the defect several days after surgery.

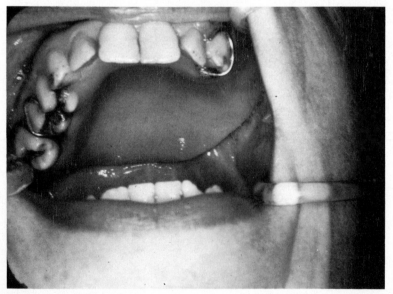

FIGURE 6–97   View of the temporary prosthesis in position. This prosthesis is immediately inserted after surgery to prevent food from lodging in the nasal cavity, facilitate swallowing, improve speech, and help the wound to heal.

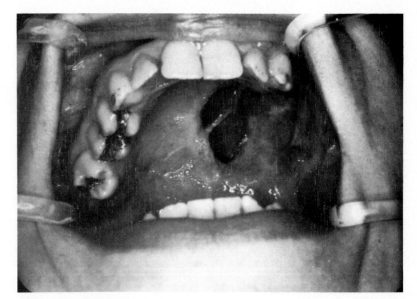

FIGURE 6–98 Palatal view five months after surgery.

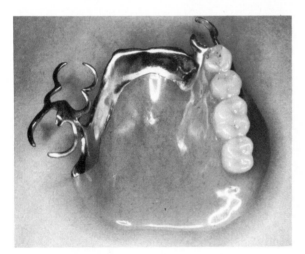

FIGURE 6–99 The oral view of the prosthesis.

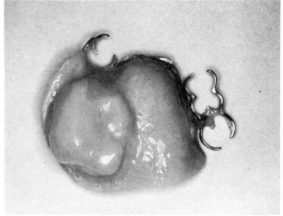

FIGURE 6–100 Nasal view of the prosthesis and obturator. Note that the obturator does not have to extend too far within the nasal cavity and is convexed so that secretion and food do not collect in this area.

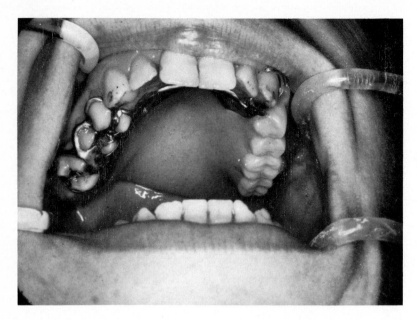

FIGURE 6–101 View of the prosthesis in position.

CASE HISTORY: J. C. B.

NAME: J. C. B.   *AGE:* 65   *SEX:* Male

RACE: Caucasian   *OCCUPATION:* Justice of the Peace

HOSPITAL ADMISSION DATE: June 15, 1965

History

This 65-year-old Caucasian male, who lost all of his maxillary and mandibular molars six years ago, was referred by his family dentist and is being admitted for exploration and biopsy of the maxillary antrum for a cystic swelling of this area.

History of Present Illness. The patient noticed approximately six to seven weeks ago that he had a lump on his hard palate that made his dentures difficult to insert. Approximately three to four weeks ago, his nose was becoming obstructed on the left side. About the same time, he began to perceive a swelling of the cheek on the left. He had a nosebleed approximately six to seven weeks ago. There has been no extensive drainage from his nose. He does have some drainage from the right nostril, but this is just mucus. His general health has been good.

Past History. The patient has had no serious illnesses, operations, or allergies.

Review of Systems. He is in good health with no chills or fever. His appetite and bowel movements are good.

Cardiovascular. Results were negative. He is able to walk up three flights of stairs and only gets short of breath. Does have some cramping in the feet at night, after being on them for eight hours at a time.

Musculoskeletal. Results were negative.

He smokes a pipe and cigars, but not cigarettes.

Physical Examination

Patient is a well-developed, well-nourished, adult male, in no acute distress.

Head.   There is an asymmetry of the face because of a swelling in the left cheek area.

Eyes.   Extraocular motions are intact. Pupils are equal and reactive.

Nose.   There is a mass pushing from the left maxillary sinus area medially, completely obstructing the left passageway. The right passageway seems normal.

Mouth.   A cystic swelling that involves the entire left side of the hard palate, alveolar ridge, and anterior third of the soft palate is present.

Neck.   No cervical adenopathy was found.

Chest.   Nothing was detected through auscultation and percussion. There was a slight increase in anteroposterior diameter.

Heart.   Rate is regular with no murmurs. There is an occasionally dropped beat.

Abdomen.   The abdomen is soft and moderately protuberant with no masses or scars.

Extremities.   The extremities are grossly normal. There is some decrease in the hair on the feet and lower legs. The posterior tibial pulses are absent bilaterally and the dorsalis pedis pulses are weak bilaterally.

Radiographic Examination.   Clouding of the left maxillary antrum and some evidence of maxillary bony destruction are present.

Impression

There is a tumor of the left maxilla with a possible malignancy change.

Operation Performed

Biopsy.

Procedure and Findings

With the patient under general endotracheal anesthesia, the face was prepared with Zephiran, as was the oral mucosa. Incision was made in the canine fossa over the left maxillary antrum. There was a moderate amount of edema. The anterior wall of the antrum had been practically destroyed, so that it was possible to enter the antrum by excising the tissue with a scalpel. Tissue was removed for biopsy. The tumor seemed to involve the floor of the antrum and the medial wall with extension into the palate and the nose. The mucosa of the nasal and oral surfaces was intact. The biopsy site was closed with #3–0 chromic catgut. The patient tolerated the procedure well and was returned to the recovery room in good condition.

Microscopic Examination and Diagnosis

Nonkeratinizing, moderately well-differentiated squamous cell carcinoma of maxillary sinus was found.

Readmission, June 22, 1965

Patient was readmitted to St. Joseph Hospital in Lancaster for a maxillectomy, following a stay at home for three days. His general condition was unchanged from the previous admission except that there was less swelling and induration in the area of the tumor.

Operation Performed (by Philip Long)

A left maxillectomy was performed.

Procedure and Findings

The patient was anesthetized and intubated lying supine on the operating table; the face was prepared with Zephiran and draped in the routine fashion. The Weber-Ferguson type of approach was used, splitting the lip in the midline and going around the ala of the nose up along the nose to the inner canthal area of the eye and then across the lid to the lateral orbital rim. When this incision was made, there was a small step placed in the upper lip. Bleeding vessels were clamped and electrically cauterized. The cheek flap was turned back, and an incision made along the mucosa and back to the area of the maxillary tubercle. A Gigli's saw was passed around the zygoma, which was severed along with lateral orbital rim. The nasal process of the maxilla was severed with a chisel.

An incision was made in the mucosa over the palate using the electrocautery. This had to extend slightly beyond the midline as it was apparent the tumor was growing to the midline and slightly beyond. The hard palate was then separated using an osteotome. The palate was cut across the attachment of the soft palate and the hard palate. Then, with an osteotome placed posterior to the maxillary tubercle, the pterygoid was separated and the maxilla was freed and removed. The floor of the orbit was left intact, although it was somewhat fragmented. The antrum was curetted of all remaining sinus mucosa on the superior and posterior areas and filled with warm, moist packing.

A split-thickness skin graft was then taken from the right thigh. This was used to line the cheek flap and also placed into the maxillary antrum area. Since the floor of the orbit seemed somewhat insecure, a strip of the temporalis fascia with muscle was swung under the eye to help give support to the infraorbital area. The skin graft was placed with sutures of silk and catgut. The cheek flap was then returned, suturing with #3-0 plain catgut and interrupted #6-0 silk for the skin. Packing was placed into the area of the defect to hold the skin graft in place and was held in this position with sutures of #4-0 silk. The patient tolerated the procedure well. There was fairly active bleeding, and he lost approximately 2500 to 3000 cc. of blood. He was given 2500 cc. of blood while in the operating room. The patient was returned to the recovery room in good condition.

Microscopic Examination and Diagnosis

1. The following were found: bony sequestra, subacute healing reaction, and marked edema of the mucosa. No neoplasm was present. (Superficial portion of specimen—squamous mucosa.)

2. There was an extensive, moderately well-differentiated, noncornifying squamous cell carcinoma extending to or close to the respiratory epithelium and to the base of the section. A secondary infection was present. (Base of specimen.)

3. Extensive neoplasm with secondary necrosis and inflammation was found. (Center of lesion.)

Postsurgical Observation

Patient was scheduled to be seen at the dental clinic shortly after his discharge from the hospital on July 1, 1965.

The patient has a defect involving the total left hard palate, alveolar ridge, and anterior two-fifths of the soft palate. A portion of the hard palate on the right is also affected. The inner portion of the cheek and antrum was lined with a skin graft. The defect appears healthy, without any evidence of recurrence. The remaining portion of the soft palate appeared to be functioning and the patient demonstrated velopharyngeal closure (this was also substantiated by cineradiography). The patient complained of food lodging in the defect and fluid loss through the nose. He also has noted a great reduction in oral pressure and flow. The patient objected to his nasality and unintelligible speech and has used pad and pencil for communication since his palatal operation. The previous dentures were ill-fitting and occlusal relationship required a major modification; therefore, it was decided that dentures were not adaptable for alteration as a temporary prosthesis.

Prosthetic Restoration

Acrylic Denture Base Obturator Without Teeth. A stock tray lined with a metal rim for an edentulous mouth was selected. This tray was modified in the area of the defect and the remaining alveolar ridge with green compound and Adaptol, and an irreversible hydrocolloid impression was made. An acrylic, perforated, custom-made tray, properly extended, was constructed over the maxillary study cast; again an alginate impression was made. An acrylic denture base with proper extension into the surgical defect was fabricated. The temporary obturator without teeth was inserted several days after the initial visit. The patient's speech improved, and problems of regurgitation, lodging of food in the defect, and general swelling were alleviated within a short time. This prosthesis was worn by the patient for six months, and he reported that he did not experience any difficulty with the denture base retention. Utilization of some of the undercut in the defective area has provided the patient with a somewhat greater base retention.

Complete Denture with Obturator and Removal of Partial Denture. After one week the patient became so accustomed to the denture base that he could partially resume his everyday responsibilities. He was asked to return periodically for observation of the defect, surrounding oral and nasal tissue, and prosthesis. Six months after initial surgery, it was felt that the patient was ready for a more permanent type of prosthesis. In November 1965, preliminary impressions were made using acrylic resin trays constructed over the preliminary casts. The maxillary impression included some of the undercut areas in the nasal region. The undercuts were blocked, and an autopolymer resin base was fabricated for the maxillary ridge and defect using a pressure cooker. Wax occlusal rims were constructed over the maxillary base and the lower partial denture frame. The vertical dimension of occlusion and centric relation were registered. The upper cast was transferred to an anatomical articulator by means of a face-bow transfer.

It has been our experience that this type of patient will tolerate the monoplane acrylic teeth better than any other kind. The teeth were arranged on the bases, and the trial setup was brought to the mouth and checked for jaw records and tooth placement in regard to static requirements and function. The positions of the maxillary anterior teeth were somewhat affected by the limited function of the upper lip following surgery.

It was decided that the obturator portion of the prosthesis should be made hollow; and proper steps were taken for this procedure in processing the denture. It was also decided that the maxillary prosthesis, including the obturator's portion, should be relined with one of the available silicone soft liners, to engage nasal undercut areas for greater retention.

The prostheses were inserted and checked for speech, border extension, obturation, retention, stability, occlusion, and weight. Minor adjustments were required. The patient was instructed in the insertion of the denture and home care. Three days later he reported that he was well satisfied with his speech, chewing ability, and all other functions of the prosthesis. He was referred to the speech department for recording and instruction.

A week later the dentures were remounted with the aid of an intraoral balancer, and occlusion was balanced and equilibrated, The patient again was reminded of the home care recommended by the manufacturer of the silicone material. He was instructed to return in two weeks and then every two months.

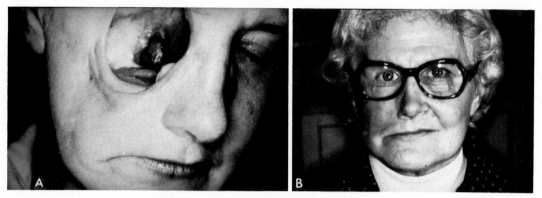

FIGURE 6–102 *A,* Facial defect. *B,* Facial and eye prosthesis in position.

DISCUSSION

Denture retention is a major problem for patients with an acquired or congenital edentulous condition and cleft.

Silicone #390 was used in this patient for extension of the obturator to engage the undercuts, with some result. The growth of fungi on the silicone liner makes it necessary to replace the material every so often. A soft liner with ideal requirements for intraoral use has not been introduced.

Close cooperation between the surgeon and the prosthodontist is necessary if the patient with an orofacial defect is to gain the full benefits of treatment.

TWO BRIEF CASES

Another patient helped by the provision of a prosthesis following cancer surgery was a woman in her fifties, a secretary. The malignancy had required excision of the antrum and the maxilla, as well as the right orbit (Figure 6–102). Immediately after the operation we constructed a temporary prosthesis that prevented food from lodging in the nasal cavity and also permitted her to speak with greater clarity than she could without such assistance. Approximately six months later we made a more permanent prosthesis, including an

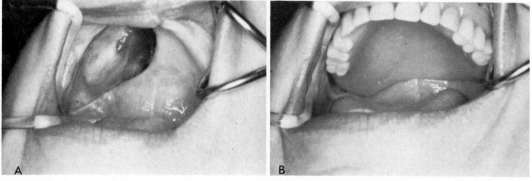

FIGURE 6–103 *A,* Palatal defect of the patient in Figure 6–101. *B,* Full denture obturator in position.

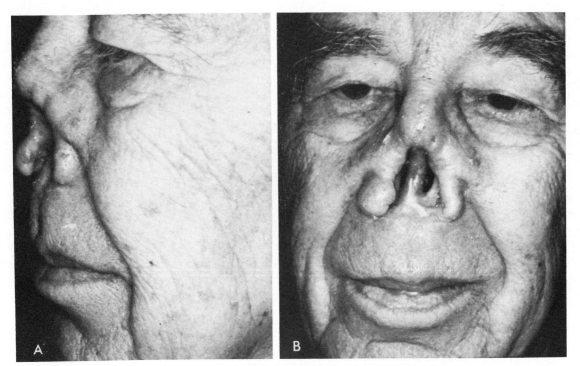

FIGURE 6–104 *A*, Profile and *B*, full face of a patient who has had nasal resection.

eye socket and artificial eye. She had been able to return to her secretarial position in a state government office soon after the surgery, and so effective was the speech part of the prosthesis (Figure 6–103) that her associates were not aware that she had suffered any impairment.

A retired Lancaster man underwent a nasal resection for cancer that destroyed the lower half of the nose (Figure 6–104). It was explained to him

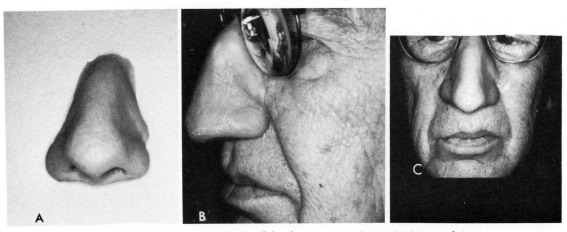

FIGURE 6–105 *A*, The prosthetic nose constructed for the patient in Figure 6–104. *B* and *C*, Prosthesis in position. Dow Corning MDX-4-4210 Elastomer was used for making the prosthesis for this patient and the patient in Figure 6–102.

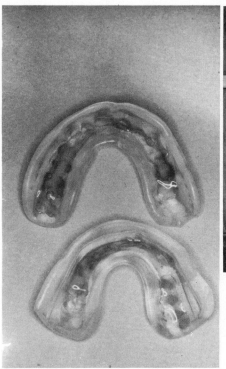

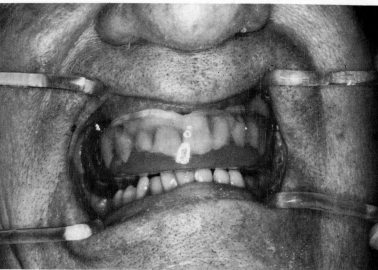

FIGURE 6–106   A, Carrier tray for viscous fluoride gel made for home use. B, Application of the fluoride gel by patient, who holds it in place for several minutes.

that a series of surgical procedures could be carried out to reconstruct a nose, but he decided on the alternative of a prosthesis (Figure 6–105). In both this and the preceding case, the prosthesis was made of Dow Corning MDX-4-4210 Elastomer.*

Radiation Caries

It should be kept in mind that cancer patients who have received radiation therapy over the oral region are prone to radiation caries. This arises from radiation-induced changes in the consistency of the saliva and its reduced quantity, from gingival recession with exposure of root surfaces, from a tendency for more plaque formation, and from dietary alterations that may occur during radiation treatments.

These patients should be encouraged to be especially conscientious about their oral and dental hygiene, which should include the local application of fluorides by the patient and the dentist. A fluoride viscous gel preparation is available and can be applied by the patient at home with a special tray (Figure 6–106).

*Dow Corning Corporation, Medical Products Division, Midland, Michigan.

References

1. Biggerstaff, R. H., and M. Mazaheri: Oral manifestations of the Ellis-Van Creveld syndrome. J. Am. Dent. Assoc., 5:1090, 1968.
2. Blakely, R. W.: Temporary speech prosthesis as an aid in speech training (abstract). Cleft Palate Bull., 10:63, 1960.
3. Broadbent, B. H.: A new x-ray technique and its application to orthodontia. Angle Orthod., 1:45, 1931.
4. Cooper, H. K.: Cinefluorography with image intensification as an aid in treatment planning for some cleft lip and/or cleft palate cases. Am. J. Orthod., 42:815, 1956.
5. Cooper, H. K.: Recent trends in the management of the individual with oral-facial and speech handicaps. Am. J. Orthod., 49:683, 1963.
6. Cooper, H. K., R. E. Long, J. A. Cooper, M. Mazaheri, and R. T. Millard: Psychological, orthodontic, and prosthetic approaches in rehabilitation of the cleft palate patient. Dent. Clin. North Am., p. 381, 1960.
7. Cronin, T. D.: Method of preventing raw area on nasal surface of soft palate in pushback surgery. Plast. Reconstr. Surg., 20:474, 1957.
8. Dorrance, G. M.: Lengthening of the soft palate in cleft palate operations. Ann. Surg., 82: 208, 1925.
9. Gibbons, P., and H. Bloomer: A supportive-type prosthetic speech aid. J. Prosthet. Dent., 8:362, 1958.
10. Gillies, H. D., and W. K. Fry: A new principle in the surgical treatment of congenital cleft palate, and its mechanical counterpart, Br. Med. J., 1:335, 1921.
11. Gonzalez, J. B., and A. E. Aronson: Palatal lift prosthesis for treatment of anatomic and neurologic palatopharyngeal insufficiency. Cleft Palate J., 7:91, 1970.
12. Grabb, W., S. Rosenstein, and K. Bzoch (eds.): Cleft Lip and Palate, Boston, Little, Brown, p. 629, 1971.
13. Harkins, W. R.: Cleft palate prosthetics. In Goldman, H. M., S. P. Forest, D. L. Byrd, and R. E. McDonald: Current Therapy in Dentistry, vol. 2, St. Louis, C. V. Mosby, 1966.
14. Ivy, R. H.: Editorial: Some thoughts on posterior pharyngeal flap surgery in the treatment of cleft palate. Plast. Reconstr. Surg., 26:417, 1960.
15. Lancaster Cleft Palate Clinic Booklet, revised edition, Lancaster, Pa. 1968.
16. Lang, B. R., and L. J. Kipfmueller: Treating velopharyngeal inadequacies with a palatal lift prosthesis. Plast. Reconstr. Surg., 43:467, 1969.
17. Mazaheri, M.: Prosthetic treatment of closed vertical dimension in cleft palate patients. J. Prosthet. Dent., 11:187, 1961.
18. Mazaheri, M.: Indications and contraindications for prosthetic speech appliances in cleft palate. Plast. Reconstr. Surg., 30:663, 1962.
19. Mazaheri, M.: Prosthondontics in cleft palate treatment and research. J. Prosthet. Dent., 14:1146, 1964.
20. Mazaheri, M.: Cleft palate prosthetics. Curr. Ther. Dent., 3:315, 1968.
21. Mazaheri, M., and R. H. Biggerstaff: Standardized sectional laminagraphs of the temporo-mandibular joint. J. Prosthet. Dent., 5:489, 1967.
22. Mazaheri, M., R. L. Harding, and R. H. Ivy: The indication for a speech-aid prosthesis in cleft palate habilitation. Proceedings of the Third International Congress of Plastic Surgery, Washington, D.C., October 1963. Excerpta Medica International Congress, Series 66, Amsterdam.
23. Mazaheri, M., R. L. Harding, and S. Nanda: The effect of surgery on maxillary growth and cleft width. Plast. Reconstri Surg., 1:22, 1967.
24. Mazaheri, M., and F. A. Hofmann: Cineradiography in prosthetic speech appliance construction. J. Prosthet. Dent., 12:571, 1962.
25. Mazaheri, M., and R. T. Millard: Changes in nasal resonance related to differences in location and dimension of speech bulbs. Cleft Palate J., 2:167, 1965.
26. Mazaheri, M., R. T. Millard, and D. J. Erickson: Cineradiographic comparison of normal to non-cleft subjects with velopharyngeal inadequacy. Cleft Palate J., 1:199, 1964.
27. Mazaheri, M., S. Nanda, and V. Sassouni: Comparison of midfacial development of children with clefts and their siblings. Cleft Palate J., 4:334, 1967.
28. Mazaheri, M., and P. P. Sahni: Techniques of cephalometry, photography and oral impressions for infants. J. Prosthet. Dent., 3:315, 1969.
29. Millard, R. T.: Wide and/or short cleft palate. Plast. Reconstr. Surg., 29:40, 1962.
30. Mills, L. F., J. D. Niswander, M. Mazaheri, and J. A. Brunella: Minor oral and facial defects in relatives of oral cleft patients. Angle Orthod., 38:199, 1968.
31. Pruzansky, S., and E. F. Lis: Cephalometric roentgenography of infants: sedation, instrumentation and research. Am. J. Orthod., 44:159, 1958.
32. Swain, E. D.: Artificial vela and obturators. Dent. Rev., 2, 1888.
33. Veau, V., and S. Borel: Division Palatine; Anatomie, Chirugie, Phonetique. Masson et Cie., Editeurs, Paris, 1931.

Chapter Seven _____

The orthodontic management of the patient with cleft lip and/or cleft palate has received considerable attention in recent years, almost to the point of being classed as a subspecialty in itself. It must be constantly borne in mind that the objectives and responsibilities of the orthodontist managing these cases with oral-facial anomalies and communicative disorders are in essence identical to those laid down for the specialty of orthodontics as a whole:

> Orthodontics is that area of dentistry concerned with the growth, guidance, correction and maintenance of the dentofacial complex, with special emphasis on developmental disturbances and those conditions that cause or require movement of teeth. The area of orthodontic practice includes the diagnosis, prevention, interception and treatment of all forms of malocclusion of the teeth and the associated alterations in their supporting structures; the design, application, and control of functional and corrective appliances; and the guidance of the developing dentition to attain optimum occlusal relations in physiologic and esthetic harmony with other facial and cranial structures.[25]

To this basic definition by the American Association of Orthodontists might be added the goal of providing these orofacially "crippled"[19] patients a structural and functional oral apparatus conducive to the acquisition and maintenance of socially acceptable speech. Also required is the integration of services with other concerned specialists on the team. There is special emphasis on growth and development of the craniofacial and dento-alveolar complexes, and the orthodontist is presented with a unique opportunity to apply and contribute his knowledge and training to the total rehabilitation effort.

The integrated team concept of cleft palate management was introduced and developed by the senior author, H. K. Cooper, Sr., himself an orthodontist. In the 1930's, realizing the scope of the problem and his own limitation as an orthodontist, he organized a small team that eventually became the Lancaster Cleft Palate Clinic. The early history of the Clinic is related in the opening chapter of this volume.

ORTHODONTICS AND ORAL ORTHOPEDICS

HERBERT K. COOPER, SR.,
ROSS E. LONG, SR.,
ROSS E. LONG, JR.,
and J. MICHAEL PEPEK

This milieu of integrated services in which the orthodontist finds himself when involved in cleft palate management has been specifically described by Cooper[20] as follows:

> An unrelated step-by-step series of procedures is not true integration. The greatest good cannot be achieved by having one specialty after another, under the guise of a correlated program, attempt to solve the problem with the method peculiar to the specialty. True integration starts with a meeting of the minds of the individuals who first examine the patient together and then agree on a program for treatment. (page 28)

and

> ...The responsibility falls on members of all professions to keep the services which they render in proper balance with the sum total of necessary and desirable services ... (page 28)

This latter concept has been schematized by Cooper[20] (Figure 7–1) and emphasizes the point that the orthodontist is just one spoke of a very large wheel. At various points in time in the overall treatment of the patient, his role on the team may fluctuate from primary to secondary or ancillary, but his input is continuous and integral to the smooth operation of the group. It should also be evident that because of his interest in and knowledge of craniofacial growth and development, from birth to adulthood, the orthodontist's "spoke" on the team wheel probably comes around to a point of primary importance just as often, if not more so, than many other members of the team.

As one of the team members concerned with the craniofacial and dento-alveolar growth and development of patients with clefts, the orthodontist must be aware that while there are specific problems peculiar to the cleft population, the problems faced are gradually changing, as treatment methods are improved in *all* the specialties involved. The mutilated, orofacially disfigured, and dentally handicapped individuals who

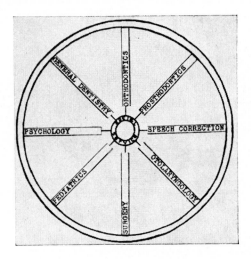

FIGURE 7-1 Integration of services in the treatment of cleft lip and cleft palate. (From Cooper, H. K.: J. Am. Dent. Assoc., 47:27–32, 1953. Copyright by the American Dental Association. Reprinted by permission.)

confronted the orthodontist at the turn of the century caused Kingsley[70] and Case[15] to recommend discontinuation of surgical intervention. Such an extreme step was not taken, but the facial growth disruption documented by Graber[43] and illustrated by Cooper[18, 20] (Figure 7–2) prompted interaction of surgeon, prosthodontist, and orthodontist to evolve better surgical techniques. These led ultimately to the contrasting and favorable growth trends seen in recent cleft populations, including those treated at the Lancaster Cleft Palate Clinic.[65, 76, 83, 88] As a consequence, the problems originally considered "endemic" in this group of patients, and that faced the orthodontist, have changed from the almost untreatable gross skeletal discrepancies of years ago to more localized dento-alveolar growth disturbances, very amenable to corrective orthodontic and orthopedic measures. This is not to deny the occurrence of major skeletal imbalances in the cleft palate population, but merely to put it in its proper perspective in light of more recent post-surgical results.

PHILOSOPHY OF ORTHODONTIC MANAGEMENT

In most approaches to the discussion of cleft palate orthodontics, specific treatment timing, methods, modalities, and mechanisms are presented as they relate to the technical management of cleft palate malocclusions. As the profession continues to improve its techniques, today's methods or fads may become tomorrow's curiosities. The philosophy upon which various management procedures are based, however, and the means used to establish the philosophy transcend the day-to-day changes in approach.

Forty years of orthodontic experience and interaction at the Lancaster Cleft Palate Clinic and H. K. Cooper Institute have been responsible for the evolution of just such a philosophy-generating concept.

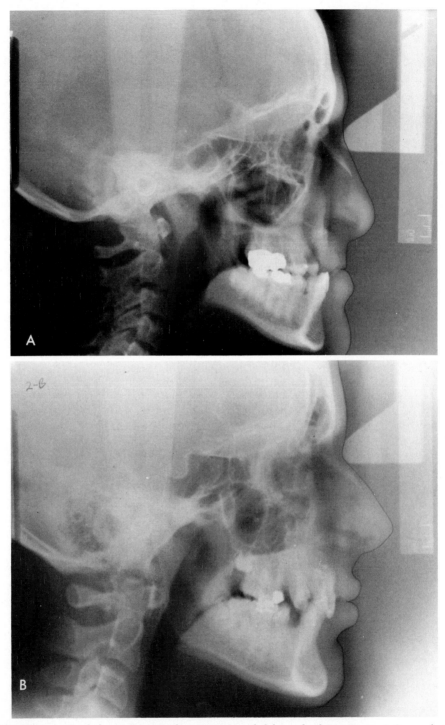

FIGURE 7–2   Cephalometric x-ray of postoperative cleft lip and palate patients. *A*, Severe facial deficiencies due to traumatic surgery; *B*, Acceptable facial profile following less traumatic surgical techniques.

Overview of Problem

First and foremost is the need to establish a broad but flexible overview of the total scope of the problem. It is obviously necessary for the orthodontist to be well-versed in the biomechanics of tooth movement and in the ratios, dimensions, angles, and patterns of normal and abnormal facial growth. This is essential in his management of malocclusions in non-cleft patients. But if he is to integrate his services effectively with others in the treatment of those with clefts, he must also understand the total problem relating to the congenital defect as well as to the rehabilitation challenge.

Specifically, a working knowledge of such aspects as incidence, etiology (genetic and environmental), embryogenesis, and neonatal anatomy and physiology enhances the ability of the orthodontist to interact with the team geneticist and the pediatrician. Discussions with the plastic surgeons demand a familiarity with the anatomical deviations and the techniques of lip and palate closure. It will also be helpful if he has a knowledge of the normal and cleft speech mechanisms and of hearing aspects, so that he can participate with the speech, audiology, and otolaryngology members of the team. All of these, plus a broad insight into the general dental, maxillofacial prosthetic and prosthodontic, and social service problems, are prerequisites for the orthodontist's successful interaction with the rest of the team.

Interaction with Other Team Specialists

A second major premise upon which the orthodontist should build his philosophy is that his interactions with other specialists must be both prospective and retrospective. The former involves proper diagnosis, treatment planning, and prognosis, and should be self-evident. The latter, while less frequently considered, is no less important, and it is the best way in which improvements in all rehabilitory techniques can be evolved. The orthodontist, because of the longitudinal nature of his concern with the patient's growth and development, not infrequently finds himself in a position to provide other team specialists with a retrospective evaluation of their current therapeutic methods. The most notable example, of course, is with regard to the surgeon's methods and timing of lip and palate repair as related to subsequent growth and development of the craniofacial and dento-alveolar complexes. (See Chapter 2.) Additionally, he might offer information regarding effects, if any, of speech therapy or tongue placement therapy on the teeth and jaws.

It is equally important for the orthodontist to make a retrospective evaluation of his own work with regard to such things as: (1) the degree to which alignment or normalizing of underlying hard tissues (dental and/or skeletal) enhances surgical repair of overlying soft tissues or (2) the degree to which establishment of normal dento-alveolar structure and alignment facilitates speech therapy measures.

All of these types of interactions presuppose that all phases of treatment are being adequately and objectively documented *longitudinally*,[154, 156] a requirement of special importance to the orthodontist in his record-keeping. Without such long-term serial documentation the innumerable possible confounding variables, many of which have been neatly outlined by Dickson et al.,[32] can so muddle the data gathered as to make them meaningless for retrospective interactions.

But one must be aware of certain problems in the handling of longitudinal data. Even if one confines the evaluation to his own longitudinal records, he finds that there is such a wide variability in craniofacial features in the cleft population, from the time of birth on, and so many new variables are added by surgery of the lip and palate, that it is difficult for the orthodontist to sort out from these many variables the factors that are responsible for his own orthodontic results. When one adds to this the variations in technical skills among different surgeons and different orthodontists, it can be seen that longitudinal results drawn from other centers and applied to one's own team and patient population may lose much of their usefulness so far as contemporary methods of documentation are concerned.

An important requisite to successful retrospective interaction is that the orthodontist be willing to compromise his own approach to treatment when it affects the ability of others on the team to render their services successfully. Thus, the plastic surgeon is usually the one best qualified to determine the amount of orthodontic/orthopedic preparation he requires prior to his surgery to facilitate his own techniques. As another example, the speech specialist may be better qualified to determine the degree to which oral hard tissues may be affecting the patient's speech acquisition or correction. The orthodontist may therefore be advised to maintain a sufficiently flexible philosophy to be able to adjust his treatment accordingly, so long as he does not jeopardize his own long-term results.

Acquisition of New Knowledge

Another rule for developing a philosophy of orthodontic management of cleft cases is to maintain a receptive interest in the acquisition of new knowledge about craniofacial growth and development as developed by related basic sciences and to augment or alter one's approach as influenced by that new knowledge. As examples, several such developments can be cited that indirectly enhanced the orthodontist's chances of obtaining satisfactory results. Studies by Scott and Sarnat, emphasizing the possible role of the cartilaginous nasal septum in facial growth[149, 150] and illustrating the consequence of septal damage,[146, 147] significantly altered surgical attitudes in the handling of the premaxilla and septal stalk in bilateral cleft lip and palate cases. Further analysis of this concept led to the de-emphasis of the postnatal importance of the cartilaginous septum and instead stressed other factors.[78, 100] Of these, the realization of the importance of soft tissue "functional matrices"[99] in craniofacial growth instilled new significance into the application of Wolff's Law of Bone Transformation (as described by Sir Arthur Keith)[69] to surgical approaches. And the importance to the orthodontist of an esthetic *and* functional lip repair by the surgeon became increasingly apparent through the observations of Harding and Mazaheri of our Institute[54, 87] and of others.[49, 50, 121, 123, 124, 129, 144, 157, 158, 160] As a final example, studies that clearly implicated palatal scarring on or near the alveolar ridges as being responsible for arch deformation[73] exerted considerable influence on subsequent orthodontic treatment[142-144] and resulted in additional precautions or changes in palatal surgery.[27] In short, the orthodontist must base his approach not only on his own observable, longitudinal clinical results but also on the acquisition of sound, relevant basic science data.

Determination of Cost/Benefit Analysis

Still another concept in the philosophy of treatment useful for all forms of orthodontic diagnosis and treatment planning, but especially relevant to the cleft palate problem, is the cost/benefit analysis. Labeled "therapeutic modifiability" by Moorrees and Grøn[97] and recommended for all forms of diagnosis and treatment planning,[1] it must be a cornerstone of consideration for cleft palate orthodontic rehabilitation. While the label used is recent, the concept is not; it was expressed by Kingsley[70] in 1880 as follows:

Much of the success in treating irregularities will depend upon a correct diagnosis and prognosis. . . . It is not a question of the ability to bring one or more teeth into the line of a regular dental arch, so much as it is, will the result, when obtained, be *permanent and justify the means used?* (page 40) (emphasis added)

Others have presented this same concept more recently, with specific reference to cleft palate orthodontic management:

Maximum efficiency should be the paramount consideration in cleft lip and palate therapy; otherwise it may happen that these children are subjected to continuous treatment from birth to adulthood.[155]

and

The multidisciplinary treatment required is considerable, and can be a heavy burden on both cleft patient and his family. The orthodontic treatment takes by far the greatest amount of time and, consequently, if one is to relieve the strain on the cleft individual of time consuming treatment, the orthodontic procedure should be considered first.[5]

Thus, the philosophy of management generated by the orthodontist cannot be limited to the pure environment of orthodontic ideals, desirable as that may be. It must also weigh the anticipated result against the amount of improvement actually achieved and the total investment in terms of time, cost, effort, and possible untoward consequences of that treatment. With regard to the latter, it is obvious that the cleft palate patient is usually subjected, in his rehabilitation course, to a long, extensive series of operations, examinations, and appointments from the other team specialties alone. Frequently travel to a treatment center is prohibitive, in terms of finances, time, and distance. Total treatment costs can be exorbitant. Most significantly, the patient's own psychological attitude and cooperation toward his rehabilitation may be at stake.

While it is conceivable that a particular approach to orthodontic management could produce dependably excellent results, it is equally probable that the best approach may involve a compromise of ideal orthodontic objectives with other, more important considerations to the patient. A desire to "normalize" these afflicted patients orthodontically at the earliest possible age is laudable, but it must be tempered with consideration for the long-range therapeutic "modifiability" of the problem at hand and the means available to correct it. Perhaps the suggestion often offered to patients with these anomalies, to "accept with serenity the things we cannot change, have the courage to change the things we can, and the wisdom to know the difference,"[20] might on occasion be equally well applied to the orthodontist planning a total course of treatment for the cleft palate patient, given the potential limitations imposed on any ideal treatment objectives.

Recognition of Variability in Cleft Population

We would emphasize again that in building an orthodontic philosophy one must appreciate the tremendous variation in the cleft population regarding size, shape, and form of the affected facial structures;[18, 124, 157] the individual response to various modes of treatment;[3, 121, 124] and the inherent growth potential.[12, 108, 129, 161]

The important concept propounded by Ricketts that "the cleft palate occurs in patients exhibiting a variety of facial patterns" and "the cleft defect, with ensuing influences, is superimposed on a basic morphologic pattern"[129] means that the unpredictability caused by variability in facial types and growth patterns in the normal population will also be present in the cleft population and will be further complicated by the cleft condition.

What this demands of any philosophy of orthodontic management is that regardless of the specific approach utilized, it is impractical to attempt to treat all cases alike with the expectation of achieving uniform results. As expressed by Robertson and Fish:[132]

> Because the anatomic variations in clefts of the lip and palate are so numerous, it is to be expected that no rigid formula of treatment will be successful in all instances. However, to determine the most suitable treatment program for any type of case, adequate long-term records are essential and the records must be capable of accurate analysis to permit a valid assessment of the treatment procedure under review. (page 290)

Two conclusions then evolve from this point. First is the reappearance of a need mentioned earlier, namely, good longitudinal documentation. Second is the inference that since one single treatment method cannot be expected to give equally satisfactory results, it becomes mandatory for the orthodontist to arrive at two further realizations. One is the need to maintain a flexible and adaptable philosophy of treatment, capable of handling the great variety of problems seen. The other is the need to be able to discern the types of problems most amenable to each of those treatment formulas available so that the appropriate approach *for the individual case* may be selected.

As a straightforward example (Figure 7–3), it should be obvious that mandibular prognathism in the cleft patient could result from one of several possible mechanisms, each requiring precise differentiation and calling for different approaches to treatment. Thus, the severe lack of vertical maxillary development often seen in older cleft palate populations, presumably the result of some disturbance of dento-alveolar development (see page 390), leads to overclosure of the mandible and consequent Class III appearance. Alternatively, in another patient it is conceivable that a true Class III mandibular growth pattern may exist beneath the *superimposed cleft,* so that even if the maxillary growth pattern approximates normality in all dimensions, a Class III skeletal profile will still result. However, the former case, with normal mandibular proportions, requires prompt attention to mechanics geared to increase maxillary vertical dento-alveolar development, while the latter must be handled in the mandible, either as soon as possible with some form of extraoral orthopedics or postpubertally by some form of mandibular surgery. In either case, the two variables must be differentiated so that the appropriate treatment approach can be instituted. One single mode of handling Class III skeletal relations will not produce equally satisfactory results in both cases.

While in this example the differential diagnosis involved is a fairly straightforward matter of longitudinal lateral cephalometric analysis, other types of problems may not have available such dependable objective means of differentiation. In the latter cases, i.e., "gray" zones in which there are no reliable characteristics for predetermination of the variables affecting outcome, the orthodontist must develop an approach based on the other aspects mentioned previously. He must weigh the potential changes in the long-range "therapeutic modifiability" of a problem if it is treated incorrectly, inadequately, or unnecessarily.

The considerations just mentioned provide the orthodontist with an approach to concrete treatment philosophies, which, regardless of changes in specific techniques, offer the greatest chance of successful rehabilitation and meaningful team interaction. With this in mind it now becomes possible to examine the most frequently encountered orthodontic problems in the cleft palate patient and to outline the methods of treatment presently employed at the H. K. Cooper Institute for dealing with those problems.

DIAGNOSIS

DATA COLLECTION

A major part of all orthodontics is diagnosis — determining the nature of the problem, the essential basis for deciding what to do about it and when to do it. Because of the complicating factors brought into the picture by the cleft, diagnosis becomes an even more complex undertaking with these individuals. We shall therefore devote a major portion of this chapter to diagnostic considerations. And as with non-cleft orthodontic diagnosis, the first step in outlining the problems is the gathering of records. A major difference in the cleft population, however, is that in most instances the record collecting begins at birth. The social service personnel assist in this task, and as soon after birth as possible the dentist examines the infant and makes oral impressions for upper and lower study models, as well as facial casts. Details of these procedures are given in the chapter on Prosthodontic Care, which also outlines the methods of making full mouth panoramic radiographs; periapical and bitewing films, when necessary; and facial and intraoral slides. Height/weight records are made, and to provide further information about skeletal maturation, hand/wrist films may be taken. These procedures have been described elsewhere,[84, 85] and while they require considerable teamwork and experience, they are readily and reliably accomplished (see Figure 6–1, page 271).

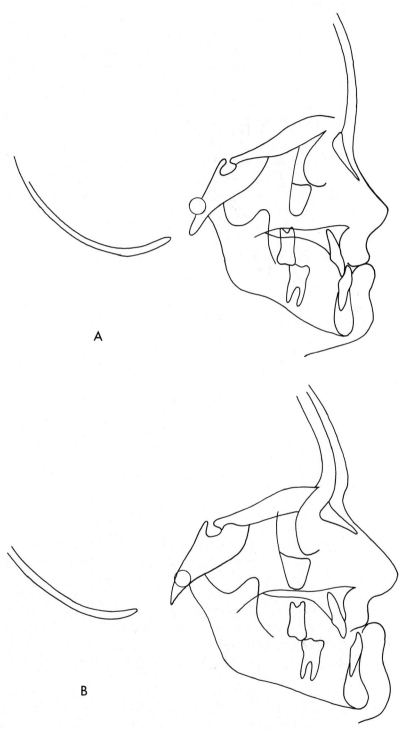

A

B

FIGURE 7–3 Two class III cleft profiles. *A*, Due to mandibular over-closure: *B*, Due to true mandibular prognathism.

Because of the importance of keeping good longitudinal data, as mentioned previously, these records are collected every six months to the age of two years, then every year after that. These records thus become a valuable and essential resource for later treatment by the team orthodontist at the center, for management of referral cases to be handled later by a private orthodontist outside the center, and for the previously discussed purposes of prospective and retrospective evaluation of treatment.

Once adequate records have been collected, the same methodical process of analysis and diagnosis employed in non-cleft orthodontic treatment is carried out for these cleft palate cases. Moreover, in the diagnosis of cleft-related orthodontic problems the need for a thorough, organized approach is even more critical because of the numerous possible problems and etiologies, each requiring serious consideration. To this end the recent development of a "group classification system" for describing and rating malocclusions by Ackerman and Proffit,[1] with its accompanying recommended data base, provides just such a system. While other methods can be utilized with equal success, the Ackerman-Proffit system constitutes a convenient framework within which to describe the orthodontic problems most frequently encountered. Their data base plan is divided into three main segments: (A) patient history, (B) examination of the patient and the panoramic radiograph, and (C) systematic description of the occlusion and analysis of the orthodontic records. We shall present here the topical outline of each segment before discussing the elements in detail.

Data Base

Patient History

1. Medical-dental.
2. Social and behavioral.
3. Somatic growth, development, and maturation.
4. Genetic and family history.
5. Habits.

Medical-Dental. A well-kept, up-dated medical and dental history in these cleft patients is a necessity. (See chapter on Prosthodontic Care.) Of primary importance is the accurate description of the type and extent of cleft present at birth and a record of the timing and type of surgery performed to correct the defect. The former is relevant because of the well-established differences in growth patterns and dimensions between isolated cleft palate (CP), complete unilateral cleft lip and palate (UCLP), and complete bilateral cleft lip and palate (BCLP)[54, 65, 76, 88, 108, 144] (to be detailed later). Other useful correlations are the tendency for mandibular arch underdevelopment in the CP group[87, 108] and the variations in frequency of dental abnormalities depending on cleft type.[68, 72] Information regarding severity of the cleft and timing and type of surgery is necessary not only for estimating the probable severity of the resulting arch deformity but also for retrospective evaluation of the effects of various types of lip and palate repair on subsequent orthodontic management.

Since the frequency of anomalies associated with cleft lip and/or palate ranges from 10 to 25 per cent,[41] an accurate medical history also becomes a useful tool in picking up other abnormalities that may affect orthodontic treatment. Although the portion of that 10 to 25 per cent in which there is an actual bearing on orthodontic therapy is probably small, such things as mental retardation and neuromuscular or skeletal tissue anomalies can easily be recognized as potential complicating factors in achieving treatment objectives. All have been known to occur in association with facial clefting. (For an excellent summary table, see Gorlin and Pindborg.[41])

Additional facts in the medical and dental histories relevant to orthodontic therapy would include frequent upper respiratory infections, enlarged tonsils or adenoids, or other forms of nasal obstruction known to be common in cleft palate patients. Some of these conditions may predispose to mouth breathing or to abnormal tongue posture.

Finally, it is important to discover any medical or dental problems that may be unrelated to the cleft itself but which may influence orthodontic treatment.[1] Items such as phenytoin (Dilantin)-related gingival hyperplasia in an epileptic patient, or trauma to teeth or jaws resulting in fracture, devitalization, pathological resorption, and so forth must all be given the same consideration as in the non-cleft patient.

Social and Behavioral. Although recent improvements in total cleft palate rehabilitation by integrated teams of specialists have avoided or greatly alleviated any psychosocial adjustment problems these patients may have had as a result of their clefts, it is not uncommon to find several behavioral characteristics that must be taken into account in orthodontic treatment planning. A long history of surgical, dental, and speech appointments may be coupled with the actual oral discomfort of repeated surgical procedures, appliances, and oral examinations. There may be embarrassment over unattractive facial or dental appearance. These factors not infrequently place patients in a category of low "dental appreciation." While some studies have shown no significant increases in caries indices for cleft patients,[81] common clinical impressions[144] would substantiate that this low dental appreciation often manifests itself as extremely poor oral hygiene and a poor prognosis for cooperation in maintaining a clean mouth during orthodontic therapy. Even with a positive dental attitude, proper oral hygiene often becomes a difficult task because of extremely malposed teeth.

Of equal concern is the prognosis for patient cooperation throughout a prolonged, extended period of treatment. The familiar orthodontic colloquialism of "burning out" such cooperation over extended treatment time becomes a very real problem in the cleft patient whose cumulative treatment history starts from birth and includes the sum total of all his cleft-related appointments. In general, sufficient cooperation can be elicited in the cleft patient to carry out most orthodontic procedures, but the orthodontist must be alert to the aforementioned possibility and must be willing to adjust the treatment plan accordingly.

Somatic Growth, Development, and Maturation. A growth assessment of the cleft patient can generally be obtained by a combination of clinical evaluation, serial height/weight data, dental age, and skeletal age using hand/wrist films, if necessary. In addition to recording information about age, sex, and race, several other pertinent points of information are necessary. With the opportunity to collect serial height/weight data, important information is available to the orthodontist for evaluating skeletal maturation, especially with regard to adolescent-age treatment. On the average, we have found that children with a cleft do not differ significantly from non-cleft children in their height and weight, although there may be a slight lag in infancy (perhaps related to surgical trauma or initial feeding

MALES

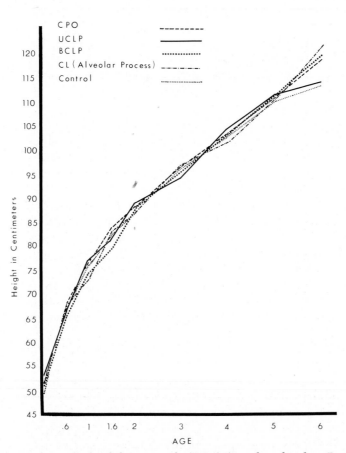

FIGURE 7–4 Height graphs for cleft vs. normal—(B-6:0). (Based on data from Ranalli, D., and Mazaheri, M: Height-weight growth of cleft children birth to six years. Cleft Palate J., *12*:400–404, 1975.)

Illustration continued on opposite page

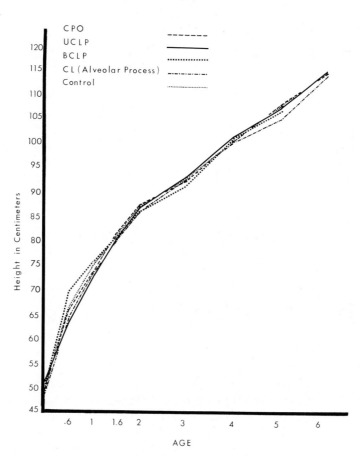

FIGURE 7–4 *Continued.*

problems), which is eliminated in early childhood by "catch up" growth[127] (Figure 7–4). This, however, may vary in other cleft palate clinics, depending on the care provided, with a resultant tendency toward smaller stature.[144] Whatever the case, different cleft types do not seem to differ from one another in height/weight growth,[127] and thus it cannot be generally considered as representing a significant factor in cleft malocclusions.

With regard to skeletal maturation as determined by hand/wrist films, there appears to be a tendency for cleft patients to exhibit lower skeletal ages[91] than the established normals,[47] indicating the possibility of a delayed maturation. This trend seems to be most marked in those with complete bilateral and unilateral clefts of the lip and palate, and it should be kept in mind when planning treatment around specific growth/time intervals. Finally, while data on dental age of the cleft population are inconclusive, most clinical impressions from this and other[107, 108, 144] centers indicate the frequent occurrence of delayed dental development and retarded eruption. Such aspects must be considered in terms of possible serial extraction, initiation of active treatment, and so forth. These matters are discussed in more detail in the chapter on Craniofacial Growth.

Genetic and Family History. The importance of this portion of the data base to cleft palate orthodontic diagnosis lies not in an attempt to determine a possible genetic role in the clefting itself nor in a desire to offer genetic counseling to the family. These aspects fall under the purview of the team geneticist and family counselor. (See chapter on Genetics.) Rather, the pertinent information required here relates to any hereditary pattern that may exist in facial morphology or growth trend. As detailed previously, the concept of a cleft superimposed upon an underlying skeletal growth pattern that may vary from Class I to Class II to Class III, as in the non-cleft population, carries with it certain implications for orthodontic treatment planning. The orthodontist, by a study of the family history, can utilize knowledge of the inherited facial growth pattern in his management of cleft-related problems.

For example, the positive family history frequently seen in Class III-growers would be an essential guide early in the treatment planning stages of a cleft patient with associated maxillary sagittal hypoplasia. Such a combination would require immediate attention and extraordinary corrective efforts (e.g., extraoral chin cap traction or orthognathic surgery) and would probably alter other plans for dento-alveolar masking of the skeletal dysplasia. A history of skeletal Class II pattern with the same cleft-related maxillary hypoplasia would, however, provide skeletal bases more compatible with a purely orthodontic correction. In either case, thorough treatment planning calls for as accurate a determination of these approaches as is possible.

Habits. The role of habits in the etiology of malocclusions in the cleft population is not significantly different from that in the non-cleft population (Figure 7–5). The main concern is that since the normal dento-alveolar growth and adjustment mechanisms appear to be already compromised by cleft-related problems, these oral habits may more severely aggravate the situation than would otherwise be the case. Thus, while tongue-thrust should generally not be considered an etiological factor in malocclusion until after puberty,[119] its pre-pubertal occurrence in cleft patients with

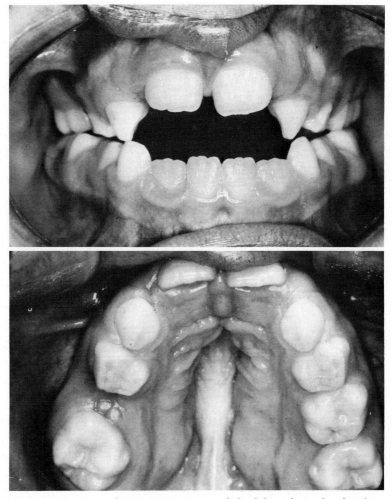

FIGURE 7–5   Anterior open bite in postoperative cleft of the palate related to finger-sucking habit.

disturbed vertical dento-alveolar development not only may be increased by this cleft-related dysplasia but may in turn worsen the vertical under-development. Consequently, the "habit" of a *normal* developmental stage becomes, in the cleft population, a potentially serious problem demanding early orthodontic intervention. A similar case could be made for orthodontic consideration of finger- or thumb-sucking habits or of prolonged use of pacifiers by these patients.

Clinical and Panoramic Radiograph Examinations

This segment deals with the actual detailed clinical examination of the patient, utilizing a single panoramic radiograph to aid in determining the status of unerupted dental units and their bony support. We shall describe the examination under the following four subheadings:

1. Facial esthetics.

2. Intra-oral soft tissue.

3. Muscle balance and function.

4. Dental structures.

Facial Esthetics. The evaluation of the head and face of the cleft palate patient is often a useful means of acquiring a preliminary idea of the structural basis of the presenting malocclusion. In clefts of the palate only, with no involvement of the lip or alveolar process, the facial esthetics are usually close to normal. Lip thickness and contours, being unaltered by the cleft, appear normal. There is the possibility, however, with an extensively scarred palate, that a slight generalized maxillary underdevelopment may result,[66] leading to a straight or mildly concave mid-facial profile. While only marginally noticeable during childhood, continued growth of the mandible and nose will be inclined to worsen this tendency. Also, with the frequent association of isolated cleft palate with mandibular hypoplasia, as in Pierre Robin syndrome,[41] the opposite facial esthetics may result. While this problem seems to improve with age,[87, 144] it may be of sufficient severity to alter or compromise treatment objectives. Other potential problems, such as asymmetrical facial balance or deviations between the dental and facial midlines, are generally unremarkable in the isolated cleft population.

Complete cleft of the lip and palate, on the other hand, with involvement of lip, nose, and premaxilla, usually presents significant facial esthetic deviations. While evaluation of the appearance of the lip and nose repairs themselves do not fall under the purview of orthodontic treatment planning per se, the esthetic effects of altered tooth position on those soft tissue structures do warrant consideration. (Further discussion of this subject will be found in the chapters on Surgery and Prosthodontic Care.)

In both unilateral (UCLP) and bilateral (BCLP) clefts, the forward rotation and/or positioning of the premaxillary segment at birth manifests itself as a somewhat protrusive midface in early childhood. This effect seems to be more prominent in severe bilateral cases. With the continued molding action of lip repair, however,[86, 87, 121] this tendency is reduced, and with further growth of surrounding tissues, coupled with more potentially severe maxillary growth deficits than were evident in isolated cleft palate, the lower facial esthetics tend to straighten and frequently become concave (Figure 7–6). This trend is not as prominent in unilateral cases.[47]

In bilateral cases, further frequent findings are a tethered nasal tip with less forward projection, a thin upper lip and protrusive lower lip, and a generally retrusive soft tissue profile.[52] However, the frequent problems with mid-facial asymmetry in the unilateral patient are less frequent in these bilateral cases. Finally, although maxillary vertical *underdevelopment* is a commonly recognized problem,[56, 65, 66, 108, 118, 144] excessively *long* lower face height when evaluated *in repose* is a common facial esthetic finding among these more severe cleft types.[56, 65, 76] Presumably the result of a mandibular postural adjustment for lowered tongue posture[89, 129] caused by either a constricted, scarred, obliterated palatal vault[55, 145, 157] or a mouth-breathing pattern resulting from a collapsed nasal cavity[144, 160] or enlarged adenoidal masses,[10, 128] this finding emphasizes the need for evaluating these patients in occlusion and in repose[144] (Figure 7–7).

Intra-oral Soft Tissue. The most important consideration here, in the

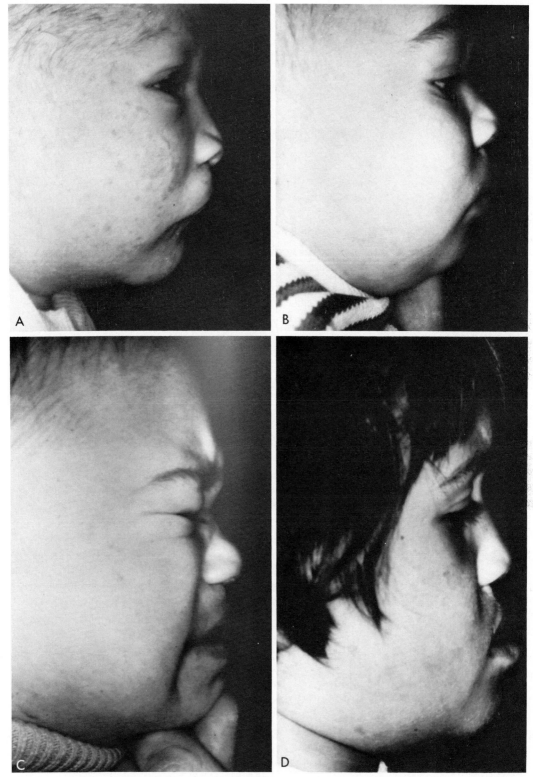

FIGURE 7–6   Profile changes in unilateral cleft of the lip and palate showing (A) initial protrusive maxilla (0:6 year) and (B) convex profile (1:0 year) changing to (C) a relatively straight profile (2:0 years) and then to (D) a concave profile (6:0 years) with growth.

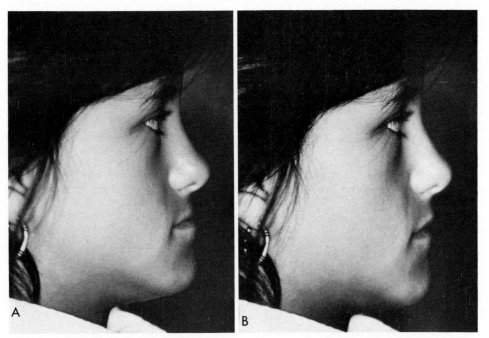

FIGURE 7-7   Profile of patient with same pseudoprognathic face in (A) centric occlusion and (B) same patient in repose.

cleft population, is an estimate of the extent, location, and severity of palatal and alveolar scarring, a subject to be discussed in detail in the chapter on Surgery. While at present there exists no reliable, objective means to quantify this scarring, clinical evaluation can frequently provide a clue as to the possible response of a palate to expansion, the degree of retention required afterward, the impediments to tooth movement, and the possible cause of altered tongue posture, all affecting reasonable treatment objectives. In addition, as in non-cleft diagnosis, careful assessment must be given to soft tissues potentially leading to altered mandibular posture or function. Thus, hypertrophy of tonsils and adenoids as a result of frequent upper respiratory infections seen in cleft children may force a mouth-breathing pattern, with its concomitant alterations in tongue position and mandibular posture.[10, 128] In relation to this, careful thought must also be given to soft palate form and function, inasmuch as hypertrophy of lymphatic tissues may nonetheless be vital to the patient in achieving adequate velopharyngeal closure. A third soft tissue component of the cleft condition involves possible abnormal or scarred frenal attachments, especially in the area of the cleft in UCLP and BCLP. Frequently the labial vestibule is shallow or obliterated and may affect the configuration of any appliance contemplated (i.e., long vertical loops in the archwire would be contraindicated). Careful attention must also be paid to monitoring gingival signs of developing periodontal disease related to poor oral hygiene. This is especially important in the line of the cleft, where abnormal tooth position may make proper home care impossible.

Muscle Balance and Function.   Of all the details of the clinical examination of the cleft palate patient, an analysis of function of the oral structures is most important. Of prime concern to the cleft palate orthodontist is the diagnosis and interception of developing functional problems, from early childhood through stabilization of the adult dentition. The very frequent occurrence of severely malposed teeth, dental anomalies, and skeletal dysplasias predisposes the cleft patient to a myriad of functional alterations in terms of mandibular closure, tongue function, and respiratory patterns.

The problems of mouth-breathing and tongue function and posture have already been mentioned. Other frequently occurring functional problems include lateral deviations of the mandible in closure caused by mild bilateral maxillary constriction of the deciduous or permanent dentition. This creates a cuspal interference with full centric occlusion in the centric relation position. To compensate, the patient may shift his jaw laterally to achieve maximum intercuspation, but in doing so he produces the clinical appearance of a unilateral crossbite in centric occlusion[144] (Figure 7–8). This is

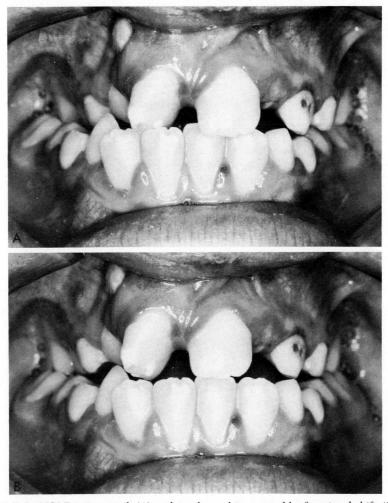

FIGURE 7–8   UCLP patient with (A) unilateral crossbite created by functional shift. (B) Same patient in centric relation exhibiting mild bilateral maxillary constriction.

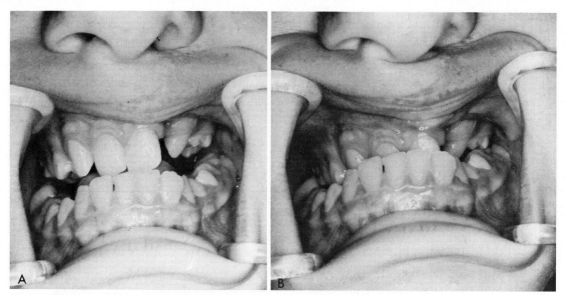

FIGURE 7–9 (A) Centric relation and (B) Centric occlusion of a UCLP patient with a pseudo class III relationship and a negative overjet due to a functional shift forward.

most frequently seen in CP and BCLP populations and must be differentiated from the true unilateral posterior crossbites seen in UCLP patients on the side of the cleft.

Also often observed in early mixed dentition of cleft patients, especially UCLP and BCLP cases, is an anterior functional shift of the mandible because of incisal interference with full intercuspation. The frequent lingual eruption and inclination of the maxillary permanent incisors, coupled with the aforementioned maxillary underdevelopment, create the need for this shift, resulting in a pseudoprognathism and negative overjet incisal relationship (Figure 7–9).

Further common functional problems in cleft cases with lip involvement center around problems of lip muscle tonus and function. The relationship of lip pressure to tooth position has been defined for the non-cleft population,[9, 120] and the significance of this aspect in cleft cases with free premaxillae or otherwise discontinuous alveolar ridges has been mentioned previously.

The problems just mentioned represent only the most frequent functional difficulties in the cleft population and should not be considered all-inclusive. Constant attention must be paid to function throughout all age groups, with careful differentiation of rest positions, centric relation, and centric occlusion. Regardless of the exact nature of the functional deviation, the need to detect and intercept these problems as soon as they become manifest, in order to prevent additional compensatory growth adjustments, is widely recognized.[24, 35, 66, 107, 110, 123, 143, 144, 157, 158, 160]

Dental Structures. Clinical and panoramic radiographic findings in reference to dental morphology and tooth number assume additional significance for the cleft patient because of the well-known increase in incidence of dental abnormalities in the cleft population.[68, 72] To cite spe-

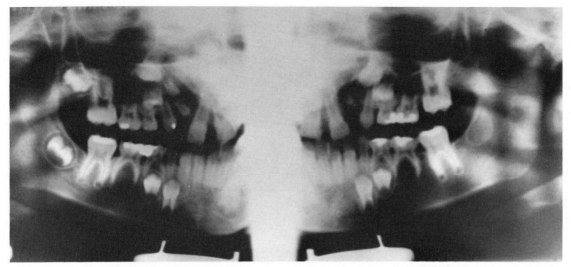

FIGURE 7-10 Panoramic radiograph of patient with BCLP. Note the calcification anomalies of the maxillary central incisors, the supernumeraries in the line of cleft, and the congenitally missing second premolars and lateral incisors.

cific examples, the common occurrence of supernumerary primary teeth in the vicinity of the cleft, as well as a high incidence of congenitally missing permanent maxillary lateral incisors and maxillary and mandibular second bicuspids (Figure 7-10), needs to be accurately determined prior to treatment planning because of the possible effect of these findings on normal exfoliation and eruption of teeth and on extraction decisions. (More details concerning anomalies may be found in the chapter on Prosthodontic Care.)

Hypoplasia, hypocalcification, and other morphological irregularities are also frequently present, especially in central incisors of BCLP patients and in bicuspids in all cleft types. Long-range treatment planning must take these into consideration, particularly with respect to extraction decisions and eventual prosthodontic contributions. Of special importance is the common occurrence of these abnormalities even in cases not involving the alveolar ridge, and in the mandibular dentition as well.[72]

As with all orthodontic patients, those with cleft palate must be closely monitored to detect and control caries and thus prevent needless loss of teeth. Such senseless consequences of hygienic neglect may seriously compromise orthodontic objectives. For example, maxillary arches that are already underdeveloped because of the cleft may suffer a further decrease in usable arch length if deciduous molars are lost prematurely. Caries may also lead to further loss of permanent tooth structure in jaws already marked by multiple congenitally missing teeth.

Analysis of Diagnostic Records

Prior to itemizing the most often seen cleft problems in the diagnostic records, it is important for the orthodontist to understand the basic dentoalveolar and craniofacial developmental potential in the cleft condition that is *not* influenced by external intervention. This is to enable him to differentiate, in handling the *postoperative* case load, between those growth-related problems inherent to the cleft condition itself and those developing as untoward results of therapeutic measures.

In general, all children with clefts appear to be born with varying degrees of lateral displacement and distortion of parts,[3, 26, 87, 142, 157, 159] presumably caused by abnormal muscle pull or cartilage-mediated development. They also have varying degrees of tissue deficiency.[26, 125, 157] If left untreated, these children seem capable of achieving reasonably normal skeletal and dental relationships at adulthood.[7, 64, 92, 112, 113] Whether this indeed represents "normal" craniofacial growth or is rather the result of uncompromised compensatory mechanisms of growth is a moot point. What is important for the orthodontist is to realize that many of the orthodontic problems arising in the cleft population, at least as far as present day techniques are concerned, are the result of the treatment rather than the defect itself, as Graber pointed out in 1949.[43]

Specific examples and exceptions to this should be noted. First, it appears that isolated clefts of the palate, with an intact alveolar ridge, have the best chance for achieving normal, stable adult craniofacial and occlusal dimensions and relations.[64, 92] Second, in clefts involving the alveolar ridge (UCLP and BCLP), the adult occlusion tends to be normal in all dimensions, with the exception of minor collapse or rotation of the free end of the lateral cleft segment or segments that lead to a one- or two-tooth crossbite in the area of the cleft. This same localized site may similarly be slightly underdeveloped vertically, resulting in lateral open bite in the cleft area.[64] Finally, in cases of BCLP, the premaxilla tends to maintain its anterior displacement, resulting in somewhat *convex* adult profiles.[112, 113] In no cases of these unoperated clefts is there evidence at maturity of generalized maxillary underdevelopment or collapse, either skeletal or dento-alveolar With these concepts in mind as a baseline for comparison, the following problems can be evaluated in the proper perspective as specifically related to their post-surgical development.

1. Intra-arch alignment and symmetry.
2. Profile/esthetics.
3. Transverse problems.
4. Anterior/posterior (sagittal) problems.
5. Vertical problems.

Intra-arch Alignment and Symmetry.   Figure 7–11 illustrates representative upper and lower arch forms at birth in UCLP, BCLP, and CPO. This is included to emphasize the point made previously about the unoperated condition and to serve as a baseline to observe subsequent development of arch form disturbances. The process of lip repair in UCLP and BCLP patients results in a generalized reduction in cleft width and maxillary arch width dimensions and begins a gradual process of reshaping the distorted arches:[3, 4, 54, 86, 121, 124, 129, 143, 158, 160] The same effect is continued, though to a lesser degree, by palatoplasty,[3, 54, 86, 87, 124, 129] and although the interim maxillary arch growth rates are near normal,[54, 86, 87] they are superimposed on the lags associated with cheiloplasty and palatoplasty. The degree to which this segment alignment continues is at present unpredictable,[3, 124] and by the time the deciduous dentition erupts, about 50 per cent of the maxillary arches in UCLP and BCLP show varying degrees of asymmetry, especially

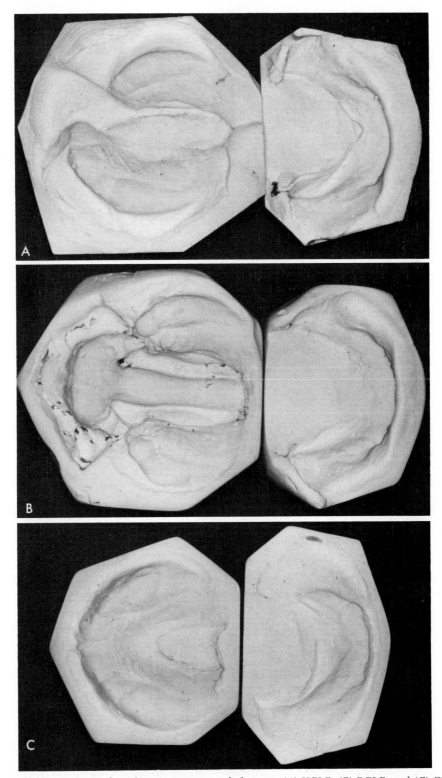

FIGURE 7–11 Examples of representative arch forms in (*A*) UCLP, (*B*) BCLP, and (*C*) CPO patients, prior to surgical intervention.

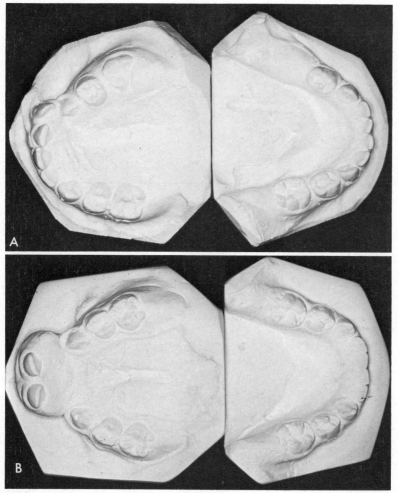

FIGURE 7-12   Arch forms of (A) UCLP and (B) BCLP patients at the primary dentition stage. Note the slight medial collapse of the lateral segment(s).

related to the site of the cleft.[3, 54, 86, 87, 124] Characteristically, this is limited to some degree of medial displacement of the lateral segment or segments. Except for the segmental collapse at this early age, the dental alignment, on the whole, tends to be fairly unremarkable. Minor rotations or other malpositions of primary cuspids or lateral incisors in the cleft site are the only additional findings. In general, isolated CP cases seem not to show these problems at this stage (Figure 7-12), and even with the potential deviations just outlined, the deciduous dentition in all cleft types appears to be less adversely affected than at later stages.

It is with the eruption of the permanent dentition that the majority of intra-arch malalignments appear. Using contemporary surgical procedures, the basal maxillary segments themselves seem to show no increase in the amount of collapse with further growth. But when there is superimposed upon the initial deviations previously mentioned the additional problem of distortion in the eruption of the developing permanent dentition, a worsening intra-arch situation is created. This is most apt to be the result of a continuum of scar tissue across the palate, incorporating the supracrestal periodontal fibers,[142–144] and this can result in severe lingual inclination of both posterior and anterior permanent teeth. This accentuates any pre-existing arch asymmetries (especially in UCLP and BCLP), and the consequent reduced arch perimeter tends to lead to more crowding problems than would have been indicated by examination of the primary dentition.[66] This crowding is, in turn, further aggravated by loss of usable alveolar arch length because of the cleft ridge. As with the non-cleft crowded dentition, the teeth most severely involved in this alignment problem are those erupting into the arch last. Thus, the cleft patient frequently exhibits second bicuspids in severe linguo-version, creating the typical "hourglass" collapse and permanent cuspids impacted high in the cleft (Figure 7–13).

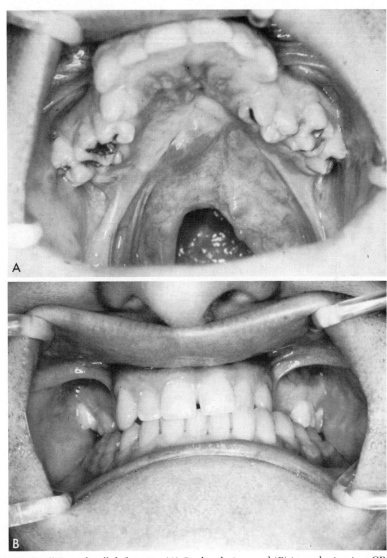

FIGURE 7–13 "Hourglass" deformity: (A) Occlusal view and (B) in occlusion in a CPO patient with bicuspids positioned lingually and a continuum of scar tissue across palate.

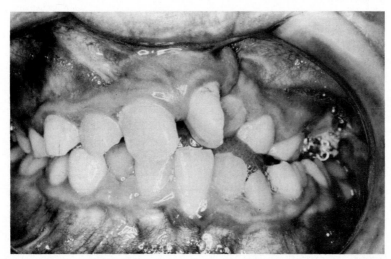

FIGURE 7–14   Severe rotation of the permanent incisor adjacent to the cleft in a UCLP patient. Such rotations with and without severe lingual inclination are a common sequela in clefts involving the alveolar ridge.

Severe rotations of permanent incisors are extremely common when clefts involve the alveolar ridge (Figure 7–14). This, coupled with the occasionally severe lingual inclination, especially in BCLP cases, results in an increasing distortion of arch form and alignment in the permanent dentition. It should also be noted that while the arch problems just mentioned are the ones commonly presented by the cleft population, improved surgical techniques and care for these patients are reducing the severity and extent of these deviations.

As far as mandibular arch symmetry and alignment are concerned, there seems to be no significant difference between the problems of the cleft and the non-cleft populations, with the exception, of course, of the hypoplastic mandibles associated with isolated CP in Pierre Robin syndrome. The only recurring developments worthy of special mention are an apparent tendency for the mandibular dento-alveolar complex to show compensatory adjustments to the maxillary arch deviations described heretofore.[163] Thus, severely lingually inclined mandibular buccal teeth are frequently noticed in cases of serious maxillary constriction, unilaterally and asymmetrically, as the case may be.

Profile/Esthetics.   These considerations of the diagnostic records closely coincide with those mentioned previously under the section on Clinical Evaluation; they need not be covered again.

Transverse Problems.   Skeletally, all cleft infants start life with excessive maxillary width dimensions. The greatest maxillary width occurs in the child with bilateral cleft lip and palate (BCLP), with decreasing degrees of severity usually seen in children with unilateral cleft lip and palate, isolated cleft palate, and down to the normal child. The situation can be expressed as follows: BCLP>UCLP>CP>normal. The situation undergoes the changes already described following lip and palate repair, however, so that by the time of the full deciduous dentition the maxillae have rotated medially and the maxillary width dimensions among these children are reversed, with the

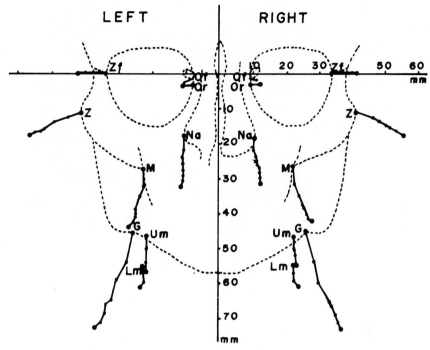

FIGURE 7–15   Posterior-anterior composite of growth direction from birth to 6:0 years in UCLP patient. Midline structures are essentially downward with the midface vertical and slightly lateral. Note that on affected (left) side vertical component predominates, leading to molar crossbite. In the mandible the main thrust of growth is vertical, with a lateral component. (From Ishiguro et al., Cleft Palate J., *13*:104–126, 1976.)

BCLP the narrowest, as follows: BCLP<UCLP<CP = normal.[65] While this tendency is usually responsible for only mild crossbites in the deciduous dentition of UCLP and BCLP patients, and very few at that, the subsequent skeletal growth pattern predisposes to more severe transverse problems. Specifically, a purely vertical growth direction, bilaterally in BCLP and on the affected side in UCLP (Figure 7–15) with no lateral component, as in normal,[65] means that although the maxillary breadth does not constrict further, it *does* become narrower relative to the mandible, as the latter continues to express its normal width potential. However small this may be, it does contribute to aggravating the transverse skeletal discrepancy with age. This growth pattern also implies that even if the upper arch is expanded by the orthodontist early in the primary dentition and is held in that position, its subsequent inability to keep pace with the mandibular growth in the lateral dimension will lead to a recurrence of the crossbite at a later time. Thus a re-expansion will invariably be necessary, not because of a progressive maxillary skeletal collapse but because of an incompatibility in growth direction.[6]

Dentally, the most commonly seen developments transversely are those described on page 374, in which posterior teeth eruption paths are deflected lingually.[142–144] This, in turn, carries with it two important consequences. First, in severely scarred cases, the dento-alveolar constriction compounds the skeletal dysplasia just outlined and can lead to full posterior crossbites (Fig-

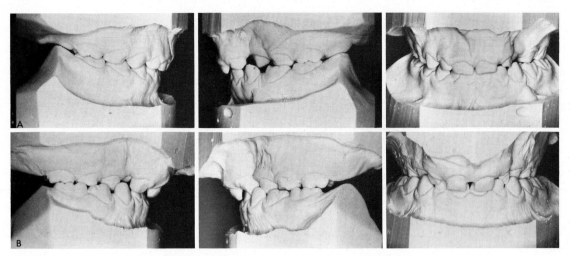

FIGURE 7–16   (A) Unilateral posterior crossbite in the primary dentition in the UCLP patient;
(B) bilateral posterior crossbite in the primary dentition.

ure 7–16) even in isolated CP patients with near-normal maxillary width.
Second, even mildly affected cases can sufficiently handicap the normal
dento-alveolar adjustment mechanism so that the developing skeletal
dysplasia cannot be compensated, thereby also resulting in progressively
more severe posterior crossbite.

Hence it can be easily realized that transverse problems in isolated CP
are usually more dentally related[27] and consequently appear less severe,
while UCLP and BCLP, with both skeletal and dental components, can be
potentially handicapping. It is also evident that if surgery is performed
judiciously and if the palatal scarring adjacent to the alveolar ridge is
minimized or eliminated, these cases should show increasingly well-com-
pensated marginal transverse skeletal discrepancies.

Anterior/Posterior (Sagittal) Problems.   The expected *skeletal* findings
in this dimension seem to follow those described for the transverse
dimension, at least in the first few postnatal years. Before describing them,
though, it is important to consider the great variability and uncertainty
injected into antero-posterior (a-p) skeletal evaluations by the gross displacement and distortions of those landmarks usually employed for determining
sagittal skeletal development and relations (i.e., ANS, A, PNS), especially in
UCLP and BCLP.[77] Thus, it must be remembered that it is possible to obtain
measures of tremendous maxillary protrusion (i.e., in a severe BCLP case) and
excessive maxillary length as measured from the most anterior point on the
premaxilla to the tuberosities, when, practically speaking, there is a
deficiency in useful maxillary a-p dimension. Thus, the reconciliation of a
skeletally "protrusive" maxilla, as measured on lateral cephs using SNA for
example, with a dental Class III relationship may often require consideration
of these components separately.

At birth, maxillary length and protrusion are such that BCLP>UCLP>CP
= normal,[54] primarily because of the aforementioned premaxillary displacement in the first two cases (see Figure 7–11). Cheiloplasty then begins a

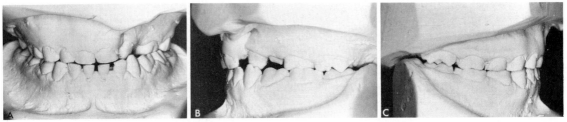

FIGURE 7–17 (A) Frontal view of patient with UCLP: exhibiting (B) class III molar relationship on the side of the cleft and (C) edge-to-edge molar relationship on the nonaffected side.

reduction and remolding of the deformity in UCLP and BCLP and seems concomitantly to produce a temporary lag in antero-posterior growth rates.[54, 83] Although this rate seems to accelerate again shortly thereafter, the combination of lag and remodeling produces maxillary a-p dimension and position, such that BCLP>UCLP = CP = normal.[54, 87] This same trend is continued following palate repair, so that at the time of the primary dentition BCLP> normal≥UCLP≥CP.[54, 87] While this generalization probably varies greatly from population to population[56, 76] and the tremendous midfacial hypoplasias of years past[43] have been much alleviated by improved surgical techniques that minimize trauma to the nasal septum and circumoral soft tissues, substantial a-p orthodontic problems are still occasionally seen in the primary dentition stage. Of these, Class III molar relationships, especially on the affected side in UCLP[101] (Figure 7–17), and anterior crossbite[163] are corresponding *dental* symptoms of greatest concern to the orthodontist. It has been suggested that the main problem at this stage is a retroposition of the maxillary buccal segment,[101] perhaps as a result of the scar-mediated "maxillary ankylosis" as proposed by Ross.[142] This seems entirely reasonable in light of the fact that most measurements of maxillary excess or protrusion seem to be directly related to cases with premaxillary involvement,[14, 54, 76] while those using premaxillae not involved in the cleft (i.e., CP) show the true nature of the retrusion.[76] Paradoxically, however, the incidence of anterior crossbite in the primary dentition seems to occur equally as often, if not more so, in UCLP (20 to 40 per cent) than in the other types of clefting[53, 101, 163] (Figure 7–18). This can be most easily explained by calling on the aforementioned (see page 380) scar continuum from palate to supracrestal fibers adjacent to the teeth,[142-144] deflecting the anterior teeth lingually in their eruption.[53] Also contributing to this loss of normal labial eruptive development could be a tight or unyielding lip repair.

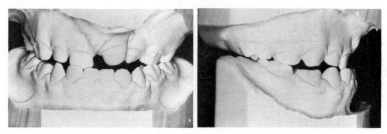

FIGURE 7–18 A UCLP case in the primary dentition exhibiting anterior crossbite.

Using these premises, two further deductions can then be made. First, it is to be expected that this lingual inclination will be more severe in those cases requiring surgical repair of clefts involving the premaxilla (UCLP and BCLP). Of these, the one being least protrusive to start (UCLP) would be the one most severely affected by a retruded dental eruption pattern of the anterior teeth. Further, since CP, with unaffected anterior dento-alveolar adjustment mechanisms, seems able to compensate for the developing "maxillary ankylosis" and BCLP, with the greatest initial premaxillary protrusion, can mask the ankylosis even without dental compensation, both of these types show correspondingly fewer anterior crossbites in the primary dentition.

The second logical consequence of this appraisal is that, as with the transverse problems, the antero-posterior discrepancies tend to worsen with age.[6, 142] The a-p maxillary growth pattern has little or no anterior component (any evident forward component probably being a function of premaxillary involvement).[54, 76, 88] The situation is compounded by the normal anterior expression of mandibular growth and a more severe lingual-deflection effect on the permanent incisors.[6, 143] All this presents a problem of progressing severity through the pubertal growth spurt, and it has been labeled as the major growth challenge facing the cleft palate orthodontist.[142]

That these antero-posterior discrepancies should continue to worsen through the mixed and early permanent dentition can be explained for the

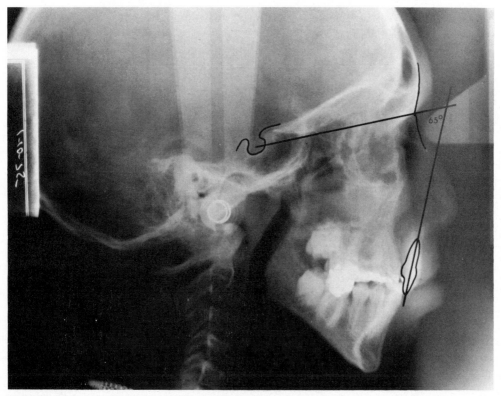

FIGURE 7-19   Maxillary incisor to SN angle of 65° seen in BCLP patients — the result of deflection of permanent incisors and tipping of premaxilla as a whole.

most part by the fact that the *dento-alveolar* development of the permanent dentition adds increasingly to the underlying *skeletal* dysplasia. Upper permanent incisor to sella-nasion angles of 70° to 80° (normal 103° to 106°) (Figure 7–19), seen especially often in BCLP cases, can certainly lead to a significant increase in the amount of anterior crossbite in the mixed and permanent dentition[6, 107–110] (Figure 7–20), especially when superimposed on a skeletal retrognathism. The overjet relationship of the primary anteriors seems to have little control over this subsequent development.

Due consideration must be given to adjacent skeletal structures, since maxillary retrusion is only *relative* to the *surrounding* bones. Although the influence of the cleft on the cranial base has not been agreed upon,[30, 76, 141] it would appear that, in general, the cranial base itself has little or no significance in the analysis or treatment of cleft palate orthodontic problems. On the other hand, mandibular growth and posture are intimately involved. While most linear dimensions of the mandible tend to be normal in all types of clefts,[56] at least during childhood, the mandible in rest position is frequently measured as being retrusive relative to the cranial base, (i.e., lower SNB angles). This seems to arise as a result of a measurably increased gonial angle in all forms of clefting,[56, 76] presumably the result of the postural problems of the tongue outlined on page 376. While there may be a tendency for mandibular underdevelopment in some older cleft populations,[56] this would not appear to be a consistent enough finding to warrant consideration.

What must be given constant consideration, however, is the position of the mandible at the time of record-taking.[144] The aforementioned postural and morphological adjustments, dropping the mandible down and concomitantly back, may mask a maxillary hypoplasia by producing a generalized retrusive

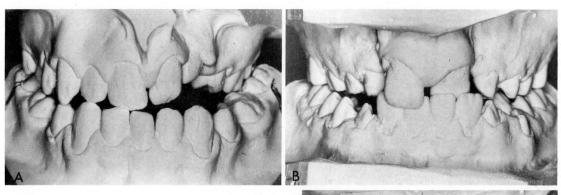

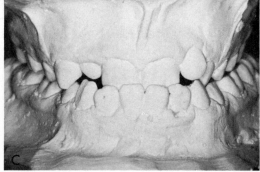

FIGURE 7–20 Examples of anterior crossbites in the permanent dentition of (A) UCLP, (B) BCLP and (C) CPO patients.

profile[52] relative to the cranial base, with close-to-normal ANB values. On the other hand, problems in maxillary *vertical* development (to be described later) may lead to a mandibular overclosure in maximum intercuspation, swinging the mandible up and forward, and thereby producing antero-posterior discrepancies (as revealed by ANB or facial convexity angles) of greater magnitude than exist in actuality. Since this change is itself the consequence of a dysplasia in another dimension, the rest position of the mandible is probably the most important baseline from which the orthodontist should analyze these antero-posterior problems.[144]

Vertical Problems. *Skeletal* problems facing the cleft palate orthodontist analyzing this third plane of space seem in general to follow the trends seen in the transverse and antero-posterior dimensions. Tremendous variability is injected into determinations of vertical development by the distortion, inconsistency, and potentially unrelated behavior of the standard landmark points (A, ANS, PNS) to the surrounding skeletal elements with which the maxilla is to be related.[77] Thus, overall clinical judgment must on occasion be employed to discern when an increased upper anterior facial height reading in BCLP (i.e., Na-ANS or A) is, practically speaking, a true skeletal vertical excess or is rather a function of a downward and backward rotational displacement of the free premaxillary segment following lip and palate surgery. Likewise, the postural variations of the mandible in these cleft cases (see page 378) may generate excessively long *or* short total anterior face heights, depending on the position of the mandible when evaluated (Figure 7–21).

Nonetheless with these considerations fully weighed, a general characterization of the development of vertical orthodontic problems in the cleft patient is possible. Of all the discrepancies of growth in the cleft patient, vertical dysplasias tend to become manifest at a much later time in the patient's development. The excess vertical maxillary skeletal measurements seen in the first few years of life would appear to be a genuine developmental hyperplasia, and not the result of the previously described premaxillary rotation. The latter possibility can be ruled out because the greatest discrepancy seen at this age is in CP cases with no such premaxillary involvement.[65] Near-normal vertical growth increments during the primary dentition[76] also support the clinical finding of no significant vertical component to these early cleft malocclusions.

It seems that vertical contributions to the fully expressed cleft palate orthodontic problem arise during development of the mixed dentition. The typical finding at this age is a progressively decreasing rate of maxillary vertical development, so that during the mixed dentition years, the patient changes from the initial excess facial height characteristic of earlier years to significantly deficient vertical dimensions by the time of the early permanent dentition.[56, 88] Further, UCLP and BCLP show the additional effects of the premaxillary involvement and increased severity of down-and-back premaxillary rotation. In BCLP, for example, the isolated premaxilla appears to be largely alveolar bone and consequently the lingually deflected eruption of permanent incisors (see page 382) results in a deflected premaxilla, A point, and ANS. As a result, the palatal plane in these cases shows a definite cant, with less vertical development posteriorly and tipped down anteriorly[56, 88] (Figure 7–22).

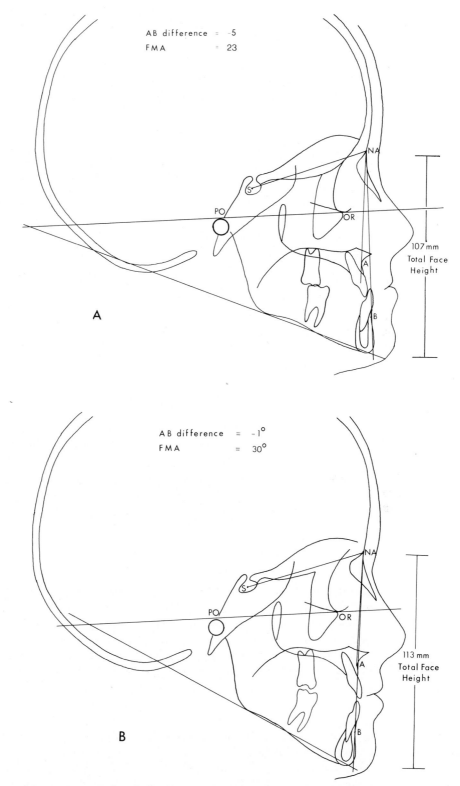

AB difference = -5
FMA = 23

107 mm
Total Face
Height

A

AB difference = -1°
FMA = 30°

113 mm
Total Face
Height

B

FIGURE 7–21   Lateral cephalometric tracing in (A) full occlusion and (B) rest position illustrating changes in SNB, ANB, and FMA angles and in anterior facial height.

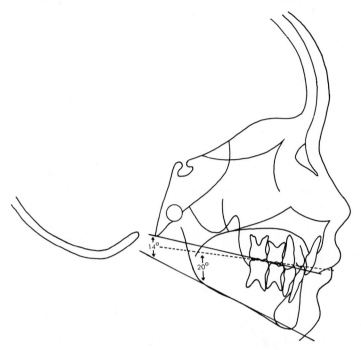

Figure 7–22. Lateral cephalometric tracing of BCLP patient with the cant of the occlusal plane caused by a tipped-down premaxilla. Occlusal plane taken as a line running through the bisection of the molars and the bisection of the central incisors (solid line) and occlusal plane taken as the plane of buccal occlusion (dotted line).

Another interesting paradox in cleft palate orthodontics is that in spite of this developing maxillary vertical hypoplasia, the total face height, *in repose*, is often found to be *normal* or *excessive*.[56] This can be most directly related to an increase in lower anterior face height as a result of the altered mandibular posture and the associated increase in the gonial angle, described earlier (see Figure 7–21).

Whatever the etiology of the postural change may be (see page 374), the resultant lower tongue position,[89] down-and-back mandibular rotation, and deficient vertical development of the upper jaw result in the aforesaid total face height dimensions, as well as an excessive freeway space.[145] Normally, the dento-alveolar complex would compensate for this. Once again, however, as was evident in the other dimensional problems, this crucial normalizing influence seems to be disturbed, thus aggravating the basic vertical skeletal dysplasia. Whether the impeded vertical eruption[118] is due mainly to the interposition of the altered tongue posture between the dental arches[129, 144] or is related to the alveolar scarring hypothesized by Ross[142–145] to account for transverse and a-p dento-alveolar distortion is not easily discernible. However, the final result and its ramifications are readily visible and represent the most common vertical problem facing the orthodontist.

Several additional vertical discrepancies often appear that, although of a more localized nature, must nonetheless be analyzed and treated appropriately by the team orthodontist. Since the maxillary problems are obviously most severe and consequently require the most careful analysis, it is frequently forgotten that there are also mandibular components of most of the cleft palate malocclusions. The major skeletal alteration has been mentioned. The dento-alveolar changes that take place do so because this adjustment mechanism in the lower jaw, unaffected by scarring, can partially adapt to deviations in the vertical development of the antagonistic maxillary arch. Thus, the finding of excess vertical dento-alveolar development in the lower arch[118, 163] is not an infrequent one, especially with focal exacerbations in the area opposite the alveolar cleft site in UCLP and BCLP.

Finally, mention should be made of one more annoying dento-alveolar vertical problem that is often difficult to correct, namely, the local disturbances in the vertical eruption of teeth adjacent to a cleft involving the alveolar ridge (especially permanent cuspids and laterals). These are seen in unoperated cleft populations (see page 380) and also are invariably evident in operated cleft populations. This eruption disturbance may be compounded by the effects of arch crowding, but its presence in operated as well as unoperated cases suggests that it may be a characteristic of the defect itself, and not the result of the surgical intervention. In either case, this problem tends to resist treatment, probably as the result of a basic insufficiency of stable bony support upon and through which the teeth can erupt. An especially extreme variation of this disturbance is seen in cases of BCLP in which the combination of deficient vertical eruption of the teeth distal to the cleft and normal but deflected eruption of the incisors in the downwardly rotated premaxilla causes a significant vertical discrepancy within the maxillary occlusal plane (Figure 7–23). Again, this vertical "step" at the cleft requires substantial effort to correct.

All of the disturbances just detailed, while contributing to the total malocclusion in their own right, can also interact in various ways to either aggravate or alleviate the total malocclusion. The Ackerman/Proffit group classification system[1] very nicely accommodates just such a description, and the schematic interconnecting Venn diagrams of that system certainly serve to stimulate such a unified three-dimensional analysis.

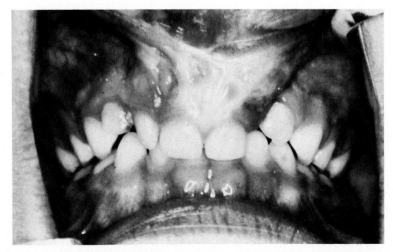

FIGURE 7–23   Occlusal plane with a severe step from the tipped-down premaxilla to the lateral segment in patient with BCLP.

The nidus around which these three-dimensional interactions most closely revolve is the gradually developing vertical problem. The antero-posterior and transverse consequences of a decrease or loss of vertical dimension, as seen by the prosthodontist in edentulous mouths, for example, are well known. Analogous consequences are exhibited by the cleft palate patient with varying degrees of vertical maxillary hypoplasia. The resulting overclosure of the mandible to occlusal contact tends to rotate "B" point and Pogonion forward (see Figure 7–21). The concomitant increase of SNB and facial convexity angles and decrease in ANB difference (even frequently becoming negative) all serve to describe this vertically induced change toward a relative mandibular prognathism. If this trend is superimposed on the maxillary antero-posterior deficiency usually evident in the cleft patient as described heretofore, a more severe Class III skeletal and/or dental problem is produced, the profile becomes more concave, and the cleft-related midfacial hypoplasia is accentuated.

An opposite antero-posterior ramification of this vertical dysplasia relates to the lowered tongue and mandible posture in *rest* position and the increase of the mandibular gonial angle. The downward and backward mandibular

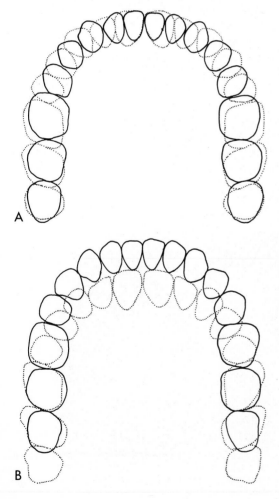

FIGURE 7–24 Superimposition of a maxillary arch (dotted line) over a mandibular arch (solid line) (*A*) with ideal anterior and buccal overjet and Class I molar relationship(s). (*B*) The same maxillary and mandibular arch with the maxillary arch moved posteriorly into a Class III molar relationship. Note that the maxilla in a retruded position produces crossbites in the anterior and posterior segments even though the arch dimensions are the same.

rotation involved in this development tends to decrease the anterior prominence of "B" point and Pogonion and in so doing decreases SNB and facial convexity angles and increases the ANB differences (see Figure 7–21). While elongation of the facial profile is one of the results of all this, it occurs while simultaneously masking the antero-posterior jaw imbalance, which can occasionally be considered a favorable interaction in the orthodontic management of these patients.

The third dimension, transverse, shows equally significant effects of vertical and antero-posterior changes because of the well-known fact that as maxillary buccal teeth are forced to occlude increasingly far back on the diverging mandibular arch, they must concomitantly expand in width to maintain proper buccal overjet (Figure 7–24). Given a cleft palate problem with maxillary transverse dimensions already diminished, the dento-alveolar adjustment mechanism compromised in its ability, and then mandibular overclosure and forward rotation to occlude with a maxillary arch already retruded, one can realize the tendency for the transverse relations to be subsequently worsened.

The net result of this complex interaction is that in occlusal contact the *vertical* deficiency tends to accentuate the *antero-posterior* discrepancy between jaws, and then both problems serve to create a worsening *transverse* imbalance. It also follows that with the tendency of transverse and antero-posterior cleft-related malocclusions to worsen with age, and with the later onset of the vertical problem during the mixed and permanent dentition (see page 390) and its superimposition on the other two already present, the substantial increases in the severity of malocclusions seen at this age are the rule rather than the exception. Further, the orthodontic condition of the primary dentition usually cannot be used as a milestone for estimating this degree of worsening, inasmuch as it is impossible at that stage to evaluate the magnitude of the future vertical problem and its potential effects on other pre-existing problems.

In general then, cleft palate orthodontic diagnosis must evaluate potential problems in all three planes of space, with both skeletal and dental components. It must take into account features both common to and unique for the various types of clefts, as all tend to get worse with further growth and development. While this section of the chapter has explored some of the more commonly expected findings, it has not assumed to cover them all. Nor has it implied that the problems itemized occur all the time in all patients. Rather, as surgery and team treatment continue to improve, the severity of the problems can only be expected to decrease dramatically as it has over the past 25 years. To be sure, there are ever-increasing numbers of cleft patients presenting with malocclusions more characteristic of the non-cleft individuals (Figure 7–25), though they are still in the minority. For that reason we have not dealt with them in this chapter, which has focused rather on the cleft palate orthodontic problems most commonly seen today. In describing the latter in such detail—the malocclusions definitely complicated by the cleft itself—we may have appeared to some readers to have overstated their severity and incidence. On the other hand we would not want to minimize the many potential ramifications of cleft palate malocclusions, for regardless of the improvements in cleft palate rehabilitation, these complex malocclusion

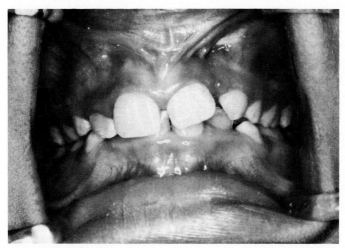

FIGURE 7-25   Intraoral photograph of UCLP patient with a malocclusion that is more typical of the non-cleft population.

conditions still constitute the greatest challenge faced by the orthodontist working in this field.

TREATMENT: MODES AND TIMING

To be complete, any chapter dealing with orthodontic management of cleft palate patients should contain some description of specific treatment methods. However, two points need to be re-emphasized to develop a proper perspective prior to dealing with this topic. First, as every orthodontist knows, there are usually *several different methods for the treatment of a particular problem, each of which can produce equally satisfying results when appropriately applied.* There are few, if any, "absolutes" in orthodontic therapy; so one is seldom justified in taking the stance that of the many approaches available, there can be *only one way* to treat any particular problem. Second, as mentioned previously in this chapter (see page 365), the tremendous variability that pervades the entire scope of cleft palate orthodontics, involving both the patient and the specialists organized to treat him, makes it unwise to limit one's thinking to *one* particular treatment technique for *all* cleft populations. Consequently, the treatment to be described represents those techniques and approaches *presently* employed at the H. K. Cooper Institute. It is representative of 40 years of orthodontic experience in best coping with the problems presented in *our* cleft population. It does *not* represent a panacea for achieving universally superior orthodontic results in *all* cleft populations, because at present *no* such panacea appears to exist. However, it is felt that, given the basic philosophy of this Institute, described previously, the treatment approach and techniques to follow do produce the most uniformly satisfactory results in our clinic at present, with special due consideration to the "intangibles" of cost/benefit limitations that lie at the heart of every cleft palate orthodontic problem.

The concept of treatment timing, or when to begin active orthodontic intervention, is a major consideration in dealing with the non-cleft patient. It assumes an equally, if not more, important role in cleft palate orthodontics. The topic has received enormous attention in the literature, and it is very clear that the issue finds little agreement from author to author and center to center. The basic range of suggested times for orthodontic intervention has been outlined with considerable clarity by Fishman[35] as follows:

1. Pre-dental (1 to 18 months of age)—prior to eruption of primary molars.
   a. Pre-surgical.
   b. Post-surgical.
2. Deciduous dentition (3 to 6 years)—after full eruption of primary dentition.
3. Early mixed dentition (7 to 9 years)—after or during eruption of permanent maxillary incisors.
4. Late mixed and early permanent dentition (from 9½ years on).

Each of these stages will be considered separately.

Pre-dental Treatment

Interest in correcting the cleft-related orthodontic problems at as early a stage as is reasonably possible reached its ultimate expression in the mid and late 1950's with the recommendation by McNeil[90] and Burston[14] to align the distorted maxillary arch segments orthopedically in early neonates, prior to any surgical repair. Since that time, the topic of *pre-surgical orthopedic intervention* has generated considerable and often heated debate about the virtues of such treatment and has noticeably polarized various factions of the cleft palate orthodontic community, with still others modifying the initial concept to take up some position in mid-ground.

In its presently used form, the approach has taken on a multi-faceted appearance from center to center. Some of the variations recommended in the literature include simple passive holding appliances[60–62, 95, 136, 164] as opposed to more active orthopedic movement,[13, 80, 82, 131, 132, 134, 135, 140] additional elaborate extra-orally activated controls of pinned appliances,[38, 39, 80, 125] and the use of these pre-surgical measures with[11, 40, 46, 59, 94, 136-140, 165] or without[60–62, 130-132, 134, 153] primary bone grafting, or with periosteoplasty.[39, 57, 58] The rationale and/or suggested advantages for the use of this type of appliance and intervention at this age include:

1. To facilitate feeding.[45, 60, 63, 82, 106, 140]
2. To help establish normal tongue posture.[13, 45, 60, 82, 111]
3. To provide a psychological boost to the parents.[13, 45, 63, 82, 106, 111, 140, 151]
4. To assist the surgeon in his initial repairs.[13, 45, 63, 67, 82, 111, 116, 130, 164, 165]
5. To stimulate palate bone growth.[13, 82, 106, 111, 116]
6. To restore the orofacial "functional matrix."[60, 62, 82, 114]
7. To help decrease the number of ear infections.[82]
8. To expand or prevent collapsed segments.[13, 60, 61, 63, 82, 114, 116, 140, 164, 165]
9. To reduce the need for later orthodontic treatment.[13, 62, 111, 137, 164]
10. To allow soft tissues to grow more before surgery.[63, 106]

11. To guide tooth eruption.[61]
12. To improve esthetics.[116, 140, 164]
13. To re-establish proper sutural growth patterns early, when the sutures are most responsive.[39, 79]

While all of these can be considered as lofty objectives for *any* type of proposed approach to treatment at this pre-surgical stage, it remains the responsibility of the proponents of the particular approach to establish that that approach is a reliable means to attain those objectives. As stated by Robertson[131] ". . . the burden of proof lies with those who advise the introduction of a new technique, or the adaptation or modification of an older method."

At the H. K. Cooper Institute the present method for dealing with the problems seen pre-surgically in cleft cases does *not* include *any* form of maxillary orthopedic intervention. Although the suggested favorable consequences of pre-surgical orthopedics, as just listed, can be considered desirous objectives of our own philosophy of treatment, the existing forms of pre-surgical orthopedics, as described in the literature, *do not* seem, at present, to provide a better means of achieving the desired objectives than does our own present approach. This seems especially evident when the total, long-range benefits are evaluated in relation to the "costs" invested to attain them.

Although similar approaches have been taken by other authors before,[122, 162] it behooves each center to weigh the pros and cons of this aspect of cleft palate orthodontics/orthopedics on the basis of its own total treatment philosophy. We ourselves place heavy emphasis on *minimizing* total active orthodontic intervention, limiting it to what is required to achieve the optimum results. And we feel that properly timed and executed surgery of the cleft structures promotes restoration of form and function to as near normal as can reasonably be expected. Therefore, our present approach precludes any active orthodontic/orthopedic therapy at this stage. Rather, the patients are monitored continuously as the natural remolding effects of restored functional matrices act in the manner described by Wolff's Law.

While the shortcomings of such an approach in producing uniformly satisfactory results are not denied, this mode of treatment does have the advantage of not adding "cost" in terms of extra treatment time, financial outlay, or any of the other considerations mentioned previously in the discussion of "therapeutic modifiability" (see page 364). Nor is it enough for the proponents of pre-surgical orthopedics to demonstrate equal or marginally superior results, since the additional "costs" of this early intervention must bring about sufficiently reliable, improved, and long-term benefits to offset the definite disadvantages of additional treatment. With these aspects in mind, it becomes possible to establish the basis for our own specific rationale at the Institute for questioning the claimed advantages of pre-surgical orthopedics.

FIRST, the proposal that a pre-surgical prosthesis assists in feeding implies that there is a significant problem in this regard. If a major feeding problem can be documented, this point probably remains valid. However, given the many other means to facilitate feeding (special or altered nipples, infant position, eye-droppers, and so forth), data on our own population of patients provide no evidence that feeding is a major problem with regard to the child's growth.[127] The occasional exceptions to this rule, involving either slow weight gain or the mother's psychological problems, are easily handled with a removable plate designed specifically to help in feeding. But to apply to all patients a treatment method needed only for the occasional exception to the rule would appear to us to constitute overtreatment.

SECOND, to suggest that these early appliances promote "normal" tongue posture and swallowing patterns implies that a definite problem may occur in the future that is directly related to tongue problems at this pre-dental age. There is strong support for the notion of long-range orthodontic problems related to postural alterations of the tongue from collapsed nasal cavities, hypertrophied adenoids, or mutilated collapsed palatal vaults (see page 374). But the relationship of tongue posture in the unoperated condition to these problems is cloudy at best. Additionally, interaction with the speech pathologists at the Institute has revealed no sound evidence to support the theory that abnormal tongue habits affecting speech can be directly related to positional problems developed before eruption of the baby's teeth. Finally, the attempt to "normalize" tongue habits at this early age would probably be a monumental task in light of the fact that throughout the first decade *abnormal* tongue swallowing habits are the rule rather than the exception.[119] To attempt to "normalize" the problem, then, presupposes a definition of "normal" for the very young infant, which may be "abnormal" in later years.

THIRD, to say that early active orthopedic intervention has psychological advantages for the parents presupposes the failure of those team members whose specific role is to deal with parental psychological adjustments. Further, the argument that this early treatment makes the parents feel *involved* in their child's rehabilitation or that it provides frequent opportunities for waiting-room group therapy must be weighed against the possible psychological *disadvantages* of potential overtreatment or of requiring the parents to live with a child with an unrepaired lip for several months longer than they would otherwise have had to do.

FOURTH, with regard to assisting the surgeon in executing a better repair of the lip and/or palate, it has been our philosophy to leave such decisions up to the surgeon himself. It is the surgeon's responsibility to determine the conditions under which his own methods of surgical repair can be best carried out, with due consideration to esthetics and function, and then to recruit team assistance when needed to create those conditions. In our clinic, the surgeon (R.L.H.) has not expressed the need for pre-surgical orthopedics to provide conditions beyond which he can obtain with his own techniques. (See chapter on Surgery.) As a result, this reason for early treatment is unnecessary. It is clearly recognized, however, that other surgeons, working at other centers under other conditions, may justifiably request orthopedic intervention by the orthodontist. If such a request arises, serious consideration would have to be given to pre-surgical orthopedics as a means to fulfill that request. It is very clear, however, that the present lack of good long-term objective evaluation of surgically related parameters suggests that more work is needed in this area to determine if certain selected cases or problems might, in fact, benefit from such orthopedic therapy.

FIFTH, the desire to stimulate bone growth of the palatal shelves was one of the initial bases upon which McNeil[90] first proposed early pre-surgical orthopedics. However, the finding of apparent bony shelf growth following pre-surgical orthopedics[106] must be interpreted cautiously, since significant shelf growth has also been documented following lip repair *only*.[86] Thus it becomes imperative, if this supposed advantage of pre-surgical orthopedics is to be considered valid, not only to document the presence of bony shelf growth but also to establish amounts of growth beyond what would have occurred without the pre-surgical treatment. At present, such documentation does not appear to be available.

SIXTH, the degree to which pre-surgical orthopedics restores the orofacial functional matrices to normal doubtless depends on one's interpretation and application of that theory to the cleft patient. At this Institute, it is felt that the closest approximations of normalcy in orofacial functional matrices occur when the cleft soft tissues are repaired in as physiologically normal a fashion as possible. Attainment of good muscle continuity and function across the lip and an intravelar veloplasty to re-attach abnormal insertions of the velopharyngeal musculature are regarded as the treatment of choice in attempting to restore orofacial function. Further, it is felt that the degree to which skeletal form will subsequently be returned to normal is directly related to the success of our surgical repairs in restoring these orofacial muscular matrices (Figure 7–26). The artificial mechanical displacement of distorted skeletal parts to an idealized form, while perhaps esthetically pleasing, does not necessarily return normal function to still abnormally structured musculature. Further, the relationship of tongue

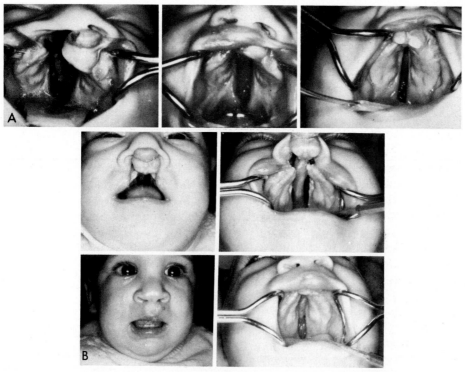

FIGURE 7–26 (A) UCLP patient and (B) BCLP patient before and after lip repair, showing molding effect of segments without presurgical orthopedics.

function to the use of these appliances is felt, as we mentioned earlier, to be tenuous at best.

SEVENTH, the improvement of middle ear infections purportedly resulting from use of pre-surgical orthopedic appliances, if valid, can certainly be seen as a beneficial consequence. The importance of this problem is fully appreciated. At present there do not appear to be any sound, objective data available, however, to document a positive relationship between early appliance therapy and improved middle ear conditions. Until such data appear, the prevention or management of middle ear problems at this Clinic is based on the assumption that the primary etiological factor involved is the abnormal structure, attachments, and function of auditory tube cartilage and musculature. Further, any symptomatic treatment required during the course of management is left to the discretion of the otolaryngology member of the team. At this Institute no need has been expressed to augment his repertoire of management techniques with early appliances.

The EIGHTH and NINTH proposals for pre-surgical orthopedics, to prevent or realign collapsed arch segments and, as a result, to reduce the need for later orthodontic treatment, are probably the primary objectives of this form of treatment. They are the ones that require most careful evaluation. The use of pre-surgical appliances to achieve these objectives is at present not employed at this Clinic for several closely interrelated reasons. First, as with the discussion on bone growth stimulation, one must assess the average baseline results attainable through lip repair only. Excellent reviews of such a comparison are provided in the literature[2, 4] and need not be repeated here. We shall only say that most of the well-documented, longitudinal data available to date seem to place the incidence of no crossbite or a minor one-tooth (canine) crossbite in the primary dentition at about 50 to 60 per cent without the use of *any* pre-surgical orthopedic appliances (Figure 7–27), both at this Institute[87] and at others.[6, 53, 124] Since in this Clinic the simple one-tooth minor crossbites are not considered serious enough to warrant primary dentition correction, they are from a practical standpoint appropriately included in the group of no-crossbites. Soft tissue profile[52] and skeletal measures[65] on our cleft population without pre-surgical treatment also reveal no significant demonstrable deficiency at this stage.

Thus, using crossbite as our baseline for evaluation, in our opinion less than half of the total cleft population would sufficiently benefit in this respect from any additional mode of therapy. This is not to deny that the existence of a potentially serious problem in those other 40 to 50 per cent might call for continued improved efforts. However, one limiting factor at present in the application of any improved techniques to these 40 per cent is the inability to reliably predict before therapy which of the cases will require this additional treatment and which will not.[124] Such a limitation is understandable in light of the tremendous number of variables (see page 365) potentially affecting the ultimate outcome, only one of which *may* be pre-operative cleft width.[74] Moreover, the present state of the art includes *no* dependable way to integrate and evaluate the additional contributing variables of the surgeon's ability, surgical technique, timing of surgery, inherent growth potential, response to scarring, pre-operative maxillary size, shape, form, and so forth.

As a result, to insure that the 40 per cent predisposed to significant primary dentition crossbites are reached with any proposed preventive

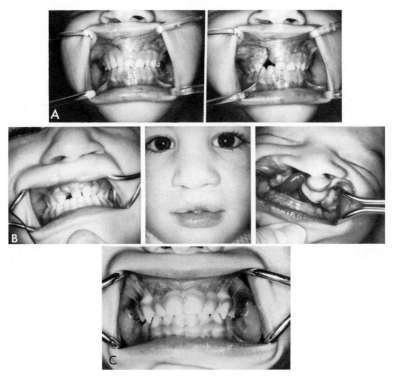

FIGURE 7–27   Results of lip and palate repair in (*A*) UCLP, (*B*) BCLP, and (*C*) CPO patients in
the primary dentition, showing good occlusion without presurgical orthopedics.

orthopedic measures, essentially *all* of the patients must be subjected to the
treatment. At this Institute, such an approach is considered serious
overtreatment, especially in patients and families already frequently pressed
to their limits of endurance by the sum total of team treatment. If on the other
hand, reliable means of detection are ever developed to sort out this group of
patients, then serious thought would have to be given to applying early active
appliances that may have proved successful for the interception of this
developing malocclusion. To date, such a prospect has not appeared.
Recognizing the heterogeneity of the pre-operative cleft condition, it
certainly would seem to be a worthwhile endeavor, however, to devote more
research effort toward accumulating good long-term data, clinical and
experimental, which would provide a means of detecting pre-surgical
conditions that might benefit from such orthopedic therapy.

Moreover, we reject pre-surgical orthopedics as a means of preventing
arch collapse or lessening future orthodontics because we do not believe
enough success has been achieved toward these two goals to warrant its use,
at least in its present form. While several reports offer data to show a decrease
in the number of primary dentition crossbite problems following pre-surgical
orthopedics,[45, 46, 60, 62, 74, 106] the percentage improvement, if reliable, does not
seem to justify the means. Even if a generous reproducible result of only 20
per cent remaining primary dentition crossbites is granted, essentially only
half of those original 40 per cent needing additional measures are being aided

by this procedure, while five or six out of every ten will have been treated unnecessarily. If this is further complicated by the added finding of tremendous variability of results and not infrequent reports of results only equal or *inferior* to those without pre-surgical intervention,[2, 4, 28, 101] this mode of treatment becomes even more dubious.

We have seen no evidence that the present forms of pre-surgical orthopedics in any way reduce the overall need for future orthodontic treatment or can result in significantly improved, stable orthodontic results. The primary limitation at this point is the absence of any well-controlled, long-term, longitudinal results through the permanent dentition stage, and this is in spite of the fact that the technique itself has been in common usage since the late 1950's. The main point of contention here is that for pre-surgical orthopedics to become an accepted measure at this Institute, its long-range "benefits," in terms of improving the quality or decreasing the amount of orthodontic treatment later, must significantly outweigh the "costs" of additional treatment in these early stages, both financial and otherwise. With the lack of data on which to make this judgment at present, our stance to date is based on theoretical, experiential, and experimental considerations presently available. Of these, a few can be cited.

First, analysis of the developing problem, as described earlier in this chapter, makes it clear that our interpretation of the "natural" course of events for these malocclusions is that they will become progressively worse with age (an interpretation not unique to this clinic).[142-144] This, plus the fact of the later onset of vertical problems with the erupting permanent dentition and the compounding detrimental effects of these problems on the transverse and sagittal discrepancies, suggests that a beautifully aligned arch in the primary dentition does not preclude the possibility of the development of potentially severe malocclusions in the mixed and permanent dentition. Further, the lack of influence of pre-surgical orthopedics, as presently employed, on these vertical problems makes such a possibility even more likely. This conclusion has also been substantiated in the literature.[6, 145]

A second consideration of ours is that while it has been suggested that this early pre-surgical treatment of arches makes correction and/or retention of crossbites easier than correction at a later time, this has not been substantiated by any *objective* evaluation. Also, our own experience has not provided any indication that this is valid to a degree to justify the pre-surgical treatment.

Finally, in our attempts to limit the total amount of time during which any of our cleft patients must be undergoing active treatment to that necessary to achieve optimum results, one further finding deserves comment. Since it would appear that to a first approximation, there is no significant correlation between the severity of a given malocclusion and the duration of orthodontic treatment required to correct it,[48] it seems to us at present that unless early pre-surgical intervention can eliminate or reduce the subsequent permanent dentition malocclusions to a point at which little or no orthodontics is required, the gains of minor localized improvements here or there in the malocclusion will probably not reduce the full-banded treatment time. To us, this makes such early orthopedics marginally successful at best, in this regard.

The TENTH "advantage" attributed to pre-surgical orthopedics is based on the premise that its use means that surgery is delayed for several months,

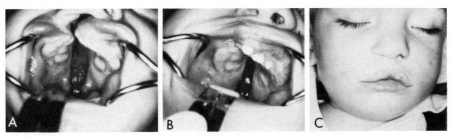

FIGURE 7–28   A UCLP child (*A*) before lip repair, (*B*) after lip repair, and (*C*) at the time of primary dentition, illustrating esthetics resulting from lip repair only.

thus allowing tissues to grow more prior to surgery. While such a consequence of pre-surgical orthopedics cannot be refuted, at present, from a surgical standpoint, no such desire has ever been expressed to the orthodontists by the surgeons at the Institute. Further, if such a delayed approach were necessary, we at present see no need to use pre-surgical orthopedics as the means to effect that delay.

The rejection of the ELEVENTH and TWELFTH objectives outlined for this early intervention (guiding tooth eruption and improving esthetics) is based on our feeling that the problems attacked are not of sufficient magnitude to warrant the added treatment at this stage. In general, at this Institute, the eruption of the primary dentition into relatively acceptable alignment seems not to be a problem of any consequence (see Figure 7–27). As was outlined in the "diagnosis" section, the main problem areas at this early stage do not include significant dental components, but if they did, it is felt that through our constant monitoring the situation could be dealt with easily once it developed. Likewise, any improvements in facial esthetics that may accrue from pre-surgical orthopedics are difficult, at best, to document. This is especially true in light of the beneficial molding action of good surgical repairs of the lip and palate on the previously distorted facial skeleton (Figure 7–28).

The THIRTEENTH stated goal of pre-surgical orthopedics is the re-establishment of the proper sutural growth patterns at an early age, when the sutures are most responsive. We agree that abnormal sutural growth patterns in the circum-maxillary system[79] are not in themselves an unexpected finding. Given the well-accepted responsive nature of facial sutures to alterations in the forces applied to them extrinsically, however,[96] it is difficult to see why a simple restoration of the circumoral musculature would not produce the same effects on the sutures as would pre-surgical orthopedic appliances. Although histological documentation of this is not found in the literature, the argument that pre-surgical orthopedics can provide sutural growth-controlling influence not resulting from physiological cheiloplasty has similarly not been proved. Until it is, we have chosen to reject the significance of this alleged advantage.

Having thus analyzed all available aspects of this mode and timing of treatment, our present position on the subject is basically similar to that expressed by various surveys of the state of the art.[154, 156] The present lack of good long-term evaluations of the effects of this form of therapy makes it difficult to evaluate the benefits to be derived. Further, it is our opinion that, while acknowledging the existence of orthodontic problems that would greatly benefit from improved techniques, both surgical and orthodontic/orthopedic, documentation of the results of the present forms of pre-surgical orthopedics does not offer a solution to these problems sufficient to warrant their universal use. Further research is needed to determine whether or not their application on a limited and selected basis is justifiable.

One other procedure occasionally recommended for pre-dental stages of orthodontic/orthopedic treatment is that of bone grafting the cleft alveolar ridge, either at the time of initial lip repair or shortly thereafter. It can be stated categorically that at this center *no* form of primary bone grafting is employed. With our present philosophy of allowing lip and palate repair to mold the segments naturally without any pre-alignment by active treatment, the use of bone grafts would be self-defeating by not allowing the freedom of segment movement.[54] Also, it appears to us that the procedure can be potentially damaging. Following the initial publications by Nordin and Johansen[102] and Schmid,[148] the number of centers that have tried the procedure and subsequently discontinued it because of disappointing and/or detrimental results seems to be increasing.[28, 34, 60–62, 67, 71, 101, 116, 130, 135] In addition to its apparent inability to add any particular degree of stabilization to the arch, the high incidence of growth problems in the anterior part of the arch (decreased SNA, primary incisor crossbite) and the problems with future orthodontics involving the graft site[34] have all prompted the widespread conclusion that there is little, if any, value to the procedure to offset its potential disadvantages,[8, 154, 156] Whether or not those cases still being managed with routine primary bone grafts but with techniques supposedly different from those of the studies just cited,[94, 136, 138, 140, 165] or whether the more recent technique of periosteoplasty introduced by Skoog[152] and presently used as a primary procedure at several centers[39, 57, 58] will show significant improvement in results remains to be established by long-term follow-up. Until then, the technique as a primary procedure appears to us to be of dubious enough benefit to be rejected as a mode of treatment.

Deciduous Dentition Treatment

As with active pre-dental orthodontic intervention, treatment at the primary dentition stage has received considerable attention and has demonstrated a wide variety of philosophies from center to center, ranging from routine full banding[117] to routine expansion[35, 121, 123, 157, 158, 160] to treating only severe functional deviations[143-145] to no routine treatment whatsoever.[5, 6] It has been suggested that proper alignment and/or expansion of the primary dentition will (1) proceed more rapidly because of better suture response at a younger age,[35, 160] (2) improve the alignment of permanent tooth eruption,[35, 108, 117, 158] (3) unlock stunted alveolar growth in the cleft area,[35, 157, 158] (4) improve speech development,[35, 121, 123, 157, 158] (5) allow normal tongue posture and/or nasal breathing,[121–123, 157, 158] and (6) reduce the need for future orthodontics.[35] At this Institute, the desirability of these objectives is fully appreciated, but the practical usefulness of attaining them all through routine primary dentition treatment seems questionable.

The general lack of severity of the problems in the deciduous dentition, and the onset of more difficult problems with the eruption of the permanent dentition, all described previously, tend to diminish our enthusiasm for active treatment at this early stage. This is especially true in view of the certain need for later full-banded orthodontics, regardless of the treatment given in the deciduous period. There seems to be little proof that the nature of the primary dentition can sufficiently facilitate normal eruption and position of the permanent dentition of these cleft palate cases in a manner that will ease future orthodontic problems. The main skeletal changes that have been documented for primary dentition treatment seem to be related only to elevated mandibular posture and decreased gonial angle, presumably the result of tongue posture changes.[145] However, these two changes are not considered desirable in all cases, in that both remove the masking effect of the lowered mandibular posture on any developing antero-posterior maxillary

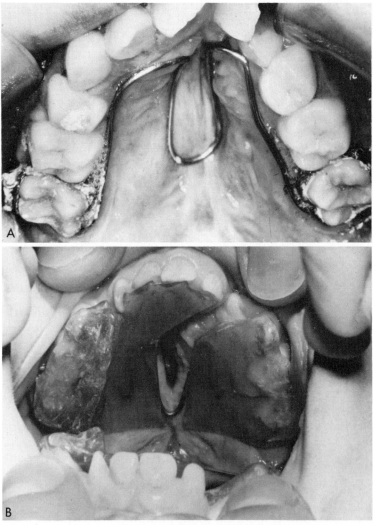

FIGURE 7–29 (A) A fixed maxillary palatal appliance (W arch). (B) A removable maxillary appliance (courtesy of Dr. William Posnick of the University of North Carolina School of Dentistry) that can be used in the primary or early mixed dentition for correction of maxillary constriction.

deficiency and may even tend to accentuate it in the new rest position. Consequently, early expansion is not carried out routinely in this clinic for this purpose.

Speech considerations for early palatal expansion in the primary dentition at the H. K. Cooper Institute are primarily placed at the discretion of the team speech pathologist, as discussed in the chapter on Speech. In general, it is felt that only in the more severely collapsed cases in this stage of development does the possibility of a resulting speech disturbance warrant orthodontic intervention. While such cases are extremely rare in our view, it must be stressed that only close cooperation between orthodontic and speech personnel will reveal those cases.

In general, the majority of those few cleft palate cases that are subject to active primary dentition orthodontic therapy involve some type of *functional* mandibular shift as a result of developing dento-alveolar incompatibility between the arches. Most often this is seen as a lateral shift into a complete unilateral crossbite, as a result of a mild bilateral maxillary arch constriction (see Figure 7–8) or a slide forward into a negative overjet relationship, as a result of incisal interference from lingually tipped maxillary central incisors (see Figure 7–9). It is deemed important to treat these cases early to prevent consequent permanent growth disturbance from making future orthodontic treatment more difficult.

Generally, the treatment mode of choice at this clinic for these early cases needing expansion is a simple form of fixed maxillary lingual appliance (i.e., either a W-arch or an Arnold expander). These are preferred over the removable split palate type of appliance because of the occasional cooperation problems, missed appointments, and lost appliances, which, coupled with the extremely rapid rate of relapse, make treatment with removable appliances frustrating to the orthodontist. However, it is realized that equally satisfactory results can be obtained with many different methods (Figure 7–29) and often the mode and exact timing of orthodontic correction of these early functional problems may be determined by speech therapy or other considerations.

Anterior functional crossbites, on the other hand, can be readily and simply managed oftentimes with a removable inclined plane on the lower incisors or a maxillary Hawley retainer with lingual finger spring (Figure 7–30). The need to go to fixed banded appliances for these cases is minimal.

Following expansion, these few treated cases need continuous retention through the mixed dentition stage and almost invariably require re-expansion in the permanent dentition, for reasons previously discussed. Once again, both fixed and removable retainers have been used here with equal success, depending on the particular case. Although it has been proposed that arch expansion at this stage is achieved more readily[123] or with more stability than at later stages,[61] in our own experience we have not found this to be true to a degree that would justify *routine* primary dentition expansion. We prefer that, if possible, most simple crossbites, anterior and/or posterior, with *no functional component,* be left alone.

One final aspect of primary dentition treatment that frequently demands attention is the high incidence of primary supernumerary teeth in the line of

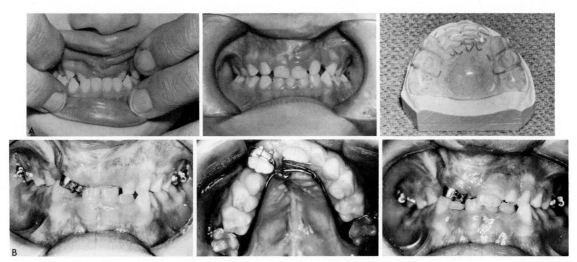

FIGURE 7–30   Correction of anterior crossbite in the primary dentition using (*A*) a removable appliance (courtesy of Dr. William Posnick of the University of North Carolina School of Dentistry). Early mixed dentition correction of anterior crossbite utilizing (*B*) a fixed appliance with finger spring.

the cleft. It is desirous to identify these teeth early and to make a decision as to their removal. While in most cases they should be extracted to avoid crowding or possible interference of permanent successor eruption paths, the possibility of retaining these extra teeth to maintain the associated alveolar bone[118] must be entertained when appropriate.

Mixed Dentition Treatment

Treatment during the mixed dentition years has also been described amply in the literature.[5, 35, 66, 107–110, 143, 144, 157] As opposed to earlier forms of treatment, however, the approach to the problems at this stage appears to be fairly uniform, and the treatment provided at this clinic can be said to coincide fairly well with that described elsewhere. While we find ourselves intervening more during the mixed dentition than in the previous two stages, such intervention is not *routine*. Rather, the severity of the particular problem dictates the need for correction during the mixed dentition years. Any problem that can be delayed without esthetic, psychological, functional, or speech detriments is most often simply monitored until full banding permanent dentition treatment is undertaken. In essence then, it becomes a judgment call on the part of the orthodontist, in conjunction with other specialists. Due consideration must be given to maintaining a positive balance between beneficial results and the possibility of "burning out" prematurely the cooperation much needed later during permanent dentition treatment.

The problems that frequently do present with sufficient severity to warrant correction are the following:

1. Posterior crossbite.
2. Malposed permanent incisors.
3. A-P molar discrepancies.

4. Serial extraction.

5. Detection of dental anomalies.

Posterior Crossbite. The very prevalent problem of progressively increasing posterior crossbites must be re-evaluated once again and dealt with appropriately. The severity of the crossbite, along with any possible functional correlates, dictates the need for, or choice of, treatment. In general, when deemed necessary, crossbites are corrected as previously described. Additionally, however, there is the occasional minor crossbite that, *by itself,* would be considered insufficient to demand correction but that may be treated nonetheless if another more severe problem does warrant mixed dentition intervention. Both problems can then be dealt with simultaneously. As with expansion at all ages in these cleft patients, once completed, full-time retention is required. This is because the posterior expansion, with no mid-palatal suture system to fill in bone and consolidate the expanded segments, is very unstable. The stretched palatal scar tissue can then cause collapse of the unsupported segments to original dimensions in a matter of days if retention is not used. Also, it must be realized that the possibility still remains that permanent dentition re-expansion will be needed, even if the case is retained, as continued growth, coupled with a three-dimensionally aggravated maxillary hypoplasia, continues to result in transverse incompatibility (Figure 7–31).

Malposed Permanent Incisors. A second oft-encountered situation is that of severely rotated and lingually inclined maxillary anterior teeth

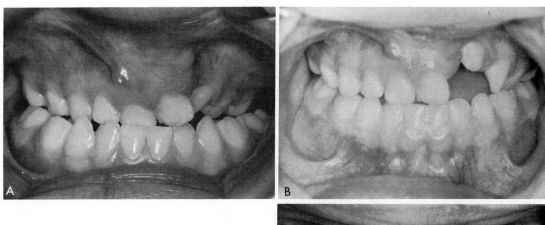

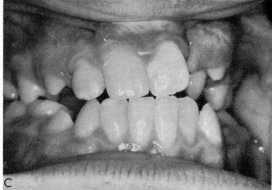

FIGURE 7–31 (*A*) Posterior crossbite in the mixed dentition and (*B*) after expansion. (*C*) Same patient in late mixed dentition with recurrence of crossbite. (Courtesy of the University of North Carolina School of Dentistry.)

(centrals especially) in UCLP and BCLP (see Figure 7–14). In severe cases, the resulting position makes the teeth a potential hazard for lip injury and predisposes them to fracture. It also often leads to anterior crossbites and forward shifts of the mandible for accommodation. The malposition can be an esthetic and psychological handicap and may create a tendency to speech articulation errors. If any of these consequences are deemed imminent as a result of this distorted incisor positioning, a partial-banded approach is undertaken. Usually banding permanent molars, cuspids (if bandable), and incisors in the maxillary arch and placing light-looped or straight-arch wires with any needed auxiliaries or elastics will suffice to align these teeth (Figure 7–32). Occasionally molar occlusal coverage with an acrylic plate is required

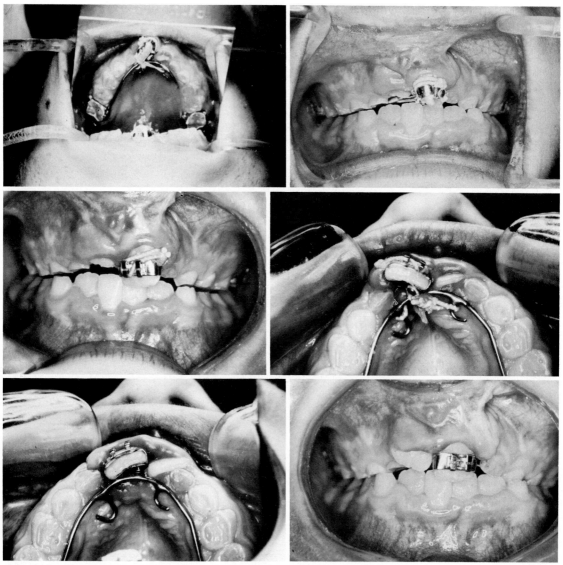

FIGURE 7–32   Correction of severely rotated maxillary incisor in the early mixed dentition in UCLP patient.

to expand the incisors labially over the anterior crossbite, while less severe cases may be treated entirely with a maxillary Hawley retainer and finger springs. As with the posterior expansion, once alignment is attained, full-time retention is advisable.

A-P Molar Discrepancies. A third developing problem frequently handled at this stage is an early, severe antero-posterior molar discrepancy. Thus, as with usual non-cleft population treatment plans, full Class II molar relationships are often fitted with headgears during this mixed dentition stage. The usual regimen is a cervical pull appliance with 12 to 16 ounces of force per side, to be worn 12 to 14 hours per day. Care must be taken, however, not to start this type of potentially orthopedic force upon a maxilla that is already tending toward severe antero-posterior hypoplasia, and one should avoid impacting unerupted second permanent molars. Excluding these precautions, though, rapid correction is usually achieved, with the added benefit of helping to extrude the maxillary molars. Such extrusion initiates therapy to correct vertical deficiencies while further masking a potential maxillary insufficiency. In the opposite case of early Class III molar relationships, if it appears that there may be a mandibular overgrowth component, chin cup therapy has been used at this center with varying degrees of success (high pull, directed through the condyles, 2 to 3 pounds per side, to be worn 14 to 16 hours per day). At present, however, this cannot be considered one of the more commonly used approaches at this Institute.

Serial Extraction. The fourth decision often facing the cleft palate orthodontist at this stage is the dilemma of whether or not to start serial extraction procedures on developing crowded arches. Basically, the procedures followed at this clinic are patterned after the early descriptions by Dewel.[30, 31] It must be emphasized, however, that in dealing with these cleft cases the application of serial extraction procedures is not always as clear-cut as it can be in non-cleft, skeletal Class I, crowded, certain-arch-length-discrepancy cases. This is because of three main confounding variables. First, the effective arch length is often difficult to determine accurately, owing to the cleft in the alveolar ridge and the difficulty in predicting how much additional alveolar bone can, or will, be generated as teeth adjacent to the cleft attempt to erupt. Furthermore, in addition to the problems inherent in accurately determining at this stage whether or not extractions will be required, it is also difficult to establish which permanent teeth should be removed, if extraction does, in fact, become the treatment plan. Maxillary permanent cuspids may occasionally have to be the teeth chosen for removal because of the improbability of bringing those that are erupting high into the cleft down into occlusion with sufficient alveolar bone on their mesial root surface to guarantee their usefulness or long-term survival in the mouth. Likewise, the high incidence of missing or grossly underdeveloped laterals and bicuspids requires that serial extraction procedures not be carried out into the permanent dentition without due consideration for already missing teeth.

The second consideration in cleft palate serial extraction planning is that early commitment to such a sequence, which usually leads to alignment of the dentition on their respective basal bones, may remove the possibility of later masking the often-seen skeletal disproportions by dento-alveolar compensation. As a result, occasional cases that *might* have been handled adequately by orthodontic masking of a moderate skeletal imbalance in the permanent dentition must instead be committed to an orthognathic surgical procedure to correct the dysplasia.

The third complicating factor of concern in serial extraction is the delayed and often distorted eruption patterns of the maxillary permanent teeth in these individuals. Retarded eruption may mean that the timing so essential to serial extraction success may have to be juggled so that primary teeth are not extracted prematurely, resulting in a further slowing of the permanent successor eruption. Additionally, the scar-deflected eruption paths, described thoroughly before, imply that the self-correcting adjustments of permanent tooth eruption, often desired in serial extraction, may not occur to an appreciable degree.

Because of these complicating factors, serial extraction procedures in early, crowded, mixed dentition cases are often begun as an "open-ended" procedure, whereby primary cuspids are removed to alleviate incisor crowding (especially in the lower arch) and primary first molars may be removed, when appropriate, to hasten the eruption of first bicuspids. However, the plans for permanent dentition extractions remain flexible until a more accurate determination of the situation can be made.

Detection of Dental Anomalies.   The fifth and final major determination to be made at the mixed-dentition stage is actually an extension of that just reviewed. To help in the future treatment planning, especially with regard to extractions and possible prosthodontic intervention, the mixed dentition stage is a good time to begin accurate detection of all the various dental abnormalities to which these cleft cases are often heir. Extractions are often unusual and determined in part by possible hypoplasia or hypocalcification. Maxillary central incisors, often abnormally formed, especially in BCLP cases, must be evaluated for their possible use as fixed bridge abutments. When in doubt about their usefulness, the policy of this clinic is generally to proceed to align and maintain them until later times, when more definitive treatment plans can be formulated. With the free premaxilla largely composed of alveolar bone,[66] their early removal may often lead to a subsequent loss of this bone and a resulting anterior bony defect that is often difficult to conceal.

Permanent Dentition Treatment

The principles and techniques of permanent dentition treatment of cleft palate cases are no different from those used in non-cleft orthodontics. There are, however, several methods that are employed more routinely in the cleft population, with its unique and often characteristic problems.

One concept of immediate importance is the initial recognition of orthodontic limitations in executing this usually final active phase of treatment. While the number of maxillary basal arches or dentitions mutilated by repeated surgical procedures is fortunately declining, the occasional existence of such a case requires that the orthodontist be aware of the orthodontic limitations and the prosthodontic capabilities. In this clinic, these cases are often best treated with a minimum of orthodontic movement, if any at all, to position the teeth favorably for full coverage and an overlay denture. (See chapter on Prosthodontic Care.) In less severe cases, the orthodontic

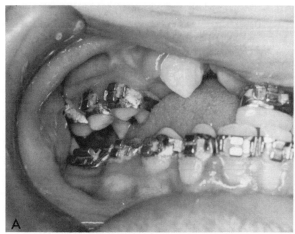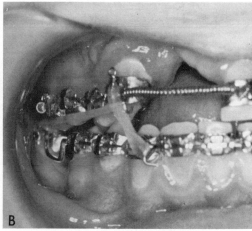

FIGURE 7–33   UCLP patient with (A) ectopically erupted cuspid approximating alveolar cleft and (B) cuspid positioned in arch with full banded orthodontic appliance. (Courtesy of the University of North Carolina School of Dentistry.)

limitations may be confined to hopelessly malposed or malformed teeth in the cleft area, while the prognosis for the rest of the arch is more favorable.

A second concept is the frequent use of treatment plans that start out with no detailed and specific long-range procedure in mind, but rather with a flexible series of tentative decisions that are continually modified as treatment progresses and response to treatment is evaluated. Coincident with this is the procedure labeled "therapeutic diagnosis,"[1] in which treatment is initially based on a tentative diagnosis of the problem and is subsequently modified as response to treatment is monitored. As an example, maxillary permanent cuspids are often seen erupting or apparently impacted high in the cleft. Whether the basic defect here is simply a failure of vertical eruption and alveolar bone development because the collapsed maxillary segment has been "locked" into a restrictive position, as has been suggested,[157, 158] or whether this represents a basic limitation of alveolar bone development inherent to the cleft itself, is not easily determined.

In such cases, and in many cleft cases seen, prior to any definitive, rigid decisions about total treatment plan, initial therapy is started on the maxillary arch only. It includes basically just palatal and/or dento-alveolar expansion and initial light-looped or twist-arch wires to initiate alignment and leveling (Figure 7–33). As such treatment progresses and some of the more gross transverse problems are alleviated, it often becomes apparent whether or not the "high" cuspids can be brought into arch form with any type of favorable prognosis. Based on such "therapeutic diagnostic" measures, a more accurate definitive treatment plan can subsequently be formulated.

The specific appliances used at the H. K. Cooper Institute for permanent dentition treatment include a full-banded strap-up of either Begg or Edgewise appliances, depending on the operator. Both have been used with equal facility and success. Palatal expansion devices at this stage are invariably of the fixed variety. Because of the often unique nature of the cleft maxillary constriction, with the anterior portion of the lateral segments collapsed more severely than the tuberosity level (Figure 7–34), a wide assortment of

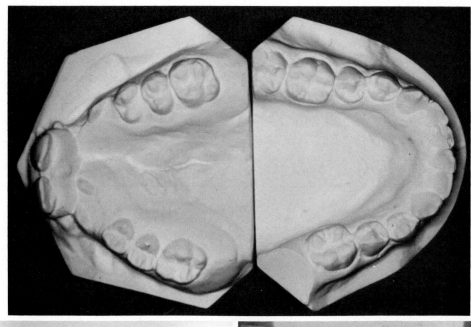

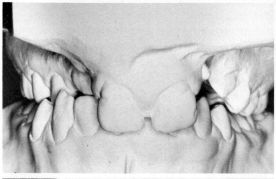

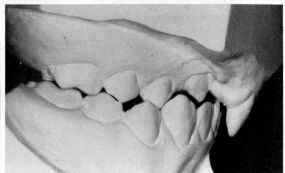

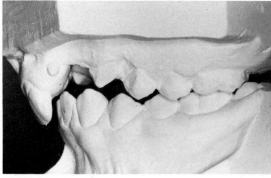

FIGURE 7–34 Model of typical permanent dentition occlusion in BCLP patient showing mild arch collapse in cuspid region leading to crossbite in same region.

appliances has been designed, some more or less specifically for the cleft patient.[144] At this clinic, if disproportionate anterior-to-posterior collapse is a major concern, an Arnold-expander with splint lingual tube is on occasion used, while more generalized maxillary constriction is handled equally as well as Hy-Rax®, Haas-type, or W-arch expanders. The choice usually depends on the operator's preference. Also, owing to the nature of the expansion, with most resistance coming from palatal scar tissue that only very slowly seems to be able to reorganize to a new, expanded position, and with no compensatory sutural bony deposition to stabilize the expansion, some form of fixed, transverse palatal stabilizing arch is often used throughout the remainder of treatment to insure that the expansion is maintained.

Finally, the orthodontist should be forewarned that not infrequently the initial expansion may open oro-nasal fistulae (Figure 7–35), which will lead to increased hypernasality and possible nasal regurgitation of liquids, potentially upsetting patient and parents. It has been our experience, however, that these fistulae are not produced by the expansion itself, but were pre-existing defects concealed by bunched palatal scar tissue. In either case, parents should be forewarned of this possibility.

A third problem that requires attention early in the treatment planning stages of permanent dentition therapy is one that is becoming increasingly important to the cleft palate orthodontist. Specifically, since the popularization of surgical correction of hypoplastic maxillae by Obwegeser,[103-105] the refinement and application of this approach to the cleft palate patient,[17, 29, 115] coupled with the procedures available for true mandibular prognathism in these patients,[36, 126] have opened up new avenues of treatment available to the orthodontist. It also, however, has placed new emphasis on precise diagnosis of the major etiological and contributing factors that create a particular cleft

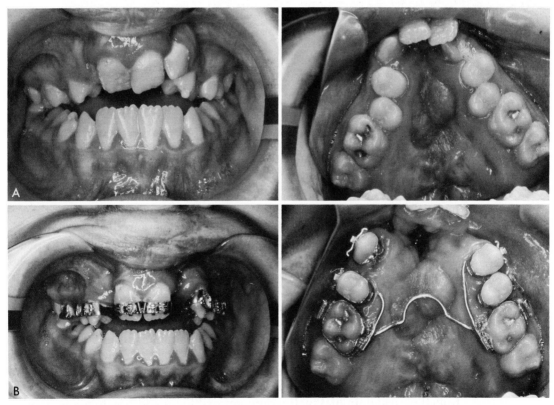

FIGURE 7–35 BCLP patient (A) before and (B) after expansion, with an oronasal fistula uncovered by maxillary expansion. (Courtesy of the University of North Carolina School of Dentistry.)

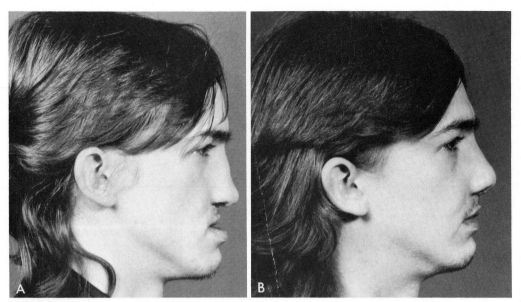

FIGURE 7–37 Profile of cleft prognathism (*A*) before and (*B*) after treatment with surgery and orthodontics. (Courtesy of the University of North Carolina School of Dentistry.)

Another surgical adjunct to permanent dentition orthodontic treatment, which is increasing in popularity at this Institute and is opening additional avenues to orthodontic management, is the use of secondary bone grafting in the cleft alveolus (Figure 7–38). While the use of such grafts at earlier ages (e.g., 5 to 7 years) seems not to be as successful,[119] their use from later mixed dentition stages through the permanent dentition appears to be a stable, reliable procedure with no serious untoward consequences. With this possibility open for consideration, the orthodontist not only has more "ammunition" in his battle for stability, but also has available a means to save otherwise hopelessly positioned teeth (cuspids especially) in the region of the cleft. Evidence indicating the ability to move teeth into and through such grafts[8] further enhances this possibility.

The net effect of the procedures available through joint orthodontic-surgical-prosthodontic efforts requires an early cooperative determination of the individual potentialities and limitations in each case, so that the remaining permanent dentition orthodontic treatment can be appropriately outlined.

Once definitive plans are made, the mechanics of treatment follow normal orthodontic procedure. Of particular interest, perhaps, are several modes of therapy that find nearly universal application in the cleft palate patients. Namely, because of the gradually developing vertical deficiency and the benefits to be derived in all three dimensions by encouraging further vertical maxillary development, headgears to hold anchorage are most uniformly of the cervical or low pull variety, and the prolific use of *inter*-maxillary elastics is accepted and encouraged. Also, it is not uncommon to have lingual root torque requirements in the maxillary incisor region, which require extraordinary means to approximate. Most notably, in BCLP cases whose original defect may have included a severely protruding premaxillary segment that

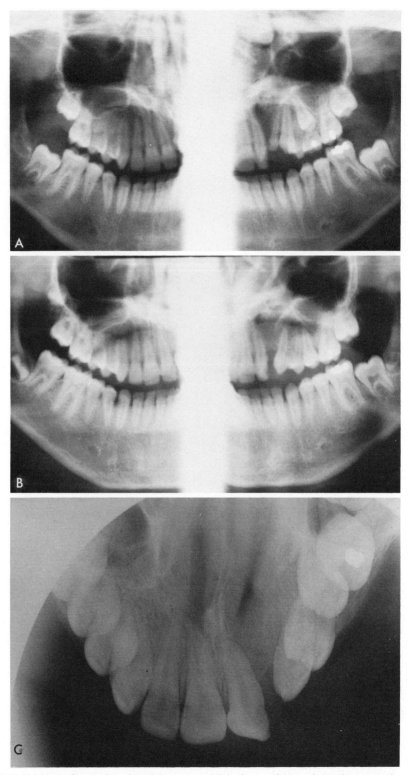

FIGURE 7–38   Radiographs of UCLP patient (*A*) before and (*B* and *C*) after secondary bone graft to alveolar ridge. (Courtesy of the University of North Carolina School of Dentistry.)

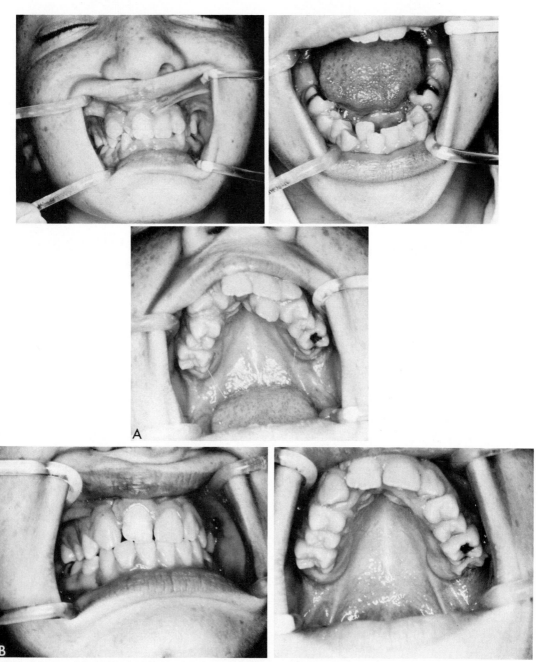

FIGURE 7–39 (A) Before and (B) after orthodontic treatment of a severe malocclusion in a patient with a cleft of the lip and alveolar process showing acceptable orthodontic results.

underwent an undesired down and back rotation following lip repair, the lingual inclination of the premaxilla itself, coupled with the serious lingually deflected eruption paths of the permanent central incisors, can produce situations requiring nearly 40 to 50° (see Figure 7–19) of lingual root torque to the centrals. While this is clearly an impossibility by itself, it must be remembered that the torque to the teeth will also probably result in a certain degree of premaxillary torque or repositioning. When using the Edgewise approach, such torque requirements usually demand the use of torquing auxiliaries in addition to that normally generated in the arch wire. Further, as lingual root torque and/or premaxillary rotation occurs, the case must be carefully observed for signs of root resorption or perforation of the root apices through the premaxillary palatal alveolar bone. If such a development arises, the remaining problem may be handled by the use of vomer resection and surgical premaxillary alignment stabilized with alveolar grafts.

While these are the most notable characteristics of permanent dentition treatment encountered in this particular clinic setting at the present, they are by no means the only ones seen. Nor may they even be the major ones at other clinics with different approaches to treatment from birth to adulthood, nor the major ones that will be seen in the future as techniques and management improve. Nonetheless, they, along with others outlined in the literature, should be borne in mind by the orthodontist contemplating cleft palate treatment, so that he might have available to him a source of treatment techniques equal to the challenge at hand (Figure 7–39).

Retention

In cleft palate patients, the period of orthodontic retention is invariably longer than for the non-cleft patient and may even become a full-time life-long necessity if the orthodontist would hope to maintain his correction. The reasons for this have been touched upon heretofore, and basically they involve a lack of bony stability, contracture of stretched or new scar tissues, and the frequent need to have finished treatment at a compromised goal of inherently less stability than an ideal occlusion.

Most frequently, this phase of treatment becomes the joint responsibility of both orthodontist and prosthodontist, as an appliance is made to serve both as a retainer and a prosthetic replacement for missing dental units. Such appliances can be either fixed or removable. The latter may be favored at this stage for several reasons. First, with the patient near maturity and hopefully with improved dental appreciation and pride in his own appearance, cooperation is usually sufficiently reliable so as not to be a concern. Also, removables may be more easily adapted to potentially changing situations, especially when it is felt that a speech aid is needed as well. In such instances, the appliance may serve a three-fold role in the cleft patient's rehabilitation: retention, prosthetic replacement, and speech aid (Figure 7–40). However, the ideal type of retention/stabilization for these patients, when possible, is fixed anterior bridgework that spans the cleft and thereby unifies the free segments. The success of such an approach, both esthetically and functionally, is often enhanced with alveolar bone grafts to bridge the bony segments and to support any secondary lip or nose revisions planned by

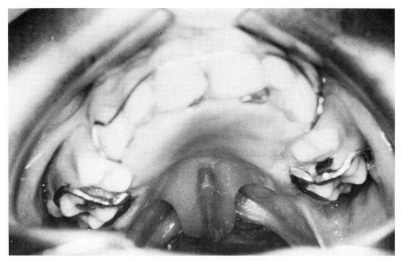

FIGURE 7–40 Removable retainer that is also used as a speech aid appliance.

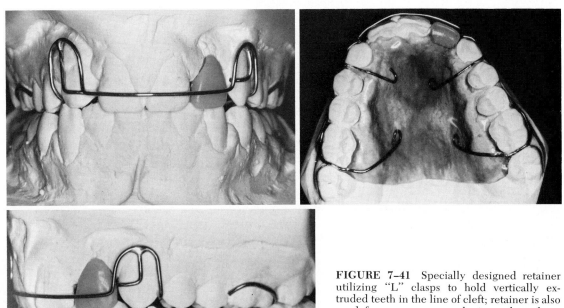

FIGURE 7–41 Specially designed retainer utilizing "L" clasps to hold vertically extruded teeth in the line of cleft; retainer is also used for temporary prosthetic tooth replacement.

the surgeon. As a result of these interactions, it should be obvious that the orthodontist must work closely with the prosthodontist and surgeon through-out treatment and into retention, so that the final stages of treatment can provide the best foundation for maintaining the desired end result.

Other aspects of retention that may involve the prosthodontist and/or surgeon include the management of any oro-nasal fistulae that may have been uncovered during orthodontic treatment, maintenance of incisor correction, and post-surgical fixation and retention following orthognathic surgery. Because of these many variables, appliance design follows no standard pattern, other than to say that *rigidity of construction* is a crucial characteristic. In this sense, tooth positioners probably have little value at present in retaining all aspects of cleft palate orthodontic correction. Also, while the rigidity of the maxillary appliance itself will retain transverse and antero-posterior correction, oftentimes extra effort in clasp, bow, and attachment design must be utilized to maintain vertical corrections, especially in the teeth related to the cleft (Figure 7–41). In general, each plan of retention becomes both highly individualized and the product of input from speech, surgical, prosthodontic, and orthodontic team members.

CONCLUSIONS

Cleft palate orthodontics and oral orthopedics provide a unique opportu-nity for the orthodontist to apply all of his training in biomechanics, growth and development, facial and dental esthetics, and artistic positioning. Moreover, he must utilize that knowledge and those tools if any degree of success is to be expected. While many of the problems endemic to the cleft population have etiologies unique to the clefting malformation and its subsequent treatment, the keys to the solution or alleviation of those problems are not unique, but lie within the realm of orthodontics for all types of patients.

Of the problems seen at this Institute and the methods of treatment employed here, the following are considered the most significant: (1) the dento-alveolar and skeletal irregularities are largely the result of the surgical procedures used to repair the cleft; (2) the malocclusions seen generally have both dento-alveolar *and* skeletal components, and the contribution of each to the specific malocclusion may vary from cleft type to cleft type and from patient to patient; (3) the dysplasias usually involve all three planes of space, with vertical deficiencies acting to accentuate transverse and sagittal problems; (4) the dento-alveolar component of the malocclusion seems to be most marked in the permanent dentition, owing to the deviant eruption pattern of the permanent teeth, which results in a problem that tends to increase in severity with age; (5) as a result of the factors just mentioned, while primary dentition may appear close to normal, the cases almost always require active orthodontic treatment at later stages, regardless of prior intervention; (6) the discouraging lack of reliable data on the long-term results of pre-surgical orthopedic therapy, especially after more than 20 years of its use at various centers, characterizes that approach as still experimental and not justifiable for widespread use at this time; and (7) the persistence of frequently severe malocclusions in the cleft population demands that continued effort in basic and clinical research be emphasized and applied to improve our present modes of therapy.

Perhaps the only time-proven and truly unique aspect of orthodontic treatment is the degree to which it must be integrated into an overall plan for *total* patient rehabilitation, involving specialists of many and varied backgrounds and training. Therein may lie the most important key to successful treatment of these patients, without which even the most ideal orthodontic result attained in a cleft patient otherwise totally unrehabilitated can only be considered, overall, as a failure by the team, the patient, *and* the orthodontist. On the other hand, the proper utilization of such a team concept by the orthodontist in his treatment approach can make possible rehabilitory results previously unattainable by dedicated clinicians working alone.

References

1. Ackerman, J. L., and Proffit, W. R.: Diagnosis and planning treatment in orthodontics. *In* Graber, T. M., and Swain, B. F. (eds.): Current Orthodontic Concepts and Techniques. Philadelphia, W. B. Saunders Co., 1–110, 1975.
2. Aduss, H.: Management of the maxillary segments in complete unilateral cleft lip and palate: maxillary orthopedics. *In* Georgiade, N. G. (ed.): Symposium on Management of Cleft Lip and Palate and Associated Deformities. St. Louis, C. V. Mosby Co., 47–57, 1974.
3. Aduss, H., and Pruzansky, S.: Width of cleft at level of the tuberosities in complete unilateral cleft lip and palate. Plast. Reconstr. Surg., *41*:113–123, 1968.
4. Aduss, H., Friede, H., and Pruzansky, S.: Management of the protruding pre-maxilla. *In* Georgiade, N. G. (ed.): Symposium on Management of Cleft Lip and Palate and Associated Deformities. St. Louis, C. V. Mosby Co., 111–117, 1974.
5. Bergland, O.: Treatment of the cleft palate malocclusion in the mixed and permanent dentition. Trans. Eur. Orthod. Soc., 571–574, 1973.
6. Bergland, O., and Sidhu, S.: Occlusal changes from the deciduous to the early mixed dentition in unilateral complete clefts. Cleft Palate J., *11*:317–326, 1974.
7. Boo-Chai, K.: The unoperated adult cleft of the lip and palate. Br. J. Plast. Surg., *24*:250–257, 1971.
8. Boyne, P., and Sands, N.: Combined orthodontic-surgical management of residual palato-alveolar cleft palate. Am. J. Orthod., *70*:20–37, 1976.
9. Brader, A. C.: Dental arch form related with intra-oral forces: PR = C. Am. J. Orthod., *61*:541–561, 1972.
10. Brader, A. C.: A cephalometric x-ray appraisal of morphological variations in cranial base and associated pharyngeal structures. Angle Orthod., *27*:179–195, 1957.
11. Brauer, R. O., and Cronin, T. D.: Maxillary orthopedics and anterior palate repair with bone grafting. Cleft Palate J., *1*:31–42, 1964.
12. Brodie, A. G.: Behavior of normal and abnormal facial growth patterns. Am. J. Orthod., *27*:633–647, 1941.
13. Brogan, W. F., and McComb, H.: The early management of cleft lip and palate deformities. Aust. Dent. J., *18*:212–217, 1973.
14. Burston, W. R.: Early orthodontic treatment of cleft palate conditions. Dent. Practit., *9*:4156, 1958.
15. Case, C. S.: A Practical Treatise on the Technics and Principles of Dental Orthopedia and Prosthetic Correction of Cleft Palate. Chicago, C. S. Case Co., 1921.
16. Collito, M. B.: Management of the maxillary segments in complete unilateral cleft lip patients. *In* Georgiade, N. G. (ed.): Symposium on Management of Cleft Lip and Palate and Associated Deformities. St. Louis, C. V. Mosby Co., 58–61, 1974.
17. Converse, J. M., Wood-Smith, D., and Coccaro, P. J.: Surgical positioning of the maxilla. *In* Georgiade, N. G. (ed.): Symposium on Management of Cleft Lip and Palate and Associated Deformities. St. Louis, C. V. Mosby Co., 228–237, 1974.
18. Cooper, H. K.: Cleft palate: dentistry's opportunity. J. Am. Dent. Assoc., *42*:37–47, 1951.
19. Cooper, H. K.: Crippled children? Am. J. Orthod. Oral Surg., *28*:35–38, 1942.
20. Cooper, H. K.: Integration of services in the treatment of cleft lip and cleft palate. J. Am. Dent. Assoc., *47*:27–32, 1953.
21. Cooper, H. K.: Ministry of service. Am. J. Orthod., *52*:599–607, 1966.

22. Cooper, H. K.: Oral aspects of rehabilitation. J. Am. Coll. Dent., 52:52–59, 1960.
23. Cooper, H. K.: Recent trends in the management of the individual with oral-facial and speech handicaps. Am. J. Orthod., 49:683–700, 1963.
24. Cooper, H. K., Long, R. E., Cooper, J. A., Mazaheri, M., and Millard, R. T.: Psychological, orthodontic, and prosthetic approaches in rehabilitation of the cleft palate patient. Dent. Clin. North Am., 4:381–393, 1960.
25. Council on Orthodontic Education of the American Association of Orthodontists: Orthodontics: Principles and Policies, Educational Requirements, Organizational Structure. St. Louis, American Association of Orthodontists, 1968.
26. Coupe, T. B., and Subtelny, J. D.: Cleft palate, deficiency or displacement of tissue? Plast. Reconstr. Surg., 26:600–612, 1960.
27. Crikelair, G., Price, R., and Cosman, B.: Hourglass maxillary collapse in repaired post-alveolar clefts of the palate. Cleft Palate J., 9:13–17, 1972.
28. Derichsweiler, H.: Early orthodontic treatment of the cleft palate patient as related to the prevention of jaw abnormalities. In Hotz, R. (ed.): Early Treatment of Cleft Lip and Palate. Berne, Hans Huber Medical Publishers, 132–138, 1964.
29. DesPrez, J. D., and Kiehn, C. L.: Surgical positioning of the maxilla. In Georgiade, N. G. (ed.): Symposium on Management of Cleft Lip and Palate and Associated Deformities. St. Louis, C. V. Mosby Co., 222–227, 1974.
30. Dewel, B. F.: Serial extraction in orthodontics: Indications, objections, and treatment procedures. Int. J. Orthod., 40:906–926, 1954.
31. Dewel, B. F.: Serial extraction: Its limitations and contraindications in orthodontic treatment. Am. J. Orthod., 53:904, 1967.
32. Dickson, D. R., Grant, J. C. B., Sicher, H., DuBrul, E. L., and Paltan, J.: Status of research in cleft palate anatomy and physiology. July, 1973 – Part 1, Section III, maxillary growth and development. Cleft Palate J., 11:486–492, 1974.
33. Dignam, P. F.: Orthodontic treatment in the late mixed and permanent dentition for the cleft palate patient. Trans. Eur. Orthod. Soc., 575–578, 1973.
34. Fish, J.: Effects of bone grafting on orthodontic tooth movement in children with cleft lip and palate. Br. Dent. J., 135:373–376, 1973.
35. Fishman, L. S.: Dentistry's responsibility to the cleft palate patient. N. Y. State Dent. J., 35:467–479, 1969.
36. Georgiade, N. G.: Mandibular osteotomy for the correction of facial disproportion in the cleft lip and palate patient. In Georgiade, N. G. (ed.): Symposium on Management of Cleft Lip and Palate and Associated Deformities. St. Louis, C. V. Mosby Co., 238–241, 1974.
37. Georgiade, N. G. (ed.): Symposium on Management of Cleft Lip and Palate and Associated Deformities. St. Louis, C. V. Mosby Co., 1974.
38. Georgiade, N. G., and Latham, R. A.: Intra-oral traction for positioning the pre-maxilla in the bilateral cleft lip. In Georgiade, N. G. (ed.): Symposium on Management of Cleft Lip and Palate and Associated Deformities. St. Louis, C. V. Mosby Co., 123–127, 1974.
39. Georgiade, N. G., and Latham, R. A.: Maxillary arch alignment in the bilateral cleft lip and palate infant using the pinned coaxial screw appliance. Plast. Reconstr. Surg., 56:52–59, 1975.
40. Georgiade, N. G., Pickrell, K. L., and Quinn, G. W.: Varying concepts in bone grafting of alveolar palatal defects. Cleft Palate J., 1:43–51, 1964.
41. Gorlin, R. J., and Pindborg, J. J.: Syndromes of the Head and Neck. New York, McGraw-Hill Book Co., 1964.
42. Grabb, W. C., Rosenstein, S. W., and Bzoch, K. R. (eds.): Cleft Lip and Palate. Boston, Little, Brown and Co., 1971.
43. Graber, T. M.: Craniofacial morphology in cleft palate and cleft lip deformities. Surg. Gynecol. Obstet., 88:359–369, 1949.
44. Graber, T. M., and Swain, B. F. (eds.): Current Orthodontic Concepts and Techniques. Philadelphia, W. B. Saunders Co., 1975.
45. Graf-Pinthus, B., and Bettex, M.: Long-term observation following pre-surgical orthopedic treatment in complete clefts of the lip and palate. Cleft Palate J., 11:253–260, 1974.
46. Graf-Pinthus, B., and Bettex, M.: Maxillary segmental stability in cleft lip and palate subjects. Cleft Palate J., 6:54–58, 1969.
47. Greulich, W. W., and Pyle, S. D.: Radiographic Atlas of Skeletal Development of the Hand and Wrist. Stanford, Stanford University Press, 1959.
48. Grewe, J., and Hermanson, P.: Influence of severity of malocclusion on the duration of orthodontic treatment. Am. J. Orthod., 63:533–536, 1973.
49. Hagerty, R.: Cleft lip repair, its orthodontic significance. Angle Orthod., 27:1–10, 1957.
50. Hagerty, R., Andrews, E., Hill, M., Calcote, C., Karesh, S., Lifschiz, J., and Swindler, D.: Dental arch collapse in cleft palate. Angle Orthod., 34:25–35, 1964.
51. Hall, A. M.: Some orthodontic problems associated with cleft lip and palate. Br. J. Orthod., 3:239–243, 1976.

52. Hanada, K., and Krogman, W.: A longitudinal study of postoperative changes in the soft tissue profile in bilateral cleft lip and palate from birth to six years. Am. J. Orthod., 67:363–376, 1975.

53. Handelman, C., and Pruzansky, S.: Occlusion and dental profile with complete bilateral cleft lip and palate. Angle Orthod., 38:185–198, 1968.

54. Harding, R., and Mazaheri, M.: Growth and spatial changes in the arch form in bilateral cleft lip and palate patients. Plast. Reconstr. Surg., 50:591–599, 1972.

55. Harvold, E. P., Vargervik, J., and Chierici, G.: Primate experiments on oral sensation and dental malocclusions. Am. J. Orthod., 63:494–508, 1973.

56. Hayashi, I., Sakuda, M., Takimoto, K., and Miyazaki, T.: Craniofacial growth in complete unilateral cleft lip and palate: a roentgenocephalometric study. Cleft Palate J., 13:215–237, 1976.

57. Hellquist, R.: Early maxillary orthopedics in relation to maxillary cleft repair by periosteoplasty. Cleft Palate J., 8:36–55, 1971.

58. Hellquist, R.: The influence of periosteoplasty on dental orthopedics. Trans. Eur. Orthod. Soc., 559–561, 1973.

59. Horton, C. E.: The prevention of maxillary collapse in congenital lip and palate cases. Cleft Palate J., 1:25–30, 1964.

60. Hotz, M.: Aims and possibilities of pre- and post-surgical orthopedic treatment in uni- and bilateral clefts. Trans. Eur. Orthod. Soc., 553–558, 1973.

61. Hotz, M.: Pre- and early post-operative growth guidance in cleft lip and palate cases by maxillary orthopedics (an alternative procedure to primary bone grafting). Cleft Palate J., 7:368–372, 1969.

62. Hotz, M., and Gnoinski, W.: Comprehensive cure of cleft lip and palate children at Zurich University: A preliminary report. Am. J. Orthod., 70:481–504, 1976.

63. Huddart, A. G.: Observations on the treatment of cleft lip and palate. Dent. Practit., 16:265–274, 1970.

64. Innis, C. O.: Some preliminary observations on unoperated hare-lips and cleft palates in adult members of the Dusan tribes of North Borneo. Br. J. Plast. Surg., 15:173–181, 1962.

65. Ishiguro, K., Krogman, W., Mazaheri, M., and Harding, R.: A longitudinal study of morphological craniofacial patterns via P-A x-ray headfilms in cleft patients from birth to six years of age. Cleft Palate J., 13:104–126, 1976.

66. Johnston, M. C.: Orthodontic treatment for the cleft palate patient. Am. J. Orthod., 44:750–763, 1958.

67. Jolleys, A., and Robertson, N.: A study of the effects of early bone grafting in complete clefts of the lip and palate—five year study. Br. J. Plast. Surg., 25:229–237, 1972.

68. Jordan, R., Kraus, B., and Neptune, C.: Dental abnormalities associated with cleft lip and/or palate. Cleft Palate J., 3:22–55, 1966.

69. Keith, Sir Arthur: Wolff's Law of Bone Transformation. In Keith, Sir Arthur: Menders of the Maimed. Chapt. XVIII, Philadelphia, J. B. Lippincott Co., 277–289, 1952.

70. Kingsley, N. W.: Treatise on Oral Deformities as a Branch of Mechanical Surgery. New York, D. Appleton and Co., 1880.

71. Kling, A.: Evaluation of results with reference to the bite. In Hotz, R. (ed.): Early Treatment of Cleft Lip and Palate. Berne, Hans Huber Medical Publishers, 193–197, 1964.

72. Kraus, B., Jordan, R., and Pruzansky, S.: Dental abnormalities in the deciduous and permanent dentitions of individuals with cleft lip and palate. J. Dent. Res., 45:1736–1746, 1966.

73. Kremenak, C. R., Huffman, W. C., and Olin, W. H.: Growth of maxillae in dogs after palatal surgery: I. Cleft Palate J., 4:6–17, 1967.

74. Krischer, J., O'Donnell, J., and Shiere, F.: Changing cleft width: a problem revisited. Am. J. Orthod., 67:647–659, 1975.

75. Krogman, W.: Lancaster Cleft Palate Clinic joins Pennsylvania State University. Am. J. Orthod., 96:675–678, 1974.

76. Krogman, W., Mazaheri, M., Harding, R., Ishiguro, K., Buriana, G., Meier, J., Canter, H., and Ross, P.: A longitudinal study of the craniofacial growth pattern in children with clefts as compared to normal, birth to six years. Cleft Palate J., 12:59–83, 1975.

77. Krogman, W., Meier, J., Canter, H., Ross, P., Mazaheri, M., and Mehta, S.: Craniofacial serial dimensions related to age, sex, and cleft-type from six months of age to two years. Growth, 39:195–208, 1975.

78. Latham, R.: A new concept of the early maxillary growth mechanism. Trans. Eur. Orthod. Soc., 53–63, 1968.

79. Latham, R., and Burston, W. R.: The effect of unilateral cleft of the lip and palate on maxillary growth pattern. Br. J. Plast. Surg., 17:10–17, 1964.

80. Latham, R., Kusy, R., and Georgiade, N.: An extraorally activated expansion appliance for cleft palate infants. Cleft Palate J., 13:253–261, 1976.

81. Lauterstein, A. M., and Mendelsohn, M.: An analysis of the caries experience of 285 cleft palate children. Cleft Palate J., *1*:314–319, 1964.

82. Lubit, E.: Cleft palate orthopedics: why, when, how. Am. J. Orthod., *69*:562–571, 1976.

83. Mapes, A. H., Mazaheri, M., Harding, R. L., Meier, J. A., and Canter, H. E.: A longitudinal analysis of the maxillary growth increments of cleft lip and palate patients (CLP). Cleft Palate J., *11*:450–462, 1974.

84. Mazaheri, M.: Specific dental responsibilities in the cleft palate team and coordinating of dental care: long-term planning. Cleft Palate J., 7:459–464, 1969.

85. Mazaheri, M., and Sahni, P.: Techniques of cephalometry, photography, and oral impressions for infants. J. Prosth. Dent.,*21*:315–323, 1969.

86. Mazaheri, M., Harding, R., and Nanda, S.: The effects of surgery on maxillary growth and cleft width. Plast. Reconstr. Surg., *40*:22–30, 1967.

87. Mazaheri, M., Harding, R., Cooper, J., Meier, J., and Jones, T.: Changes in arch form and dimensions of cleft patients. Am. J. Orthod., *60*:19–32, 1971.

88. Mazaheri, M., Nanda, S., and Sassouni, V.: Comparison of midfacial development of children with clefts with their siblings. Cleft Palate J., *4*:334–341, 1967.

89. McKee, T.: A cephalometric radiographic study of tongue position in individuals with cleft palate deformity. Angle Orthod., *26*:99–109, 1956.

90. McNeil, C. K.: Oral and Facial Deformity. London, Sir Isaac Pitman and Sons, 1954.

91. Menius, J. A., Largent, M. D., and Vincent, C. J.: Skeletal development of cleft palate children as determined by hand-wrist roentgenographs: A preliminary study. Cleft Palate J., *3*:67–75, 1966.

92. Mestre, J. C., DeJesus, J., and Subtelny, J. D.: Unoperated oral clefts at maturation. Angle Orthod., *30*:78–85, 1960.

93. Monroe, C. W.: Management of the protruding pre-maxilla. *In* Georgiade, N. G. (ed.): Symposium on Management of Cleft Lip and Palate and Associated Deformities. St. Louis, C. V. Mosby Co., 103–110, 1974.

94. Monroe, C. W.: Use of bone grafts in complete clefts of the alveolar ridge. *In* Georgiade, N. G. (ed.): Symposium on Management of Cleft Lip and Palate and Associated Deformities. St. Louis, C. V. Mosby Co., 242–247, 1974.

95. Monroe, C. W., and Rosenstein, S. W.: Maxillary orthopedics and bone grafting in cleft palate. *In* Grabb, W. C., Rosenstein, S. W., and Bzoch, K. R. (eds.): Cleft Lip and Palate. Boston, Little, Brown and Co., 573–583, 1971.

96. Moore, W. J., and LaVelle, C. L. B.: Growth of the Facial Skeleton in the Hominoidea. New York, Academic Press, 1974.

97. Moorrees, C. F. A., and Grøn, A. M.: Principles of orthodontic diagnosis. Angle Orthod., *36*:258–262, 1966.

98. Moss, M. L.: Malformations of the skull base associated with cleft palate deformity. Plast. Reconstr. Surg., *17*:226–234, 1956.

99. Moss, M. L.: The functional matrix. *In* Kraus, B. S., and Riedel, R. A. (eds.): Vistas in Orthodontics. Philadelphia, Lea and Febiger, 1962.

100. Moss, M. L., Bromberg, B. E., Song, I. C., and Eisenmann, G.: The passive role of nasal septal cartilage in midfacial growth. Plast. Reconstr. Surg., *41*:536–542, 1968.

101. Norden, E., Linder-Aronson, S., and Stenberg, T.: The deciduous dentition after only primary surgical operations for clefts of the lip, jaw, and palate. Am. J. Orthod., *63*:229–236, 1973.

102. Nordin, K. E., and Johansen, B.: Freie knochen-transplantation bei Defekten im Alveolarkam nach Kieferorthopädischer Einstellung der maxilla bei Lippen-Kiefer-gaumenspalten. Fortschr. Keifer-u, Gesichtschr., *1*:168, 1955.

103. Obwegeser, H. L.: Eingriffe am Oberkiefer zur Korrektur des progenen Zustandsbildes. Schweiz. Monatschr. Zahnheilkd., *75*:365, 1965.

104. Obwegeser, H. L.: Surgery as an adjunct to orthodontics in normal and cleft palate patients. Trans Eur. Orthod. Soc., 343, 1967.

105. Obwegeser, H. L.: Surgical correction of small or retropositioned maxillae. Plast. Reconstr. Surg., *43*:351–365, 1969.

106. O'Donnell, J. P., Krischer, J. P., and Shiere, F. R.: An analysis of pre-surgical orthopedics in the treatment of cleft lip and palate. Cleft Palate J., *11*:367–373, 1974.

107. Olin, W. H.: Cleft lip and palate rehabilitation. Am. J. Orthod., *52*:126–144, 1966.

108. Olin, W. H.: Orthodontics. *In* Grabb, W. C., Rosenstein, S. W., and Bzoch, K. R. (eds.): Cleft Lip and Palate. Boston, Little, Brown and Co., 599–616, 1971.

109. Olin, W. H.: Timing of orthodontic treatment. *In* Georgiade, N. G. (ed.): Symposium on Management of Cleft Lip and Palate and Associated Deformities. St. Louis, C. V. Mosby Co., 248–249, 1974.

110. Olin, W. H.: Timing of orthodontic treatment. Trans. Eur. Orthod. Soc., 579–581, 1973.

111. Oliver, H.: Neonatal orthodontics. Trans. Eur. Orthod. Soc., 562–563, 1973.

112. Ortiz-Monasterio, F., Rebeh, A. S., Valderrama, M., and Cruz, R.: Cephalometric

measurements on adult patients with nonoperated cleft palates. Plast. Reconstr. Surg., *24*:53–61, 1959.

113. Ortiz-Monasterio, F., Serrano, A., Barrera, G., Rodriguez-Hoffman, H., and Vinageras, E.: A study of untreated cleft palate patients. Plast. Reconstr. Surg., *38*:36–41, 1966.
114. Peat, J.: Early orthodontic treatment for complete clefts. Am. J. Orthod., *65*:28–38, 1974.
115. Pedersen, G., and Blaho, D.: Total maxillary osteotomy for cleft palate rehabilitation. Oral Surg., *39*:669–685, 1975.
116. Pickrell, K., Quinn, G., and Massengill, R.: Primary bone grafting of the maxilla in clefts of the lip and palate. Plast. Reconstr. Surg., *41*:438–443, 1968.
117. Pierce, G., Terwilliger, K., Pennisi, Jr., Y., and Klabunde, H.: Early orthodontic treatment in cleft palate children. Angle Orthod., *26*:110–120, 1956.
118. Posen, A.: Some principles involved in orthodontic treatment of operated unilateral and bilateral complete cleft palate. Angle Orthod., *27*:109–113, 1957.
119. Proffit, W. R., and Mason, R. M.: Myofunctional therapy for tongue-thrusting: background and recommendations. J. Am. Dent. Assoc., *90*:403–411, 1975.
120. Proffit, W. R., McGlone, R. E., and Barrett, M. J.: Lip and tongue pressures as related to dental arch and oral cavity size in Australian aborigines. J. Dent. Res., *54*:1161–1172, 1975.
121. Pruzansky, S.: Factors determining arch form in clefts of the lip and palate. Am. J. Orthod., *41*:827–851, 1955.
122. Pruzansky, S.: Pre-surgical orthopedia and bone grafting for infants with clefts of the lip and palate: A dissent. Cleft Palate J., *1*:164–187, 1964.
123. Pruzansky, S.: The role of the orthodontist in a cleft palate team. Plast. Reconstr. Surg., *14*:10–29, 1954.
124. Pruzansky, S., and Aduss, H.: Arch form and the deciduous occlusion in complete unilateral clefts. Cleft Palate J., *1*:411–418, 1964.
125. Quinn, G.: Orthodontic treatment for the cleft palate child. Trans. Eur. Orthod. Soc., 567–570, 1973.
126. Quinn, G., Pickrell, K., and Massengill, R.: Treatment of mandibular prognathism in cleft palate patients. Am. J. Orthod., *59*:76–86, 1971.
127. Ranalli, D., and Mazaheri, M.: Height-weight growth of cleft children – birth to six years. Cleft Palate J., *12*:400–404, 1975.
128. Ricketts, R. M.: The cranial base and soft structures in cleft palate speech and breathing. Plast. Reconstr. Surg., *14*:47–61, 1954.
129. Ricketts, R.: Oral orthopedics for the cleft palate patient. Am. J. Orthod., *42*:401–408, 1956.
130. Robertson, N.: Early treatment – a critique. Trans. Eur. Orthod. Soc., 547–552, 1973.
131. Robertson, N.: Recent trends in the early treatment of cleft lip and palate. Dent. Practit., *21*:326–338, 1971.
132. Robertson, N., and Fish, J.: Early dimensional changes in the arches of cleft palate children. Am. J. Orthod., *67*:290–303, 1975.
133. Robertson, N., and Fish, J.: Some observations on rapid expansion followed by bone grafting in cleft lip and palate. Cleft Palate J., *9*:236–245, 1972.
134. Robertson, N., and Hilton, R.: The changes produced by pre-surgical oral orthopedics. Br. J. Plast. Surg., *24*:57–67, 1971.
135. Robertson, N., and Jolleys, A.: Effects of early bone grafting in complete clefts of lip and palate. Plast. Reconstr. Surg., *42*:414–421, 1968.
136. Rosenstein, S.: A new concept in the early orthopedic treatment of cleft lip and palate. Am. J. Orthod., *55*:765–775, 1969.
137. Rosenstein, S.: Early orthodontic procedures for cleft lip and palate individuals. Angle Orthod., *33*:127–137, 1963.
138. Rosenstein, S. W.: Management of the maxillary segments in complete unilateral cleft lip patients. *In* Georgiade, N. G. (ed.): Symposium on Management of Cleft Lip and Palate and Associated Deformities. St. Louis, C. V. Mosby Co., 43–46, 1974.
139. Rosenstein, S. W.: Management of the protruding pre-maxilla: maxillary orthopedics. *In* Georgiade, N. G. (ed.): Symposium on Management of Cleft Lip and Palate and Associated Deformities. St. Louis, C. V. Mosby Co., 118–122, 1974.
140. Rosenstein, S. W., Jacobson, B. N., Monroe, C., Griffith, B. H., and McKinney, P.: A series of cleft lip and palate children five years after undergoing orthopedic and bone grafting procedures. Angle Orthod., *42*:1–8, 1972.
141. Ross, R. B.: Cranial base in children with lip and palate clefts. Cleft Palate J., *2*:157–166, 1965.
142. Ross, R. B.: The clinical implications of facial growth in cleft lip and palate. Cleft Palate J., *7*:37–47, 1970.
143. Ross, R. B.: The management of dental arch deformity in cleft lip and palate. Clin. Plast. Surg., *2*:325–342, 1975.

144. Ross, R. B., and Johnston, M. C.: Cleft Lip and Palate. Baltimore, The Williams and Wilkins Co., 1972.
145. Ross, R. B., and Johnston, M. C.: The effects of early orthodontic treatment on facial growth in cleft lip and palate. Cleft Palate J., 4:157–164, 1967.
146. Sarnat, B. G.: Postnatal growth of the upper face: some experimental considerations. Angle Orthod., 33:139–161, 1963.
147. Sarnat, B. G., and Wexler, M. R.: Growth of the face and jaws after resection of the septal cartilage in rabbits. Am. J. Anat., 118:755–768, 1966.
148. Schmid, E.: Die Annaherung der Kieferstümpfe bei Lippenkiefer-Gaumenspalten; Ihre Schadlichen Folgen und Vermeidung. Fortschr. Keifer Gesichts. Chir., 1:37, 1955.
149. Scott, J. H.: The cartilage of the nasal septum. Br. Dent. J., 95:37–43, 1953.
150. Scott, J. H.: The growth of the human face. Proc. Roy. Soc. Med., 47:91–100, 1954.
151. Shiere, F. R., and Fisher, J. H.: Neonatal orthopedic correction for cleft lip and palate patients: A preliminary report. Cleft Palate J., 1:17–24, 1964.
152. Skoog, T.: The use of periosteal flaps in the repair of the primary palate. Cleft Palate J., 2:332–339, 1965.
153. Spira, M., Findlay, S., Hardy, S., and Gerow, F.: Early maxillary orthopedics in cleft palate patients: A clinical report. Cleft Palate J., 6:461–470, 1969.
154. Spriestersbach, D., Dickson, D., Fraser, F., Horowitz, S., McWilliams, B., Paradise, J., and Randall, P.: Clinical research in cleft lip and palate: The state of the art. Cleft Palate J., 10:113–164, 1973.
155. Stöckli, P.: Orthodontic planning and treatment in combination with secondary surgical procedures in cleft lip and palate. Trans. Eur. Orthod. Soc., 564–566, 1973.
156. Subcommittee on Dentistry: Cleft lip and cleft palate: research relevant to clinical management in dentistry. Am. J. Orthod., 63:398–406, 1973.
157. Subtelny, J.: Orthodontic treatment of cleft lip and palate, birth to adulthood. Angle Orthod., 36:273–292, 1966.
158. Subtelny, J.: The importance of early orthodontic treatment in cleft palate planning. Angle Orthod., 27:148–158, 1957.
159. Subtelny, J. D.: Width of the nasopharynx and related anatomic structures in normal and unoperated cleft palate children. Am. J. Orthod., 41:889–909, 1955.
160. Subtelny, J. D., and Brodie, A.: An analysis of orthodontic expansion in unilateral cleft lip and cleft palate patients. Am. J. Orthod., 40:686–697, 1954.
161. Swanson, L. T., McCollum, D. W., and Richardson, S. O.: Evaluation of the dental problems in the cleft palate patient. Am. J. Orthod., 42:749–765, 1956.
162. Swoiskin, B. L.: Discussion of paper by S. W. Rosenstein. Angle Orthod., 33:135–137, 1963.
163. Swoiskin, B. L.: Lower arch form in unilateral cleft palate. Angle Orthod., 27:124–132, 1957.
164. Troutman, K.: Maxillary arch control in infants with unilateral clefts of the lip and palate. Am. J. Orthod., 66:198–208, 1974.
165. Wood, B.: Control of the maxillary arch by primary bone graft in cleft lip and palate cases. Cleft Palate J., 7:194–205, 1970.

Chapter Eight

Of all the burdens that cleft palate inflicts upon the individual, by far the most troublesome is impairment of speech. Its severity and duration depend, of course, upon the extent of the anatomical and physiological defect and how soon it can be satisfactorily repaired. Regardless of what other measures are taken, the knowledge and skills of the speech pathologists are essential to a successful rehabilitation. In recent decades it has become apparent that the speech pathologists can be most effective if they enter into close association with other members of the cleft palate team quite early in the life of the affected child.

HISTORICAL BACKGROUND

During the 1930s and 1940s most children who had undergone surgery for cleft palate required speech therapy. But at that time it was common practice for surgeons to wait until the age of three or four to close the palate. Naturally the child had developed his language by age four and frequently had acquired compensatory articulation habits because of a constricted maxilla and a nonfunctional velopharyngeal port. His unoperated condition made it impossible for him to impound air within the oral cavity (Figure 8–1). Nasal air emission and hypernasal resonance could not be avoided.

When surgery was finally performed, the family as well as the surgeon were often dismayed to find that a dramatic change in tonal quality had not occurred with the closing of the cleft. The child frequently continued to talk very much as he had talked before the operation, with a "cleft palate speech." In many cases this was because his maladaptive speech habits had become so ingrained that his voice sounded "familiar" and "right" to him. If he did not recognize it as abnormal, this meant that he and the speech clinician were in for a long siege of therapy.

Several types of dental prostheses were used in the 1930s and 1940s as primary treatment for separating the oral and nasal cavities; however, the cleft problem was considered an exercise for the surgeon. If and when there was a breakdown in the surgical repair, the surgeon repeated his procedures in his effort to close the palatal defect. Some of the early patient histories at

THE PROCESSES OF SPEECH: EVALUATION AND TREATMENT

JOHN E. RISKI AND ROBERT T. MILLARD

the Institute record 10, 15, and 20 surgical procedures in attempting to close the oral defect (Figure 8–2). Hypernasal voice quality and maladaptive articulation habits were associated with these multiple surgical failures. Some surgeons felt that the next logical step after surgical management failed was to refer the patient to a prosthodontist. Few speech clinicians were available to the surgeon until the team concept of cleft palate management developed.

Certainly the early surgeons had their measure of success, but the percentage of good results was not to swell until the late 1950s and early 1960s, when plastic surgeons expressed their awareness of human growth and development of the midthird of the face. With this awareness they were able to improve their techniques and to time the surgical procedures to minimize interference with centers of facial growth. Lengthening the oral tissue and utilizing a vomer flap greatly reduced the trauma to maxillary segments. More important to speech development was the improved two-stage palatal closure technique, implemented before the child reached 18 months of age. These factors had a marked influence on the development of more normal speech and voice patterns in children with a cleft palate.

H. K. Cooper realized that no one treatment procedure was a panacea. But his team concept, which he began to implement in the 1930s, emphasized the varied advantages of interdisciplinary evaluation and treatment of cleft palate. He stressed the rehabilitative management of the total person, and as professional members of the interdisciplinary team, we realized we were dealing with an integrated part of the whole person. This is the concept that has been developed and continually stressed at the Lancaster Cleft Palate Clinic

It is our purpose in this chapter to present the role of the speech pathologist as he functions as a member of this team. Actually he fills several roles. He is a diagnostician, serving with his colleagues in establishing the precise nature of each patient's difficulties and capabilities; he participates in the decisions regarding the most appropriate treatment program; he conducts research in his area; and day by day he provides speech therapy.

As a speech pathologist he is specifically concerned with the oral communication status of the child with cleft lip or palate. What happens in the speech production and learning process as a result of this defect? What must

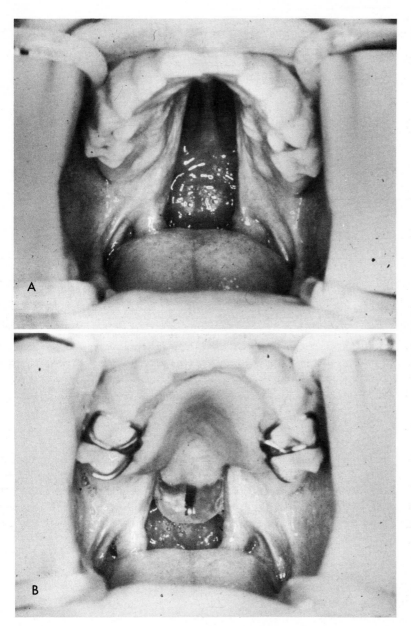

FIGURE 8-1 *A*, Preschool child with unoperated cleft of the hard and soft palate. *B*, The cleft is obturated with an appliance.

the child have, in terms of form and function, and what must he learn, if he is to speak clearly?

BEGINNINGS OF SPEECH

It is our view that to fully understand and evaluate disordered speech, the speech pathologist must first have a thorough knowledge of normal speech, or more broadly, the communication process. Communication may be regarded as the conveying of demands, requests, ideas, thoughts,

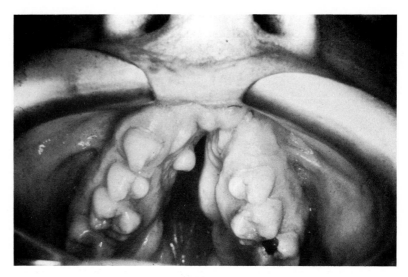

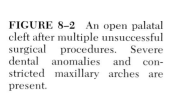
FIGURE 8–2 An open palatal cleft after multiple unsuccessful surgical procedures. Severe dental anomalies and constricted maxillary arches are present.

feelings, or opinions by a system of signs, signals, and symbols. We call this language. Oral communication is the expression of these signals and symbols in vocal form—mainly spoken words, but with occasional resort to cries and exclamations. Although a meaningful cry can be produced almost from the moment of birth, as a reflex response to an internal or external stimulus, speech is an acquired skill. And the sounds of speech must be learned aurally—through the sense of hearing—as a prerequisite to speaking them.

Learning to speak begins for the infant at a very early age, a few weeks or months after birth. While his first utterances hardly qualify as words, they become the ingredients of words. And if he has normal hearing and a capacity for learning, he possesses two of the three basic requisites of speech, the third being an adequate speech mechanism, which is the main concern of this book. Whether his vocal equipment is perfect or not, the infant employs both his ears and his voice as he becomes aware of himself and his surroundings.

He turns his head in the direction of a noise or a voice. He appears to enjoy the sounds of his own vocal play—cooing, chuckling, gurgling, laughing. As those near him respond with similar sounds, or more sophisticated ones—words—the infant begins to associate the sounds with familiar faces, and he learns to repeat certain syllables.

His first "word" usually evolves from one of his random noises. That it is often the word "mama" arises from the circumstance that the babbling labial sounds, "mum-mum-mum-mum," are among the first he makes in his spontaneous vocalizing. They are also the most visible. To the mother, whether her language is English, Spanish, Italian, German, or French, this sounds like the word she is most eager to hear. She thinks her baby is deliberately saying "mama," so she rewards him with a smile, a delighted "Go-o-o-d baby!" and another spoonful of applesauce. She may also coax out a repetition of the word "mama" by pressing the baby's lips together a few times with her fingers while she herself repeats it. The important point is that the sound, originally produced in vocal play, is now reinforced so that it soon becomes part of the child's repertoire of meaningful and useful words, his working vocabulary. In similar fashion the labial plosive sound "puh, puh, puh" becomes "papa."

By the age of nine months the infant is responding to his own name, or to the words "bye-bye" or "patacake." He listens with obvious interest to familiar words and he responds appropriately to simple requests. As his pleasure mounts at feeding time, so does his joyous vocalizing. He is soon articulating words as he babbles to himself and to others.

Briefly, this is the beginning of oral communication for the normal child, who by the time he is two years old will use a vocabulary of nearly 100 words and by the age of three will have increased it to 400 to 500. For the child with a cleft, the acquisition of a spoken language will proceed less smoothly and rapidly. Lip surgery at about 10 weeks will help to enhance the capacity to make labial sounds, but a cleft of the palate will require a great deal of attention from the various specialists participating in the habilitation of the child. The surgeon, dental specialist, speech pathologist, audiologist, social worker, and geneticist each perceive the specific dysfunction against his or her own background of knowledge and skill. Yet their success will depend in large measure upon the thoughtful integration of their skills to bring to the individual what he so urgently needs in order to achieve his full potential in today's society—the gift of speech.

SPEECH PRODUCTION

When we analyze speech, we perceive that it is the end result of several systems (Figure 8–3). It begins with respiration, which provides the power that vibrates the vocal cords. The resulting sound is modified by the resonators, namely, the walls of the pharyngeal, oral, and nasal cavities. It is further shaped by the movements of the articulators, the soft palate, the tongue, the mandible, the teeth, and the lips. Thus we arrive at the end product, fully formed speech sounds.

Let us examine the action at each of these levels in a little more detail. Respiration involves the activity of the muscles of the rib cage, abdomen, and diaphragm. During inhalation, in preparation for seven or eight seconds of speech, the contraction and lowering of the diaphragm and the movement of the external and internal intercostal muscles increase the size and volume of the rib cage, reducing the pressure on the lungs and thereby allowing air to flow into them.

Exhalation provides the necessary air pressure for producing speech. (In some foreign languages certain speech sounds are made on inhalation, but English is uttered only on the exhaled breath.) As the diaphragm and the external intercostals relax and the abdominal muscles tense, the air is expelled from the lungs. As it flows up through the trachea into the larynx, under pressure, it forces the adducted vocal cords apart and causes them to vibrate. As the air escapes and the pressure falls, the cords return to their closed position. If talking is to continue, the pressure is built up again and the cycle is repeated. This repeated cycle produces the sound we call voice.

The respiration cycle differs in breathing to sustain life from that in breathing to produce speech. Quiet breathing apportions equal time to inhaling and exhaling. In speaking, on the other hand, the breathing rate is

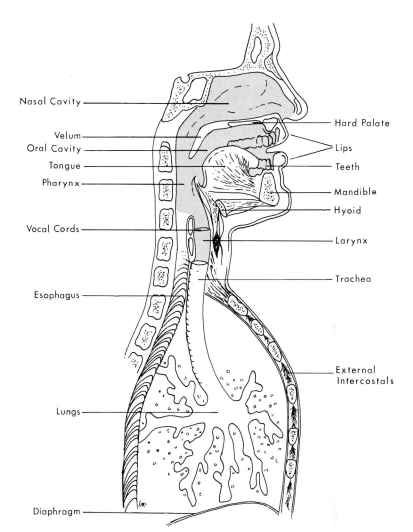

Nasal Cavity

Velum
Oral Cavity
Tongue
Pharynx

Vocal Cords

Esophagus

Lungs

Diaphragm

Hard Palate
Lips
Teeth
Mandible
Hyoid
Larynx
Trachea

External
Intercostals

FIGURE 8–3 Cross-section of human head, neck, and chest illustrating the organs of speech production.

regulated according to the air supply needs of phrase and sentence length (Figure 8–4). Since our speech takes place only on exhalation, we can devote up to 85 per cent of the cycle to exhaled talking, refilling the lungs with short inhalations in the remaining 15 per cent of the time.

The exhaled sound waves generated at the laryngeal level are not yet speech, however. As we have indicated, the sound or buzz resonates in the chambers of the pharyngeal, oral, and nasal cavities, and it is given additional selective molding by alterations in the size, shape, and tenseness of these chambers. The relative dimensions of the three sections of the pharynx—the epipharynx, the oropharynx, and the nasopharynx—are changed by the rising and lowering of the larynx (particularly noticeable in a man's "Adam's apple" as he shifts his speaking or singing pitch from high to low) and by the tension of the pharyngeal muscles. The lowering and closing of the mandible and the changing shape of the oral cavity with movements of the tongue also influence resonance, as does the shape of the hard palate in conjunction with the flexibility and mobility of the soft palate.

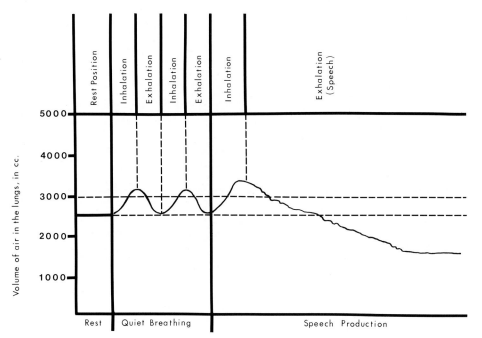

FIGURE 8-4   Graphic representation of inhalation-exhalation intervals for quiet breathing and for speech productions.

These factors determine the quality of the voice tone, the characteristic generally believed to give each person his own remarkably distinctive, recognizable, and identifiable "voice." When the resonating sound is further tuned and sharpened by the lips, teeth, and tongue, a process we call articulation, the speech sounds—vowels and consonants—issue as completely enunciated words.

It is important to appreciate at this point that in the series of complex adjustments required for speech—adjustments learned, with some variations, by the speakers of any language—a velopharyngeal incompetency can cause deviation at each level of speech production. The respiratory cycle in a speaker with VPI is influenced by loss of air during speech at the level of the larynx and the velopharyngeal valve. Vocal effort and the closed cycle of the vocal cords are increased. Resonance is influenced by nasal coupling and very probably by compensatory placement of the tongue. Articulation is influenced by the loss of intraoral air pressure and by assorted dental and occlusal anomalies.

If then, aberrations occur at these levels, and our current understanding is that they do, the speech pathologist must be aware of this and be able to evaluate speech production at each level, if necessary. He must understand normal function and the sometimes complicated interactions among the components at the several levels.

Phonology

To carry the description of the speech process on into more detailed analysis of the different oral sounds and syllables themselves, it will be helpful to consider the phonological and morphological substrata of language. Phonology is the study of the phonemes or sounds of a language. Some sounds are found only in certain languages, while others are shared by many languages. A child learns the sounds of his parents' language in a rather orderly fashion, although not all children will learn them at the same rate (Figure 8–5). The youngster first learns to distinguish and then to produce sounds of universal or large contrasts, such as vowels on the one hand and consonants on the other Gradually he masters finer or more specific distinctions, as between /s/ and /z/, which differ only in that /s/ is unvoiced and /z/ is voiced. The process of learning a phonological system usually begins in the first year of life and is completed in the eighth year. The average eight-year-old will use "adult" articulation or sound production.

The phonological system used in the English language comprises approximately 17 vowel sounds (including six diphthongs) and 25 consonant sounds. These phonemes are identified by the characters adopted as the International Phonetic Alphabet (IPA).

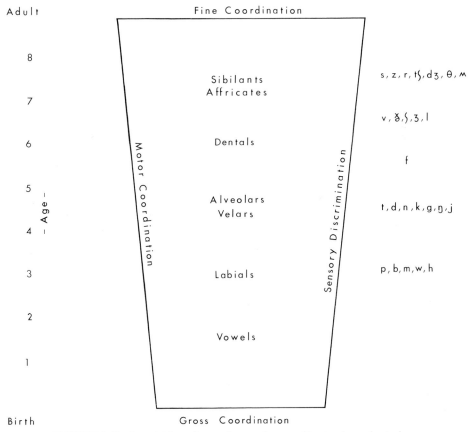

FIGURE 8–5 Acquisition of speech sounds according to chronological age.

Vowel Sounds

The vowel sounds originate with the vibrations of the vocal cords and are modified, as we have just said, as the vibrating column of air passes through the resonating chambers. A principal factor here is the movement of the tongue in the oral cavity (a resonator), which produces changes in the size of that resonator and influences what we perceive as vowel sounds. We can create 11 vowels and six diphthongs in English, primarily by the positioning of the tongue, although the lips and pharynx are also important in some sounds. We protrude or round the lips, for example, to say "oo" /u/ and retract them against the teeth to say "ee" /i/.

Table 8–1 presents a list of words that illustrate the most commonly used vowels and diphthongs in English. The symbols opposite the words are the corresponding International Phonetic Alphabet (IPA) characters for each vowel or diphthong.

As you can see by the symbols adjacent to each diphthong, a diphthong is a continuous sound made by a transition from one simple vowel sound to another.

A convenient way to describe tongue position for vowel production is by use of a quadrangle (Figure 8–6). The quadrangle graphically depicts each vowel by tongue position, and from this diagram we can see the necessary transitions for diphthong production. For example, the / ɔɪ / in boy involves moving the tongue from a mid-back position for the / ɔ / element to a high front position in the mouth for the / ɪ / element.

Tongue position is an important variable because, as we will see later, the positions of the tongue, jaw, and velum are all interrelated. In addition, a high tongue position such as in /i/ or BEET may constrict the oral cavity enough to force the resonance flow nasally. In evaluating for nasal resonance we will want to use a speech sample with vowel sounds from the four corners of the vowel quadrangle, e.g , BEET, BAT, BOOT, and BOUGHT.

Consonant Sounds

The consonantal sounds in English are responsible for most of the information we use in recognizing a word. In a way this is unfortunate, for most consonants are weaker than vowels. They are not so loud and they are of shorter duration. While all vowels require voice (vocal cord vibration), some consonants are voiced and some are voiceless. Most of the consonants, however, demand some degree of oral pressure for their production.

Velopharyngeal incompetency (VPI) may have two effects on consonantal production. If present during voiced consonantal production, it can influ-

TABLE 8-1 Pronunciation Key: American-English Vowels and Diphthongs

VOWELS				DIPHTHONGS	
beat	/i/	put	/ʊ/	bait	/eɪ/
bit	/ɪ/	boot	/u/	bite	/aɪ/
bet	/ɛ/	but	/ʌ/	bout	/aʊ/
bat	/æ/	bird	/ɝ/	boat	/oʊ/
balm	/ɑ/	sofa	/ə/	bay	/eɪ/
bought	/ɔ/			pew	/ɪu/

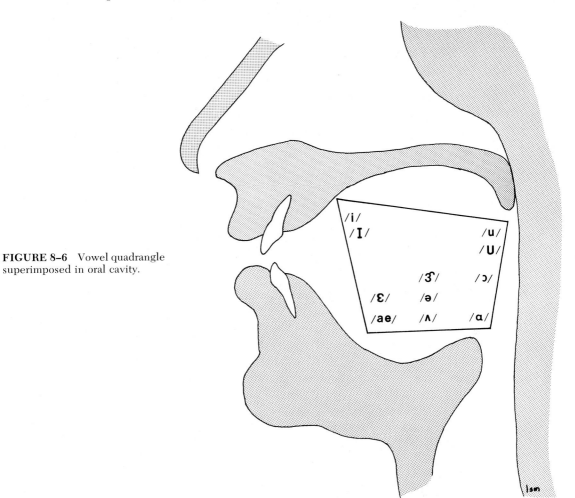

FIGURE 8-6 Vowel quadrangle superimposed in oral cavity.

ence the increase of nasal resonance. If a VPI exists during voiceless pressure consonantal production, one might perceive nasal air emission or weak consonantal production.

Although many of the IPA symbols for the consonantal sounds are identical to the graphemic characters of English, several are not. Listed in Table 8-2 are the consonantal phonemic symbols with a key word. The grapheme in the word that the phoneme represents is italicized.

TABLE 8-2   Pronunciation Key: American-English Consonants

*b*oy	/b/	*l*ove	/l/	vi*si*on	/ʒ/
*d*o	/d/	*m*e	/m/	*t*ie	/t/
*j*ump	/dʒ/	*n*o	/n/	*ch*air	/tʃ/
*f*un	/f/	si*ng*	/ŋ/	*th*is	/ð/
*g*un	/g/	*p*ie	/p/	*th*in	/θ/
*h*orse	/h/	*r*ose	/r/	*v*ase	/v/
*y*es	/j/	*s*un	/s/	*w*e	/w/*
*c*at	/k/	*sh*oe	/ʃ/	*z*oo	/z/

*Many American speakers substitute /w/, as in *w*att, for /ʍ/, as in *wh*at; therefore, /ʍ/ has been omitted.

TABLE 8–3   Place and Manner Classification of American-English Consonants

PLACE	MANNER*						
	Pressure					*Nonpressure*	
	Plosive		*Fricative*		*Affricative*		*Semivowel*	*Nasal*
	uv[1]	v[2]	uv	v	uv	v	v	v
Bilabial	p	b					w	m
Labial Dental			f	v				
Lingual Dental			θ	ð				
Lingual Alveolar	t	d	s	z			l	n
Palatal			ʃ	ʒ	tʃ	dʒ	j	
Velar	k	g					r	ŋ
Glottal		ʔ[3]	h					
Pharyngeal			ħ[4]					

*1 = unvoiced; 2 = voiced; 3 = glottal; 4 = pharyngeal fricative.

Consonants are also best summarized if plotted by place of articulation. Unlike vowels (which are all produced essentially in the same manner) consonants may be produced in various ways. Table 8–3 presents a list of English consonants plotted by manner of production and place of articulation. The place of articulation is stated on the vertical column. A bilabial is produced by articulation of the lips, a lingual alveolar by articulation of the tongue against the alveolar ridge, and so forth. The manner of production is denoted along the horizontal. When a sound is voiced, it indicates that there is vocal cord vibration during its production. An unvoiced sound has no vocal cord vibration. A plosive or affricative consonant is produced when the two articulators are brought together to close off air flow, and then released explosively. A fricative sound is produced by approximating the two articulators closely enough to cause turbulence of the air stream, but not closely enough to stop air flow. A nasal is produced when the oral cavity is occluded and the velum is lowered, so as to force the voiced sound through the nasal cavity.

The group of sounds noted as pressure sounds (plosives, fricatives, and affricates) requires velopharyngeal seal. There is evidence that these sounds cannot be learned without this seal.

VELOPHARYNX

This brings us to one of the most critical anatomical and physiological problems with which the child with a palatal cleft must contend. Normally the nasal cavity is not a resonator for speech; it is separated from the remainder of the vocal tract at the level of the nasopharynx by the valve-like action of the velum and the pharyngeal walls. But an inadequate or insufficient velopharyngeal valve may prohibit occlusion at the nasopharynx. A fistula (hole) in either the hard or soft palate may also allow introduction of unwanted air and sound waves into the nasal cavity and produce the abnormal pattern we have termed "hypernasal resonance." (The velopharyngeal valve operates to close the nasal cavity off from the lower part of the vocal tract for all English speech sounds except the nasal /m/, /n/, and /ŋ/.

"Velopharyngeal inadequacy," as we at the Clinic use the term, is the shortness of tissues in the nasopharyngeal region, an organic deficiency. "Velopharyngeal incompetency" is poor function in spite of adequate substance or tissue. Either condition may be referred to as "velopharyngeal insufficiency" or "VPI."

If a VPI exists during the early years of a child's speech development, he may, as we mentioned at the opening of this chapter, adopt compensatory or maladaptive articulatory habits. Frequently the child will learn to valve the air stream below the level of the insufficient valve. Two common compensatory articulations that result are the glottal stop /ɔ/, as in "uh huh," an audible obstruction of the air stream at the level of the glottis, and the pharyngeal fricative /ħ/. The latter appears to be produced by the approximation of the tongue and the pharyngeal wall. Glottal stops are typically substituted for oral plosive sounds, and pharyngeal fricatives for oral fricative sounds.

In view of the central importance of the velopharyngeal mechanism in the speech production of the individual with cleft palate, it will be helpful to examine the origins of our information about it before proceeding to the present-day techniques of evaluation and management.

The importance of this valve's functioning has been appreciated for several hundred years. However, the precise operation of the velopharyngeal valve is not fully understood even today. (Much of the following account is taken from the historical survey of the study of the velopharyngeal mechanism by Fritzell.[9])

Speech was first studied as a science by the ancient Greeks, who had a basic understanding of respiratory function, voice production, resonance, and articulation. However, rhetoric and public address were the fostered arts in their society, and more attention was directed to syntax and grammar than to the production of speech.

Leonardo da Vinci (1452–1519) was the first to draw the soft palate and to discuss its function. He stated that vowels were formed with the posterior part of the movable palate. Soft palate function was more correctly delineated by Fallopio (1523–1562), who observed that a perforation of the palate was detrimental to voice quality. He also noted that disease of the uvula alone does not affect voice, but that abnormalities of the soft palate must also be involved.

Not until the eighteenth century was the velopharyngeal mechanism recognized as responsible for speech quality. During that century speech sounds were analyzed and divided into nasal (/m/ /n/) and nonnasal sounds. About this time, assimilation nasality, the effect of nasal sounds on preceding or following vowels, was identified.

In the nineteenth century velopharyngeal function was first observed directly through a defect in the face. The velum and posterior pharyngeal wall were found to move actively toward each other during speech and respiration, while the lateral pharyngeal walls were active also during deglutition. Study of the velopharyngeal mechanism continued throughout this century. Interestingly enough, techniques for evaluating nasal air emission and nasal resonance were very similar to techniques used today. Observations of velar movement elevation were made then with simple, yet clever techniques, and those early observations have not been altered, but only reinforced by the most sophisticated of present-day equipment.

Nasal air emission was tested for by observing the flicker of a candle flame and the fogging of a cold mirror held under the patient's nose. Hypernasal resonance was evaluated in the late nineteenth century by pinching a patient's nose as he produced alternating /i/ and /u/ sounds. If voice quality changed when the nose was pinched, this was considered indicative of velopharyngeal insufficiency. This is the cul-de-sac test described in more detail later in the section on evaluation of velopharyngeal insufficiency.

The height of the velum during vowel production was further documented by introducing a small wire along the floor of the nasal cavity. The deflections of the wire were observed and found to be greatest for /i/ and least for /ɑ/. This was shortly confirmed in an experiment in which water was instilled into the nose during vowel production. When the individual said "/ɑ/," water passed into the oropharynx, but the water remained in the nasopharynx for the production of all other vowels.

Knowledge that a velopharyngeal gap of 20 mm.^{2} is necessary to interfere with speech production was hinted at in the nineteenth century. Rubber tubes with inner cross-sectional areas of 12.6 mm.^{2} and 28.3 mm.^{2} were introduced between the soft palate and the posterior pharyngeal wall. It was reported that the 12.6-mm.^{2} tube did not appreciably alter speech, while the 28.3 mm.^{2} tube interfered with consonant production (Passavant, 1863). A number of other unique experiments confirmed these results and refined the current knowledge of velopharyngeal physiology.

With the advent of radiographic procedures at the close of the nineteenth century and beginning of the twentieth, investigators reconfirmed many of these early observations and further advanced our understanding of speech physiology. In 1955 Cooper and Hofmann[5] first reported the use of cineradiography with image intensification (Figure 8–7). This system electronically intensifies a weak radiographic image and, therefore, allows radiographic techniques to be employed with minimal radiation dosages. Since then, cineradiography with image intensification has become a most valuable instrument for clinical and research evaluations of normal and abnormal speech physiology.

It is a valuable assessment tool because it allows dynamic rather than static observation of the speech articulators. With the use of cineradiography, we have learned that velopharyngeal function during sustained vowel production is not unfailingly predictive of function during connected speech. A sustained vowel frequently will be phonated with the valve slightly open, or closure may be attained and released. Since a primary purpose of the evaluative procedure is to recommend a treatment correcting nasal air emission or hypernasal resonance during connected speech, the best evaluative procedure would be to observe the valve during connected speech behavior.

The value of cineradiography has been further extended by taking the craniometric procedure of plotting points and distances and adapting it to use with the cineradiographic films. (A compilation of these points and measurements can be found in the Appendix of Chapter 2.)

Cineradiography does have some restrictions. It projects a three-dimensional object in only two dimensions. However, techniques of radiographic filming in the anteroposterior plane, such as frontal or basilar cineradiography, when used in conjunction with lateral radiographic techniques,

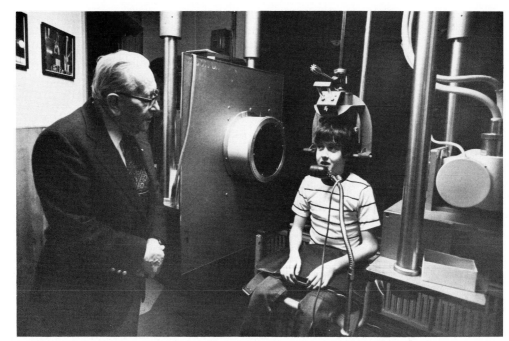

FIGURE 8–7   Dr. Herbert Cooper with the cineradiographic unit in use at the H. K. Cooper Institute.

should help provide invaluable information regarding a more complete three-dimensional velopharyngeal port function. Unquestionably the application of motion picture x-ray techniques to our studies has given us a much clearer understanding of what the speech structures look like as they are performing during speech.

It has helped us to define certain variations in velar function, for example. The fact that the velum functions differently in sustained phonation and in connected speech has both clinical and research implications. Velar elevation has been found to correlate with tongue height for vowel production. That is, both velum and tongue are higher for such high vowels as /i/ than for low vowels such as /ɑ/. Velar configuration during closure for speech sound production also appears to be dependent on the sex and age of the speaker.

As to tongue positioning for vowels and consonants, here, too, cineradiography has shed better light than did still x-ray films. It has also brought about a general appreciation of the independent yet complementary or compensatory actions between the tongue and the mandible. Cineradiographic research has shown that tongue placement for production of vowel phonemes progresses from a high, front position for /i/ as in BEET, to low, front for /æ/ as in BAT, and high, back for /u/ as in BOOT, to low, back for /ɑ/ as in BALM. More recently it has been demonstrated that velar contact with the posterior pharyngeal wall is greater for high vowels such as /i/ or "EE" than for low vowels such as /ɑ/ or "AH." Further studies have reaffirmed that the velum elevates more for high vowels than it does for low vowels.

It is interesting to note that non-cleft speakers are judged more nasal on low vowel sounds, while a cleft individual is judged more nasal on the high vowel sounds. This at first seems incongruous, and it probably represents two distinct phenomena. In the non-cleft speakers the velum is lowered and achieves less velopharyngeal contact during low vowel production. Thus, the chance for sound resonance to enter the nasal cavity is increased. However, in the speaker with cleft palate a high tongue position constricts the oral cavity and forces more sound energy into the nasal cavity.

Investigators have reported other variations of physiology and nasality judgment with regard to specific phonetic or physiological factors in non-cleft speakers. The velum has been observed to achieve a fuller velopharyngeal contact during vowel production when that vowel is in an oral consonant environment than when it is in a nasal consonant environment. There is a differentiation in the perception of nasality among oral consonants. Voiceless plosive consonants such as /p/ are judged less nasal than voiceless fricatives such as /s/. This information becomes critical when developing a speech sample to evaluate velar port function either acoustically or radiographically, an application we shall discuss later.

The materials and techniques for obtaining cinefluorographic films at the Cooper Institute have been described previously by Cooper and Hofmann[5] and by Cooper.[4] The instrumentation has been updated as technology advances, but the purpose of the system remains the same, that is, to evaluate the oral speech structures in order to plan management procedures and determine their postmanagement effects.

Warren and Hofmann[28] utilized these techniques to study the physiology of the velopharyngeal mechanism of 37 non-cleft individuals at the Clinic. These researchers demonstrated that the velum exhibits an oscillatory motion as it moves to occlude the nasopharynx and that the velum may not always maintain closure of the nasopharynx throughout phonation of an isolated sound (Figure 8–8). They found an inverse relationship between the length of the velum and velar elevation. However, they found no relationship between length of the soft palate and pharyngeal depth. They demonstrated further that velar elevation varies for sound production /i/ and /u/ and for blowing Finally, the posterior pharyngeal wall appears immobile in normal non-cleft speakers.

Physiological differences in the oral speech apparatus between cleft and[12] non-cleft individuals have been studied with cineradiography by Mazaheri, Millard, and Ericson. The velum was observed to be longer and thicker in the normal group, but there was no significant difference between experimental and normal individuals in the depth of the nasopharynx (Table 8–4). The arithmetic difference in the means of the soft palate length and the depth of the nasopharynx between the normal and an experimental VPI group was significant, however. The amount of residual velopharyngeal gap as observed in the lateral dimension did not correlate with the rated voice quality nor with the rated intelligibility of the speaker. However, the quality judgment and the intelligibility judgment were highly correlated.

Investigators at this clinic have utilized cineradiography to evaluate the optimal placement of speech appliances (Mazaheri and Millard[11]). Voice quality was judged as best when the speech bulb was positioned at the level of the pharyngeal wall activity, as determined by lateral cineradiography. The inferosuperior dimension of a speech bulb could be reduced to one fourth of the original thickness without perceptibly increasing nasal quality

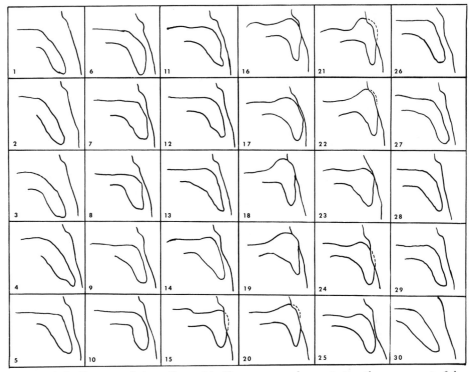

FIGURE 8–8 Tracings of cineradiographic film sequence demonstrating the movement of the velum from a rest position through the production of /pɑ:/ and back to rest. (Adapted from Warren, D. W., and F. A. Hofmann: Plast. Reconstr. Surg., 28:556, 1961.)

TABLE 8–4   Oropharyngeal Dimensions in Cleft and Non-cleft Children[*]

	CLEFT			NON-CLEFT		
DIMENSION	*Range*	*Mean*	*SD*	*Range*	*Mean*	*SD*
Soft Palate Length	27 to 40	31.2	4.654	31 to 39.5	34.6	3.153
Depth of Nasopharynx	25 to 36.5	29.4	3.674	23.5 to 31.8	27.8	2.435
Thickness of Soft Palate	5.3 to 7.9	6.5	0.215	6.5 to 13	9.2	1.521
Height of Elevation[†]	6.7[b] to 8.7[a]	2.1	4.327	1.7[b] to 7.6[a]	2.6	2.961
Height of Closure	None	None	None	9.7[b] to 7.6[a]	−1.3	4.800
Gap	1.7 to 12.5	4.9	3.641	None	None	None
Posterior Pharyngeal Wall Forward	0 to 7.7	2.0	2.391	0 to 2	None	None

[*]Obtained values, in millimeters, for seven measures for experimental subjects (N=11) and normal subjects (N=10) (Mazaheri, Millard, and Ericson, 1964).

   [†]a = value above palatal plane.

    b = value below palatal plane.

TABLE 8–5   Lateral Dimensions and Positions of Speech Bulbs (in mm.) °

| | LATERAL DIMENSION | | REFERENCE TO PALATAL PLANE° | |
	Range	Mean	Range	Mean
Original Bulb	20 to 32	26.3	Highest Point −10 to +10	+2
			Lowest Point −24 to −3	−12
Bulb High	16 to 29	24.4	−3 to +9	+1
Bulb Medium	16 to 32	24.7	−10 to +3	−5.7
Bulb Low	17 to 32	24	−16 to −4	−13

° Measurements in millimeters for inferior-superior lateral dimensions, and position relative to the palatal plane for the original and experimental speech bulbs (Mazaheri and Millard, 1965).

°+ above palatal plane.
  − below palatal plane.

(Table 8–5). Thus the weight of the bulb could be reduced. They also found that the lateral dimension of the bulb did not change with alterations in the height of placement. Therefore, the width of the nasopharynx apparently remains stable in the inferosuperior dimension.

EVALUATION OF SPEECH STATUS

The evaluation procedure has a dual purpose. The first is to identify problems that may exist; the second is to decide upon a therapeutic course of action. At times neither objective is met or fulfilled as easily as one might anticipate. Difficult questions must be answered in both the diagnostic and therapeutic areas. For example, an interdental lisp may be present as the result of either mislearned articulation or an open bite. A VPI may be treated either directly by surgical or prosthetic means or indirectly through a speech program. We feel that the identification of the problem and the decision as to which management procedure to follow can be made best by a team of trained specialists. In this section we shall present the responsibilities of the speech pathologist as a member of that team.

The human ear is still the speech pathologist's most useful tool as he carries out his main clinical and research obligation, namely, the assessment of speech. Although he has at his command a battery of instruments to help him quantify specific parameters, he must rely heavily upon his ear and his listening skills in determining the presence and the nature of the speech disorder.

In his appraisal of the voice quality and the articulatory skills of the speaker with a cleft, he will find that the most common disturbance is hypernasality. This condition is usually due to an unoperated cleft (see Figure 8–1A), a large fistula in the postoperative hard palate (Figure 8–9), or an inadequate or incompetent velar mechanism (see Figure 8–15B). However, the opposite condition, hyponasality, or some other disorder such as hoarseness,

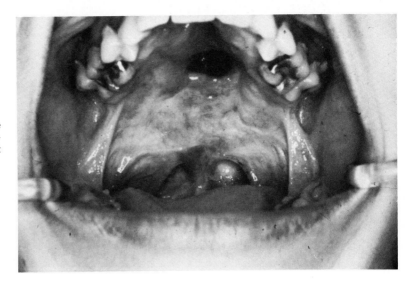

FIGURE 8-9 A fistula in the hard palate remaining after an attempt to close the palatal cleft surgically.

harshness, or "breathiness," also may be associated with a congenital oral defect. The patient's vocal resonance may be affected by some concomitant condition. Enlarged tonsillar or adenoid tissue, development of other growths in the nasal passageways, enlargement of the turbinates, gross deviation of the nasal septum—any one of these may constrict the nasal freeway and force the individual to breathe through the mouth. His vocal resonance may thus be altered to the extent that he is judged hyponasal or denasal.

It is a good idea for the evaluator to assess the patient's voice quality even before looking into his mouth. Quite often one is surprised that speech can be so good in view of the observed anatomical and physiological abnormalities of the oral region. We listen before we look in order to reduce any bias we might establish by a visual inspection of the speech structures.

A search for all the possible causes of a speech disorder may occasionally turn up environmental factors, such as parental pressure or sibling competition. Some parents put pressure on a child to do better than he is physiologically equipped to do, so in order to satisfy them he strains his voice and develops laryngeal deviation and hoarseness on top of his original hypernasality. Or if there are four or five children in the home and one has a cleft, he has to strain to be heard above the ambient decibel level—or become lost. Here again his penalty is hoarseness.

In maintaining a record of voice variations, the speech clinician charts phonemic evaluations of substitutions, distortions, or sound omissions. Free speech and reading samples are scored with reference to voice quality and intelligibility and are recorded on tape for future use. Replaying the recorded example and reviewing the diagnostic examination notes will reacquaint the speech pathologist or other member of the team with the primary problem. Such records are also useful to speech therapists or clinicians from other rehabilitation centers or from school systems in helping them to plot changes in pathology or progress in a management program.

The speech pathologist must recognize coexisting problems that may mask, complicate, or contribute to a speech disorder. Mental retardation

(MR), neurogenic dysfunction, or a hearing loss may be accompanied by VPI with hypernasality. Although the VPI can be surgically or prosthetically managed, the articulation disorders associated with MR and hearing loss will persist. Many individuals with VPI and a glottal speech pattern will retain the glottal pattern even after effective management of the VPI. There are countless other examples, but the point to be made is that during the evaluative procedure the speech pathologist must distinguish between those speech problems attributed to the VPI and those that coexist but are due to other causes and therefore can not be alleviated by surgical or prosthetic management, but will require speech therapy.

The initial step at the Clinic is to ascertain the presence of incomplete velopharyngeal closure during speech. While hypernasality and nasal emission are the more common symptoms, an inadequate speech valve is frequently signaled by nasal grimacing, glottal and/or pharyngeal articulation, "breathiness," or hoarseness. Sometimes a patient referred for hypernasality is found to be exhibiting nasal twang ("hillbilly speech"). Other voice quality anomalies, especially hyponasality (frequently heard in the speech of individuals with severe hearing losses), are often misdiagnosed as hypernasality. The speech pathologist must be able to differentiate among these voice and speech disturbances.

Approximately 24 per cent of the children who have undergone primary closure of the palatal cleft at this Clinic will subsequently demonstrate a velopharyngeal incompetency or insufficiency and will require secondary palatal procedures, i e., a pharyngeal flap or a speech aid prosthesis (Table 8–6). The underlying need for secondary surgery usually arises from an inadequacy of velar tissue. In contrast there are instances in which the velum, upon examination, appears long enough to make contact with the posterior pharyngeal wall. Examination, usually by lateral cineradiography, reveals that there is a limited range of velar movement or elevation. This is called a

TABLE 8–6   Secondary Procedures for Velopharyngeal Insufficiency*

| | NUMBER OF PATIENTS RECEIVING *No* SECONDARY PROCEDURES | | NUMBER OF PATIENTS RECEIVING SECONDARY PROCEDURES | | | |
| | | | *Pharyngeal flap* | | *Speech Aid Prosthesis* | |
Category	M	F	M	F	M	F
UCLP	37	20	8	7	0	2
BCLP	22	9	5	1	0	1
Hard and Soft Palate	30	38	7	11	3	4
Soft Palate Only	11	10	2	2	2	0
Total	100	77	22	21	5	7
Total M & F	177(76%)		43(19%)		12(5%)	

*The number of patients listed by the necessity of secondary palatal procedures for velopharyngeal insufficiency (Riski, 1977).

velopharyngeal *incompetency.* In such a case there is usually a neurological deficit, such as one observes in cerebral palsy or bulbar (flaccid) dysarthria (Darley, et al.[7]).

At the beginning of an evaluation of the velopharyngeal valve mechanism, one should establish the openness of the nasal passages. The examiner should have the patient close his mouth and breathe through his nose. He should listen for nasal air resistance as he holds first one nostril closed and then the other, recording which side exhibits the least resistance. Nasal congestion caused by a cold or allergies or crying will interfere with nasal air flow, as will a deviated septum or nasal polyps. Subsequent testing for hypernasality and nasal air emission must be interpreted in the light of any air resistance found in the nasal passages themselves.

Diagnosis of Hypernasality

The phenomenon of hypernasality or hypernasal resonance is a disturbance of voice quality, and its presence or absence can be determined, therefore, only during production of voiced speech sounds. We know that velar height varies with the height of the tongue in vowel production, and for that reason we have selected some voiced consonants and the four vowels that represent the four corners of the vowel quadrangle to construct our test words. They are BEAT, BAT, BOOT, and BOUGHT. Since the severity of the hypernasality may vary, we have devised three levels of listening criticality. These levels employ the listening tube, cul-de-sac test, and rating of oronasal resonance balance during connected speech.

The listening tube (Blakeley[2]) provides a critical test for the presence of nasality (Figure 8–10). This device consists of a length of rubber tubing about 24 inches long. On either end are nasal tips (nasal olives). The tip on one end is inserted into the patient's freest nasal passage as determined by the breathing test described earlier. The other end is held to the examiner's ear. The patient, holding the listening end to his own ear, is frequently

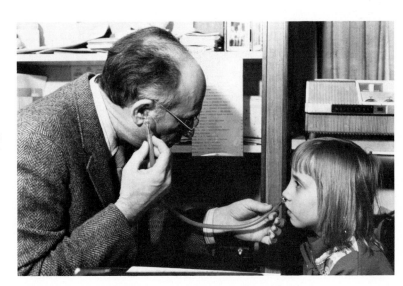

FIGURE 8–10 Examiner using listening tube to evaluate the presence of hypernasality.

amazed at the amount of nasal resonance he perceives in this way. Hypernasality is recorded as present or absent for each of the test words and during a standard test passage, e.g., BUY BABY A BIB. We have found a test of this type to be quite useful in evaluating the final stages of speech bulb or palatal lift construction or post-pharyngeal flap surgery.

Less critical is the cul-de-sac test. For this evaluation the patient is instructed to say each of the test words twice. For the first production the nares are unoccluded. For the second both nares are pinched closed by the examiner (Figure 8–11). A shift in resonance from the first to the second production is considered a positive indicator of hypernasal resonance.

Although the results of these test procedures may indicate hypernasal resonance, the most important consideration is whether resonance is perceived during conversational speech. To establish this we rate oronasal resonance on a scale of one to five; one is normal and five is extremely hypernasal. During connected speech the examiner listens for the tone quality of the vowels and the strength of /b/ or the possible substitution of /m/ for /b/.

Diagnosis of Nasal Air Emission

Nasal air emission is the air flow lost through the nasal cavities during speaking as a result of VPI. In its least severe form it may be heard as a mild snorting sound as the velum only loosely contacts the posterior pharyngeal wall. In its most severe degree it may exist as audible and interfering nasal

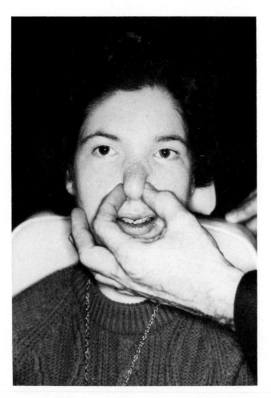

FIGURE 8–11 Examiner pinching the nostrils of a patient during the cul-de-sac evaluation. An alteration of the perceived resonance when the nostrils are pinched is a positive indication of velopharyngeal insufficiency.

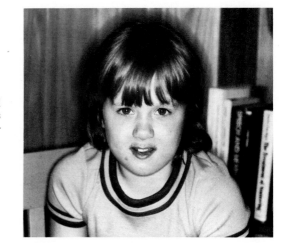

FIGURE 8–12 Patient exhibiting a nasal grimace or nasal flaring during speech production. The presence of this grimace is a positive indication of velopharyngeal insufficiency.

air flow accompanied by nasal flaring or some form of facial grimacing. Nasal flaring during speech is a positive sign that a VPI is present (Figure 8–12).

Intraoral air pressure is inversely proportionate to nasal air escape. As nasal air escape increases, intraoral air pressure decreases. Seriously diminished intraoral air pressure will interfere with pressure sound production.

Nasal emission of air also can be recognized easily by using techniques similar to those described previously for the diagnosis of the oronasal resonance balance. Again we must establish that the nasal passage is clear. Because nasal air emission is a deviation of air flow, rather than a resonance, we use a speech sample loaded with voiceless pressure sounds, such as the voiceless fricatives and plosives, as in PAPER, PEOPLE, SISTER, or SIXTY-SIX. The patient is instructed to say these words and the examiner assesses the presence of nasal air flow, using a mirror, air paddle, or a nasal listening tube (Figure 8–13). We should note that the glottal stop substitution will mask nasal air emission. Since the valve for this sound is at the level of the larynx, air flow does not reach the velopharyngeal valve.

In order to determine the effect of nasal air emission on speech articulation, the nares can be pinched shut gently by the examiner, eliminating all nasal air escape. With nares closed he listens to the energy for pressure sounds such as /p/, /t/, or /s/. If oral air flow is sufficiently increased, it would suggest that VPI may be interfering with pressure sound articulation.

Once the existence of a VPI has been established, we try to quantify several of its parameters. To accomplish this end a number of instrumentations are available, including radiography, cineradiography, sound spectrography, oral manometry, and speech sound inventories.

Radiographic Studies

Anatomical and physiological differences within the oral and nasopharyngeal regions must be evaluated as variables responsible for nasal air escape during phonation. Lateral head films can be employed to register the "gap" between the velum and the posterior wall of the pharynx, the pres-

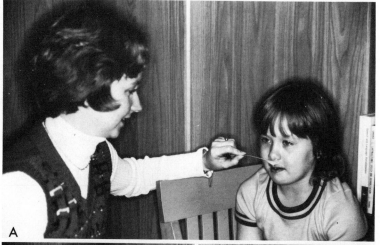

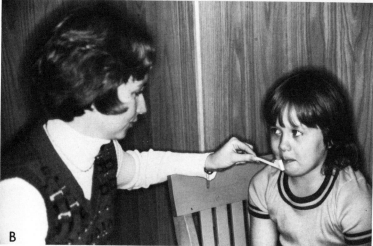

FIGURE 8–13 *A*, The deflection of the air paddle during speech production is an indication of nasal air emission. *B*, The air paddle can be used also to train oral air flow.

ence and effect of enlarged tonsils on displacement of tongue and velum, the presence and size of adenoid mass, and the configuration of the nasopharynx. Two films are taken for our evaluations, the first with the patient breathing quietly through his nose so that the velum will be in a functional rest position (Figure 8–14). A second lateral head film is exposed while the subject prolongs his phonation of the vowel /i/ in "HE." Comparing the two views demonstrates the degree of elevation and extension of the velum during phonation and reveals the extent or lack of velopharyngeal competency. Still radiographic head films are readily available to the speech pathologist wherever there are orthodontic specialists or hospital facilities within a radiology department.

Studies of the velopharyngeal valve using lateral still radiographs should be interpreted carefully. Studies completed by one of the authors (J. E. R.) with colleagues at the University of Florida (Williams, et al.[29]) have demonstrated that a VPI can be diagnosed from the production of a sustained vowel or a consonant and vowel combination recorded by still radiography. However, cineradiographic study shows that velopharyngeal closure was

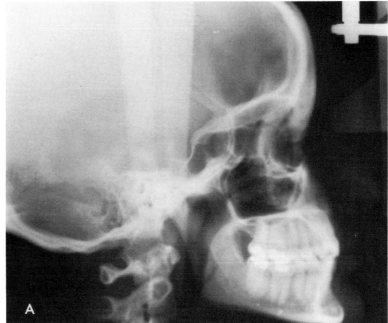

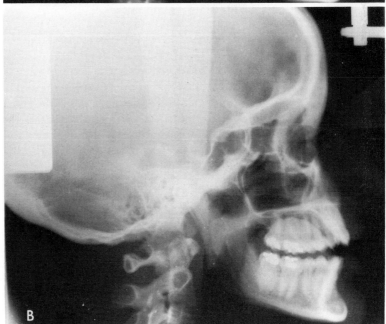

FIGURE 8–14 *A*, Lateral x-ray of adult female with normal velopharyngeal function breathing quietly. *B*, Lateral x-ray with patient phonating, showing closure is achieved.

present in connected speech (Table 8–7). In other words, relying on lateral still radiographs alone can frequently lead to misdiagnosis of VPI.

Cineradiography has become a widely used tool by the clinician and the researcher for observation and analysis of oral speech function. Its nature provides for dynamic study of structures in function.

With the refinement of cineradiographic technology and investigative procedures, we have gained a much clearer understanding of the oro-

TABLE 8–7   Diagnosis of Velopharyngeal Function Related to Speech Sample (N = 20)

SPEECH SAMPLE	RADIOGRAPHIC TECHNIQUE	VELAR PORT DIAGNOSIS	
		Adequate	*Inadequate*
"EE" (as in BEET)	Lateral Still	4	16
PEE, PEE, PEE	Lateral Still	10	10
Connected Speech	Cineradiography	13	7

Williams et al., 1976.

pharyngeal structures during function. Speech researchers have spent considerable effort studying these structures in motion for speech. The advantages of cineradiography over lateral still roentgenographs are obvious after first viewing the speech structures in motion. Moreover, cineradiography enables us to evaluate position, movement, and synchrony of dynamic structures in connected speech.

The initial step for clinical or research purposes requires definition of several important parameters, each of which has a bearing on the other. At some point a problem is observed; to the clinician in a cleft palate clinic the problem is one of velopharyngeal function. He or she has already determined that a VPI exists in a patient and now must define its parameters. The problem can be delineated in the form of several questions: Does the velum move during speech production? Is the movement appropriate for the sample of speech studied? What is the amount of velar movement or what is the residual gap between the velum and the posterior pharyngeal wall?

The nature of the problem allows the clinician to define the population as those individuals exhibiting VPI. Finally, the speech sample with which to study the problem will be defined. A knowledge of normal speech physiology directs the clinician to use pressure sounds and an assortment of vowels representing the vowel quadrangle, and these sounds will be employed in a connected speech sample. Of course, a four-year-old with a VPI may not be the most cooperative of patients or be able to repeat a long sentence. For this reason several words may be added to the sample. Care and thought should be taken in developing this sample, and it should remain standard for all cineradiographic studies of VPI. The speech sample used here consists of isolated vowels, consonant-vowel syllables, selected words, a sentence, swallowing, and blowing This sample was designed to demonstrate velar elevation and extension and posterior pharyngeal wall activity under a variety of conditions.

Observation of the velar port in speech gives us important information in the selection of the corrective procedure most suitable for an individual patient. We first observe the *appropriateness of velar movement*. The velum should be closed against or should be attempting to close against the posterior pharyngeal wall for all sound production except the nasal sounds (Figure 8–15).

We can observe the *adequacy of the velar movement*. A velum that does not move or appears to have a limited range of motion may indicate soft pal-

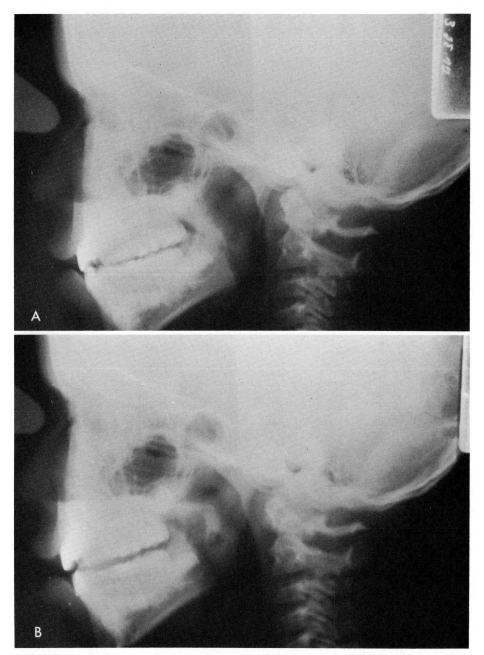

FIGURE 8–15 Adolescent girl with a velopharyngeal insufficiency. *A*, Lateral x-ray with patient breathing quietly. *B*, Lateral x-ray with patient phonating the EE in HE.

ate paralysis or paresis. A postoperative soft palate may be heavily scarred, which will reduce its range of motion.

A very important piece of information that we obtain from the cineradiographic speech examination is the size of the residual gap that remains during the optimum attempt at closing the orifice. This examination also provides detailed information important to the surgical member of the team. He can observe the point of attempted closure of the velum against the posterior pharyngeal wall, the depth of the retropharyngeal space, and the presence and thickness of adenoid pads on the posterior pharyngeal wall. (A more detailed account of the cephalometric measures used in radiographic and cineradiographic studies of the dynamic speech structures is included in the Appendix of Chapter 2.)

Sound Spectrography

In 1956 Millard's paper, "Role of the Sound Spectrograph as a Diagnostic Tool," was read before the International Congress of Logopedics, Barcelona, Spain.[13] Although the article indicated that visual displays were not easily quantified for research, he demonstrated that the patterns did have practical clinical implications.

The Kay Sona-Graph* has been employed as one of the diagnostic tools at the H. K. Cooper Institute since 1953 (Figure 8–16). A speech signal is spectrographically analyzed on a display paper referred to as a "sonagram." The patient's voice is recorded on a magnetic band within the instrument. Electrostatic markings are burned onto sensitized paper as the stylus travels upward, moving through a narrow (45 Hz) or wide (300 Hz) band-pass filter within the 80 to 8000 Hz range of the unit. The visible display is actually a three-dimensional pattern of frequency versus time related to vocal intensity.

---

*Manufactured by Kay Elemetrics, Pine Brook, New Jersey.

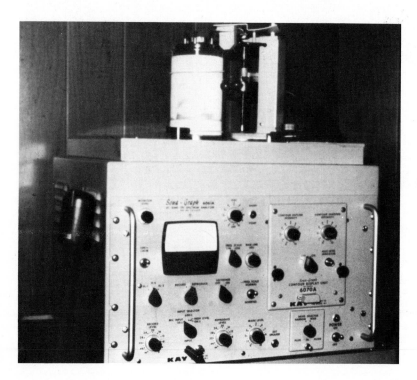

FIGURE 8–16   Kay Elemetrics Sona-Graph 6061–A.

The horizontal axis covers a period of 2.4 seconds; the vertical axis relates to frequency. Voice prints displayed on paper are read from left to right. Voiced and voiceless plosive, fricative, and sibilant consonants have distinctive patterns, as do the voiced vowels. Vowels display energy bars called formants. The second and third formant above the base bar gives identification to vowel and vowel-like sounds.

Nasality, as a voice quality disorder. is displayed with several easily discernible characteristics (Figure 8–17). The resonant (formant) frequencies for vowels are identified by their number (from low to high frequency), configuration, and location of resonance on the scale. When nasal air escape is associated with hypernasality, the vowel formants are broken and hashy, and additional resonant bars may be noted in the middle frequency range, and high frequency hashing may occur at the top of the scale directly above the vowel formants. Voiceless plosives normally illustrate "spikes" of quick energy release. High frequency hashing preceding the weak or absent plosive spike is also a sign of nasal air escape and reduced intraoral air pressure. As the subject attempts to build up intraoral pressure for the plosive, he "snorts" because of velopharyngeal inadequacy.

The speech pathologist may encounter hypernasal patients who do not exhibit the nasal emission problem. Characteristics of nasality are displayed on the sonagram in different ways. The resonant vowel bars may be increased in width and number and have "shadows," all signs of oronasal coupling. When the third formant is missing the vowel is weak. Most fre-

WITHOUT LIFT

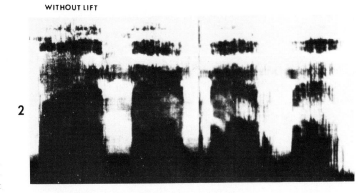

2

FIGURE 8–17 Sonagrams of the speech sample "Buy Baby a Bib" for two conditions: *with* and *without* a palatal lift speech appliance. (1) Additional resonances found with velopharyngeal incompetency. (2) Plosive spike is absent. (3) Presence of additional vertical striations indicates nasal air emission.

WITH LIFT

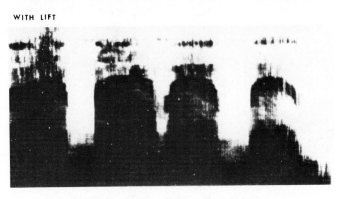

BUY BA BY A BIB

quently one notices a series of broken formants without a well-defined resonant area.

The spectrogram displays variances in production of the consonant sound elements. The characteristic spike of the voiceless plosive may be missing, may be extremely light in energy, or may have increased width (time), indicating slurring of the sound.

Fricative and sibilant sounds produce heavy, compact areas of hashing covering 1.5 to 4.5 K Hz, extending down from the top of the scale. Nasal emission reduces the oral output of sound energy, weakening the display and causing loss of density. Pharyngeal noises associated with fricative sounds are identified by several vowel-like resonant bars in the low and middle frequency range. These suggest oral resonance. The common high frequency display is lowered on the scale and broken in several energy groupings.

Although used mainly as a valuable diagnostic aid, the sonagraph is also very helpful as a training tool for clinician, parent, and patient. Sonograms made after primary or secondary surgical repair, when compared with the presurgical patterns, visualize the patient's progress in oral air control. Elimination or reduction of hypernasality can be "viewed" by patient, parent, and clinician. These sound energy images demonstrate positive differences for the patient—he can *see* his successes. The same is true for the patient following insertion of a speech aid prosthesis. He notices the spontaneous changes in his own voice immediately. He *sees* his improvement before he *hears* it. When the prosthesis is first inserted, the voice he hears within his head generally is not interpreted as a positive difference, even though the voice is different from what he's used to hearing. As Wendell Johnson said so often, it takes a difference to make a difference. Visual displays make the difference. The patient's new pattern compared with his former display and to a standard or "normal" display gives him the sense of immediate accomplishment. Patients in our residence program review their initial and final sonagrams at the end of a period of several weeks as documentary proof that their voice quality has been improved by the surgery or prosthesis, with speech therapy.

Because hypernasality varies from person to person, we must expect the sonagrams to reflect this variability in the displays. As clefts are different and nasality is different, so sonagrams are different. In summary, the primary characteristics in sonagrams of cleft patients whose voices are judged as substandard lie in the introduction of high frequency hashing over the vowel, reduction of formant intensity, broken and hashy formants, elimination of the second formant, increased number of resonant areas, and the increased band width of formants with "shadows." Weak consonants are identified by reduction of intensity, the elimination of voiceless plosives (spikes), high frequency hashing preceding plosive consonants at a time when intraoral air pressure should have been impounded, and substitution of a pharyngeal fricative.

Air Pressure Measurements

Very few treatment centers can afford the expensive research equipment necessary to validate objective measurements of nasality. Measurements of nasal air escape during blowing can be acquired with the Hunter oral manometer (Figure 8–18). However, these measurements are not always an accurate measure of nasality because there is not a one-to-one relationship between the processes of phonation and blowing. Nevertheless, comparative readings of complete exhalation with nostrils occluded and unoccluded indicate the adequacy or inadequacy of velopharyngeal closure for this test. If the velopharyngeal mechanism is functional, similar scores will be attained for the unoccluded and occluded trials. The ratio of unoccluded over occluded would be greater than 0.90. The smaller this ratio becomes the greater the amount of nasal air escape during blowing. Low ratios are also frequently associated with hypernasality and nasal air emission during speaking. Since there is not a one-to-one relationship between valve function for blowing and speaking, however, manometric measurements must be interpreted in light of the results of other tests for velopharyngeal competency. Manometric testing should be undertaken with the bleed valve of the instrument open. Invalid readings can be obtained with the valve closed, owing to the ability of the patient to build and maintain pressure with the tongue. With the bleed valve open this is not possible.

Another point should be made concerning the interpretation of these blowing scores. Certain patients have been known to elevate the tongue to create a velopharyngeal seal when blowing, a phenomenon observed by cineradiography. Under this condition the patient would score well on the manometer, but he would still have nasal emission during speech.

Articulation Testing

The articulation test is probably the most frequently used of any of the tests available to the speech pathologist (Figure 8–19). The examiner is

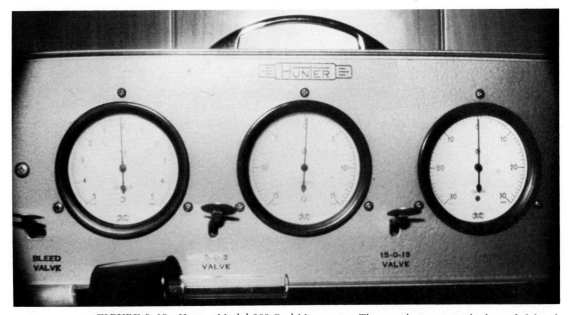

FIGURE 8–18 Hunter Model 360 Oral Manometer. The mouthpiece is in the lower left-hand corner.

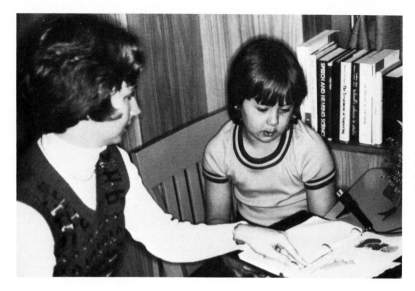

FIGURE 8–19 The examiner is testing the patient's articulation skills using the Templin-Darley test of articulation. Records of articulation proficiency are maintained and analyzed for each patient in the longitudinal series.

required to make a judgment about an individual's sound production. Unfortunately this judgment is somewhat subjective. In a center such as ours, where we are engaged in clinical research, there is a need for acceptable reliability, when several examiners are engaged in the testing. We have found that we can reduce the subjective nature of our judgments by defining the nature of each type of production and outlining the decision-making process used to arrive at each judgment.

The initial step was to agree to all possible productions that a patient will exhibit. Once that was accomplished, we set about the task of defining each of these productions. We have found the following definitions to be useful:

Sound tested: the sound under test or the desired sound.

Correct sound production: the sound produced is an acceptable production of the desired sound.

Sound omission: there is no audible characteristic of the correct sound nor any other sound present in the tested position.

Sound substitution: recognizable production of another sound without any perception of the desired sound.

Simple or typical sound substitution: the sound produced is recognized as an acceptable production of another English phoneme.

Laryngeal or glottal stop substitution: the sound produced is an audible obstruction of air flow assumed to be at the level of the glottis.

Pharyngeal fricative substitution: the sound produced is an audible fricative sound assumed to be at the level of the pharynx.

Nasal air emission substitution: the sound produced is an audible fricative sound assumed to be emitted from the nasal cavity.

Sound distortion: the sound produced is a recognizable but unacceptable production of the desired sound.

Simple or typical distortion: the sound produced is recognizable, but unacceptable, owing to noise generated within the oral cavity.

Nasal distortion: the sound produced is recognizable, but it is accompanied by nasal air emission or a hypernasal voice quality.

Pharyngeal distortion: the sound produced is recognizable, but it is accompanied by noises assumed to be generated at the level of the pharynx.

As a second step, we defined a stepwise process by which we should arrive at our decision (Figure 8–20). We were able to identify six levels in this decision-making process. A decision is made at each level before proceeding to the next. The first level is the *Testing* level. This represents the sound tested. The second level is the *Production* level. At this level a decision is made as to whether a sound in the test position was produced. The question to ask is "was the sound produced?" If the decision is that no sound was produced in the test position (for example "AT" for "SAT"), then it is a sound omission and may be so scored. If a sound is produced (for example, "SHAT" for "SAT"), we go to the next level.

The third level is labeled *Acceptance*. The decision is made whether the uttered sound is acceptable or unacceptable. If it was acceptable, it is scored; if unacceptable, we proceed to the next level.

The fourth level has been labeled the *Recognition* level. Here we begin the process of identifying and labeling the error in production. The decision must be made between substitution and distortion. The question asked is whether the desired sound can be recognized. If it can be recognized, the response is a distortion of the desired sound.

The fifth level has been termed the *Type* level. Here we make the distinction between oral and extraoral, i.e., pharyngeal or nasal productions. An oral substitution has been termed a simple or typical substitution. If a typical substitution is found, the sound is recorded using the IPA. If the decision is made that the sound is not a typical substitution, then we proceed to the sixth and final level in order to identify the production.

If the sound production has been labeled a distortion, then at the *Type*

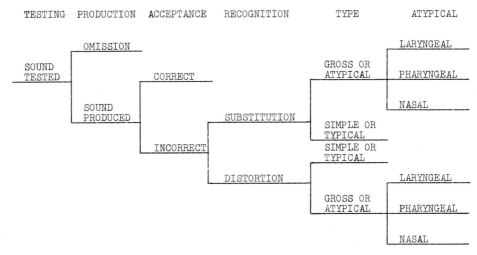

FIGURE 8–20 Sound production evaluation process.

level we decide whether it is an oral or typical distortion or an atypical one. If it has been determined that the sound produced is recognizable, but unacceptable owing to misplacement of the tongue, then it is recorded as a simple distortion. If sound is generated at levels other than the oral cavity, it is termed an atypical distortion and again we proceed to level six to identify it.

Level six has been termed the *Atypical* level because each of these substitutions or distortions is atypical for the *non*-cleft palate, or more correctly, the non-VPI population. The atypical substitutions are those produced at the level of the larynx (a glottal stop), the level of the pharynx (a pharyngeal fricative), or the level of the nasal cavity (nasal air emission). Each of these substitutions is a compensatory effort to produce an acoustically acceptable speech sound under the handicap of a VPI.

The atypical distortions are defined as recognizable sound productions accompanied by extraneous noises generated at the level of the larynx, pharynx, or nasal cavity. Just as the typical distortion of the speech sound represents a higher level error than does the simple substitution, so the atypical distortions represent a remnant of an atypical substitution pattern.

The conclusion of research on the articulation of children, adolescents, and adults with cleft palates is that, in general, they are delayed or possibly retarded in their acquisition of articulation (Bzoch;[3] Spriestersbach, et al.;[24] Counihan;[6] and Morris[16]). However, investigations have been cross-sectional in design. Extrinsic variables were difficult to control. Frequently it could not be determined whether the subjects in the studies were operated on by the same surgeon, using the same technique and the same time sequence in closing the cleft. Moll[15] and Spriestersbach and associates[25] have stated that there is a need for describing the development of articulation skills in children with palatal clefts. Philips and Harrison[17] suggested that such knowledge should help define the need and timing of speech therapy intervention.

As an integral part of the research program at the H. K. Cooper Institute, the articulation skills of every child in the cleft lip and palate research series are assessed on his birthday and six months following, from the age of three years through adolescence. In 1976 Riski and associates[20] presented a preliminary descriptive analysis of these data. They are summarized in Figure 8–21. Since this is an ongoing study, the data have been updated since the 1976 presentation.

Our studies suggest that the children in this series are delayed but not retarded in the acquisition of articulatory skills. The children with cleft palate are most deficient, compared with normals, prior to four years of age. After four the children with palatal clefts exhibit accelerated articulatory acquisition. Moreover, the articulatory skills continue improving at least until eight years of age. Further growth and study of the series is necessary to determine if and at what age these children with cleft palate achieve normal articulation.

Whereas Templin[27] reported that the articulation skills of non-cleft children become more consistent after age six, we have observed that children with palatal clefts still display a wide range of articulatory proficiency. That is, after six years of age there emerges a group of children with cleft palates whose articulation is within normal limits, while there is another group that has retained defective articulation patterns (Figure 8–22). Identification

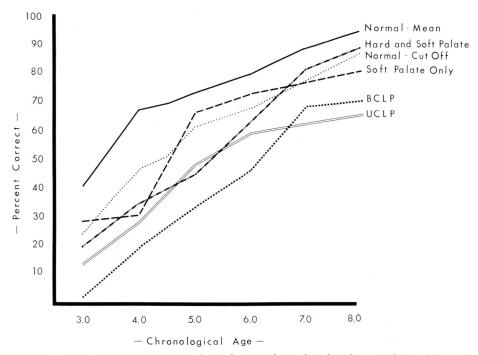

FIGURE 8–21   The mean percentage of sounds correctly produced on the Templin-Darley Fifty Item Screening Test. The mean scores for the four cleft types are compared with the mean scores for normal and to the cut-off for normal production. The cut-off represents approximately one standard deviation from the mean.

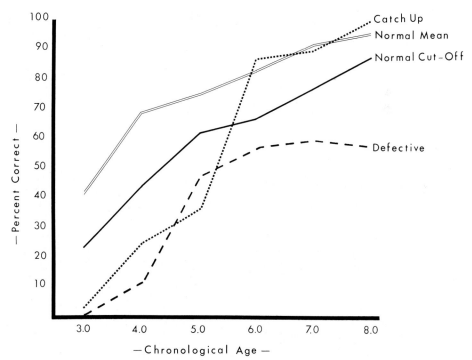

FIGURE 8–22   Graphic representation of the mean percentage of correct sounds produced on the Templin-Darley Fifty-Item Screening Test. The mean score and the cut-off for normal production are represented with the articulation profiles of two children with UCLP. One UCLP child "catches up" to normal by eight years of age, while the second demonstrates a "deficient" articulation profile through the test period.

of factors that can distinguish between these groups should serve to prompt earlier intervention and result in more effective management of speech defects associated with palatal clefts.

Oral Peripheral Examination

In assessing the cleft palate patient's speech problem, one must consider not only such internal elements of the speech machinery as the velopharyngeal valve, to which we have thus far given major attention, but also certain external, or at least more visible, features. These are of particular importance from the standpoint of articulation. It will be helpful, therefore, to conduct a thorough examination of what may be termed the "peripheral speech mechanism."

We shall begin with observation of labial fullness, contact, and maneuverability, noting the extent and thickness of scarring, the mobility of the upper lip (Figure 8–23), the presence or absence of the cupid's bow, and the asymmetry of the lip and face. Are the lips most frequently separated because the child breathes through the mouth (Figure 8–24)? Is the lower lip redundant or flaccid? Has the patient had cross lip surgery? Can the lips be extended and retracted easily?

Next, we shall study the profile. Here the relationship of the maxilla and premaxilla is important. Protrusion of the premaxilla tightens the upper lip. Deficient growth of the maxillary process results in pseudoprognathism of the mandible with a "dished-in" midthird of the face (Figure 8–25). Each of these factors or a combination of them will have an effect upon appearance, mastication, and speech.

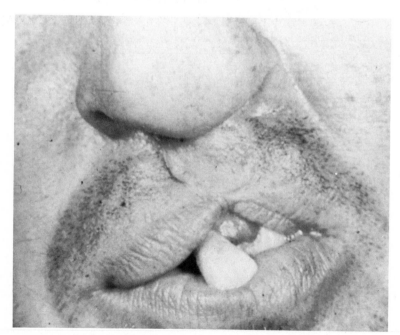

FIGURE 8–23 A patient with multiple dental anomalies and scarred upper lip with reduced mobility. Surgery and dental procedures were carried out to correct this neglected condition.

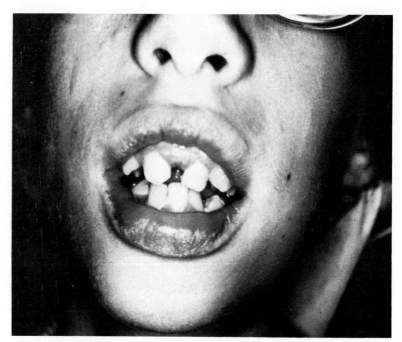

FIGURE 8-24   A facies typical of a mouth breather.

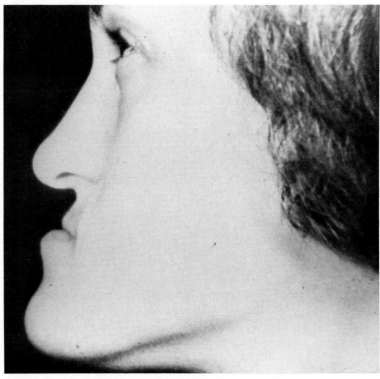

FIGURE 8-25   Mandibular prognathism.

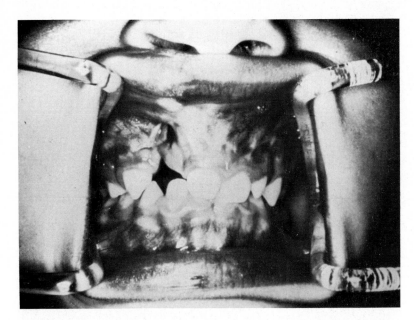

FIGURE 8–26 Congenitally missing lateral incisor on side of cleft.

   The nose may be quite flat with a broadness of one or both alae. The nasal septum of the patient with complete unilateral cleft of lip and palate most frequently veers to the unaffected side. Nasal breathing may be affected by the deviated septum, by enlargement of the turbinates, or by adenoid mass. These variables must be studied carefully because the subject may demonstrate some hyponasality and hypernasality in the same utterance. Total awareness of the structural deviations assists in providing an adequate diagnostic and treatment program.

   The absence of lateral maxillary incisors (Figure 8–26) and the presence of malformed or malposed teeth have their influence on the process of articulation. The status of the occlusion with respect to crossbite, total maxillary collapse, overbite, openbite, maxillary or mandibular protrusion, or retrusion should be observed and studied to determine how the dental condition affects consonantal articulation. A lisp on the sibilant sounds is frequently associated with missing teeth or mandibular prognathism.

   When checking the tongue one should observe it fully extended. Does the tip lateralize equally? Can the tongue be extended without the tongue blade being forced down and over the lower lip because of the lingual frenum's attachment (Figure 8–27)? How well can the patient elevate the tongue to the dental ridge for the postdental sounds? The examiner should check for asymmetry and unusual markings of the tongue's surface. If a lingual flap has been used to aid in closing a palatal cleft, a scar will remain on the tongue (Figure 8–28). The patient should be asked to produce a series of alveolar syllables (/ta, ta, ta/, /da, da, da/, /na, na, na/, /la, la, la/) and velar syllables (/ka, ka, ka/, /ga, ga, ga/). If the posterior section of the tongue fails to elevate to the palate for the /k/ and /g/ syllables, one should ask for production of /n/. Frequently the tongue position for /n/ is acceptable when /k/ and /g/ are charted as glottal. The /k/ and /g/ sounds can be stimulated by exploding an acceptable / ŋ / production.

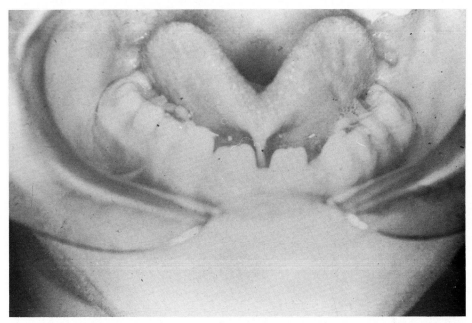

FIGURE 8–27   A short lingual frenum restricting the mobility of the tongue tip.

Mobility of the upper lip should be evaluated during speech production. A heavily scarred lip or one protruded by a premaxilla or plumped out by an anterior dental appliance may not be able to meet the lower lip for bilabial sound production. One young patient recently seen at the Institute had his upper lip plumped out by an addition to his anterior appliance (Figure 8–29). The plumping improved the esthetics of the profile, but made it most difficult for production of bilabial sounds during conversation. Labiodental sounds were substituted. Once this was recognized, the dental and speech specialists, working together, were able to reduce the plumping enough to achieve normal bilabial production and yet maintain an esthetic profile.

The examiner should indicate the status of the tonsils as "absent," "present," or "appear to be enlarged."

These authors have seen isolated cases in which enlarged tonsils appear to be restricting the upward movement of the velum. We have also seen cases in which enlarged tonsils appear to restrict free nasal breathing and force the tongue to a forward rest position. The result is a mouth-breathing pattern. One should note the color and position of the tonsils within the oropharynx and refer the patient to an otorhinolaryngologist for unusual conditions.

With adequate lighting, one should view the palate. Does it elevate symmetrically? If not, there may be a unilateral paresis or paralysis of the elevator. Do the lateral pharyngeal walls move medially?

Stimulability

Finally, it must be emphasized that evaluation is not complete unless there is a recommendation and, more important, a prognosis. For example,

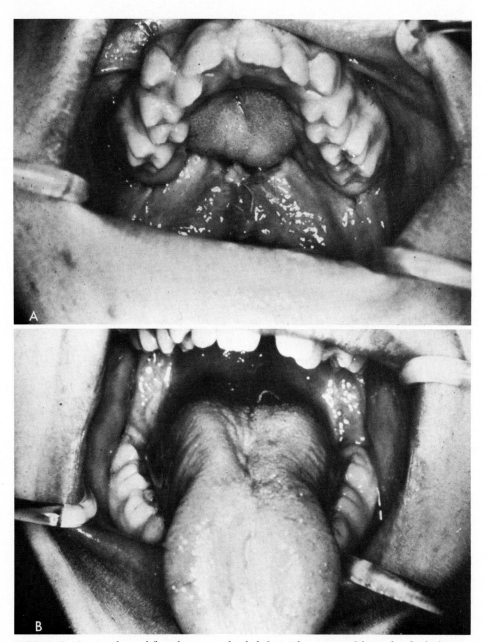

FIGURE 8–28 *A,* A lingual flap closing a palatal cleft. *B,* The tongue of this individual, showing site from which lingual flap was raised.

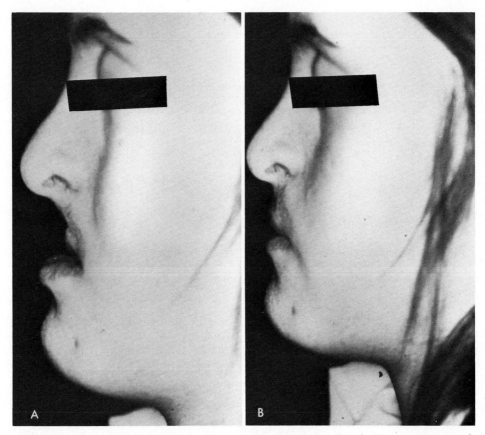

FIGURE 8-29   *A*, Profile of a patient with deficient growth of midthird of face. *B*, Patient with anterior appliance and plumper in place.

Joe is a 17-year-old with a repaired bilateral cleft lip and palate. An inferiorly based pharyngeal flap was not valving adequately. An appliance was in place to supply some anterior teeth and obturate an anterior fistula. The appliance was loose, and Joe reported that he needed to use his tongue to hold it in place. He was to be a senior in high school the following fall. His speech pattern was glottal—no oral consonants were evident in conversational speech. Moreover, the tongue could be observed resting on the floor of the mouth during speech. Further dental and surgical work were obviously necessary, but what did speech therapy have to offer this young man? He obviously had a severe speech problem—he recognized it and his family recognized it. He had not had speech therapy in three years.

Five minutes of trial therapy with Joe enabled us to make a firm prognosis that he should make progress in a speech therapy program. Joe was first asked to produce a voiceless /p/ sound. He did this without noticeable difficulty. This was followed by /t/ and /k/. Again he produced these in the initial trial. The sounds were then repeated once with the nares unoccluded and once with the nares occluded. Intraoral air pressure was present without occlusion of the nares, but it increased with occlusion.

Joe was asked to imitate /æt/ or AT. With the voiced phoneme included, the glottal pattern returned. He was asked to say /t/ again, listen to it, watch as the oral air pressure blew a paper paddle, and then to reproduce that sound at the end of the word AT. Joe was able to produce the word with oral air flow on the second trial.

Next he was asked to imitate /bæt/ or BAT. Again the first try resulted in a glottal pattern and again with a short explanation and demonstration he was able to imitate the word with the oral consonant intact and no glottal pattern.

Finally, various vowels were substituted for /æ/. Joe was asked to say the words BEAT, BAT, BOOT, and BOUGHT. Then different consonants were substituted. He was asked to imitate PAT, TAT, and CAT. He was able to do so usually on the first or second trial. This entire prognostic procedure took only five or 10 minutes.

Obviously not all cases respond this quickly; however, a surprising number will. The case in point had as severe a glottal pattern as one is likely to encounter

Summary

We must caution that no single instrument or technique can serve alone as the best method for the team of examiners and evaluators. The several approaches we have described must be employed, in conjunction with the speech pathologist's own judgment through listening and visual inspection of the patient's labial, oral, palatal, and pharyngeal structures during phonation, in order to arrive at the optimum choice of treatment procedures.

SPEECH THERAPY

Once the evaluation process has established the characteristics of the speech errors, the team of specialists turns to the question of treatment. This may involve surgery or a speech prosthesis and almost certainly speech therapy at one time or another in the total program. The severity of the velopharyngeal insufficiency, the nature of the speech problem as a whole, and the location of the patient's home in relation to the treatment facilities will all have a bearing upon the type and timing of the plan recommended for each patient.

Harding and Mazaheri have summarized in their chapters the conditions that determine the necessity for surgical or prosthetic treatment. Speech therapy may be selected to complement other measures or it may be chosen as a single treatment. In either event, certain conditions will call for speech therapy. In some situations, in which there is only a slight hypernasality, a trial period of therapy is recommended. The therapist will encourage the patient to reduce vocal effort, that is, to make the production of speech easier and therefore reduce nasal air emission and nasal resonance. Frequently, with the modification of vocal effort, the speech disturbances can be reduced or eliminated. But it is important that a patient in a trial therapy program be seen by the team at the end of the program to evaluate the results and to determine whether the patient can be dismissed or whether an alternate management procedure should be pursued.

A patient who exhibits articulatory disturbances should be considered a candidate for speech therapy. Speech disturbances may be those associated with VPI, e.g., glottal stop or pharyngeal fricative sound substitutions, or the misarticulations may be associated with an immature speech pattern, e.g., simple substitutions, omissions, or distortions. Therapy may be initiated prior to secondary procedures if any are considered.

The speech clinician should advise parents of the expected speech results from prosthetic or surgical management. Parents frequently believe that all speech problems will be alleviated with a speech bulb or a pharyngeal flap. The speech disturbances noted previously can be treated only with speech therapy. Furthermore, subtle differences in patients can demand different treatment procedures. Two patients of the same age exhibiting VPI of similar degree will be managed differently if one demonstrates hypernasality and nasal air emission while the other exhibits a glottal sound substitution in addition to the nasal distortions. The former may be successfully treated either prosthetically or surgically, while the latter will be more successfully managed with an initial period of speech therapy in an effort to reduce the coexisting articulatory malfunction.

To fellow speech pathologists we would like to emphasize that speech therapy is our main treatment method. We must use it effectively and document our results. Therapeutic records, including baselines and session-by-session "progress" reports, are a must for communicating the effectiveness of our techniques. In this respect therapy is a continuation of the diagnostic process, only now we are evaluating the results of our therapeutic efforts.

The speech pathologist must also be able to relate and interpret the pre- and post-treatment speech status of the patient to the other team members. A pharyngeal flap operation is performed or a speech bulb or palatal lift appliance is constructed to improve the quality of a patient's speech. Who, then, could be a better judge of the effectiveness of such treatment than the speech pathologist? The clear communication of quantitative information will lead to more successful management and consequently to better post-management speech.

Early Indirect Speech Therapy

Parents of children with cleft lip or palate frequently ask the question: "When will my child be ready for speech therapy?" What they are usually thinking about is speech lessons on a regular, formal basis. But we feel that "indirect" therapy can start at home during the time the child is beginning to produce speech sounds and develop language. What follows, therefore, are suggestions that may be conveyed by the speech pathologists to the parents.

The toddler cries, makes faces, points, pushes, and makes sounds to tell the parents something Are the parents alert to these early signs of communication? What do they do about these infant overtures? Parents can help promote oral communication by being with the child, by listening and talking to him, by reading to him, and by taking time to do special things to help the child.

Find time to be with the child. Make it a fun time. Share his favorite activity: cars, sandbox, puzzles, walks, dolls. Put the child's actions into words. Let him or her "help" dust, sort laundry, empty trash, wash dishes, set the table, pick up toys, work in the yard, or bake cookies. It will take longer to do the household chores, but your little helper will be learning lots of new things.

Make everyday things fun. Have your child near you so you can talk to him. Children like to play where they can see their parent.

Be a good listener with the child. You will teach him to be a good listener by example. Children hear, understand, and then talk. It takes a lot of listening before a child does talk. Make him feel good about what he says. Try not to interrupt him when he tries to tell you something.

When a child begins to talk, he needs a listener who understands him. If you don't know what he is saying, encourage him to tell you in another way. Ask him to help you by showing you what he wants. Keep in mind that a child may use a single word to represent an entire thought. In your response to him, help him to expand this thought.

Talk as you do your daily activities: driving on errands, cleaning, washing. Put what you see into words. Talk about what you are doing. Put what your child sees and hears into words. Use simple words and sentences so he can understand you. Have special "talking" times with your child.

Repeat what your child says as clearly as you can, without actually telling him he said it wrong. Never correct him when he is trying to tell you something.

Reading is one of the most pleasant experiences of childhood. The happiness of being close to a parent, hearing his voice, and seeing colorful pictures is warm and stimulating to a child.

Babies love brightly colored pictures of toys, people, and animals — things that are familiar. Toddlers, one- and two-year-olds, like to look at pictures and listen to you name each one. They learn to watch and say the words and imitate the sounds you make.

Two- and three-year-olds enjoy nursery rhymes, word play, and rhythm. They like stories about animals and people. Reading to a child of two or three may entail only pointing to and naming a picture or two on each page. The attention span of a young child is short, so keep the session within his limits. Reading an entire book word by word may be too much for a child at this age.

Three-, four-, and five-year-olds have make-believe stories as well as real life stories. Both kinds will help them to develop imagination and creative thinking. Let your preschooler tell you a story. Encourage his attempts and help him out, if necessary, by asking appropriate questions. Once the child can recognize a few words, pick them out of the text of the book. Match the word to the correct picture or have the child say the word when you point to it.

Direct Speech Therapy

We also instruct the parents to engage in some direct speech sound therapy. During early counseling sessions parents learn the type of verbalizations that will be within their child's morphological and chronological capabilities at each stage of surgical management.

Prior to closure of the palate, which will occur at 14 to 16 months, the child should be encouraged to produce words with nonpressure sounds. Production of these sounds does not require velopharyngeal closure; consequently, their production is possible prior to closure of the palate. They may be distorted by nasal resonance, but they will be perceived correctly by the family. Words and sound games in which one syllable is produced over and over, such as LA LA LA. stimulate tongue movement and promote verbal interaction between parent and child.

After surgical closure of the palate, pressure sound production should be encouraged. This requires velopharyngeal closure for correct production and thus promotes palatal movement. By the time the soft palate is closed, the child is developmentally and structurally ready to produce real words. The speech pathologist can suggest verbal word games using these sounds.

For the children who don't talk well, their first success will come from listening and pointing to the right pictures and objects. Sit at the child's eye level so he can see your mouth. Hold the object or picture beside your mouth so your child will watch as you say the word. Use only one or two pictures or objects at a time. Encourage whatever attempt your child makes to say a word.

Match objects to pictures. Play hide and seek with objects and name them as they are found. Tell one or two sentence stories about the pictures in the scrapbook. It is easier to learn sounds if they appear at the beginning of the word. Therefore, collect pictures and objects with special sounds in the initial position of their respective words. Make a scrapbook, a stack of picture cards, or a grab bag for collected objects.

The parents in our language and speech development program are reminded to keep the sessions short. Several five-minute sessions are better than one long session. Say the words often. Make the sessions fun. Use your imagination. Show happiness for your child when he tries new words. Change activities to keep interest.

Articulation Therapy

The opportunities to intervene as described earlier are not as frequent as a speech pathologist would hope. More frequently he sees the child with a cleft palate in a diagnostic clinic or in the public schools, a child prone to resonance disorders, air flow problems, and misarticulations.

The clinician desires to work with a mechanism that is capable of performing the gymnastics required to create adequate speech sounds. Nevertheless, if the subject's articulatory pattern is quite substandard for his age level and mental abilities, we prefer to attack the speech or articulation problem before trying to correct physically the velopharyngeal incompetency. Our reasoning here is that during the process of repatterning consonantal sound articulation, the patient frequently reduces the severity of hypernasality. However, it is necessary to set time limits for reaching specific goals. For school-age children with adequate hearing and intelligence and with intelligible but hypernasal speech, we suggest speech therapy for no more than a school term—less if therapy can be intensified to three sessions per week. If hypernasality cannot be controlled satisfactorily, then other measures must be employed—usually surgery.

Attempts to stimulate or increase velar and pharyngeal wall movement have been, for the most part, unsuccessful. Techniques have been used that employ electrical prosthetic stimulation, blowing, sucking, swallowing, and gagging exercises. None has been successful in increasing velopharyngeal movements. Recently, however Shprintzen and colleagues[23] demonstrated that there may possibly be two types of velopharyngeal valve action, one type for pneumatic activities such as speech, blowing, and whistling, and a second type for "nonpneumatic" activities such as gagging and swallowing. In another study Shprintzen and colleagues[24] selected four subjects with a VPI for speech who nevertheless demonstrated normal closure for whistling and blowing A therapy program in which phonation was paired with blowing resulted in increased velar movement for speech and reduced nasal air emission. At present, subject selection for this treatment is strict and dependent upon multi-view videofluoroscopic evaluation, but this type of therapy program does appear to offer promise.

Since we as speech pathologists cannot hope to increase velopharyngeal movements, except possibly under the conditions stated above, we must rely on our already available skills. We are aware that close relationships exist between articulation, perceived nasality, and intelligibility. Therefore, if we can improve one parameter, we can expect improvement in the others. For example, by improving articulation proficiency, we can reduce perceived nasality and increase intelligibility. The initial therapeutic steps are to establish oral air flow and promote oral articulator movement. The former can be aided by occluding the nostrils, the latter by facilitating labial and lingual movements. Making the sound production as visible as possible should also help. One should begin with bilabial sounds or use labiolingual contact initially for lingual alveolar production, and as the patient masters each step he should move the tongue further back to the normal alveolar contact (Figure 8–30).

Once a glottal or pharyngeal articulation pattern is identified, speech therapy can be started as soon as it is feasible. A functional velopharyngeal port is not a prerequisite to initiating speech therapy. For therapeutic purposes, pinching the nostrils will prove quite effective during short-term trial therapy.

A pharyngeal fricative is frequently found substituted for the oral fricative sounds. Like the glottal stop, it is a sound substitution unique to a VPI condition, although we have observed it as a functional problem in post-adenoidectomy patients. It should be treated by stimulating oral air flow and lip and tongue movements.

When some oral movements have been stimulated, the patient is likely to coarticulate the glottal and the oral patterns. This demonstrates learning of the new pattern, but further work is required to remove the glottal articulation.

Lateral distortion of sibilant sounds is not too uncommon in the cleft palate population. Oral air flow during sibilant production is diverted to one or both sides of the mouth because of missing or malaligned teeth. A device as simple as a straw is most useful in first identifying the direction of oral air flow and then as a clinical tool in indicating properly directed air flow (Figure 8–31).

We must use our knowledge of phonetics to establish conditions and

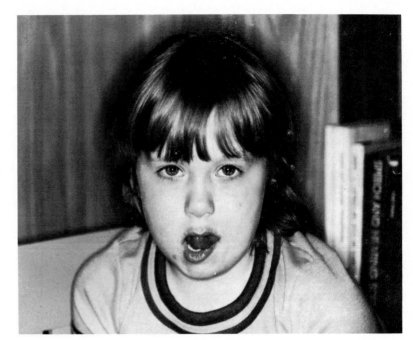

FIGURE 8–30 Patient with tongue extended to upper lip for the production of [lɑ].

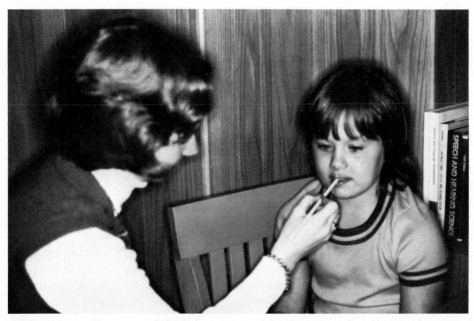

FIGURE 8–31 This straw aids both the patient and the clinician in identifying the direction of air flow for sibilant production.

movements of the speech mechanism that will facilitate improvement in the speech itself. The following hints are intended to assist the speech pathologist in carrying out a training program with the patient.

When teaching linguoalveolar sounds such as /t/, /d/, /n/, or /l/, have the patient at first extend the tongue tip to the upper lip. Once he is able to produce a labiolingual plosive, he should retract the tongue until a linguoalveolar results. Accept a compensatory placement if it is acoustically agreeable and not esthetically displeasing.

Avoid conditions that require extreme amounts of oral air pressure. "Trying harder" may prove more detrimental than beneficial, because it will usually increase the duration or the amount of pressure behind oral occlusion, either of which will force air flow nasally. Rather, one should promote easy production and light contacts. Begin with sounds that require little oral air pressure, such as /l/ and /r/. Then move to voiced plosives and fricatives and finally to the voiceless pressure sounds.

Promote articulator movement. An individual with a glottal speech pattern may exhibit very little lingual movement. Mirror work may be beneficial in imitating and encouraging lingual movement. Modify interfering facial grimaces. In general promote easy production with slow and inflected speech.

SPEECH BULB CONSTRUCTION

During the construction of the speech bulb, the speech pathologist works closely with the prosthodontist. Ideally the size of the bulb is adjusted until the patient demonstrates good oral air pressure for speech production and until unwanted nasal resonance is eliminated. At the same time, the patient must be able to breathe clearly through his nose and produce acceptable nasal sounds. The two specialists walk the fine line between good oral air pressure and the complete occluding of the nasopharynx.

The clinician should be warned that any type of nasal obstruction such as deviations of the nasal septum can interfere with his testing of the adequacy of the speech bulb. Recently a young woman with a speech appliance in place presented denasal and restricted nasal air flow on one hand, and hypernasality and reduced oral pressure that interfered with consonantal production on the other. The denasality and restricted nasal breathing were at first attributed to the speech bulb, yet both were evident even when the speech bulb was removed. Visual examination of the frontal radiograph revealed a severely deviated septum. In actuality, the restriction of air flow was in the nasal cavity, not in the nasopharynx. As a result, the size of the speech bulb was enlarged, nasal resonance was reduced, and oral air pressure was improved.

The speech pathologist's role during construction of the prosthetic speech appliance is one of continued observation and evaluation, and he relies on many of the same listening skills he used in the initial evaluation. He tests oral versus nasal air flow with a speech sample comprising voiceless pressure consonants. He tests for unwanted nasal resonance with a speech sample consisting of voiced sounds. The listening tube becomes an impor-

In group sessions the patient observes the actions and reactions of others who are already wearing speech appliances. He finds it easier to accept the situation as a member of a group than if he had been treated alone as an out-patient. In addition to speech and nonspeech exercises, we review with the youngsters the principles of good oral hygiene in caring for the teeth and the appliance.

The prime goal is to have each individual achieve intelligible speech at the socially acceptable level. While ample time must be allotted to speech therapy techniques, such as the articulation of isolated sounds, syllables, words, and sentences, attention must also be given to other aspects of communication skills. These include breath control (allowing enough inspired volume for specific situations), inflection, stress, and rate of speech. Mirrors are used to permit the child to study facial expressions often seen in cleft palate speech — "bunny nosing" and forehead wrinkling — as well as tongue placement. Paper paddles are held beneath the nostrils to give the patient a visual clue of air escape. The listening tube mentioned earlier in this chapter is also employed.

An essential part of the speech therapy program is listening. Listening is a learned art, and unfortunately too many patients with cleft palate haven't learned it. They speak without really hearing their own speech distortions, sound omissions or substitutions, glottal stops, or pharyngeal noises. To make them more aware, we encourage them not only to listen to themselves but to use video recording tapes and mirrors in conjunction with the application of their tactile sense to feel where the sounds are being made. Precise identification of the anatomical location of a problem is very important. Within this shared experience the patient can isolate his specific problems as he learns to observe the problems of other members of the group.

We would like to emphasize that there is much more to speech training than working with the speech machinery itself. Segments of the residential program are aimed at helping the individual to visualize not only his goals but his limitations and at assisting him in overcoming those limitations. For example, with puppets or dolls representing himself and his family members, the child is encouraged to participate in role-playing activities that bring out any feelings of frustration or lack of confidence that intrude in speaking situations. And since not all communication is oral, the children write letters home as part of their therapy. A certified school teacher is retained during the residence period to enable the youngsters to carry on their regular academic studies.

Trained counselors also play important roles in the program in testing, therapy, and handling personal problems. All candidates for residence therapy are screened at the outset with basic tests so that they can be selected on the basis of their needs and their ability to live and work together. Daily sessions are designed to help them accept and live with their problems and to set realistic goals as they strive to become the persons they would like to be. Some of the discussions relate to self-control and personality adjustment to the demands of daily living. Here the counselors are indispensable, for the task is too large and too complex to be handled by the speech pathologists alone. Actually the student learns to identify his speech problems with the speech pathologist and his behavior problems with his counselor. Group counseling is often carried out in closed sessions with a psychologist.

The counselors also supervise the recreation and the planned social experiences, including a certain amount of travel to nearby places of interest. Activities are designed to provide fun and entertainment and to afford leadership opportunities. The extracurricular side is very important, for many of these children, self-conscious about their appearance or speech defect, are shy and inhibited in social contacts, especially with the opposite sex. Eight weeks together in a warm and understanding environment can do much to relax these interpersonal tensions.

The resident counselors serve *in loco parentis* while the children are away from home. Each is a confidant, a leader, and an observer. He reports to other staff members regarding problems as well as improvement in the patient's behavior, his personal and oral hygiene, and his interest in carrying his newly learned speech habits outside the classroom. Weekly staff conferences are held to keep all the professional personnel informed regarding the progress — or negative reactions — of each individual.

There are, of course, a few difficulties encountered in a residential program. Some children become homesick, especially if they have been overprotected. But we have had much more trouble with parents who are upset about their youngsters' absence than we have had with homesickness among the children themselves. In any event the problem is a minor one and both child and parent adjust rather quickly. And the children may go home for a weekend or receive visits from their parents.

Perhaps the most troublesome and most persistent problem is one of financing the operation. It costs a great deal of money to maintain full-time, qualified resident counselors and to provide adequate home-like living quarters and food. Many of the eight-week sessions are conducted during the school year, and school-age children cannot be removed from the classroom for eight weeks without seriously hampering their educational programs. The expense of a certified teacher falls on the Institute because the public schools or agencies will not fund the educational activities of a private institution.

Among other special expenditures required in a residency undertaking are liability insurance, health and accident insurance, beds and bedding, furniture, ownership and maintenance of a van-type vehicle for transportation, and of course the general maintenance of separate living quarters for boys and girls and resident counselors.

Funds for the recreational activities and educational tours are furnished by the Clinic's Ladies Auxiliary. Some moneys for the residential budget come from such agencies as the Pennsylvania Department of Health, Cleft Palate Plastic Surgery Program, or the Pennsylvania Bureau of Vocational Rehabilitation. But these funds are for specific diagnostic or treatment services and the fee schedule set by the agencies does not meet the actual costs of operating a residency program. Therapy and dental treatment "line items" in the state's fee schedule are less than the usual or customary private practice fees for these services. Most of the children are affiliated with the state programs and the Clinic can be reimbursed only according to these limited schedules. Therefore it is necessary to obtain additional money, from donations or other sources, to meet our costs and bring our finances into balace.

Discouraging as the financial picture may be at times, we are thoroughly convinced that the program is worthwhile and that it and others like it deserve public support. Although the literature contains only a few reports concerning residential or intensive speech programs for children with cleft palate, those that have appeared reflect favorably upon the effectiveness of such treatment. Certainly our own evaluation efforts support that conclusion. It is not difficult to demonstrate speech improvement in children who have gone through the program when one employs before-and-after test analyses of articulation or intelligibility scores. Tape recordings, pressure-flow readings, and sound spectrographic analysis are utilized to hear, chart, and display differences in voice quality that have taken place as the result of intensive therapy.

In one study of the effectiveness of the Lancaster Cleft Palate Clinic residency program, Fricke[8] used two psychophysical procedures to evaluate the overall speech quality of the patients before and after the eight weeks of intensive speech therapy. The first method was the equal-appearing interval scale in which listeners evaluated a tape-recorded sample of the patient's speech on a nine point scale of severity in which one equals normal speech and nine equals extremely poor speech. The values between one and nine represent intermediate degrees of severity. The second method of evaluation was a paired-comparisons test. For this method listeners heard two randomly presented tape recordings of a patient, one before therapy and one after therapy. Their task was to select the one recording that represented the patient's best speech.

There was a total of 89 patients in the eight-week clinical speech programs over a period of five years. Speech therapy had stressed improvement of articulation and reduction of hypernasality. Seven trained listeners were asked to make an evaluation of recorded speech samples, based on their perception of a combination of articulatory patterns and voice quality — in other words, an overall rating of speech performance. They found that a majority of the patients demonstrated a positive change in speech behavior following the eight-week program. The results from the paired comparison tasks were regarded as showing a more favorable positive change than the results from the equal-appearing interval task.

Van Demark[27] reported the effects of a six-week intensive therapy program at The University of Iowa, finding that the students significantly improved their rating in terms of reducing articulatory defectiveness. Moreover, the results of the two articulation tests and three repeated sentence measures showed significant improvement upon post-therapy evaluation. Schendel and Bzoch[21] have reported similar increases in articulatory performance following intensive therapy in a residence program at the Florida State University at Tallahassee.

Children aged six to 12 attending 10-week sessions of a speech and language resident school at the dental school of the University of North Carolina at Chapel Hill have achieved speech improvement of 30 to 50 percentage points, according to Sandie Barrie Blackley, the speech clinician. Improvement was measured by the Whole Word Accuracy Test described by McCabe and Bradley. Gail Salling, the teacher assigned by the public school system to provide academic instruction, has reported that the youngsters, about half of whom have cleft palate, are so highly motivated and receive so much individual attention that many have made as much as a year's progress in the 10 weeks in a particular subject area.[1] The special school, which takes eight children in each session, is part of the orofacial and communicative disorders program, directed by William C. Trier, at the University.

Above and beyond all of the objective evaluations, such as the before-and-after articulation tests and the sound spectrographs, one can measure the worth of the residence programs, we believe, in the psychological gains reported by parents, teachers, and school therapists when the children return to their home communities. The improvements may be too subtle to demonstrate immediately upon completion of the eight-week residence period, but in the months and years that follow they are recognized and warmly appreciated for their lasting value to the patient and his family.

Improvement in speech intelligibility ranges from 35 to 90 per cent, depending upon the number of errors present at the beginning of the program, the patient's intellectual capacity, his level of acuity, and, most important, his degree of motivation. Those patients who continue with speech therapy programs at school have the highest rate of carry-over improvement when reevaluated six months after their session in residence. The patients who do not follow up the residency work with additional speech therapy do tend to regress after six months. However, the point of regression or back-sliding is still above their score when admitted to the intensive speech program.

In following our patients we maintain an interest in their ability to communicate effectively, to continue their education, to improve their social contacts, to become employed, and to marry. They have succeeded in a wide variety of vocations; many of them are also parents.

The goal of our residence program is to help these young people to learn about their physical differences and how to overcome their structural defects, to speak with social acceptability, and function in society. On the wall of the Clinic waiting room are these lines:

> Oh God, give me the serenity
> to accept the things I cannot change,
> the courage to change the things I can,
> and the wisdom to know the difference.

When that statement is understood by the patient, the family, the speech clinician, and all of the principals involved in the process of rehabilitation, then we can say: "We've met and handled the challenge."

References

1. ADA Newsletter American Dental Association, January 10, 1977.
2. Blakeley, R. N.: The Practice of Speech Pathology: A Clinical Diary, Springfield, Illinois, Charles C Thomas, 1972.
3. Bzoch, K. R.: An investigation of the speech of preschool cleft palate children. Unpublished Ph.D. Dissertation, Northwestern University, Chicago, 1956.
4. Cooper, H. K.: Cinefluorography with image intensification as an aid in treatment planning for some cleft lip and/or cleft palate cases. Am. J. Orthod., 42:815, 1956.
5. Cooper, H. K., and F. A. Hofmann: The application of cinefluoroscopy with image intensification in the field of plastic surgery, dentistry and speech. Plast. Reconstr. Surg., 16:135, 1955.
6. Counihan, D. T.: Articulation skills of adolescents and adults with cleft palate. J. Speech Hear. Disord., 25:181, 1960.
7. Darley, F. L., A. E. Aronson, and J. R. Brown: Clusters of deviant speech dimensions in the dysarthrias. J. Speech Hear. Res., 12:462, 1969.

8. Fricke, J. E.: Speech improvement following intensive clinical treatment. Unpublished data, Lancaster Cleft Palate Clinic, Lancaster, Pennsylvania, 1971.
9. Fritzell, B.: The velopharyngeal muscles in speech. Acta Otolaryngol. (Suppl.), 250:1, 1969.
10. Mazaheri, M., and E. Mazaheri: Prosthodontic aspects of palatal elevation and palatopharyngeal stimulation. J. Prosthet. Dent., 31:319, 1976.
11. Mazaheri, M., and R. T. Millard: Changes in nasal resonance related to differences in location and dimension of speech bulbs. Cleft Palate J., 2:167, 1965.
12. Mazaheri, M., R. T. Millard, and D. M. Erickson: Cineradiographic comparison of normal to noncleft subjects with velopharyngeal inadequacy. Cleft Palate J., 1:199, 1964.
13. Millard, R. T.: Role of the sound spectrograph as a diagnostic tool. International Congress of Phoniatrics and Logopedics, Barcelona, Spain, 1956.
14. Millard, R. T.: Training for optimal use of the prosthetic speech aid. In Bzoch, K. (ed.): Communicative Disorders Related to Cleft Lip and Palate (Revision in press), Boston, Little, Brown, 1977.
15. Moll, K. L.: Speech characteristics of individuals with cleft lip and palate. In Spriestersbach, D. C., and D. Sherman (eds.): Cleft Palate and Communication, New York, Academic Press, p. 61, 1968.
16. Morris, H. L.: Communication skills of children with cleft lip and palates. J. Speech Hear. Res., 5:79, 1962.
17. Philips, B. J., and R. J. Harrison: Language skills of preschool cleft palate children. Cleft Palate J., 6:245, 1969.
18. Project Child, Beginning to talk: How parents can help. Lancaster-Lebanon Intermediate Unit #13, 1976.
19. Riski, J. E.: Unpublished data, Lancaster Cleft Palate Clinic, Lancaster, Pennsylvania, 1977.
20. Riski, J. E., R. T. Millard, C. Watt, et al.: Longitudinal analysis of speech development in children with clefts from three to eight years. Presented at the yearly meeting of the American Cleft Palate Association, San Francisco, May 13, 1976.
21. Schendel, L. L., and K. R. Bzoch: Advantages of intensive summer training programs. In Grabb, W. C., S. W. Rosenstein, and K. R. Bzoch (eds.): Cleft Lip and Palate, Boston, Little, Brown, 1971.
22. Shprintzen, R. J., G. N. McCall, M. L. Skolnick, et al.: Selective movements of the lateral aspects of the pharyngeal walls during velopharyngeal closure for speech, blowing, and whistling in normals. Cleft Palate J., 12:51, 1975.
23. Shprintzen, R. J., G. N. McCall, M. L. Skolnick, et al.: A new therapeutic technique for the treatment of velopharyngeal incompetence. J. Speech Hear. Disord., 40:69, 1975.
24. Spriestersbach, D. C., F. L. Darley, and V. Rouse: Articulation of a group of children with cleft lips and palate. J. Speech Hear. Disord., 21:436, 1956.
25. Spriestersbach, D. C., D. R. Dickson, F. C. Fraser, et al.: Clinical research in cleft lip and cleft palate: The state of the art. Cleft Palate J., 10:113, 1973.
26. Templin, M. C., and F. L. Darley: The Templin-Darley Tests of Articulation, Bureau of Educational Research and Services, Division of Extension and University of Iowa, Iowa City, 1969.
27. Van Demark, D. R.: Articulatory changes in the therapeutic process. Cleft Palate J., 8:159, 1971.
28. Warren, D. W., and F. A. Hofmann: A cineradiographic study of velopharyngeal closure. Plast. Reconstr. Surg., 28:556, 1961.
29. Williams, W. N., C. R. Eisenbach, K. R. Bzoch, et al.: Clinical guidelines in selecting a speech sample for the radiographic assessment of velopharyngeal function. Presented at the Florida Cleft Palate Association, Gainesville, Florida, March 1976.

Chapter Nine _____

The aims of this chapter are: (1) to present an overview of the status of hearing loss in cleft palate populations, (2) to describe the test procedures at this Institute for the assessment of hearing in children with a cleft palate, (3) to present a periodic audiometric examination program for such children, and (4) to indicate the directions of research into the problems of hearing and cleft palate at this institute.

The implications of a hearing loss vary among individuals and circumstances. Factors which influence the effect of the loss upon the functioning of the organism are the degree of the loss, the age at which it was sustained, and its duration.

Temporary hearing deficiency early in life may be expected to affect the child's speech, language, voice patterns, educational and social behavior, and other avenues of adjustment. A hearing loss in early childhood may affect speech development in proportion to both the degree and the duration of the loss.[24] Researchers have reported that children with fluctuating hearing losses performed less well than expected on tasks requiring auditory reception, vocal expression, or both.[15] One researcher indicated that a hearing loss, even for temporary periods during the speech learning process, can produce articulatory errors.[34] Others have suggested that the fluctuating hearing loss that accompanies otitis media is the cause of a significant delay in language development.[12]

There is a greater tendency for temporary hearing deficiency to develop among younger children than among those who are older. This variation with age may be influenced by upper respiratory infections, chronic colds, influenza, and otitis media, which occur more frequently in children than in adults. Repeated infection of the middle ear is among the most common causes of hearing loss in children.

HEARING LOSS AND CLEFT PALATE

Children with a cleft palate are known to have a higher incidence of hearing loss, particularly when they are young, than non-cleft children. When dealing with children with a cleft of the lip or palate, however, the significance of a hearing impairment is frequently minimized or entirely overlooked because of the preoccupation with the more obvious defect.

The association of hearing loss with the cleft palate has been made for many years. Skolnik[26] listed some of the early observations: In the latter half of the nineteenth century, one paper reported the cure of deaf-mutism by treating otorrhea and congenital cleft palate, and another indicated that approximately half of all patients with cleft palates had hearing disturbances.

HEARING AND AUDIOLOGY
ELCA T. SWIGART

In 1904, "draining of milk through the ear in an infant with congenital cleft palate" was reported.

Controlled audiometric studies of hearing sensitivity of patients with cleft palates have been performed and reported in the literature, but this has been a more recent development. As late as 1940 one researcher observed that "a survey of the literature over the past ten years fails to reveal even one scientific investigation concerning loss of hearing specifically in cleft palate cases."[3]

Incidence of Hearing Loss

Research programs have been initiated to gain more information about the hearing sensitivity of individuals with a cleft of the lip or palate. Since 1940 the scientific literature has presented contradictory data concerning hearing sensitivity and cleft palate, and many issues remain controversial. The reported incidence of hearing loss varied with each study. Table 9–1 presents the results of several of the investigations, noting the investigator, date of investigation, number of subjects, range of age of subjects, criterion for determining hearing loss, and per cent of subjects demonstrating a loss. The incidence of hearing loss ranged from 0 per cent (Heller, Hochberg, and Milano) to 90 per cent (Sataloff and Fraser). It has been suggested that the variation in reported incidence of hearing loss in the cleft palate population may be due to inconsistencies in research methodology. These inconsistencies include different definitions of a hearing loss and intergroup differences among the cleft palate population with respect to the type of cleft, type of physical management, and age of subjects at the time of testing.

The criteria employed to designate a hearing loss ranged from the most severe limit (average of the thresholds of speech frequency exceeding 5 dB in the worse ear), reported by Graham and Lierle, to a more liberal limit (thresholds exceeding 30 dB at one or more frequencies from 125 to 12000 Hz) reported by Miller. In some instances the definition did not indicate whether the better ear or the worse ear or both were considered. The frequencies used in the evaluation were not always specified and the definition of a hearing loss was sometimes stated vaguely, e.g., "recognizable handicap of hearing," and "conductive deafness."

Spriestersbach and colleagues[27] recognized that these discrepancies in the reported incidence of hearing loss arose from the use of different criteria for hearing loss. They employed, therefore, three types of analyses of test results: (1) the average of the speech frequencies (500, 1000, and 2000 Hz); (2) the average of six frequencies (250, 5000, 1000, 2000, 4000, and 8000

TABLE 9–1 Investigations of Incidence of Hearing Loss in Individuals with Cleft Palate

Investigator	Date	No. of Sub-jects	Age of Sub-jects	Criterion for Hearing Loss°	Per-centage with Loss	Per-centage of Institute's Group with Loss
Berry & Eisenson[1]	1956	383	–	Recognizable handicap in hearing	60	–
Drettner[2]	1960	63	5–53	More than 15 dB in speech range (average 500, 1000, 2000 Hz)	49	30
Gaines[3]	1940	44	4–13	Loss criterion not stated (64, 128, 256, 512, 1024, 2048, 4096, 8192 Hz)	–	–
Gannon[4]	1950	50	6–16	(1) 10 dB or more in better ear (average 503, 1024, 2046 Hz)	34†	18
				(2) 10 dB or more (average 128–8192 Hz)	44†	
Goetzinger, Brooks, & Proud[5]	1960	42	16–75	More than 15 dB in speech range (500, 1000, 2000 Hz) (Used mean for all subjects in either ear; individually there were some losses)	–	–
Graham & Lierle[6]	1962	43	7–26	Average loss of 5 dB or more over speech frequencies in worse ear (500, 1000, 2000 Hz)	42†	58
Graham, Schweiger, & Olin[7]	1962	54	8–26	(1) Average loss of more than 15 dB in better ear (500, 1000, 2000 Hz)	10†	12
				(2) Average loss of more than 15 dB in worse ear (500, 1000, 2000 Hz)	26†	30
Halfond & Ballenger[8]	1956	69	8–21	20 dB or more at any two or more frequencies in either ear (125, 250, 500, 1000, 2000, 4000, 8000 Hz)	54	–
Heller, Hochberg, & Milano[10]	1969	60	3–12	(1) Acceptable range of normal	0†	–
				(2) Average 15 dB or greater air-bone gap at 500, 1000, 2000, 4000 Hz	40	–
Holborow[11]	1962	–	–	Conductive deafness	50	–
Holmes & Reed[12]	1955	26	–	Greater than 10 dB in one or both ears (average 500, 1000, 2000 Hz)	62	38
Linthicum & Body[16]	1959	58	?–15	10 or 15 dB is clinically significant; frequencies not stated	40	–
Loeb[17]	1964	108	2–42	More than 15 dB in either ear up to 6000 Hz; not stated whether average or individual frequency	42	–
Master, Bingham, & Robinson[18]	1960	172	–	More than 10 dB; frequencies not stated	49	–
Means & Irwin[19]	1954	225	3–16	(1) Fail to pass 4 out of 6 freq. (250, 500, 1000, 2000, 4000, 8000 Hz) at 15 dB	59	–
				(2) 25 dB or more at either 250, 500, 1000, or 2000 Hz or 30 dB or more at 4000 or 8000 Hz	31†	39
Miller[20]	1956	35	3–23	30 dB or greater at one or more of frequencies tested (125, 250, 500, 1000, 2000, 3000, 4000, 8000, 10,000, 12,000 Hz)	54	–
Pannbacker[22]	1969	103	3–41	15 dB or more in one ear (average 500, 1000, 2000 Hz)	53	35
Sataloff & Fraser[25]	1952	30	5–16	15 dB in at least two frequencies; frequencies not stated	90	–

TABLE 9–1   Investigations of Hearing Loss in Individuals with Cleft Palate—*Continued*

INVESTIGATOR	DATE	NO. OF SUB-JECTS	AGE OF SUB-JECTS	CRITERION FOR HEARING LOSS*	PER-CENTAGE WITH LOSS	PER-CENTAGE OF INSTITUTE'S GROUP WITH LOSS
Skolnik[26]	1957	401	–	Demonstrated hearing loss	39	–
Spriestersbach, Lierle, Moll, & Prather[27]	1962	163	2–15	(1) Average over speech frequency (500, 1000, 2000 Hz)		
				10 dB better ear	29	20
				worse ear	62	41
				20 dB better ear	12	8
				worse ear	37	26
				30 dB better ear	6	2
				worse ear	18	14
				(2) Average overall frequency (250, 500, 1000, 2000, 4000, 8000, Hz)		
				10 dB better ear	19	26
				worse ear	51	47
				20 dB better ear	7	15
				worse ear	27	27
				30 dB better ear	3	5
				worse ear	13	18
				(3) Loss at any one of six frequencies (250, 500, 1000, 2000, 4000, 8000 Hz)		
				10 dB better ear	44	79
				worse ear	74	88
				20 dB better ear	16	51
				worse ear	40	65
				30 dB better ear	7	24
				worse ear	21	38
Sweitzer, Melrose, & Morris[29]	1968	107	4–25	(1) Used 9 different definitions of a hearing loss (air conduction)		
				Better ears	1–52	–
				Worse ears	15–81	–
				(2) Air-bone gap greater than 10 dB for average of 500, 1000, 2000 Hz	78	–

*The criteria are sometimes vague because the authors were vague in their definitions of a loss.
†Interpolated from information in text.

Hz); and (3) any one of six frequencies tested. In addition, the criteria of 10, 20, and 30 dB were sequentially considered to constitute a hearing loss for each type. Thus, their investigation produced percentages of hearing loss ranging from 3.2 per cent to 74.2 per cent. They concluded that "the percentage of children with a loss varies greatly as a function of the definition of a loss."

A group of 66 children between seven and 14 years old with cleft palates was selected from the Institute's files. Their pure tone thresholds were assessed and the criterion for hearing loss of each of the investigators listed in Table 9–1 was applied. The various percentages that were obtained from the same set of thresholds are listed in the final column. Blanks occur in the column in situations in which the criteria were unclear or could not be applied to the thresholds of the 66 children. The hearing sensitivity of children with a cleft palate at this Institute appears not unlike that found elsewhere. Unspecified interrelated variables may partially account for differences that exist.

There are several texts and publications which list very comprehensive bibliographies of investigations dealing with hearing loss associated with clefts. The majority of investigators state that most individuals with a cleft palate who have a hearing loss have a bilateral, conductive type of loss.[1, 11, 25, 27, 35] Others have found, however, that the majority of children with a cleft palate had significant unilateral losses in cases in which air-bone gaps were considered.[10]

There is little agreement concerning the frequencies affected most in cleft-associated hearing loss. One researcher reported a lessened perception for both the high and low frequencies;[3] another reported that the predominant hearing loss found in people with a cleft palate is in the low frequencies;[25] and a third researcher found that the high frequencies above 8000 Hz were the most affected.[20]

Variables

There are also variables within the cleft palate population that may be relevant to the hearing loss:

Type of Cleft

One finds a discrepancy in the literature with respect to the effect of the type of cleft upon hearing loss. Many researchers report no definite relationship between hearing loss and the type or width of the cleft.[4, 8, 13] An investigator in Switzerland found that the severity of the cleft of 150 postoperative patients with a cleft palate was "parallel to the increase in severity of hearing loss."[21] Others reported a higher incidence of hearing loss in the group of individuals with clefts of the hard and soft palates than in those with clefts of the lip and palate.[18] The latter authors pointed out that this difference was most evident in the better ear.

Contrary to the foregoing, others indicate that the subjects with a cleft lip and palate have poorer hearing than the subjects with a cleft palate only.[29] Their criterion for hearing acuity was the threshold for the worse ear.

In many instances it is not clearly specified whether the better or worse ear or both were considered when the hearing of individuals with different types of clefts was compared. In addition, other variables, such as the criterion for hearing loss or the age at time of testing, were not consistent in the various investigations. Consequently, the data appear to be contradictory and the relationship between the incidence of hearing loss and the type of cleft remains unclear.

Age

A variable within the cleft palate population is the age of the child when hearing is evaluated. Several authorities see a relationship between the incidence of hearing loss among individuals with a cleft palate and age. It was generally found that there are less severe degrees of hearing loss with an increase in age. The older subjects had lower mean thresholds than did the younger ones, regardless of type of cleft.

Adults with a cleft palate appear to have only a slightly raised threshold.

In terms of the criteria of normal hearing (0 to 25 dB, 1969 ANSI Standards), they possess adequate hearing through the speech range. Some researchers question whether frequently recurring middle ear disease and hearing loss in children with a cleft palate have an ultimate effect upon hearing level in later life. They conclude that middle ear disease in people with a cleft palate runs its course before adulthood.[5] To the contrary, others feel that untreated middle ear disease will result in an increased degree of hearing loss in adulthood.[20]

In the adult cleft palate population (ages 15 to 55 years) studied at the Institute,[32] the mean air-conducted thresholds for the speech frequencies were within normal limits: 12 dB for the better and 20 dB for the worse ear. The mean thresholds for those adults with a velopharyngeal inadequacy were very similar to those for the group with cleft palates. Those with only a cleft of the lip, however, demonstrated very good hearing: their mean thresholds for the speech frequencies were 3 dB and 5 dB for the better and worse ears, respectively.

An investigation of a group of seven- to 14-year-old children with cleft palates and their non-cleft siblings at the Institute supports the view that the hearing of children with cleft palates improves with age.[30] Although the hearing thresholds of the children with clefts in this age bracket were significantly poorer than those of their siblings, both groups were within what are generally considered normal limits (25 dB, 1969 ANSI Standards) at all frequencies tested.

It is important to note that although the mean threshold for the group with cleft palates was within normal limits, there were some children who had a conductive hearing loss resulting from recurrent otitis media. It is the purpose of a rehabilitation program not only to detect these children, but to offer remedial treatment as soon as possible.

Physical Management

Other controversial questions deal with the effects of physical management of the child upon his hearing sensitivity.

Surgery. Efforts have been made to relate the surgical history of the palate to auditory acuity. Several investigators could find no relationship between the incidence or degree of hearing loss and the age at which the palate was closed.[4, 13, 26] Of the studies in which relationship was indicated, age differences among the groups at the time of audiometric examination may possible account for the findings.

Speech Appliance. There has been concern whether or not a speech appliance initiates or contributes to middle ear infection and consequent hearing loss. One group of researchers, in testing 54 patients (ranging in age from eight to 25 years) before and after insertion of an appliance, indicated that there were no cases in which the hearing loss became greater following insertion of an obturator.[7] On the other hand, another researcher cautions that the use of a prosthetic device predisposes the patient to more hearing loss than other methods of palatal closure.[17]

In the study mentioned earlier of seven- to 14-year-old children with a cleft of the palate,[30] no significant difference was found between the hearing thresholds of those who wore a speech appliance and those who did not.

Likewise, in the adult population no differences in pure tone thresholds could be found among those who wore a speech appliance and those who did not.[32]

Test Methods

The routine procedures of audiometric examination for children with a cleft lip or palate used at the H. K. Cooper Institute are as follows:

Standard Pure Tone Audiometry

An audiometer is an instrument that generates pure tones; the intensity of the tones can be controlled by an attenuator. Zero on the attenuator dial indicates the lowest intensity at which the average normal ear in controlled conditions can detect the presence of the tone 50 per cent of the time. A listener is asked to indicate when a stimulus was heard. The most frequently used signals to indicate perception of a sound are raising the hand or finger or pressing a button that lights a bulb on the examiner's control panel. Hearing sensitivity is thus measured as the intensity of the pure tone (expressed in decibels above the zero point) at which the individual signals that he or she detects it. The results of the test are recorded on an audiogram, which has two dimensions: (1) frequency of the stimulus tone along the abscissa, and (2) intensity along the ordinate.

The tones produced by the audiometer are delivered to the patient's ear through earphones for air conduction tests and through a bone oscillator for tests of inner ear functioning. The symbols 0 (for the right ear) and X (for the left ear) are used to plot the threshold points for air-conducted tones at each frequency. The symbols [and] are used to plot the masked* threshold points for bone-conducted tones at each frequency for the right and left ears, respectively.

The audiogram in Figure 9–1 shows a raised threshold (a hearing loss) for air-conducted pure tones but a threshold within normal limits for bone-conducted pure tones. The comparison of hearing sensitivity by air and bone yields information of diagnostic significance. The difficulty in this case is not with the perception of sound by the inner ear, but with the transmission of sound waves from the outer ear through the middle ear to the analyzing system of the inner ear. The type of loss shown in this audiogram is termed "conductive hearing impairment" and is characteristic of individuals with a cleft palate.

Play Audiometry

Play audiometry is a variation of standard audiometry in which the child is motivated to listen to and respond to the stimulus through various playing situations. The attention span of young children ages two and one-half to five years will not always permit the lengthy testing one can accomplish

---

*When testing by bone conduction it is necessary to employ a masking noise or sound in one ear while the other is being tested in order to rule out participation of the non-test ear.

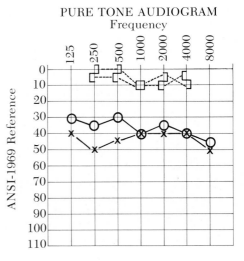

FIGURE 9-1 A typical audiogram illustrating a conductive hearing loss. The bone conduction thresholds are within normal limits, but the air conduction thresholds are raised. In this example the hearing loss results from pathology or malfunctioning of the outer or middle ear with a normal inner ear. O = right ear, air conduction; X = left ear, air conduction; [= right ear, bone conduction;] = left ear, bone conduction.

with adults. Therefore, the child is instructed to make one of a variety of responses that will keep his or her interest in the testing. At the Institute the child is seated facing the examiner in an acoustically treated room. He or she is simultaneously instructed and conditioned to perform the listening task in the following manner: The examiner places a block in the child's hand and holds the hand to the earphone. Immediately after the stimulus tone is presented well above threshold via earphones, the examiner places the child's hand holding the block into the box on his or her lap and pushes the block out of the child's hand. This procedure continues until the examiner sees that the child spontaneously initiates movement to place the block in the box after a stimulus presentation. Following conditioning, an ascending method of presenting the intensity of the stimuli is used to determine the threshold at each frequency. The results of the test are recorded on an audiogram, as in standard pure tone audiometry. Figure 9–2 shows a child being administered an audiometric examination by play audiometry.

Behavioral (Orientation Reflex) Audiometry

Auditory sensitivity can be assessed by a behavioral technique employing orientation reflexes. As illustrated by the schematic diagram in Figure 9–3, the child is placed on the mother's lap facing a camouflaged observation window in an acoustically treated room. The parent is instructed to make no response during the testing period. One of two speakers is located approximately three feet away at a 90-degree angle to the left of the child's face; the other speaker is located at a 90-degree angle to the right of the child's face. Under each speaker is a small light bulb that can be illuminated for reinforcement at the discretion of the examiner. The examiner and a trained observer are in the acoustically treated control room during all testing.

Various sounds are introduced via either of the loudspeakers. The 12 stimuli include five familiar sounds (cup and spoon, squeeze toy, rattle, small horn, and large horn), a 1000 Hz pure tone, white noise (a wide band of frequencies at approximately equal intensity), and five vocal stimuli (the child's name, "buh," "kuh," cat's "meow," and the examiner's imitation of a baby's cry). Each stimulus is repeated at an increased intensity level until

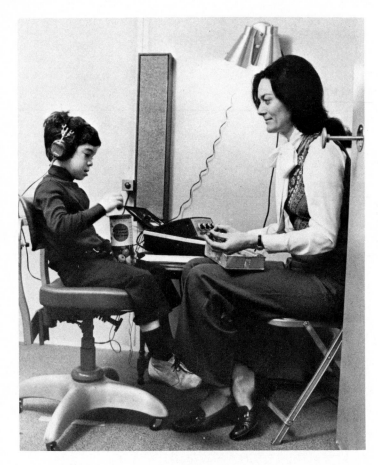

FIGURE 9–2   Audiologist tests young child's hearing by play audiometry. The child has been conditioned to place blocks in a box when he hears a sound.

the examiner observes the child making a response. A "response" is defined as any change in the child's behavior that both the examiner and the trained observer agree was evoked by the stimulus. The intensity level at which the child responded to each stimulus is recorded, as is the type of response.

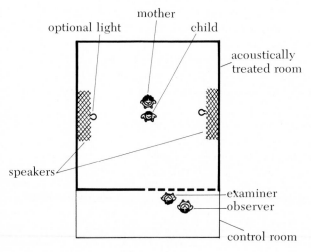

FIGURE 9–3   Schematic diagram of testing area for orientation reflexes.

Some of the most frequent acceptable responses include: (1) turning of the head in the direction of the sound source; (2) movement of the eyes in the direction of the sound source; (3) movement of the eyes up from a lower position or in a searching manner; (4) cessation of movement; and (5) cessation of vocalization.

The mean of the three lowest thresholds (the three best responses) is used to indicate the approximate threshold for the better ear. It should be remembered that the sound field test used in behavioral audiometry is a bilateral test and yields information only about the status of the better hearing ear.

Behavioral audiometry is a very subjective method of assessing auditory sensitivity. Although variations of this method are in common use with very young children, it is difficult to determine what the test is measuring.

Since children with a cleft palate typically have a relatively flat audiogram (the extent of hearing loss is approximately the same at all frequencies), an attempt was made to compare the results of behavioral audiometry with those of play audiometry for children two and one-half, three, or three and one-half years old.[31] Audiometric examinations were administered to 236 children, first by a behavioral technique employing orientation reflexes, and, secondly, by standard pure tone audiometry. For each child the means of the three lowest thresholds obtained from 12 sound field stimuli were compared with the means of the pure tone thresholds for the speech frequencies in the better ear. Of the behavioral means, 63 per cent fell within ±5 dB of the standard means; 86 per cent of the behavioral means fell within ±10 dB of the standard means; and 93 per cent of the behavioral means were within ±15 dB of the standard means. Age made little difference in the variation between the results of the two tests.

It was concluded that if used with children with a cleft palate, the behavioral audiometric examination just described was a good indication of the pure tone average for the speech frequencies for the better ear. The usefulness of the behavioral audiometric procedure lies in the fact that information may be gained indicating whether or not the child's hearing is sufficient for the acquisition of speech.

Impedance Audiometry

In simplest terms, measures of acoustic impedance tell something about the "opposition" encountered by an acoustic wave as it passes through the middle ear to the inner ear. These procedures indicate whether or not the middle ear is functioning normally.

Each of three basic measurement techniques is used to evaluate the status of the middle ear:

Tympanometry. Tympanometry is a method of measuring changes in acoustic impedance at the plane of the ear drum by measuring changes in air pressure in the ear canal. Acoustic impedance is at a minimum in the normal ear when the air pressure in the middle ear is equal to the air pressure in the ear canal. Thus, by systematically raising and lowering the air pressure in the ear canal and recording the impedance, one can obtain a graphic portrayal of the relationship between pressure in the external canal and impedance at the plane of the ear drum. Patients with otitis media or poorly functioning eustachian tubes will produce a graph different from that produced by the normally functioning middle ear. Since otitis media and poorly functioning eustachian tubes frequently accompany cleft palate, tympanometry is particularly applicable in the evaluation of this population.

Reflex measures. Contraction of the stapedius muscle increases the impedance of the middle ear. In the normal ear, the stapedius muscle will contract when the ear is stimulated with a sufficiently intense sound. For pure tones, this response occurs at a specific range above the hearing threshold level. A method of measuring hearing level is thus provided through this involuntary response to the presentation of the acoustic stimuli. This is a useful procedure in the evaluation of very young children with a cleft palate, because it requires no voluntary response.

Static compliance. Compliance refers to the mobility of the ossicular chain in the middle ear. (Acoustic impedance is a term frequently found in literature and refers to the inverse function of compliance.) Static compliance is derived from the difference of two measurement values. The first measurement is made with a specific positive pressure in the ear canal, and the second measurement is made with a pressure in the ear canal which equals the pressure in the middle ear. The latter pressure permits the tympanic membrane to be in its most compliant, or mobile, condition. The difference between these two measurement values indicates the static compliance of the middle ear. This test is particularly applicable to the cleft palate population, since it helps identify perforated tympanic membranes or indicates the patency of ventilating tubes in the tympanic membrane.

Impedance audiometry is useful with children because the tests can be administered rapidly and easily and require no voluntary response. Impedance audiometry is especially useful in the identification of middle ear pathology so frequently associated with cleft palate. Although these tests are not a substitute for pure tone threshold testing, they can provide substantial information about the ear. The procedure for administering impedance tests may be found in many audiology textbooks published within the last few years. Figure 9–4 shows a child prepared for impedance audiometry.

Tests for Special Problems in Hearing

The tests described earlier are administered routinely. It is sometimes necessary to administer a variety of specialized tests to identify the site of lesion, to select candidates for operative procedures, or to determine the existence of nonorganic hearing problems. Speech audiometry is also frequently used to assess the patient's speech reception threshold or speech discrimination ability. These specialized tests can be found in any book dealing with diagnostic audiology, such as *Modern Developments in Audiology*,[14] by James Jerger, or a *A Handbook of Clinical Audiology*,[15] by Jack Katz.

Program of Periodic Hearing Examinations

The high incidence of ear disease in children with a cleft palate has been well documented.[23, 28] Ear pathology and hearing sensitivity are frequently related, but there is not always a positive correlation between the

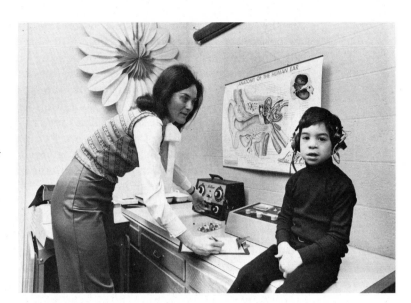

FIGURE 9–4   Testing a child for acoustic impedance.

two. In an investigation of 864 ears at the Institute, Swigart and Stool[33] found a wide diversity in the condition of the eardrum as viewed otoscopically with respect to hearing status. They are in agreement with others that pathological change is not always an indication of the degree of hearing loss.[2, 10, 25, 36] Conversely, it cannot be assumed that just because a child's ears *appear* normal, the hearing sensitivity is also within normal limits. This absence of a one-to-one relationship between hearing loss and middle ear pathology necessitates audiological and otological examinations on a periodic schedule when dealing with children with a cleft palate.

At six months of age each child with a cleft lip or palate is scheduled for the first audiometric examination. This age for initiating a test program was selected for two reasons: (1) by six months of age the orientation reflex is well established in the normally developing infant, and (2) the children are recalled at this age for treatment and examinations by the other members of the Institute team.

When children appear at the Institute for this sixth month appointment, the parents are given a flow chart listing all the professionals they will see that day. First on the list is the audiologist. It is important to evaluate a young child audiometrically before he or she is seen by the other specialists. This arrangement prevents the child from entering the environment of the hearing test when tired or apprehensive from contact with new faces. It also gives the audiologist an opportunity to inform all his or her colleagues of the child's hearing status by attaching a note to the flow sheet. Information concerning hearing sensitivity is especially valuable to the otologist and the speech pathologist. When a significant hearing loss exists, all disciplines should be aware of the problem.

Although many professionals are aware of the relationship between hearing loss and cleft palate, individuals associated with those with a cleft palate are usually unaware of a hearing loss in the patient. This is common in a situation in which a mild to moderate hearing loss occurs. The child with a mild loss has to concentrate more on what is being said, but with effort he

Chapter Ten _____

PATIENT SERVICES _____

The purpose of the patient services department is to initiate a close relationship between the patient, family, and Institute, obtain accurate patient information, explain financial costs to the family, provide individual or family counseling when needed, and facilitate the collection of vital data for clinical and research purposes. A caseworker performs these functions because he or she is well equipped to handle the emotional sensitivity involved. The following two cases illustrate the need for and the kind of flexibility necessary to insure that the immediate needs of the patient and the family are met.

When Johnny Jones* was brought to the Institute for a diagnostic evaluation to determine the full extent of his cleft lip and palate, he was just 10 days old. His parents had had an opportunity, while mother and baby were still confined in the hospital, to talk with the obstetrician, pediatrician, and other hospital personnel about Johnny's birth defect. Having been assured that the necessary care and treatment were available to them, their immediate anxieties were alleviated and they were prepared to begin participating in their son's habilitation.

The initial interview, therefore, was concerned mainly with explaining the services available and clarifying the financial issues involved. Johnny progressed nicely, had lip surgery at about seven weeks of age, and developed into a healthy, strong little boy. There was no further direct contact between the caseworker and family until two years later, at which time it was necessary to update the family information for our records.

In contrast with Johnny's case was that of Jamie King, whose mother became hysterical and at times irrational when she saw she had given birth to a child with a cleft lip and palate. She would speak to no one while in the hospital. At the time of Jamie's first visit to the Institute at two weeks of age, Mrs. King appeared distraught, disheveled, and totally exhausted. She was tearful throughout the interview and interjected many questions regarding survival of the baby. She said that she had already returned Jamie to the hospital on several occasions because she was unable to feed him and couldn't stand his crying. Mrs. King was insistent in her demands for immediate surgery to alleviate feeding problems and "make him less ugly to look at." Counseling sessions were arranged twice a week to help her understand her feelings. The immediate focus of counseling was to teach the mother how to feed the baby so that the necessary weight gain to allow lip surgery at the

*Patients' real names have not been used in this section.

PHILIP STARR
AND KITTY HEISERMAN*

earliest possible time would be achieved. Feeding instructions and demonstrations were given by the caseworker.

Daily phone calls to the caseworker were made by Mrs. King to ask questions, report on Jamie's daily progress, and just to talk. Because all criteria could be met, lip surgery was performed at four weeks of age, which led to a second period of crisis for Mrs. King because of her fears that crying would "tear out sutures and leave an ugly scar." She again returned Jamie to the hospital for several days of care, and attention was then focused on this aspect of Mrs. King's behavior. She was helped to recognize Jamie's need for consistent maternal care and, within three weeks after the removal of the surgical sutures, was able to assume full-time responsibility for the care of her son.

These two case histories span a range from an easy situation to the most difficult; most families fall somewhere in between. They illustrate, however, the need for different and flexible service approaches by the caseworker.

The usual procedure with nearly all families is to present a brief background history of the Institute at the first visit and to supplement this with a brochure that describes the history and the treatment programs in greater detail. The caseworker reviews with the family the outline of services and discusses the age levels at which the various treatments and tests may begin. The clinicians who will be directly involved with the patient's treatment and the team approach are discussed. Cooper's philosophy of "not only treating the child with a hole in his mouth, but treating the whole child" is explained.

These conversations emphasize the need for monitoring the child's physical and emotional growth and development at regular intervals. The distinction between monitoring and the actual presence of a problem is made. The value of regular monitoring for early identification of a possible problem area is stressed and assurance is given that the Institute has available the necessary treatment services when, and if, needed.

During these discussions, great care is exercised to avoid creating undue alarm and anxiety over problems that may never arise. This prevents the parents from becoming immobilized with fear over their child's future growth and development.

Many questions are usually asked during the initial interview. The most frequent is, "What caused my baby to have a cleft?" The second most com-

---

*Deceased January 5, 1978.

499

mon is, "Will all my children be born like this?" The caseworker must reply truthfully, "I don't know." The implications concerning heredity are discussed briefly and the family is then offered the consulting services of the geneticist, who can more competently and accurately determine and define the inheritance factors and risk rates for future births.

When rapport is established early in the treatment program, parents are more apt to seek out the caseworker at future appointments to discuss such concerns as the child's physical growth, delay in speech, hearing problems, physical appearance, mental development, inability to cope with the school situation, and many family problems not specifically related to the patient's treatment. When these concerns are openly discussed, proper referrals to various Institute staff members are made and the parents are encouraged to seek ongoing family counseling if necessary (Figure 10–1).

At this point, great emphasis is placed upon the family's participation in the habilitation process as well as the Institute's role in the treatment and care of the child, with a goal of total rehabilitation of the patient and family. The importance of keeping appointments is stressed. Each patient appointment is scheduled several weeks in advance; since the visit requires the time of a great many staff members during a three- to four-hour period, it is important that each family strive to keep all scheduled appointments. Families are asked to notify the Clinic if a problem arises, so that the canceled visit can be rescheduled and the time assigned to others.

The family is also told that certain aspects of clinical information gathered over the years will be translated into research data. In some instances, they may be asked to participate in specific projects. Their full cooperation and participation is elicited during the initial interview, with the assurance of anonymity and confidentiality. The effectiveness of this approach is documented by the excellent cooperation received by the social research department for two studies. In 1970 a study of adult patients with cleft lip and palate resulted in an 83 per cent participation of those contacted, and a study of teen-agers in 1975 resulted in 72 per cent participation.

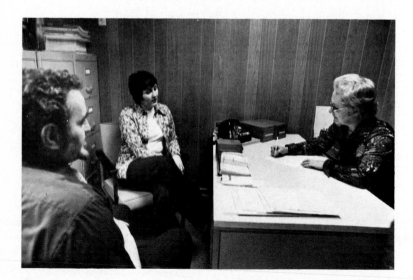

FIGURE 10–1 Phil Starr and Kitty Heiserman with a parent.

A standard intake form (Figure 10–2) is completed that provides the necessary information for an immediate overall view of family composition and financial status. With this information, the caseworker is now ready to discuss the cost ramifications of the patient's care and determine if the family will be able to meet these expenses.

Most parents automatically assume that their medical insurance will cover all costs. Each individual insurance policy, however, is written to cover only those services for which the subscriber has agreed to pay. The policy may have riders attached that prohibit payment for some specific condition existing at the time of purchase or may have a required waiting period before that condition is covered. A newborn infant is not usually covered by medical insurance before the expiration of the 28-day neonatal period, but on August 1, 1975, the governor of Pennsylvania signed Act No. 81, which abolishes the exclusionary provision of the neonatal period. Section 1 of Act No. 81 reads, "the health insurance benefits or health services applicable shall be payable with respect to a newborn child of the insured or subscriber from the moment of birth."

Industrial group insurance may have specific criteria to be met, such as length of employment before dependent children are eligible for coverage, existing conditions at time of coverage, and the employee's contribution toward payment of premiums for medical and dental coverage for dependent children. Many policies stipulate nonpayment for outpatient care except for emergency treatment resulting from an accidental injury.

There is a definite distinction between medical and dental insurance coverage. Dental insurance coverage is usually limited to the filling or crowning of teeth, extractions, those x-rays necessary to facilitate fillings and extractions, cleaning and polishing of teeth, endodontics, periodontics, and oral surgery pertaining to surgical removal of teeth. During the past three years there has been increasing coverage for prosthodontics and orthodontics, but for the most part, this is on a limited basis, such as 50 per cent of the total cost or a maximum lifetime benefit ranging from $300 to $500.

Although there is increasing recognition by insurance companies that cleft lip and cleft palate are congenital birth defects and should be viewed as medical problems, there are still some companies that define any abnormality in the oral cavity as a dental problem. Sometimes the family provides us with a medical insurance claim form that is completed for the initial diagnostic evaluation, but the claim is rejected on the basis that the services rendered were dental in nature and not applicable under medical insurance. A claim form for dental insurance is then completed, but the claim is again rejected on the basis that no actual dental treatment was performed and diagnostic services should be charged against medical insurance. As a result, the patient's parents are totally confused and feel cheated because they must now pay personally for services that they believed were legitimately purchased under their insurance contract. This has also resulted in a great deal of unnecessary duplicate claims and report writing.

Payment by insurance companies for services provided at the Institute has varied greatly. Just recently one patient received full payment for a prosthesis under dental insurance coverage, another patient received full

Program _____

DATE _____

LANCASTER CLEFT PALATE CLINIC

Initial Report _____

INFORMATION FORM

Supplementary _____

Patient's Name	Last	First	Middle	Birthdate	Sex	Race

Address		City	State	Zip	Phone

Medical Reason for Referral	Public Assistance Case Number

Patient	Father	Social Security Information		Wife	Other
		Mother	Husband		

Name of Insurance Carrier	Insurance Information	Policy or Certificate Number

Name of Insurance Carrier		Policy or Certificate Number

Family Composition (List Name)	Relationship to Patient	Birthdate	Type of Occupation

Approximate Annual Income _____

Checking and Savings Account _____

Stocks and Bonds _____

Date of Parents Marriage: Present _____ Other _____

Highest Grade Attained in School by FATHER _____

Signature _____

A PRIVATE NON-PROFIT TREATMENT CENTER

MEMBER OF THE AMERICAN HOSPITAL ASSOCIATION

LCPC 2:6/72

FIGURE 10–2

payment for a prosthesis under major medical coverage, while still another patient was reimbursed only minimally under his dental insurance coverage for the prosthesis.

It has been our experience generally that medical insurance will not make payment for speech therapy. In a few instances an exception was made because the need for speech therapy was associated with, or a direct result of, disease or accidental injury and was part of the total physical therapy recommended by the attending physician for the complete rehabilitation of the patient.

Some families have no medical insurance at all and many have very limited coverage. The latter are usually the lower income families who cannot afford to pay the cost of premiums for more extensive medical and dental insurance and cannot afford the costs for care of their child with a cleft lip or palate. In Pennsylvania, we are extremely fortunate in having a Department of Health that recognizes the total implications of cleft lip and palate: it is a congenital birth defect and costs for treatment and rehabilitation would be a financial burden for most families. In order to assure every family who resides in the state an opportunity to obtain the best possible care for a child with a cleft, a separate program called the Cleft Palate Program (CPP), under the Division of Maternal and Child Health, offers the necessary financial assistance to those families in need.

During the initial interview the caseworker explains to the patient's family the availability of the Cleft Palate Program, how it may aid them with financial payment for services, and how the initial application is completed in order to register the child for this program. If the family elects to apply for financial assistance in the Cleft Palate Program, the caseworker will then assist in completing the social-financial information form required by the Department of Health and forward it to the appropriate office, where an evaluation determines the family's eligibility. Many families are accepted immediately in the program and are given full coverage for all treatment at the Institute. Some families are considered financially able to share the costs for services and are placed on a "parent participation" program. This means that the family will be expected to pay up to the assessed amount in any one calendar year. Each family is offered the opportunity to challenge the parent participation level assessed, but few do. A third outcome that may result from the state's evaluation is, of course, that the family's economic status is such that there is no need of financial assistance. In these instances the state will pay for the initial diagnostic evaluation only. Regardless of the state's determination of financial assistance for the family, a rotating card file is kept so that each family is offered the opportunity to renew its status in the Cleft Palate Program every two years as required by the Department of Health. However, any family may request a reevaluation at any time if there have been any changes in the total family picture, such as unemployment.

There is no direct relationship between the Cleft Palate Program and public welfare. A patient's family may or may not be receiving public assistance money, and may or may not be receiving health care through medical assistance. Families composed of a mother, father, and three children, whose income may make them ineligible for public assistance and medical assistance, may still meet the criteria for total or partial coverage for care of their child on the Cleft Palate Program.

Some adults view their cleft lip or palate as a vocational handicap and feel that extended treatment such as reconstructive surgery, a new prosthesis, and additional speech therapy would enhance their employment potential. When the patient expresses this concern to one of the Institute staff members or to the caseworker, a referral is made to the Bureau of Vocational Rehabilitation (BVR), a division of the Department of Labor and Industry. If the patient meets the eligibility criteria of BVR, it can provide the following: (1) diagnostic evaluation, both medical and vocational; (2) counseling to develop a vocational rehabilitation plan; (3) physical restoration; (4) vocational training; (5) vocational placement in cooperation with employers, agencies, and training facilities; (6) occupational tools and placement equipment for small business enterprises if the establishment of such is feasible; and (7) follow-up for all services provided. Any adult who is in need of continuing care can make inquiries through the regional BVR office.

Financial assistance for payment of treatment costs for non-cleft patients is sometimes available through interagency referrals. Dental care may be financed through the Easter Seal Society for non-cleft patients who are registered with that agency for orthopedic care. Weekly speech therapy programs are sometimes funded for non-cleft patients who are under the care of local mental health and mental retardation agencies. There are many alternative sources for financial funding and it is the caseworker's responsibility to investigate all possible resources. Visits are made to local community agencies to inform them of the kinds of services available at the Institute and obtain from them information about their own agency that may be helpful in making patient referrals.

There are persons who, for religious or personal reasons, may refuse to apply for financial assistance from any source. Lancaster County, the site of the H. K. Cooper Institute, is widely known for its large Amish population. Since these people believe in absolute separation of church and state, they are opposed to state aid and refuse to accept it. They prefer a "private payment status," indicating that if financial problems arise their family and church will help them.

Families who feel their income level is too high to qualify for state financial assistance sometimes refuse even to make application because they do not wish to share personal information regarding their socioeconomic status. Every family, however, is offered an opportunity to seek some financial help. When the family of the patient with a cleft lip or palate is on a private payment status, all costs for treatment are discussed and payment programs are arranged that do not overburden the family budget.

Many follow-up procedures are performed by the patient services department. One of these functions is the follow-up of missed appointments. When the appointment secretary has been unsuccessful with the routine procedures of encouraging families to keep scheduled appointments, the patient is referred to the caseworker. The family is then contacted to reemphasize the need for continuing care and to determine the reasons the family has failed to keep the appointment. In October 1974, we undertook a review of the appointments missed during the previous 10 months. Of the 4595 appointments scheduled from January 2 through October 31, 616 or 13.4 per cent were not kept, which compares favorably with the figures reported in the literature. Our findings also indicated that the patients who missed all their scheduled appointments tended to be older, were significantly more highly educated and of a higher socioeconomic status, and lived farthest from the Institute. Our longitudinal patients (those seen at regular intervals beginning shortly after birth) have a better record for keeping scheduled appointments than do other patients with cleft lip and palate.

Delinquent accounts are referred to the patient services department for follow-up. This often results in obtaining new information about the family, such as changes in financial status, loss of job for the primary wage earner, illness or death in the family, or separation or divorce of parents. In cases of extreme hardship, information is provided as to how and where the family might seek temporary financial assistance. In these instances, payment programs are arranged or revised so that the patient is not deprived of needed treatment.

It has been our experience that overdue accounts are the result of the family's financial difficulties. With the exception of possibly half a dozen cases, the families have expressed satisfaction with the quality of care provided; thus, our clinical experience does not support the notion that payment delinquencies are due to dissatisfaction with services provided.

Essentially, the functions of the patient services department are twofold: first, to perform the necessary services in order to obtain adequate information for the Institute in regard to admissions, record keeping, and payment for treatment; second, and most important, to initiate and promote the kind of rapport necessary to involve the patient and family in the total habilitation program. The ultimate goal for the patient, though it may be 20 years in process, is to facilitate the ability to participate in meaningful and rewarding societal tasks and relationships.

PSYCHOSOCIAL ISSUES

The family is a universal societal institution organized principally to provide a stable and secure framework for the care and rearing of the young. Each society expects parents to socialize their children so that they will become responsible adult citizens. To accomplish this objective, the parents must guide their children's growth and development, specifically, help them master tasks at appropriate age levels, such as learning to talk in early childhood or learning to get along with peers in middle childhood.

In our constantly changing society it isn't easy for parents to facilitate the mastery of these developmental tasks. If the child has a cleft lip or palate, the assignment is even more difficult. The essential question of concern to parents and to the professional people involved is this: How does the child's physical condition, requiring surgical, dental, and other treatment services, affect growth and development? Does the child with a cleft lip or palate have similar or different social and emotional experiences at different age stages compared with non-cleft youngsters?

AGE-RELATED CHALLENGES

The age-related challenges facing a child with a cleft will be the basis of this analysis. At each age level, we will specify the main psychosocial issues and the research evidence known about these issues. Moreover, we will outline the focus of the social worker's role at each age level.

Prenatal Stage

In the prenatal stage, the key issue for the prospective parents concerns the risk of having a baby with a cleft. For a couple with no familial history of clefts, the risk rate is that of the general population (one in every 600 or 700 live births in the Caucasian population and one in every 2000 births among blacks).[18] For this couple at this stage, there is no role that the social worker can play.

For a couple with a known family history of clefting, however, the risk rate can be established. After the geneticist has done this, the social worker may join with him or her to counsel the couple and to help them understand what the risk rate means. Depending upon the family's history, the risk of reoccurrence of a cleft can range from 2 to 17 per cent. Therefore, the likelihood of having a baby born *without* a palatal cleft is *at least* 83 per cent. It should be emphasized to them that these figures are based on population studies and that there is *no* way to forecast whether their own baby will be born with a cleft.

At this stage, the couple should also be informed of the services available to enhance the physical and emotional growth and development of a baby with a cleft lip or palate. At the Institute, an "Are You Aware" letter from the staff is distributed to the couple to familiarize them with our services:

"ARE YOU AWARE?"

We believe that many of our patients with cleft conditions and their families are unaware of all the services that our Institute (Clinic) provides. As you know, the staff of the Institute specializes in providing services for cleft lip and/or cleft palate patients, to meet the needs of people with oral and facial problems. We provide for these patients a complete range of *dental services* including orthodontic and prosthodontic replacement of missing oral-facial parts. *Plastic surgeons* are available to perform various surgical procedures. *Speech pathologists, speech scientists, audiologists* and *otolaryngologists* are available to help with speech and hearing problems. A *geneticist* is available to counsel families concerning the possibility of occurrence and/or reoccurence of a baby with a cleft condition. A *social worker* is available to help with either a personal/marital or family problem.

We are *not* suggesting that each one of you is in need of all these services at this time. We just want you to be aware of them if and when the need arises.

Our social service personnel will be pleased to discuss financial arrangements for services.

If you have any questions concerning our services, please feel free to call our caseworker at (717) 394-3793. We hope this information will be of help to you.

The Staff

With an understanding of the risk of reoccurrence of a cleft and the availability of treatment, the couple is now in a position to decide whether to risk having another child. A review of all new cases at the Institute for a 10-year period (1965–74) revealed that having additional children after giving birth to a child with a cleft varied among parents, depending upon the cleft-type in that child. Among parents of children with a cleft lip only (CL), 29.5 per cent had additional children. Thirty-eight and six tenths per cent of the parents of a child with cleft lip and palate (CLP) and 37.1 per cent of the parents of a child with cleft palate only (CP) had additional children. We also found that those parents not having additional children tended to be older, had higher education levels, and already had larger families than those who did produce additional children after the birth of a child with an orofacial cleft. The question of what impact rearing a child with a cleft has upon a couple's decision to bear additional children is unclear and needs further exploration.

First Year

At birth, one key issue is the parents' reaction to having given birth to a baby born with a cleft lip or palate. There seems to be agreement in the cleft palate field that most parents respond with profound shock.[24, 26, 31] At the Institute, Slutsky interviewed 66 mothers to elicit attitudes and impressions related to the birth and early care of a child with a cleft.[24] He reported that 80 per cent of the mothers reacted to the birth of such a child with strong feelings of shock, hurt, disappointment, helpless resentment, and, in some cases, hysteria. They had lost the perfect baby nurtured in their dreams and had received instead a "damaged" child. Slutsky reported that most mothers recover from this painful reaction within a short time and develop greater acceptance of the child's birth defect. Clifford and Crocker suggest that immediately informing parents that surgery can remedy the cleft lip or palate helps facilitate their recovery.[4]

The first year of the child's life brings the family in direct contact with two other significant issues: feeding the child and paying for the services needed. In regard to the former, the social worker supports the pediatrician's recommended program. For example, a mother who became hysterical when she had to feed her baby was helped by a two-avenue approach. First, the social worker demonstrated to the mother that her baby could be fed without having most of the food come through the nose. Second, the importance of feeding the baby was emphasized by explaining that the plastic surgeon could not operate and remedy the cleft lip until the infant weighed at least 10 pounds.[5]

Providing the needed services to patients and their families is expensive. The cost is quite prohibitive for most families and is a cause of great concern. All states have accepted the principle that lack of money should *not* interfere with the ability to receive the services needed. At the Institute, it is an important responsibility for the social worker to be familiar with the various governmental programs and to assist families in applying for the appropriate state aid if they so desire. Therefore, all new patients are seen by a social worker as part of the diagnostic evaluation.

At the same time, an analysis of the family's current level of functioning (e.g., its occupational and social adjustment) is also undertaken to assess its ability to take advantage of opportunities and resources.[11] Here the social worker can help the parents with any interfering emotional problem and facilitate the parents' or family's participation in the child's treatment program.

One to Six

Between the ages of one and six, four main developmental issues are speech, hearing, and intellectual and social development. In this section we shall discuss the last two, as speech and hearing are covered in other chapters of this volume.

To measure the intellectual capacity of children with orofacial clefts and to determine whether their interpersonal relations are appropriate for their age level, we at the Institute tested these children at six-month intervals from the age of six months to 24 months on the Bayley Scales of Infant Development. The findings suggest that there are no statistically significant differences in the mental and motor functioning of the children with orofacial clefts as compared with the Bayley norms at each age period.[27]

Philips and Harrison report the only other study of children solely in the age range between one and six.[17] While the children with clefts obtained Peabody scores that increased at each age interval, their scores were always significantly lower than those for the non-cleft subjects.

In the area of interpersonal relations, our study of infants with clefts suggests that our subjects tend to be more passive in responding to sensorimotor stimuli as measured by the Bayley Scales for Infant Development.[27] A possible explanation for this passivity is provided by the findings of Starr and Fisher.[28] In their study of preschool children with orofacial clefts, they found that parents of children with clefts discussed sexual topics significantly less often with their children than did parents of non-cleft children. It is possible that parents of children with cleft lip or palate are overprotective and therefore less willing to discuss sexual topics with their children. Smith and McWilliams[25] and Spriestersbach[26] have made similar speculations. Presently, there is no empirical evidence to support these suggestions.

It is clear that some parents of preschool children with clefts need assistance to avoid overprotecting their children, which itself may produce the delayed social development. These parents tend to protect their children from other children and from experiences in which the children may suffer disappointment, discomfort, or injury. Unfortunately, these are the kinds of experiences that provide the children with an opportunity to grow mentally. In the last analysis, the parents are rewarding dependency. This is an area in which the skills of a social worker may be utilized. These parents can be helped to recognize that their overprotective attitude is adversely affecting their child's social and emotional growth and development. Parental understanding is achieved when the parents finally realize that their child is no longer a helpless, deformed baby and does not have to be so dependent on them.

Identifying Behavioral Problems

In a large facility like ours it is sometimes difficult to know which patients and families could benefit from the kind of counseling we have been discussing. We have found it helpful, however, to employ certain research findings to identify patients who might be regarded as high risks, in the sense of becoming more asocial. These are the children who we feel are most in need of our services. For example, in part of our study of preschoolers with orofacial clefts, we spotted six children who seemed to be having difficulty in their behavioral functioning. This assessment was based on the mothers' completion of the Missouri Children's Behavior Checklist.[23] This checklist is a set of 70 descriptions of children's behavior organized in a "Yes" or "No" fashion. The reason for using this particular checklist is that it is behaviorally referential and does not call for subjective conclusions by the rater.

Some examples selected from the full list follow:

Aggression (19 items)
1. Fights
2. Hurts animals
3. "Picks on" weaker or smaller children

Inhibition (14 items)
1. Prefers to be with children younger than self
2. Is apathetic or underactive
3. Does not try new situations

Activity Level (10 items)
1. Moves constantly, "gets into everything"
2. Becomes more active or more talkative in groups
3. Does not finish task, said to have "short attention span"

Sleep Disturbance (nine items)
1. Cries out in sleep
2. Complains of bad dreams
3. Walks in sleep

Somatization (eight items)
1. Complains of pains in the head
2. Vomits when things do not go his way
3. Worries a great deal about health

Sociability (10 items)
1. Expresses appreciation for others' acts
2. Talks easily with adults other than parents
3. Sought out by others, others say they like him.

The six children in our study were identified as having problems in three or more of the following areas: aggression, activity level, inhibition, sociability, somatization, or sleep disturbance. Because of this, appointments with the parents were made to ascertain whether the day-to-day experiences were actually those that we were able to identify in the questionnaire. Since the parents confirmed the reliability of our analysis, individual counseling was initiated to facilitate the healthy emotional growth and development of their children.

In addition, the parents of preschoolers with orofacial clefts were asked if they would be willing to meet with other mothers to discuss common child-rearing problems. Of the 30 mothers asked, 20 indicated such a desire. Because of this interest, we held several monthly meetings with this group of parents. Among the topics for these meetings were "Being Parents Isn't Easy," "Social Behavior of Preschoolers," and "Language and Speech Development." Two of the meetings were led by one of our speech therapists. The positive response of the parents to these programs led us to plan future meetings with the parents of children of this age group and other age groups. It should be noted that the orientation of these meetings has been educational and not therapeutic. The ideas discussed focus on helping the parents to be more effective by emphasizing specific child-rearing skills.

Six to 12

From the ages of six to 12, three key pyschosocial issues are intellectual development, school achievement, and social adjustment. The parents want to know whether their children have the ability to learn, whether they are actually learning in school, and whether they are developing socially in a "normal" manner.

For intellectual developmentas measured by an IQ test, Ruess compared children with clefts between seven and 12 years of age with their closest sibling in age.[20] The children with clefts scored significantly lower on the verbal and full scales of the Wechsler Intelligence Scale for Children (WISC); there were no significant differences on the performance scale.

While this is the only study we found that reports data solely for this age group, there are numerous studies for overlapping age groups. Reviews of research studies by Ruess,[21] Ross and Johnston,[18] and Goodstein[9] suggest a mild to moderate degree of intellectual impairment for children with clefts. Furthermore, the intellectual impairment seems more pronounced in the verbal than in the performance area. Another study that might be linked to intellectual development deals with creativity.[25] The children with clefts were significantly less creative on six of the 14 indexes of creativity as well as on the overall index when compared with non-cleft children after controlling for the variables of IQ, sex, race, and the family's socioeconomic status.

The second developmental issue for this age group is academic achievement. Drillien[7] and Ruess[20] both report results indicating no significant difference between subjects with and without clefts with respect to achievement in school. Their findings suggest that despite mild intellectual impairment as measured by intelligence tests, children with clefts can learn and achieve as well as their non-cleft classmates. These results can be best explained by two facts: first, while the subjects with clefts scored significantly lower than non-cleft subjects on IQ tests, their scores were within the "dull normal" range; second, IQ tests really measure the acquisition of abilities rather than a subject's capacity for learning and applying knowledge.[30]

Studies of the social adjustment of children with clefts are inconclusive. Impressionistic reports indicate that some children with clefts are rather maladjusted and disturbed.[22, 32] Various pencil and paper projective personality tests arrive at opposite conclusions.[33, 35]

These findings, coupled with IQ and school achievement tests, suggest that a key psychosocial responsibility of the social worker is to help parents of a child with a cleft to be realistic in their expectations. For example, a social worker helped the mother of a nine-year-old girl with a cleft palate to confront the child's teacher and discuss the latter's "abusive" approach with her child. After several discussions, the teacher recognized that her impatience and undue demands had interfered with the child's learning. These contacts eventually led to a change in the teacher's approach to the child and an improvement in the girl's performance in school.[19]

Adolescence

The next age period is that of adolescence (13 to 18 years of age). A crucial psychosocial issue here is interpersonal relations, focusing on dating and marital planning following puberty. Despite the importance of interpersonal relations, Goodstein's[10] review of the literature on orofacial clefts revealed no research that focused solely on adolescents.[10] Some studies included teen-age subjects, but it is not possible to determine whether the findings pertain only to the adolescents or to some combined age groups. The seriousness of this omission is further supported by Westlake and Rutherford's observation that the literature on other handicapped children suggests that difficulties in adjustment increase with age.[34]

At the Institute, we assessed 72 teen-agers with repaired clefts in regard to their attitude toward their cleft condition, their self-esteem, and their behavioral adjustment.[29] The questionnaires were self-administered and the teen-agers completed them at the Institute after being examined or interviewed by the clinical staff.

The questionnaires consisted of a list of statements, some expressing a positive view toward the cleft condition, others a negative view. The teen-agers were asked to score their reactions to each statement on a scale of one to six, ranging from strong to weak agreement. If they strongly agreed with a positive statement, such as "Cleft condition or not, I'm going to make good in life," they gave themselves a score of six. If they strongly disagreed with a negative statement, such as "Because of my cleft condition I have little to offer other people," they also marked down a high score. The individual scores were added up for each person and then compared, to determine the degree of agreement within the group.

On the basis of cleft type, there were no differences in attitude scores. That is, teen-agers with cleft lip did not, as a subgroup, have a better attitude score than those with cleft lip and palate or cleft palate only.

The 10 items in the list of 50 on which the whole group were most often in agreement, on the basis of high scores, were as follows:

1. Cleft condition or not, I'm going to make good in life. (Positive)
2. There are many things a person with my cleft is able to do. (Positive)
3. Because of my cleft condition, I have little to offer other people. (Negative)
4. Almost every area of life is closed to me because of my cleft condition. (Negative)
5. Life is full of so many things that sometimes I forget for brief periods that I have a cleft condition. (Positive)

6. A cleft condition may limit a person in some ways, but this does not mean he should give up and do nothing in life. (Positive)
7. In just about everything, my cleft condition is annoying me so that I cannot enjoy anything. (Negative)
8. Because of my cleft condition, I can never do most things that normal people can do. (Negative)
9. There are times I completely forget that I have a cleft condition. (Positive)
10. A cleft condition is the worst possible thing that can happen to a person. (Negative)

The 10 items in the list on which there was the least agreement among the teen-agers, as indicated by their low reaction scores, were as follows:

1. A cleft condition changes one's life completely. It causes one to think differently about everything. (Negative)
2. The most important thing in this world is to be physically normal. (Negative)
3. My cleft condition, in itself, affects me more than any other characteristic about me. (Negative)
4. I am unable to enjoy social relationships as much as I could if I didn't have a cleft. (Negative)
5. I believe that physical wholeness and appearance make a person what he is. (Negative)
6. With my condition, I know what I can and cannot do. (Positive)
7. I get very annoyed with the way people offer me sympathy. (Positive)
8. I want very much to do things my cleft condition prevents me from doing. (Negative)
9. More than anything else, I wish I didn't have this cleft condition. (Negative)
10. Good physical appearance and physical ability are the most important things in life. (Negative)

In sum, teen-agers with orofacial clefts are in agreement about their ability to succeed.

There was, however, a significantly wide range of attitudes, regardless of cleft type, within the entire group of 72. Thirteen, or one-sixth, scored high in responses that connoted a favorable emotional state—a positive attitude—with respect to their defect. Another thirteen gave responses that revealed an extremely negative attitude. The remaining two-thirds fell somewhere in between.

Not surprisingly, those whose collective scores on the questionnaire statements placed them in the "favorable" or "positive" category (the top sixth) were consistent in having a higher self-esteem and were lower (better) in such negative characteristics as aggression, hyperactivity level, somatization (conversion of mental states into bodily symptoms), and sleep disturbance.

The 13 students whose attitude scores placed them in the negative group were identified as potential high-risk individuals, in danger of becoming more and more asocial. Our concern about them, based at first on their own questionnaire responses, was confirmed in interviews with parents, and we then initiated counseling.

This study is another example of how the social worker can be brought into contact with youngsters most in need of help in their efforts to achieve independence and mature interpersonal relations with both sexes. The importance of these issues is underscored by the findings of Clifford and Bentz that teenagers with clefts perceive their parents as having less pride in them than "normal" adolescents.[3]

To help the teen-agers and their parents, brief treatment is offered to both parties. The parents must be encouraged to give their children more freedom, while the teen-agers must be shown how to assume more responsibility for their behavior.[12] If these assistive procedures fail, family members are referred to an appropriate facility in their area for long-term counseling.

Adulthood

The functioning of adults with orofacial clefts has also been assessed to determine how well they are taking their places as members of society. In relation to the formal education and level of employment achieved, there is no significant difference between the adults with clefts and their comparison groups.[6, 13, 15, 16]

At the Institute a follow-up study of patients with orofacial clefts who were between the ages of 24 and 54 was undertaken in 1970–71 under the direction of John Peter. This study was based on survey returns for 196 subjects with clefts, their 190 siblings, and 209 random control subjects.

The three groups were compared with respect to educational levels, high school dropout rates, and college attendance or completion, with results indicating near unity of educational attainment for all groups. In regard to employment, the results revealed that adults with clefts functioned within normal limits. There was little difference between the three groups in longest continuous employment in one job or the average number of jobs held.

McWilliams and Paradise reported that a significantly larger number of patients with clefts remained single than did their nearest siblings in age.[13] Peter and Chinsky found that adults with clefts married significantly later and had more childless marriages.[14] We assume that these behavioral patterns are indicators of interpersonal difficulty for adults with orofacial clefts.

Taken together, these studies suggest that in the somewhat structured role situations of education and employment, the adults with clefts are doing as well as those without, but that in the areas of interpersonal relationships, they are experiencing more difficulty. Birch and Lindsay's clinical report of the wide-ranging maladjustment problems for adolescent and adult patients supports these empirical conclusions.[2] With the adults, the role of the social worker is to build upon the positive attitudes of the patients with clefts to achieve as complete a normal functioning as possible in each case.

Summary

This has been a review of our current knowledge regarding the age-related changes observed in patients with clefts and their families from the prenatal stage to adulthood, and the social worker's role in relation to these changes. We do not want to create the impression that every patient must have the service of a social worker for each age-related psychosocial issue. We would, however, like to leave the reader with the idea that some patients and their parents are experiencing some difficulty at various ages and could benefit from the services provided by a social worker.

CASE HISTORIES

The following notes from our file of case histories will further illustrate the way in which a social service staff can help patients and their families to cope with the psychological and social problems that so often complicate the management of a handicap. Sensitive and patient attention to these aspects can contribute much to the whole team's efforts to achieve satisfactory rehabilitation.

MALE WITH A CLEFT OF THE LIP ONLY (#1)

Robert had been referred to the Cooper Institute by his family's pediatrician at the age of two months for evaluation and treatment of an incomplete cleft of the lip and alveolus on the left side. The hard and soft palates were not involved. At the age of three and one-half months, Robert Harding, staff plastic surgeon, successfully closed the cleft with a triangular flap cheilorrhaphy, and the patient's parents enrolled the child in our longitudinal series, which meant he would be seen at the Institute regularly on a semiannual basis.

He was brought in for these visits and examined each time by the dentist, the radiology technician, the audiologist, and the speech therapist. Except for periodic updating of the family situation, the social service staff was not active with the family until Robert was four years old.

At that age, the mother completed the Missouri Children's Behavior Checklist, a 70-item description of the child's behavior. On the basis of her rating, we noted that Robert scored atypically high on aggressiveness, activity level, and difficulty in sleeping. We discussed his behavior with both parents, who expressed concern about his sleep disturbance but did not feel he was hyperactive or too aggressive. They expressed more concern about the behavior of Robert's eight-year-old brother, Jerry. They were particularly worried that Robert would soon be imitating Jerry's behavior.

In spite of his age, Jerry was still experiencing difficulty with bed wetting. The parents were also upset over Jerry's school performance and they felt strongly that both problems were related to poor intellectual functioning. An intelligence test, however, revealed that he was in the upper range of average intelligence; moreover, he was a pleasant child who related well to the examiner. After discussing other possibilities, the parents agreed to visit their local Family and Children's Service for an evaluation of Jerry and themselves.

That agency, after assessing the situation and observing that all family members were exhibiting signs of emotional problems, recommended family therapy. The parents, however, refused to continue visits to the agency and they no longer maintain contact there.

At this same time, Robert was given another evaluation at the Cooper Institute, and because of his unintelligible speech, he was referred for speech therapy at the age of four and one half. Since the parents had declined help at the Family Service agency, our social service staff undertook to work with them and to help them recognize that they were in need of assistance, including psychological counseling. An encouraging development was their attendance at group meetings at which parents of preschool children with orofacial clefts discussed suggestions on child care.

MALE WITH A CLEFT OF THE LIP ONLY (#2)

This patient was referred to the Cooper Institute at five weeks of age for evaluation and treatment. He was diagnosed as having an incomplete cleft on the left side of the lip; the evaluation also revealed some evidence of dental anomalies. Consequently, the family accepted the recommendation of enrolling him in our longitudinal series.

The cleft of the lip was closed surgically by the staff plastic surgeon when the patient was four months old. The operation performed was a cheilorrhaphy and the results of the surgery were satisfactory.

After the initial evaluation, the patient's mother called and was somewhat upset. Her husband, who had an incomplete cleft of the lip that had never been repaired, had become increasingly depressed after the birth of the child and had very little to do with him. He didn't want to take the baby outside for others to see and he discouraged visitors at home. His wife was afraid of the possible impact on their marriage and on the child's development.

The patient's mother was reassured that her husband's reaction was quite common and that once the baby's lip was repaired surgically, the father would probably be more willing to associate with him. We also questioned her as to whether he might be feeling guilty about the child's cleft, and indicated that we would arrange for her husband to see our geneticist at the time of the next Clinic visit. We supported her during this trying time by calling weekly and also helped her *not* to place additional pressure on her husband during this difficult period.

In our discussions with her by telephone after the successful closing of the lip, she indicated that her husband's attitude had improved somewhat. He was spending some time with the baby and beginning to enjoy being a parent, but he was still refusing to allow others to see the baby, since this embarrassed him.

Monthly phone calls were made to support her and to provide suggestions to help her cope with her husband. At the time of their one-year appointment, both parents were interviewed at the office. They agreed that things had significantly improved since the husband had gained a better understanding of the multifactorial etiology of cleft lip and palate. He is now more attentive to the baby and shares in the responsibility of child care.

FEMALE WITH A CLEFT OF THE SOFT PALATE ONLY

This baby girl had been diagnosed at three weeks of age as having a cleft of the soft palate; there was no cleft of the hard palate or lip. Social service became actively involved with this family when the baby was five months old, at the request of a public health nurse who was concerned about the mother's apparent inability to care properly for the child. The baby had not gained weight and the nurse suspected she might be malnourished. The mother was only 16 when the child was born, and school records indicated that she was mildly retarded and had attended special education classes much of the time she was in school.

Social service arranged for the mother and baby to be seen by our staff pediatrician, who indicated that although the baby was small, its development was normal. The social worker explained to the mother how to use a special feeder that was approved by the pediatrician, and the public health nurse reported soon thereafter that there was general improvement in the baby's well-being.

However, because of her apparent need for more knowledge about child care and homemaking, the young mother was referred to a local center for training in these skills, a move that was successfully implemented and supported by us. The mother also continued to visit the Clinic at regularly scheduled intervals, and to assist in her transportation, a retired couple volunteered to drive her and the baby to the Clinic. They had no children of their own and were eager to keep in touch with the family to provide help.

After months of delay because of repeated colds, the child underwent surgery for closure of the palate at 18 months of age. Healing proceeded satisfactorily, but many problems demanded continued attention by the social service staff, others at the Institute, and several outside agencies that had been helping the family. At one point, a conference was held that involved all of these groups. For a considerable period the baby suffered from a severe and persistent rash on the buttocks, and our pediatrician examined the child and prescribed for her. There were also personality problems, including expressions of resentment and hostility by the mother toward one of the nurses who was making weekly home visits.

Although the mother attended the homemaking and child care class once a week, some of those who were working with her were concerned about her constant assertion that she wanted to have another baby. They were doubtful of her ability to care for two children, particularly if the second one should also be born with an orofacial cleft. Several consultations were held on this matter, including one with our geneticist.

Meanwhile, both parents were treated by the Cooper Institute's dental department for extensive restorations and dentures. Because of their limited income, arrangements were made by us to have these services paid for by the Bureau of Vocational Rehabilitation. At a two-year checkup of the child, it was learned that the father was recovering from pneumonia. The physician felt there was a strong likelihood, in view of the nature of the man's work, that he would suffer from repeated respiratory problems. He therefore recommended a change of employment, and we arranged with the Bureau of Vocational Rehabilitation to counsel the father regarding a new job.

This family presents the kind of problems that social service departments so often encounter and find challenging, if not frustrating. They are not complex in a technical sense, but they involve educational gaps, personality difficulties, and the need for constant but tactful supervision and care.

MALE WITH A CLEFT OF THE HARD AND SOFT PALATE

The patient was first seen at the Cooper Institute at the age of two and one-half months. He had been referred by the family's physician for evaluation. Examination disclosed a cleft of the soft palate and the posterior third of the hard palate. The parents were informed that clefts of this type are usually closed surgically when the baby is one year old, but the mother was much concerned about feeding problems, the kind of food to give, and how to clean out food lodged in the cleft. Our caseworker offered suggestions on feeding, explained the services available at the Institute, and solicited the parents' cooperation in the longitudinal research study.

In spite of our assurances, the mother became quite anxious and was sure that everything that *could* go wrong would be visited upon her child. We again reassured her, emphasizing that our specialists would monitor the baby's development and would be available to provide treatment at the earliest possible moment if it was needed.

We telephoned the mother every month to continue our reassurance, to confirm that the child's development seemed good, and to assist with suggestions on feeding. With the passing of time the mother's anxiety diminished. We continued these contacts until the time of surgery, when the baby was 13 months old. Surgical closure was effected with relaxing bilateral incisions, and the results were satisfactory. The surgery eased the feeding problems that the mother had been experiencing and also helped her to appreciate the value of the regular monitoring of the child's growth and development. At the time of this writing, the child was doing nicely and the parents were quite satisfied with his development.

MALE WITH A CLEFT LIP AND PALATE

The patient, a professional man in his thirties, was referred to us for evaluation of his cleft lip and palate and for help with his speech. He also wanted consultation concerning secondary surgical repair. At the Cooper Institute it was agreed that he would benefit from speech therapy, and he was referred to a therapist in his home community in another state. The decision was also made to reline his upper and lower dentures and to perform cosmetic surgery. Both the prosthetic and surgical recommendations were to be implemented by our staff members.

During the initial interview with the social worker, the patient indicated he had great difficulty in relating to people and that because of this he was dissatisfied with his present job. He was experiencing rejection by new acquaintances, even in his attempts to establish meaningful contact at church. Although he was sure he was highly qualified for numerous professional positions, he felt that because of his speech defect he had not been accepted for them. The patient also expressed great concern about the fact that his speech impairment and his voice quality had resulted in a lack of female friends.

Although he was already involved in a psychological counseling situation in his home city at the time he visited the Cooper Institute, he felt it was of minimal benefit to him. His counselor had recommended vocational counseling, but the patient had rejected this. During our interviews we supported his involvement in counseling and also urged him to seek the recommended vocational guidance. When he suggested that a move to another area might be helpful, we pointed out that his problems were of a personal nature and that he couldn't run away from them.

Some time later the patient telephoned to say he was seeing a speech therapist on a regular basis and that the treatment was progressing nicely and his speech was improving. He was also exploring the availability of vocational counseling and had decided against moving to another area. At this time, secondary surgical repair was arranged. One month after surgery he again contacted us to inform us that he was extremely pleased with the surgical results.

We shall continue to be active in this case in an effort to be of supportive help when needed.

References

1. Backus, O. J.: Speech defects. Bull. Natl. Assoc. Secondary School Principals. 32:127, 1948.
2. Birch, J. R., and W. K. Lindsay: An evaluation of adults with repaired bilateral cleft lips and palates. Plast. Reconstr. Surg., 48:457, 1971.
3. Clifford, E., and E. Bentz: When I was born: a comparative study of normal and clinical sample. Paper presented at the American Cleft Palate Association Meeting in New Orleans, Louisiana, February 1975.
4. Clifford, E., and E. C. Crocker: Maternal responses: the birth of a normal child as compared to the birth of a child with a cleft. Cleft Palate J., 8:298, 1971.
5. Cooper, H. K., Sr., et al.: Team management for the cleft lip and cleft palate patient. H. K. Cooper Institute booklet, 1974.
6. Demb, N. E., and A. L. Ruess: High school drop-out rate for cleft patients. Cleft Palate J., 4:327, 1967.
7. Drillien, C. M., T. T. S. Ingram, and E. M. Wilkinson: The Causes and Natural History of Cleft Lip and Palate, Edinburgh, Livingstone, 1966.
8. Fogh-Anderson, P.: Inheritance of Harelip and Cleft Palate: Contribution to the Elucidation of the Etiology of the Congenital Clefts of the Face, translated by E. Aageson, Copenhagen, Arnold Busck, 1942.
9. Goodstein, L. D.: Intellectual impairment in children with cleft palates. J. Speech Hear. Res., 4:287, 1961.
10. Goodstein, L. D.: Psychosocial aspects of cleft palate. In Spriestersbach, D. C., and D. Sherman (eds.): Cleft Palate and Communication, New York, Academic Press, pp. 201–224, 1968.
11. Hamilton, G.: Theory and Practice of Social Casework, New York, Columbia University Press, 1956.
12. Josselyn, I. M.: The Adolescent and His World, New York, Family Service Association of America, 1952.
13. McWilliams, B. J., and L. P. Paradise: Educational, occupational and marital status of cleft palate adults. Cleft Palate J., 10:223, 1973.
14. Peter, J. P., and R. R. Chinsky: Sociological aspects of cleft palate adults: I. Marriage. Cleft Palate J., 11:295, 1974.
15. Peter, J. P., and R. R. Chinsky: Sociological aspects of cleft palate adults: II. Education. Cleft Palate J., 11:443, 1974.
16. Peter, J. P., R. R. Chinsky, and M. J. Fisher: Sociological aspects of cleft palate adults: III. Vocational and economic aspects. Cleft Palate J., 12:193, 1975.
17. Philips, B. J., and R. J. Harrison: Language skills of preschool cleft palate children. Cleft Palate J., 6:108, 1969.
18. Ross, R. B., and M. D. Johnston: Cleft Lip and Palate, Baltimore, Williams & Wilkins, 1972.
19. Rouillon, M.: Social service. In Stark, R. G. (ed.): Cleft Palate: A Multi-Discipline Approach, New York, Harper & Row, pp. 284–298, 1968.
20. Ruess, A. L.: A comparative study of cleft palate children and their siblings. J. Clin. Psychol., 21:354, 1965.
21. Ruess, A. L.: Convergent psychosocial factors in the cleft palate clinic. In Lencione, R. M. (ed.): Cleft Palate Habilitation: Proceedings of the Fifth Annual Symposium on Cleft Palate, Syracuse, New York, Syracuse University Press, pp. 53–70, 1968.
22. Schwekendek, W., and C. Danzer: Psychological studies in patients with clefts. Cleft Palate J., 7:533, 1970.
23. Sines, J. O., J. D. Pauker, L. K. Sines, and D. R. Owen: Identification of clinically relevant dimensions of children's behavior. J. Consult. Clin. Psychol., 33:728, 1969.
24. Slutsky, H.: Maternal reactions and adjustment to birth and care of cleft palate child. Cleft Palate J., 6:425, 1969.
25. Smith, R. M., and B. J. McWilliams: Creative thinking abilities of cleft palate children. Cleft Palate J., 3:275, 1966.
26. Spriestersbach, D. C.: Psychosocial Aspects of the Cleft Palate Problem, vol. 1, Iowa City, Iowa, University of Iowa Press, 1973.
27. Starr, P., R. Chinsky, H. Canter, and J. Meier: Mental, motor and social behavior of infants with cleft lip and/or palate. Cleft Palate J., in press.
28. Starr, P., and M. J. Fisher: Intrafamilial dimensions of preschoolers with oral-facial clefts. Paper presented at the meeting of the American Cleft Palate Association in San Francisco, 1976.
29. Starr, P., and K. J. Heiserman: Acceptance of disability, self-esteem and behavior of teenagers with oral-facial clefts. Rehabilitation Counseling Bull., 20:198, 1977.
30. Stott, L. H., and R. S. Ball: Infants and preschool mental tests: review and evaluation. Monogr. Soc. Res. Child Develop., 30:1, 1965.

31. Tisza, V., and E. Gumpertz: The parents' reaction to the birth and early care of children with cleft palates. Pediatrics, 30:86, 1962.
32. Tisza, V., B. Silverstone, G. Rosenblum, and N. Hanlon: Psychiatric observation of children with cleft palate. A. J. Orthopsychiatry, 28:416, 1958.
33. Watson, C. G.: Personality adjustment in boys with cleft lip and palates. Cleft Palate J., 1:130, 1964.
34. Westlake, H., and D. Rutherford: Cleft Palate, Englewood Cliffs, New Jersey, Prentice-Hall, 1966.
35. Wirls, C. J., and R. R. Plotkin: A comparison of children with cleft palate and their siblings on projective test personality factors. Cleft Palate J., 8:399, 1971.

Chapter Eleven ─────────────────────────────

In this chapter, we shall give some insight into the place of high-speed electronic computers in the management of the patient with a cleft palate at the H. K. Cooper Institute. It is not our intent to make the reader an expert in the use of computers, but rather to acquaint him or her with the specific techniques we have been able to apply successfully and to provide an overview of the general procedures. This will give the reader some idea of the directions in which to pursue the subject further.

Modern computers have made important inroads in data analysis for medical and clinical research. They have not only assisted in keeping accurate records and preparing reports in a timely manner, but they have greatly improved data analysis and reduction in a complex research environment. It is necessary to look at the different areas of the Clinic where data originate, and then at the specific approaches and techniques that have been used in them. We are particularly concerned with the following topics:

Plastic Surgery: type and extent of cleft (lip, palate, or both), age at repair (lip, palate), type of operative procedure, success of function and cosmesis.

Dental Division: x-ray films, cineradiography films, dental casts, clinical evaluations of dental anomalies.

Growth and Development: appraisal of pre- and postoperative growth in bony and soft tissue structures.

Speech and Hearing: speech and sound inventories, voice quality ratings, cinefluoroscopic studies, tape-recorded speech samples, language test scores.

Genetics: genetic information and pedigrees.

Social Work: socioeconomic data, behavioral factors, vital statistics.

Medical Division: physical information on patient, such as height and weight, nutritional information, comprehensive medical history.

Some of the foregoing information lends itself readily to computerization, and some does not. In general, any information that can be quantified — counted or measured with some sort of scale — is adaptable to this tech-

THE USE OF COMPUTERS IN THE ANALYSIS OF CLEFT PALATE CLINIC DATA

PAUL W. ROSS

nique. Subjective information, such as a clinical evaluation, can only be placed in the patient's data file with a cross-reference to a complete written report in a manual filing system.

At the heart of any computerized data base or information system, there is initially a good manual records system. It has often been said that computers do not solve problems, people do. With this in mind, our primary goal has been to establish protocols for consistent collection of data and recording of patient information. The clinician must be sensitive to the needs of research, and the researcher must be aware of the reality of day-to-day clinical practice.

Our primary reason for developing a computerized data base has been the compelling need to deal with a large volume of information on patients and to do so in a consistent and rational manner that would produce the necessary information not only for research studies but for management of patients.

The data obtained in our clinical environment can be classified into two categories: serial data and cross-sectional data. Serial data are gathered when a patient or a group of patients is seen at regular intervals, depending on the research protocol. Various measurements are made, as in the test of speech and hearing, and the same tests may be repeated at intervals, such as six months or a year. Cross-sectional data, on the other hand, represent the state of the patient at one moment in time.

Updates and corrections are made on the record as circumstances dictate, with no retention of outdated information. An example would be the date that the patient last visited the Clinic. This information could be used to generate a list for "call-ins" of any patients who had not returned when they were scheduled.

The two foregoing types of data are used to answer two different classes of questions. The cross-sectional data can be used for determining the differences and interrelationships between two or more different subsets of the Clinic population. Serial data, on the other hand, are used to answer questions about the changes in a group of patients with respect to time; for example, are certain craniofacial measurements statistically different by seven years of age for certain modes of clefts compared with those of normal individuals?

Problems with data occur if one researcher wants to perform a study based on a large combination of factors and with information from many diverse sources within the Clinic.

X-RAYS AND CINERADIOGRAPHY

As noted in the chapter on craniofacial growth, the x-ray film of the human craniofacial complex can be digitized with standardized landmarks by well-established procedures. The digitized points are in the form of X–Y coordinates in terms of "counts," relative to the center of the digitizing screen, with an appropriate scale factor to convert the "counts" to distances in centimeters.

The error band of the measuring system is on the order of three counts, so that points can be located within 0.6 mm., or about the width of the pencil lead used in producing the tracings from the x-ray films. The usual procedure is to agree beforehand upon a suitable set of points for a particular study and then digitize these points for a set covering as many as 177 landmarks.

The 177 landmarks represent a number of specific craniofacial structural details; many of the landmarks are endpoints for linear measurements, planes, angles, and ratios. For example, the midpoint of the sella turcica (Sella or S) on the lateral head film is 95; the most anterior point of the nasofrontal suture (Nasion or N) on the same head film is 58. The anterior cranial base, S–N, thus becomes 95–58. As another example, the deepest point on the maxillary bone below the anterior nasal spine on the lateral head film is Point A, or 133. Accordingly, N–A, or 58–133, may be thought of as one measure of upper facial height. The angular relationship between S–N and N–A is an important measure of the relation of midface to cranial base: the angle S–N–A becomes 95–58–133. In any particular study in which S–N, N–A, and angle S–N–A are important, the computer program will include the appropriate instructions, e.g., to calculate the dimensions and angles by specific numbers given as input parameters. More than that, S–N, N–A, and angle S–N–A may be retrieved for each age, cleft type, and sex. Finally, we may program the computer to plot the results in respect to age-related changes for a single individual, boys, girls, or cleft-type, and this will demonstrate how these three parameters progressively and interrelatedly change with time.

Each card set produced by the digitizer contains not only the point pairs, but information regarding the patient's date of birth, identifying number, sex, cleft-type, and the date of the x-ray. This information is repeated on each card, and the cards are sequentially numbered for control purposes.

DATA-BASE MANAGEMENT SYSTEMS

In such a complex system, it has been necessary for us to establish rigid control and verification procedures to insure the validity and accuracy of the data, as at this time well over 2000 x-ray films have been digitized, representing some 350 patients. A data-base management system has been developed to index and retain these data for various current and future research activities.

Without getting into too specialized an area for the purposes of this book, some basic material on data-base management systems should be discussed. These management systems have been developed by the scientific and industrial communities in the last decade, with the advent of high-speed computing systems.

It became apparent some years ago that many data requirements often overlapped — that the data required by one researcher were often the same as a portion of the data being kept by another. It is generally conceded that data in a research organization should not be duplicated, because of the complexity of keeping more than one set of records up-to-date. There is always the danger that someone may not make the necessary corrections and the integrity of all of the data will be in question. Which set is right?

For the main file of x-ray films, the set of digitized points was selected to cover the mass of our current and anticipated research needs for major craniofacial landmarks of soft and hard tissue. A number of limited subsidiary data sets have been constructed for pilot projects, but subsets of the main point set are satisfactory for the majority of our investigations.

Inherent in any computerized data-base management system are three programming systems:

1. Update, deletion, and change in the data base.
2. Extraction of data that meet some specified criteria.
3. Calculations and reports from the extracted data for purposes of research and analysis.

In respect to the x-ray system, these general requirements have been met by the development of a series of programs utilizing either the COBOL or FORTRAN computer languages, using the American National Standard versions of these languages. This permits these programs to be transferred to other computer organizations for easy implementation.

The updating, deletion, and alteration of data in the master x-ray file are done with a program that adds records to the file and a separate program that deletes erroneous records from the file. Subsidiary programs have been written to check the sequence of cards to be added and to give a catalogue of records currently stored on the file. The data are stored on a conventional magnetic computer tape.

The extraction of specific data is done with a series of generalized extraction programs. The extraction of a subset of the file is defined in terms of cleft-types, certain patients, or specific x-ray films of certain patients taken on specific dates. These are expressed as suitable parameters, the extraction program is run, and a magnetic disc file is produced with the the desired sets of digitizations.

This subset of the main data file is then ready for further processing by one of a series of calculation and analysis programs, as follows:

1. Plot each x-ray film to scale on the printer, for inspection.
2. Plot a series of x-ray films on an overlay basis for evaluation of growth characteristics of specific landmarks.
3. Calculate the distances between specified points and retain the results.
4. Calculate the angles between specific point triplets and retain the results for further analysis.
5. Subject the data calculated in the foregoing programs to a generalized set of descriptive statistics as a guide for more extensive analysis.
6. Compare any two groups of measurements by a t-test for detection of possible differences of means. The suitability of this test is governed by the well-known limitations of the method.

In the development of the foregoing calculation and analysis programs, which are in standard FORTRAN, a primary consideration was to make the input and output data formats compatible with the various programs. We have found that this greatly eases the development of future programs and eliminates the necessity for reworking large numbers of programs to allow for minor changes in the system. Data appear either as card images of the digitization process, or in a standardized form from the output of the distance and angle calculation programs. The parameters for running each program of the analysis system must, of course, be specific to a particular program, but the general form of the output data is standardized so that it is possible to use data analysis programs such as the SPSS or BIOMED systems.*

The presentation of numerical data from information on growth is a difficult problem; the resulting information is not readily interpreted by the simple inspection of tabular data. A more successful procedure that we have used extensively is to plot the movement of craniofacial landmarks over time (i.e., successive x-ray films) of a particular patient or group of patients. To avoid the cumbersome use of digital plotters, a series of programs was developed that plots the digitized points on the computer's high-speed printer. Since a resolution of 10 points to the inch for the horizontal axis and six points to the inch for the vertical axis is possible, it is easy and convenient to evaluate gross morphological changes and, at the same time, note any general trends or pinpoint portions of the data that warrant more detailed study.

CLINIC CENSUS AND DENTAL SURVEY

With the development of both our longitudinal Research Series and our cross-sectional study of Clinic patients, we have found it useful to develop an overall data base that gives current information about the Clinic population, both active and inactive. At this stage it deals with some 50 specific

---

*See selected bibliography for documentation information.

items for each patient. The system is seen as the nucleus for a more general approach to the management of our patient records. For the time being, the file is in the form of a series of card-images, with up to six cards per patient, and a system limitation of 99 cards per patient. Each card is appropriately coded and contains information concerning a specific area of Clinic interest, such as date of birth, date of last addition of information to the file, socio-economic status, and location of residence.

As pointed out earlier in this book, we secure a great deal of special information on each of the 350 children enrolled serially in our Research Series. This special information is gathered by the surgeon, the prosthodontist, the speech pathologist, the audiologist, the geneticist, the growth researcher, and others. For each of these specialists the census and survey data become a common denominator, containing the patient number, name, date of birth, cleft-type, and other information. These basic data will be the source of common background knowledge of each child for each specialist, and it will also contain the date and age of the patient each time he or she is seen.

The data bases set the framework for interdisciplinary research: each researcher in his or her field has access to the census and survey bases. Let us say, for example, that a child was seen at three, six, nine, 12, and 18 months of age, and thereafter seen annually from two years. Cleft-type is known, as are times of lip and palate closures. Each time the child was at the Clinic, appropriate data were recorded by *each* specialist and made available to *each* researcher. If a speech researcher formulates a problem in the relation between form and function of oropharyngeal tissues as related to cleft-type, time of repair, and changes with age, obviously such a problem will bring together all data gathered by the surgeon, prosthodontist, and growth researcher. Thus, speech, surgery, dentistry, and growth and development all unite in a common effort. Any researcher in any area can, via the computer, call upon *all* data that will aid in a total rehabilitative approach for each patient.

Each computer card contains the patient number. The updating program is keyed to card-type and patient number, and updates are done by simply submitting a card with the appropriate columns changed. For the deletion of data, a special symbol is inserted in any field to be deleted, and the field is cleared to blanks.

The development of extraction and analysis programs at present consists primarily of programs that list the contents of specific card-types in alphabetical order with appropriate column headings and record counts. The file has been incorporated into our statistical systems. This approach has been deemed sufficient for research sample studies, in which it is necessary to obtain a subset of the Clinic population for a particular research study or treatment program.

Several typical sample studies conducted with Clinic data have involved counting and cross-tabulation operations for data that meet some set of criteria, such as cleft-type, date of birth, or sex. For more involved studies, it will be necessary to develop more generalized data-base extraction programs.

STATISTICAL METHODS AND SYSTEMS

The Clinic data are of such a diverse nature that a wide range of statistical methods have been applied to them. The reader is referred to the chapter on statistics for a more detailed explanation of the applicability of particular techniques.

It is possible, however, to make a number of general statements about the requirements placed upon a system from a computerization viewpoint. A number of standardized statistical "packages," such as the BIOMED and the SPSS packages, have been used with great success. These generally available statistical packages are a series of programs with provision for input parameters that describe the layout of the data to be analyzed and the particular tests that are desired. Such statistical packages have been well tested and use techniques adequately described in their accompanying documentation. This documentation is well suited for the individual who is not deeply versed in complex statistical procedures or computer techniques.

With a minimum amount of effort, it is possible to formulate a set of program parameters to give an extensive analysis of the data. With the more sophisticated systems, such as SPSS, the parameters form a "language" to retrieve and store data files and to separate them into subfiles for various studies. The majority of commonly used statistical procedures are available, and these features allow the researcher to obtain a rapid overview of the data as a guide to the application of higher level techniques with the same system.

Unfortunately, the packages do not always contain the necessary procedures to perform all desired tasks. Therefore, it has been necessary to modify or develop a number of specialized programs of statistical analysis for such topics as analysis of variance with repeated measures for unequal cell size, Cochran's "Q" test, and linear modeling. Fortunately, there are a number of excellent texts that give the computational procedures in such a form that programs may be easily developed in the FORTRAN language.

Another useful alternative is to obtain programs from other research organizations or universities. These should be obtained in the form of cards, test data, test output, and program listings. They are often available for the cost of materials and shipping.

TECHNICAL CONSIDERATIONS

It would be inappropriate to recommend any particular make of computer suitable for biomedical research purposes. It is possible, however, to make some general statements about the requirements that such systems should meet. These specifications concern both hardware and software, or programming, and deal with those features that are considered essential and those that might also be highly desirable for research efforts, based upon our experience and particular environment.

The essential requirements include those features that support the development of large-scale data bases, such as disc or tape drives in sufficient numbers to handle at least a million characters of information. We do not think that exclusively card-oriented systems are satisfactory, because they have a limited capacity for data storage, are not easily handled, and have limited programming capabilities.

Disc storage systems are preferred over tape systems, as the data-base management systems that can be constructed in that environment are much more efficient if they can have access to records on a random basis, instead of on a sequential basis, as with tape and card storage systems.

From a software or programming viewpoint, the system chosen should at least be capable of supporting a FORTRAN IV language processor. The vast majority of research computing, both in medical fields and in the scientific community in general, is done in FORTRAN. For this reason, it is often possible to exchange programs with other institutions with a minimum of difficulty in adapting the programs from one system to another. This is due to the wide use of FORTRAN and the fact that it is usually well standardized among the manufacturers of various computer systems. A large number of texts on computer programming are now available, and most statistical procedures can be formulated in a manner readily translated into computer programs.

Another language found very useful for data manipulation, in comparison to computational problems, is COBOL. This language is more like English than FORTRAN is and has found great applicability and acceptance in the industrial community. COBOL programs are generally more efficient for the processing of data files, as COBOL compilers are usually optimized for data handling, whereas FORTRAN compilers are optimized for calculational efficiency. On more sophisticated computer systems, it is often possible to write a program utilizing both languages in order to produce an optimal computational and data-handling environment.

In addition to having a language system such as FORTRAN, and perhaps COBOL, it is highly desirable to have some kind of utility sorting program for organizing data. In simpler systems, this can take the form of a mechanical card sorter, which is inexpensive but slow. In the more sophisticated systems, sorting is done by a special utility program. Most COBOL compilers support special commands that enable the sorting to be initiated from within the program itself.

In the past few years, there has been a growth of so-called "time-sharing" computer systems, in which a number of users may access a common computer from typewriter-like terminals. These systems, in the larger versions, will support all the language and system capabilities just discussed and, in addition, will have an on-line text editor, which allows the creation and alteration of data much in the way that the batch computer user would punch a deck of cards. Alteration of programs and data then becomes very convenient. It has been estimated that such systems, even though more costly, will tend to increase the overall efficiency of the research staff by a factor of two to three, as the results of computations are quickly available at a deskside terminal on an interactive basis.

THE FUTURE

In preparing a work of this nature, it is easy to see where we have been and where we are, but it is quite a chore to look forward to see where the use of computers is taking us. Some trends can be discerned, and lessons can be drawn from our past experiences that will serve to guide our steps in the future.

The first conclusion that can be drawn is that the use of computers is not a substitute for careful research design and the planning of experiments. It is simply not possible to "give the data to the computer" and have it produce an answer, because there is no substitute for a complete understanding of the research problem.

The techniques of other fields show strong possibilities of application to our own field. As an example, the computerized image-enhancement techniques used in the space program appear to be useful in the analysis of x-ray images. These x-ray images are filled with "noise" from various skull structures, and the contrast is often low. By image-enhancement techniques, similar to the manipulations conducted during photographic printing, it is possible to locally increase or decrease the contrast, to improve the rendering of areas and contours of special concern.

Some interesting trends have been developing in the area of "minicomputers"—those inexpensive small-scale systems that are very useful for such tasks as on-line data acquisition and reduction and limited amounts of computation. It appears that these systems are capable of handling some of the types of problems to which we have addressed ourselves. It is also possible to interconnect them to larger systems via telephone lines, so that the minicomputer functions as an "intelligent terminal" in direct communication with a larger system, to handle problems that are too big or complex for it alone.

From a viewpoint of system software, it appears that there will be an increase in the use of generalized statistical packages and data-base management systems, as part of the standard software complement provided by the manufacturer of the computer system. Whether there will be any wide standardization of these systems (such as SPSS) is open to some question, since the various features of these systems are strong competitive points for the individual computer manufacturer. Because the government is a large user of computers, standardization in the past has often come out of government initiative for transferability among various federally or state-owned systems.

A Selected Bibliography

Beyer, W. H.: Handbook of Tables for Probability and Statistics, 2nd ed., Cleveland, Chemical Rubber Co., 1968.

Bruning, J. L., and B. L. Kintz: Computational Handbook of Statistics, Glenview, Illinois, Scott, Foresman, 1968.

Dixon, W. J.: BMD: Biomedical Computer Programs, Berkeley, California, University of California Press, 1974.

Dorn, W. S., and D. D. McCracken: Numerical Methods with FORTRAN IV Case Studies, New York, John Wiley & Sons, 1972.

Draper, N. R., and H. Smith: Applied Regression Analysis, New York, John Wiley & Sons, 1966.

Kirk, R. E.: Experimental Designs: Procedures for the Behavioral Sciences, Belmont, California, Brooks/Cole, 1968.

McCracken, D. D.: A Guide to FORTRAN IV Programming, 2nd ed., New York, John Wiley & Sons, 1972.

McCracken, D. D., and U. Garbassi: A Guide to COBOL Programming, 2nd ed., New York, John Wiley & Sons, 1970.

Nie, N., C. Hull, G. Jenkins, et al.: Statistical Package for the Social Sciences, New York, McGraw-Hill, 1975.

Winer, B. J., Statistical Pinciples in Experimental Design, 2nd ed., New York, McGraw-Hill, 1971.

Chapter Twelve

The finest team cannot win many games against strong opponents without a "game plan," a master design assigning each player a specific task and coordinating all individual skills toward the same goal. Similarly, the investigation of challenging scientific research hypotheses must be guided and coordinated by the necessary first step of an "experimental design."

Three interrelated phases are involved in the research process: the experiment itself, the design, and the analysis. The data and the design should not be slighted in the rush to do the analysis. This is an error commonly made by experimenters who hurriedly seize upon an analysis formula found in an elementary statistics textbook or conveniently supplied as part of a computer software package. Experience has shown that such an approach, paying insufficient attention to the basic data and to the problem the data supposedly model, may at best yield the right answer to the wrong problem. Overemphasis on formulae may even, more embarrassingly, produce the *wrong* answer to the *wrong* problem. In short, while biomedical computer packages may be a valuable source to be used in analyzing data, they are not and cannot be a substitute for statistical consultation and careful construction of an experimental design.

THE PROBLEM

The first step in the development of an experimental design, the problem, must begin with a clear and precise statement—the so-called "real problem." What *is* the problem at the H. K. Cooper Institute? The problem is intimately related to the goal to be achieved. Here at the Institute, our major orientation—indeed our every effort—is the total rehabilitation of the child with a cleft, both as an individual and as a member of a family and a community. When we use the term "total rehabilitation," we speak not only of the extent of the treatment, but the quality of it. Each of the disciplines—plastic surgery, dentistry, speech, otolaryngology, audiology, and others—has as an individual goal the best treatment for the patient. The goals and methods of treatment, however, must necessarily be determined by sound clinical appraisal and judgment. Equally critical, the separate goals must be achieved in concert and harmony.

Within one discipline the best treatment of the patient's total rehabilitation may not make for optimal treatment in another area or discipline. For example, the best surgical procedure for closure of a cleft lip, which looks at only form and appearance (cosmesis), may not provide maximal function for

THE STATISTICAL APPROACH TO RESEARCH

JOSEPH A. MEIER
HARRY E. CANTER

aid in sucking, eating, speech, or labiodental relationships in terms of amount of scar tissue. A cosmetically acceptable lip repair must also provide for full restoration of lip function, especially that of the musculature around the mouth.

In an overall evaluation of the cleft lip and palate situation, several important observations can be stated:

1. *The problem* is to achieve the goal of total rehabilitation of the patient.
2. This total rehabilitation of the patient involves the aggregate of many goals and hence individual subproblems that determine the most effective or best treatment within each discipline.
3. The various subproblems in the several disciplines are related to one another in the sense that separate treatments within the realm of form and function must complement each other.
4. Sound clinical appraisal and judgment must first be exercised and can only result from the careful and detailed analysis of *all* clinical data gathered by each clinician who has given the full measure of care to the child with a cleft.

As is well known, the extent of clefts ranges from a notched or split uvula or a notched lip to a complete bilateral cleft of soft palate, hard palate, alveolar process, and lip. This range in itself necessitates a major consideration in our clinical data: *variability.* We may resolve part of the problem by the classification of cleft-types, i.e., soft palate, hard palate, lip, unilateral, bilateral, and so forth; but that is only a first step, for such a classification must be broken down in terms of the extent or degree of severity of the cleft. This means quantification and leads to measurement. On our x-ray head films, lateral and posteroanterior, and on our dental models, all gathered longitudinally for some 350 of our children, we can begin to look at and assess changes in the pre- and postoperative hard and soft tissues. This brings in degrees of change in form and function with time.

Let's look at a relatively simple problem of evaluation, closure of a cleft lip only: (1) To begin with, how severe is it? Just a notch? Partway up to the nostril? Up to the nasal floor? Unilateral? Bilateral? Here, one observes a discrete set of variables; (2) At what age will surgical closure be performed? (this is a reasonable constant); (3) What kind of procedure will be used to close the lip? Here, clinical judgment is basic; (4) Was the lip closure successful? For what—form and appearance or function?

At once, what was thought to be a relatively simple problem takes on a considerable degree of complexity, for there are not only many *sets* of variables, but *subsets* as well. All of these variables, in varying degree, will affect the final judgment of whether the closure was completely or partially successful, and even the word "partially" is in itself a qualification. There is another problem centering around the variables, for some are more important than others. If we recognize this, then we must assess kind and degree of importance, i.e., we must *rank* the variables in order of importance.

All the data made available by the clinicians who render their services to the child with a cleft become a matter of case history record. These records, in turn, are the raw data for research, for the H. K. Cooper Institute has two arms, a division of clinical services and a research division. When we evaluate clinical service one cannot say "success" or "failure," "better" or "best," unless these value judgments have been tested via the statistical assessment of *all factors* involved.

Communication within the team is enhanced tremendously by a statement defining the dependent and independent variables to be observed. Let us give an example of a dependent variable in the clinical field. Suppose we are studying craniofacial growth in cleft cases; this becomes a dependent variable, with such factors as cleft-type, sex, and age as independent variables, i.e., factors that in one way or another influence the course of craniofacial growth. Are all such variables measurable? Measurement is usually thought of as the assignment of numbers indicative of quantity to some object or trait that we seek to assess. For example, in the case of surgery of the lip, how do we measure the appearance of the lip pre- and postoperatively to evaluate a given surgical procedure? Do we simply state the appearance to be good or bad? Perhaps appearance of the lip can be rated on a scale. If a four-point scale were used, a rating of one might be associated with the worst appearance and a rating of four with the best appearance.

A rating of one (worst) might involve such items as a visible scar, an asymmetry, much scar tissue, an obvious notching of the vermilion, a faulty "cupid's bow," or other problems. A rating of four (best) would be the reverse of the above: a scar of greatly reduced visibility, symmetry, little or no scar tissue, no notching, a perfect "cupid's bow," and so on. In a four-point scale, is the difference in appearance between a pair of patients receiving a rating of one and two, respectively, the same as the difference in appearance between a pair of patients receiving a rating of three and four, respectively? Certainly the numerical differences are the same, but is the significance the same? So far, such a one-to-four rating scale is largely subjective; we are hoping to objectify it.

Moreover, how do we measure the lip profile? As a cupid's bow? The measurements or numbers assigned will hopefully lend themselves to the arithmetic operations of addition, subtraction, multiplication, and division, but this is not always the case! The scientist must often think in terms of several different levels of measurement to be defined and discussed later in this chapter), often referred to as *measurement scales.*

Independent variables or factors that may affect the dependent or response variable should also be listed once the problem is clearly defined. The number of independent variables listed usually increases very rapidly. The problem is not merely one of listing variables, but rather of deciding which ones are basic and important. Some common sense plus good practical experience will often help make this decision. On the other hand, we should be careful not to presuppose or prejudge the answer. Statistical techniques, called screening methods, are available for "sifting out" potentially important variables from a large initial set of independent variables.

The level of measurement associated with each independent variable is also of special importance. Even to a nonstatistician, the sex of a patient does not lend itself to the same degree of measurability as does, say, height or weight. We can quantify the two latter dimensions precisely. In a sense we can do this for sex on a simple numerical basis, i.e., assign a *one* for a male and a *two* for a female. In this way we can categorize sex in a way analogous to the categorization of height and weight (or any other mensurational variable).

When measurement scales are discussed later in this chapter, we will be defining four levels or scales of measurement. Imagine a problem with 20 different independent variables, each variable with one of four possible scales of measurement. What happens to the arithmetic when certain types of mathematical analyses are carried out? Putting it all into a computer will not help! Computer scientists know only too well that if nonsense is put into a computer, one can be sure of a nonsensical output.

The statement of a problem and the selection of variables and their corresponding levels of measurement are at best a compromise. There are many choices that can be made, and there is no one "best" choice resulting from "the strategy." Any given statement of a research hypothesis and its associated variables and their levels of measurement is called a mathematical model for a "real problem." There are many mathematical models for the same problem. The guiding principle in selecting a model should strike a compromise between mathematical applicability and mathematical tractability.

Obviously, the more variables we include, the more refined the measurements and the more applicable the model. We feel that the model should closely simulate the real problem. But introducing more variables will most certainly make the mathematical solution of the problem less tractable, not only from the point of view of statistical design, but also from the computational aspect necessarily associated with any given model.

Some years ago a paper discussing strategy in experimentation contained the following statement pointing up mistakes we are apt to make in doing research:

> We aren't always bold enough;
> We are apt to get in a rut;
> We are too easily fooled by the error;
> We don't always eliminate the unimportant variables first;
> And we don't always know when to quit.

THE DESIGN

With an increase in experience and the maturity it brings, the researcher becomes quite proficient in selecting the variables to be tested, suggesting possible relationships and explaining tentative underlying mechanisms of an unexpected result. However, somewhere in the middle of the problem is usually a faulty testing procedure. Time is lost, money is wasted, and in many instances valuable bits of information remain obscured—all because techniques of experimental design have not been utilized earlier. Statistics tell researchers where to place their shots in experiments involving many variables and give mathematical tools for tallying the score.

Doing research can be compared to working with a so-called "black box," which has a number of dials that can be adjusted. Each dial represents an independent variable or factor. If the box has a meter—the dependent variable or response—that is affected by the settings on the dials, one is tempted to take the box apart and study each intrinsic component in great detail to see how it interacts with the other components to produce a change in the meter reading! That would be basic research, but what if it should be impossible to take the box apart? One could still study the box from the outside by doing empirical research. The investigation would then be termed a phenomenological study: one moves the dials and observes what happens to the meter reading.

Medical research, in particular work with the cleft palate complex, possesses many of the phenomenological characteristics of the black box. Obviously, we do not imply that treatment of any patient, especially the patient with a cleft palate, can be dehumanized to the level of dealing with a black box. Rather, we intend the analogy to emphasize the problems associated with doing research on the *whole* patient with a cleft palate. The variables are many, and basic understanding of the underlying mechanisms producing the cleft palate complex is relatively slight. We can't "take the patient apart." However, the very excellent treatment provided to date testifies to the fact that the situation is not hopeless. A phenomenological study of the patient has and will continue to provide many answers related to treatment. With well-designed experiments and passage of time, we will achieve even clearer glimpses of what is inside the black box that represents the entire cleft palate complex. In the meantime, we can very productively observe and measure the many related variables and in turn predict their effects both individually and jointly by use of these experiments.

Let us take the black box idea and apply it to the cleft problem. If the total craniofacial complex takes the place of the black box, then, via x-ray films, we can take the complex apart. We can look at bones, muscles, tissues, and, by the use of cineradiography, we can observe how the components function interelatedly. With this last procedure, we can, quite literally, look at *both* form and function. In an analogous sense, the craniofacial complex has its meters and dials, which become the many factors that act upon one another. The interesting fact that emerges is that the meter and dial relationship may change, depending upon the focus of analysis. If we assume that speech is the object of interpretation, it then becomes a meter. The dials may then be considered as the type and extent of cleft, surgical repair of lip or palate, age-related changes, velar integrity, and so on. The setting (the effect) of each one of these dials, i.e., the expression of each factor, will combine to establish the meter reading of speech. If we focus on the psychosocial development of the child with a cleft, it becomes the meter, the reading of which will be determined by the dial settings of cleft-type, surgical repair, speech effectiveness, age, family milieu, peer attitudes, and so forth.

After a certain amount of reflection the researcher realizes that an immediate problem is to determine *how* to adjust the dials. There are many ways this can be done. The classical method suggests that only one dial be moved while the others are kept at a constant setting. In a real situation this approach is referred to as one-factor-at-a-time experimentation. It has great appeal and at first appears to be a very logical and precise way of conducting an experiment, since it allows for each variable to be studied separately. However, it can be demonstrated readily that this approach is inefficient; most serious of all, it frequently presents the risk of missing concealed and essential information. For example, what if the dials did not act independently of each other? How would one then choose the "constant" setting for the other dials? Is it really possible to maintain any number of variables at a constant level? If, indeed, one were fortunate enough to achieve results with the one-factor-at-a-time approach, the findings would apply only within the constant setting of the other dials. In a real life situation the cleft palate patient hardly exists in a completely or even partially constant environment.

Another testing procedure might involve setting each dial at random or by intuition and then reading the meter, and is often called the "shotgun approach" in actual experimentation. Usually it does not produce much if any understanding of the phenomenon being investigated. Most of us are not lucky enough to hit upon useful information in this way; moreover, data of this sort are not readily analyzed mathematically. The approach amounts to consulting the statistician after the data have been collected and then presenting him with the impossible task of analyzing the results. One often hears reference to a "gold mine" of data accumulated in files and resulting from a totally undesigned sequence of experiments. Many sad researchers and clinicians find out only when it is too late that the apparent "gold" turned out be only "fool's gold."

A statistically designed experiment with the black box would consist of adjusting all dials simultaneously but systematically. No dial would remain constant, nor would any dial adjustments be selected at random. For example, if we picture a black box with three dials, it may be decided in advance of experimentation to select two settings—a high setting (H) and a low setting (L)—for each of the three dials. The settings are referred to as *levels*. Every possible combination of the dial settings or levels would define eight possible experiments: LLL, LHL, HLL, HHL, LLH, LHH, HLH, and HHH. The notation LLL defines an experiment in which each of the three dials is set at the low setting, whereas LHL indicates an experiment in which the first and third dials are set at low while the second dial is maintained at the high setting. In actual experimentation with the black box, one would conduct the eight experiments in random order. The resulting eight meter readings would supply data that could be analyzed statistically.

Only data that are randomly distributed statistically will yield statistical information. Utilizing the data from the eight experiments (relatively few trials), one could determine how each dial affects the meter reading. More important, one could determine if the dials act independently or influence the meter reading jointly. In other words, the influences of the dials on the meter reading may interact with each other. For example, the effect of dial one may change depending upon the settings of dial two and dial three. Clearly, information of this type would begin to shed some light on the inner mechanisms of the black box. The one-factor-at-a-time approach would be totally inadequate to determine interaction effects.

Consider the simple example in which we want to answer the question of the relation of surgical procedure to cleft-type: procedures A, B, and C in the repair of cleft lip only (CL), cleft palate only (CP), unilateral cleft lip and palate (UCLP), and bilateral cleft lip and palate (BCLP). This can be done only by handling the clinical data in a research situation, a situation that calls for the skills of the statistician. Each operative procedure must be handled in terms of the entire group of children (the sample) who received that procedure. Further, each group of children in a given category of cleft-type must be sorted out. Then we are ready to pose several questions about our two major sets of samples, e.g., "Which operative procedure has been most successful for which cleft-type?" A setup something like this would initially be drawn up:

CLEFT-TYPE	OPERATIVE PROCEDURE		
	A	B	C
CL	–	–	–
CP	–	–	–
UCLP	–	–	–
BCLP	–	–	–

This arrangement means that each operative procedure can be tested against each cleft-type. It is only an outline, of course, and all variables under cleft-type and operative procedure must be spelled out and tabulated. This means either ordination (e.g., yes and no, or scaling, as 1, 2, 3, 4) or quantification (e.g., measurement in millimeters or angles, or the calculation of ratios).

Now let's look at a specific problem in which an experiment initially involved detecting differences between operators working with a digitizer (OSCAR) to measure distances between osteologic points in the tracing of the head film based on craniofacial cephalometry. In considering experimental designs that might answer this question, it was discovered that enough data existed for a more sophisticated study. In fact, it was possible to use a design with five factors replicated four times. The factors were tracer, sex, cleft, age, and operator. The tracer was the individual who did the cephalometric tracing, and the operator the one who used the OSCAR digitizing equipment. Each factor was held at two levels. There were two tracers and two operators, and the male and female patients were six months and 24 months of age. The soft and hard palates and unilateral cleft lip and palate were studied. With regard to sex, age, and cleft, there were four sets of patients matched according to these factors. For example, there were four patients that were male, six months old, and had a cleft of the hard and soft palate. Each patient was traced by each tracer and each tracing was digitized by each operator. The data were then subjected to an analysis of variance. Six different measurements were studied: (1) basion to nasion, (2) basion to sella, (3) basion to ANS, (4) nasion to sella, (5) nasion to ANS, and (6) sella to ANS. The measurements were those defined by sella, basion, nasion, and ANS (see the chapter on craniofacial growth for definitions).

Analysis of the data associated with the study indicated no operator difference and nonsignificant variation between tracers. However, sex and age were important factors in each measurement studied. While the cleft alone was a significant factor in only three of the measurements, it was discovered that the cleft was involved in several interaction terms. For example, a sex and cleft interaction indicated that the sex and the cleft of the patient produced a joint effect on the length of anatomical measurement. As a result, the influence of the sex factor would vary depending upon the type of cleft incurred by the patient. As a pilot study, analysis of the design raised questions as to the importance of sex and age factors in future and more refined growth studies.

The previous discussion focused upon the importance of the planning and the design of an experiment. What could have been a rather limited study to investigate operator differences became a rather sophisticated study involving a number of other factors. Data were utilized to their fullest and sophistication was made possible through statistical planning.

As a second example, an interesting follow-up study to the same pilot experiment was the analysis of *growth trends* in components of craniofacial morphology. Craniofacial growth of anatomical segments in 15 male and 15 female subjects — five in each of three types of cleft — was observed: cleft of the soft and hard palate, unilateral cleft lip and palate, and bilateral cleft lip and palate. Growth of anterior cranial base length, upper facial height, and palatal length for each of the 30 subjects was observed longitudinally, beginning at six months of age and every six months after that until age 24 months.

Owing to the fact that the primary objective of the study was to investigate the growth process of patients with a cleft, repeated measurements on patients had to be taken. Factorial experiments in which the same experimental unit (generally a subject) is observed under more than one treatment condition require special attention.

The combinations of the factors of sex, type of cleft, and age of patient had to be carefully selected in order to meet the requirements of a design for a factorial experiment with repeated measures. The primary objective of the design was to allow for analysis of the data in order to determine the presence of trends in craniofacial growth and how these trends might be influenced by the factors of sex and type of cleft, considered singly. Here again, another advantage of the designed approach was that it allowed for the effects of the factors on growth to be considered in combination with each other, thus permitting the determination of any *interaction effects* that might be underlying or identified with the process of craniofacial growth. Finally, and of no less importance, the design took into account subject heterogeneity, a situation that occurs with many problems in biobehavioral research.

Some specific questions that could be answered as part of the design were:

> *Question 1:* "Is there a trend in craniofacial growth data?" This question can be rephrased — "Are the means for growth influenced by changes in the age of the patient?"
>
> *Question 2:* "Is the trend of growth means linear or nonlinear?"
>
> *Question 3:* "Is the trend of growth means with respect to the age of the patient the same for females as for males?"

Question 4: "What differences, if any, exist among the trends of growth means for the various types of cleft?" If real differences do exist (a so-called cleft age interaction), then further questions can be asked concerning the nature of the difference or interaction. The graphs of trends are known as *profiles,* and the following questions could be posed:

(a) "Are differences between the shapes of profiles due to the 'linear part' of sex-age interaction?"

(b) "Are differences in profile due to differences between nonlinear or curvilinear trends?"

Although the first aim of the design was to detect and describe the nature of any trends in growth with respect to time, other questions not directly involving trend were capable of being considered.

Question 5: "If all growth data involving females—regardless of the levels of the associated variables (type of cleft and age of patient)—are averaged and compared with the average of similar male data, will there be a significant difference in group means?"

Question 6: "Will the difference between group means of female and male growth data be influenced by or dependent upon the type of cleft?" While group means for male and female growth data might significantly differ for clefts of the soft and hard palate, they may not differ if considered for bilateral clefts of the lip and palate. In the event such differences should exist, there is said to be a significant interaction between sex and cleft-type.

A third example is drawn from the study of mandibular movement under various speech conditions while the patient is asked to perform various speech tasks. The experimenter measured the position of the jaw (vertical and horizontal measurements) from cine films of four subjects for 10 speech tasks under three separate speech conditions. The primary interest was to evaluate the differences in jaw positions for any one of the speech tasks in each of the three conditions. Some questions asked by the speech pathologist were:

Question 1: "Does the range of mandibular movement differ statistically over the conditions?"

Question 2: "Does the total time of movement vary statistically over the conditions?"

Question 3: "Does the vertical or horizontal position of the mandible at one point (such as at the beginning of the utterance) differ statistically over the conditions?"

A significant outgrowth of discussion with the statisticians was the fact that *each one* of the four subjects would receive all combinations of speech tasks and speech conditions. An experiment of this type required a so-called *randomized block factorial design.* The detailed nature of this design is unimportant to us here. However, an important observation is the fact that the design was distinctly different from the completely randomized factorial and the repeated measures designs discussed in the first two examples. Each design was characteristic of each problem and made it possible to achieve statistical evaluation of some real questions. Collection of data was planned in advance of experiments designed to answer specific questions.

As Mendenhall[1] points out, one might think of experimentation as communication between nature and scientist. The message about the natural phenomenon is contained, in garbled form, in the experimenter's sample data. Imperfections in the measuring instruments, lack of homogeneity in experimental material or patients, and many other factors contribute background "noise" (static) that tends to obscure nature's signal and cause the observed response to vary in a random manner. The design of experiments is a very broad subject concerned with methods of sampling that reduce the variation in an experiment, amplify nature's signal, and thereby acquire a specified quantity of information.

THE ANALYSIS

The analysis, the final step in the problem, is for all practical purposes a logical consequence of the first two steps, namely, the experiment and the design. A well-designed experiment anticipates and prepares for the analysis.

Earlier in the chapter reference was made to the four levels of measurement. To provide a clearer understanding of how these levels relate to design and analysis, we will now define the four levels and consider a few real examples of data analysis of each.

Frequently the only kind of measurement that is possible is a categorization such as the following:

1. A patient is a boy or a girl.
2. Patients have cleft lip only, cleft palate only, or cleft lip and palate.
3. Patients have hearing loss in the right ear only, left ear only, or both ears.

Measuring or assigning numbers to reflect certain qualities gives rise to our first level of measurement, in which the data are said to be nominal, categorical, or qualitative—all of which, for our purposes, are synonymous. We shall use the term "nominal." To further illustrate, a group of five patients is given a paragraph to read while a listener concentrates on a certain word or sound in the paragraph. The listener must judge whether the patient can say the word or sound satisfactorily, and a one (1) will be recorded to indicate a satisfactory result, with a zero (0) for unsatisfactory. Results might look like this:

PATIENT	RESULT
1	1
2	1
3	0
4	1
5	0

Note that each patient is scored as success or failure. All successes are equivalent in value; there are no degrees of success.

One of the most common uses of nominal data arises when two or more groups with clefts are examined, with each person being assigned a number according to some quality he or she possesses. Data are then summarized in a table as follows:

| | RACE | |
CLEFT-TYPE CODE	*White*	*Black*
Cleft of soft palate only	3	1
Cleft of soft and hard palate	0	4

The values in the table represent the number of patients in the various categories. There are a variety of ways to analyze such data, but each method depends on a set of assumptions. Small samples require different methods than large samples. In the preceding example each patient is independent of every other patient with regard to race and cleft-type.

Suppose that instead of race we make an analysis of attitude; we might ask the patient, "Do you think your cleft will be a permanent handicap?" The question is asked before and after treatment, and the answer will be yes or no. The data are still nominal and the table looks similar, but the assumption of independence is altered, and thus a different analysis must follow:

TABLE 12–1

CLEFT-TYPE	PRETEST	POSTTEST
Cleft of soft palate only	3	1
Cleft of soft and hard palates	2	2

In this table, 3, 1, 2, and 2 represent the number of "yes" answers. Actually, the data would have to be displayed in a different way to be analyzed, as in Tables 12–2 and 12–3.

TABLE 12–2   Cleft of Soft Palate Only

		PRETEST	
		Yes	No
Posttest	Yes	1	0
	No	2	1

TABLE 12–3   Cleft of Soft and Hard Palate

		PRETEST	
		Yes	No
Posttest	Yes	1	1
	No	1	0

In Table 12–2 we see clearly that in the group with clefts of the soft palate only, there was 1 yes/yes, 0 no/yes, 2 yes/no, and 1 no/no. Observe also that for the group in Table 12–3 there are actually only three patients and not four, as appear in Table 12–1. We see that one patient said "yes" in the pretest and "yes" in the posttest, and so he was counted twice in Table 12–1, making it appear that there were four patients. However, this patient may be a strong-minded individual who never changes an opinion; therefore, the assumption of independent responses is lost.

More than once we have alluded to the fact that a primary problem in biomedical research is quantification of responses. Nominal data play a major role here since even the most difficult factors to measure — such as quality of speech, nasality, or quality of surgical results — can at least be categorized as satisfactory or not satisfactory. Quite a few statisticians have been devoting considerable time developing new techniques for analyzing such data. Some people feel it is foolish even to try to quantify more precisely than categorization. After all, many "normal" people do not speak perfectly, hear perfectly, or look beautiful.

We now turn our attention to the second level of measurement in which again numbers are used for categorization, but in addition the order or ranking has significance. Such data are called "ordinal" or "ranking" data. Newborn babies are given a number called the Apgar score (based on a 10-point scale) that estimates the general health of the child. Various rating scales have been devised to reflect speech intelligibility and nasality. Sociologists use a socioeconomic status scale. Psychologists and psychiatrists have used rating scales to evaluate patients for years. Class rank in high school has been a criterion in education. In a sense, any ranking scale can be thought of as a refinement of simple categories, and so it is reasonable to expect that more elaborate and precise methods of analysis are available. This is, in fact, the case; however, care must be taken, since ordinal scales have the appearance of ordinary positive whole numbers that possess mathematical properties not necessarily true with the ordinal scale. For example, suppose some individuals are each rated according to the following scheme:

1. Dead
2. Poor health
3. Fair health
4. Good health
5. Excellent health

A room contains 10 such people, of whom five are dead and five are in excellent health. What would one say is the average health of the people in the room? Would you calculate: $(1 + 1 + 1 + 1 + 1 + 5 + 5 + 5 + 5 + 5) \div 10 = 3$? The conclusion would be that the average state of health is fair. Certainly the dead, if no one else, would disagree.

An average may have no real meaning if one is using a rating scale. Everyone knows that in the set of numbers 1, 2, 3, 4, and 5, the difference between 1 and 2, 2 and 3, 3 and 4, and 4 and 5 is the same, i.e., $(2 - 1) = (3 - 2) = (4 - 3) = (5 - 4) = 1$. In the forementioned rating scale the difference between 1 and 2 is the difference between life and death, while the difference between 5 and 4 may be simply a trick knee. We do not have an *equal interval scale*. An equal interval scale is one in which if any two pairs of differences are numerically equal, then the differences are physically equivalent as well. Since having an equal interval scale permits the comparison of differences and a number of other statistical methods of analyses, many researchers try to prove, argue, or at least hope that the rating scale they are using is equal interval and proceed with crossed fingers. All the world's computers, calculations, and tables will not undo the basic error in this approach.

Sometimes, instead of assigning a patient a number from a rating scale, the researcher wishes to rank the subjects from low to high, perhaps on speech intelligibility. If there are only a few subjects, it may be possible to rank them in a consistent manner, but ranking 50 or 60 is an altogether different matter. The question of whether or not it is even possible to rank them consistently needs to be studied. One approach is to examine the subjects in pairs and to look for inconsistencies. For example, suppose there are three subjects; then, the possible pairs are (1,2), (1,3), and (2,3). What would one conclude if the study yielded the following:

    1 better than 3
    3 better than 2
    2 better than 1

Obviously there is an inconsistency. On the other hand, if 1 were rated better than 2, then the correct ranking would be: 1st (1); 2nd (3); and 3rd (2). This is the basic idea in what is known as the *method of paired comparisons*. M. G. Kendall and also H. A. David have developed much of the statistics needed for this procedure.

Ordinal data can be treated as if they are nominal data simply by ignoring the order aspect. Similarly, the next level of measurement, which has some further refinements, can be treated as a ranking scale. Many times data from a higher level of measurement are ranked before being analyzed, since the ranking methods require less in terms of population assumptions (normality, equal variances, and other factors). Techniques for analyzing data of these first two levels of measurement are usually called *nonparametric statistics*.

When measurements are taken from dental models or x-ray films of the craniofacial complex, the resultant data have a quality not found in an ordinal scale. Not only is it evident which numbers are larger or smaller, but also the magnitude of the differences is known. Although the unit of measurement may be centimeters or millimeters, the ratio of the differences between two points is constant. For example, suppose the distance from point A to point B is 3 cm., and from point B to point C is 5 cm. If millimeters were used to measure these distances, they would be 30 mm. and 50 mm., respectively; but $3/5 = 30/50 = .6$. Ratios of intervals remain invariant under change of units. Data from this level of measurement are called *interval data*, and all ordinary arithmetic operations are applicable. Means, standard deviations, standard error of the mean, and the classical statistical tests, such as t-tests and Pearson product-moment correlations, may be applicable provided the other assumptions are met (e.g., normality). There is no true zero for these data. Digitizing points from an x-ray film requires choosing a zero point, but it is arbitrary.

If there exists a true zero, such as in height, weight, income, time for recovery, and I.Q., the fourth level of measurement, called a *ratio scale*, is applicable. Ratio data are the highest level of measurement, and, provided assumptions for the design are met, all the well-known methods of analysis are available with their use. Literally hundreds of designs, multiple comparison procedures, multivariate regression analyses, and many more techniques can be used.

In summary, the classes of data or levels of measurement are: nominal, ordinal, interval, and ratio. It is always possible to move from a higher level to a lower level of measurement, but not from lower to higher. Many biomedical research problems must use only the first two levels and accompanying nonparametric analyses. Recognition of the kind of data and the level of measurement to use is second only to defining the problem as the most important initial step in research and design.

Reference

1. Mendenhall, W.: Introduction to Probability and Statistics, 4th ed., North Scituate, Massachusetts, Duxbury Press, 1975.

Chapter Thirteen

It has been a guiding principle of the Lancaster Cleft Palate Clinic that in treating an oral or facial impairment it is treating the whole person. Each member of the Clinic team may at any point in the program have his attention focused on one twist in the tangled skein of anatomical, physiological, and often emotional troubles. But all are working toward that single, clearly defined goal: helping an individual to achieve his full potential in life.

As H. K. Cooper has often remarked, the attainment of that goal depends at the outset upon a feeling that one's appearance and speech are normal. Much of this volume has been devoted to measures that the clinicians and therapists employ to bring their patients as close as possible to those desired norms of face and speech. And it is their conclusion, based on follow-up observations of thousands of patients, that most of them either reach that normal state or at least attain a level, with respect to appearance, speech, and social adjustment, that the patients themselves consider acceptable.

But for many the victory was won only after years of quiet, sometimes painful inner struggle. The person with a facial or oral defect wrestles through childhood and the teen-age years, and even in some cases on into young adulthood, with problems of a peculiarly poignant and private kind. He confronts challenges that are not always noted in the charts. We feel, therefore, that a review of the Institute's cleft palate experience would not be complete without the voices of some of the patients themselves. They provide a helpful insight into how they perceived themselves in a world that so often didn't understand them. They tell how they coped and how their outlook and their lives changed as they finally overcame their communication handicaps.

Members of the Clinic staff have been fortunate in having maintained close contact with many of their patients over a long period of time. Some have lived continuously in or near Lancaster. Others have kept in touch by letter or have returned to the Clinic community from other parts of the country for revision of speech appliances, or just to visit relatives or members of the Clinic staff, with whom they have become friends.

FROM THE PATIENT'S POINT OF VIEW
Some Reflections on How Their Lives Have Been Affected by the Handicap and by Its Correction

STEVEN M. SPENCER

We recognize that children with clefts born in recent years, when clinics for the total care of patients with a cleft palate have been more accessible than in the past, probably experience less emotional trauma in their social encounters at school and elsewhere. But the stories of these older patients, told from the perspective of maturity, should serve to remind us that the springs of stress and discomfort are ever present and may be touched off if the overall problem is not handled with skill and thoughtfulness. Here, then, are some recollections and reflections obtained from a number of Clinic "alumni" in recent interviews.

FLORIST AND GREENHOUSE OWNER

Allan Steffey (Figure 13–1) was 14 when he was first seen at the Lancaster Clinic in 1939. Born in 1925, he had undergone surgery for repair of a cleft lip in infancy, but efforts to close a palatal defect were unsuccessful and had, in fact, made his situation worse. His speech throughout childhood was extremely nasal and difficult to understand.

Fifty-one years old at this writing, married and the father of six, Steffey is a successful florist, with a greenhouse near Lancaster. But he remembers how shyness and withdrawal marked his early years.

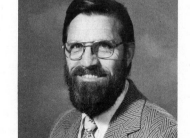

FIGURE 13–1   Allan Steffey

545

"We went to the Mennonite Church every Sunday, and I should have had friends there. But the minute church was dismissed, I was out in the car. I didn't talk to anybody. I had no close friends at all.

"At home I had a happy childhood. I was the fourth in a family of eight children. My parents were very understanding, and I had all the love and security I needed. But I was bashful and quiet when there was anybody around I didn't know.

"I used to go with my mother on Saturdays to the city market in Lancaster, where she sold dressed chickens and home-baked cookies for extra household money. I remember how often a customer would ask me the price of a chicken and I'd tell her, and she'd turn to my mother and ask, 'What did he say?'

"The thing that kind of got me the most . . . anybody who had an interest in what I was saying would ask me to repeat it, and maybe the third time he'd smile and nod his head. But I knew very well that he didn't know what I was saying.

"My teacher in the one-room school in our country village north of Lancaster was a very understanding person. She put forth much effort to help me. She didn't allow anyone to make fun of me. It was just a small group and I gradually got to know them and they knew me. My trouble came when I moved on to junior high school. There I just crawled into a shell and talked only when spoken to.

"About this time, when I was a teen-ager, I remember saying to my mother, 'If there had to be something wrong with me, why couldn't it have been a clubfoot or a bad leg. Anything is better than not being able to talk, not being understood.' But I long since learned that was foolish thinking."

Life began to offer more promise when Allan entered high school. There his history teacher, Paul R. Diller, took an interest in him, and Diller's wife, Genevieve, the speech therapist at the newly established Lancaster Cleft Palate Clinic, put him in touch with Cooper. Mrs. Diller recalls those days. "Many times cleft palate children are considered dull, just because their verbal response is poor. I think Allan was sometimes afraid of this. But my husband recognized that Allan had ability."

Because the results of the early surgery had made further efforts at repair of the palate impossible, Allan became one of the first patients for whom Cooper fitted a speech appliance. "At first it felt like a mouthful of mush. I could hardly keep from gagging. But he told me to try to keep it in place until I got home. I managed to stick it out during the half-hour trolley ride, but I almost vomited."

For three years Allan took speech lessons with Mrs. Diller in a small group that met late every Tuesday afternoon. "Improvement seemed gradual to me and to those I was with all the time. But for people I hadn't talked to for some months or years, it was quite a remarkable thing. And it certainly changed me. I'm sure I couldn't have gone through high school otherwise, and I couldn't possibly be in this business. I would never have talked on the telephone, for instance."

A measure of Allan's success was the speech he made at his high school graduation in June, 1943. Cooper and Mrs. Diller sat proudly in the audience, taking it all down with a bulky, early model recording instrument.

Since most doctors and dentists were unfamiliar with the cleft palate speech appliance in those days, Cooper took Allan Steffey with him to meetings to demonstrate it, an experience that also helped bolster the young man's self-confidence. "Dr. Cooper would introduce me just as a friend and he made sure I got to talk to a lot of people. Then, when he had everybody together he would say, 'Allan, would you take your appliance out and talk to them again? The effect was quite dramatic." Allan also went into the Clinic on occasions to talk with parents of children who needed a speech appliance but who were hesitant until they saw what could be accomplished with it.

In his own home, however, he performs no with-and-without demonstrations. "My wife and children have never heard me talk without my appliance. I take it out just to brush my teeth. It's really a part of me. And I haven't spoken without it for a long time."

The improvement in Allan Steffey's speech during high school years brought with it the emergence of a relaxed and outgoing personality. He met his wife-to-be while she was in nurse's training, and they were married when he was only 20. He now converses easily with his flower shop customers and participates in church activities, including the teaching of a Sunday school class of older teen-agers. "I have a rich, full life, a happy life," he says. "I enjoy people and I think people enjoy me. I have lots and lots of friends, and it's hard for them to believe I ever was in a shell."

HIGH SCHOOL TEACHER

When first seen at the Lancaster Cleft Palate Clinic in 1942, Edward Crumrine (Figure 13–2) was 17. He had been born with a complete (type IV) cleft of the palate and a bilateral cleft of the lip. Eight operations in infancy and early childhood had included removal of the premaxilla. This left him with an extremely flat upper lip. The shrunken appearance of his face and his poor speech (he had difficulty with all sounds) had "warped his personality, and developed in him a feeling of inferiority," to quote an early report. "He shunned all social contacts."[1]

There were, however, frequent antisocial contacts. Crumrine, now a history teacher in a York, Pennsylvania, school, recently president of the Teachers Association, and a calm and amiable man, remembers that as a youngster he often reacted to taunts by fighting. "If anybody mentioned my lip or my speech I would punch him in the mouth. I wasn't very big and I usually lost. I worked in a grocery store when I was just a little kid, for 25 cents a week. There was a fellow who used to hang around there, and every now and then

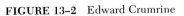

FIGURE 13–2 Edward Crumrine

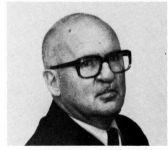

he would tease me and mimic my voice. It was just kid stuff, but I'd get mad and tackle him. He was bigger than I was and he'd get me down and then let me up and do it again. But I was a fighter. That was the way I handled the thing. Of course, eventually you get to the point where you dislike everybody.

"To show what kind of a mental state I developed, one day a man came into the grocery store and he asked me something about my lip, and I turned away from him. He meant no harm. He said, 'I think maybe I know somebody who could help you.' But I refused to talk to him, and he left. Years later I sometimes wondered — though it is highly unlikely — if that man could have been Dr. Cooper, or someone who knew Dr. Cooper."

Eddie had repressed his belligerency by the time he got to high school. There, he recalls, "I simply retired into the background. I had a general feeling of withdrawal and self-consciousness. This is a period when social life is so important to young people. But I just went to classes and that was it. Dancing, clubs, that sort of thing, forget it. That I didn't need. And during that period my grades went down. In general, I wasn't doing a very good job of it, socially or academically.

"It was partly because I was bashful about reciting. I remember one teacher who took me aside when we were doing oral reports and said I could write the assignment out instead, if I preferred. But I said, 'No, I'll do it.' Of course, I was scared to death. But I'm not so sure that's abnormal. I think all kids at that age are apt to be a little fearful of reciting."

Eddie's parents were much concerned about him. "They tell me I wanted to quit," Crumrine says. "I don't remember that. But I do know that I wanted desperately to join the armed forces. I wanted to get out of school and into the action. I was 17 and some of my friends were going into a Navy program. I found out that in some places the Navy was taking people with my problem, but not here in York, and I couldn't understand why our people were so obstinate. I think that was the big disappointment of my life."

At this time, however, Eddie was referred by a York doctor to the Lancaster Clinic, and there his rehabilitation began. Following a staff examination and numerous intelligence and personality tests — he had a high I.Q. — dental work was undertaken and thimble crowns were placed on the remaining upper teeth to permit construction of a speech appliance. This was so designed as to build out the lip and cheeks and correct the dished-in deformity. Plastic surgery in the lip area was performed several years later, and the result, a more normal contour of the face, demonstrated what could be achieved through cooperation of dentist and surgeon. The obturator, first of many that Eddie would have, permitted him to control the nasality of his speech, which was further improved by several years of speech lessons in Mrs. Diller's small class.

"We were of all ages in that group. Even two mature ladies, 'plain people,' who wore their little bonnets. Everyone was very helpful, glad to see others in the class succeed. The most helpful thing was the psychological support we received there."

Staff members at the Clinic encouraged Eddie to finish high school and enter Franklin and Marshall College, where his social adjustment improved. He joined a fraternity, was on the dean's list, and was frequently invited by Cooper to accompany him to meetings. "I would help him set up his movie screen and stuff," Crumrine recalls, "and I am sure, as I look back on it, that it was part of Dr. Cooper's plan—'Eddie's being useful.' He also encouraged me to make speeches, and of course to many people this was more impressive than if I had been a guy with a brace on his leg, because speech was supposed to be my difficulty. I remember enjoying the experience, the applause and the whole bit.

"I once gave a talk about the Pennsylvania Rehabilitation Bureau because I was getting aid through it. Many then felt that the aid should be given mainly to older people. I tried to point out that young children should get this help, so they wouldn't have to go through what I had gone through in my younger years. There were an awful lot of years that I guess were wasted for me, and if I had had the confidence when I was in my teens that I have now, why things wouldn't have been that way for me.

"All through college Dr. Cooper encouraged and assisted me, and he wanted me to go into law. I attended law school for a year in Philadelphia, but I didn't like it and decided on teaching instead." In Philadelphia, however, he met an attractive girl who became his wife. They have an equally attractive daughter, now in college.

At the time of the daughter's birth, neither parent gave much thought to the possibility that cleft palate, which is sometimes hereditary, might be passed on. The daughter arrived without blemish. "It never occurred to me when I was pregnant," Mrs. Crumrine said. "But it happened that the woman who shared my room in the hospital maternity section did have an infant with what I think was a cleft palate—they brought in a bottle with a special nipple. And I became a worrier later on. If I had had another pregnancy I might have . . . ." She left the sentence unfinished.

Crumrine had been equally unconcerned. "I didn't look for trouble then, I guess. Had we had another child I might have given it more thought. But I'm not particularly worried even now, about grandchildren. I see what is being done today [referring to the improved surgery, prosthetic work, speech training, and all-around care]. To me it looks now more like a nuisance than a great problem. They get them so young that a lot of these psychological things we've been discussing—I doubt that they occur." They do occur, of course, if the child is not brought into a proper corrective and rehabilitative program early.

As to his outlook on life, Edward Crumrine is aware that it underwent a complete change some time after those bitter teen-age years when, as he said, "you got to the point where you disliked everybody."

"For a long time my attitude was that there might be some good people in the world, but most of them were bad. I'll never forget my best friend chewing me out for that one day. He said, 'You know, that takes a lot of guts for you to say, considering all that these people have done for you.' He really nailed me down with it. And as I said to Jenny Diller, when we were talking about this a couple of years ago, my attitude now would be just the opposite. I think most people are all right. And I am just completely changed. I accept things.

"What changed my outlook? I think it may have been World War II, when I was so desperate to get in and so disappointed when I didn't. I was very much upset. I didn't want to be in college. I even did some investigating to see if I could get into the Canadian army. But then 'J' day came and the war was over. No more battles to be fought. And I think eventually it dawned on me, 'You know this is what happens. You get frustrated. You get angry and mad, and these things come to an end.' As the Scriptures say, 'This, too, shall pass.' I've sort of developed this attitude. I rarely get discouraged, or tired. I don't know whether that was the turning point or not."

TEACHER OF PSYCHIATRIC NURSING

John Bergey (Figure 13–3) was 24 at the time of his initial visit to the Lancaster Clinic in 1949. He had been troubled ever since early childhood by an awareness that his speech was difficult to understand. He was born on a Pennsylvania farm in 1925, the second in a family of seven children. His cleft lip had been repaired in infancy and two operations had been performed on his cleft palate by a competent plastic and maxillofacial surgeon in Philadelphia. But the defect had been too wide to permit complete closure; he was left with an inadequate velopharyngeal valve and a very nasal speech. Although he had managed to go through school and was in college at the time of his first visit, he was discouraged about his vocational prospects.

"In church and Sunday school, before I was old enough for public school, there was the problem that the teachers couldn't understand me, though they tried very hard," Bergey remembers. "That always bothered me a lot. In public school the teasing wasn't as bad as I know it could have been, because it was a small country school in Bucks County and many of the pupils were relatives and church friends, whom I had known before. But some children did mimic me and they'd ask 'How come you talk so funny?' That would stand out as the most disturbing question all through my childhood."

He received some help at a dental and maxillofacial clinic in Philadelphia during his high school years and then went on to a small Mennonite College in Kansas. "I got along all right there," he recalls, "and really enjoyed it. However, it was a daily concern to me that I couldn't speak better and even look a little better, because I was still in my late teens, very interested in girls, and yet I felt hesitant about asking them out." Nevertheless, he did overcome his shyness, had a number of girl friends, and met his future wife there.

In college he had taken a premedical course, but on his return home to

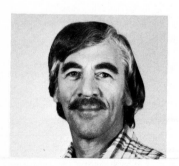

FIGURE 13–3 John Bergey

Pennsylvania he wasn't sure he wanted to follow through in that direction, largely because of fear that he'd be unable to communicate effectively. "So I was looking around for work as a truck driver. I couldn't find it. Then a friend offered me a job as a sales clerk in a shoe store. This was a real break, a tremendous boost for my self-confidence—just the realization that someone would offer a person in my situation a job of that kind, where I would be talking to people all day long."

At about the same time, John Bergey made his first contact with the Lancaster Clinic, where he was fitted with a speech appliance and started on a program of speech therapy with Mrs. Diller.

"One thing we were learning was to drink through a straw, which helped us concentrate on the muscles at the back of the throat. During the 25-mile drive back to my home from Lancaster each week, after my lesson, I would practice those muscle exercises, partly by singing a lot. And one day—I remember it so well—I noticed that I could make a completely different sound if I just let the throat muscles tighten around the speech bulb. The following week, back in Lancaster, I said to Mrs. Diller, 'You know, when I was driving home last time I could tell that something entirely different was happening. I could sense that I was controlling those muscles so well.' She said 'Well, do it now. Let me hear you.'"

John Bergey then demonstrated what we have often noticed, namely, that those who have been speaking with "cleft palate speech" for many years are not sure just how they sound to others, or exactly what is expected of them as "normal" speech.

"Well, I'm a little confused," Bergey told her. Then, in his usual nasal voice, he said, "I'm not sure whether hyou hwhant mhe to htalk like hthis? or [in clear, crisp syllables] do you want me to talk like this?"

The effect on Mrs. Diller was electrifying. She ran across a narrow street to Cooper's office and brought him back to hear for himself this sudden, spectacular change. Bergey repeated his question, first in one voice and then in the other. Cooper, who up to that time had felt John was not progressing as rapidly as he should, was astounded. "Eureka! You've got it!" he exclaimed. "Now why don't you use it?"

This exchange, whenever she thinks of it now, reminds Mrs. Diller of the scene in "My Fair Lady" in which Eliza Doolittle finally masters "the rain in Spain" and Professor Higgins shouts, "By George, she's got it!"

"That's exactly the way we all reacted."

"It was an exciting moment," Bergey recalls. Excerpts from Mrs. Diller's entry in his chart that day, December 6, 1949, reflect this excitement: "A most thrilling experience.... What a change in the whole speech picture! Delightful! We recorded the change (on a disc record) and assigned this new way of speech for him to use."

John's family and his girlfriend, hearing his "new speech," could hardly believe their ears. "When I came back to the shoe store the next day," Bergey remembers, "and showed my employer and the other clerks I could talk differently, they were really amazed. They no longer had to ask me to repeat. They could understand exactly what I was saying, and they encouraged me tremendously.

"Being in a religious family I had prayed often that somehow God would help me to correct my speech problem, that He would remove this thing from me. During adolescence it was a real crisis. But I never dreamed that this was the way it would happen.

"The Clinic staff often used the Twenty-third Psalm for recording our progress in speech therapy, and after my big improvement I was really moved by the sentence, 'He restoreth my soul.'"

With the improvement in his speech came a fresh boost to his vocational aspirations. As he recently remarked, "Dr. Cooper and his staff were largely responsible for changing my self-concept as well as my physical deformities; and also my career and direction in life were significantly changed during my days at the Clinic." He got a night job in a hospital while continuing to work days in the shoe store. Instead of resuming plans to enter medical school, he decided he wanted to "take care of patients in an even more personal way than a doctor does." So he enrolled in the School of Nursing for Men, at the Institute of the Pennsylvania Hospital, where he gained experience in psychiatric nursing.

He was married the year he graduated from the school and went to Yankton College in South Dakota for his bachelor's degree and to do psychiatric nursing in a nearby state hospital. He obtained a master's degree in nursing education at the University of Pittsburgh and for many years has been on the faculty of Fresno State College in California, teaching psychiatric nursing.

Calling on his personal experience and his skill as a psychiatric nurse, John Bergey has been able to provide expert counseling to other cleft palate patients and to parents of children with this problem. Doctors have referred patients to him for demonstration of the speech appliance and for advice. "They really have been quite encouraged by what I could do for them," he says.

PRE-MED STUDENT AND RESEARCH ASSISTANT

Rita Anichini (Figure 13–4) was born in Italy in 1952, with a bilateral cleft of the lip and palate, involving the maxilla. Surgery was performed on the lip during infancy, and the first operation on the palate was done at the age of six. She was first seen by Harding and Mazaheri in Rome in 1967 during an International Congress of Plastic Surgery, and she came to Lancaster in May, 1968, at the age of 16, mainly for further facial surgery. Subsequently, the family moved to New York City, where Rita, at this writing, is a student at Columbia University, planning for a career in medicine.

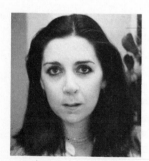

FIGURE 13–4   Rita Anichini

Like so many children with a cleft palate, Rita emphasizes that her parents were always extremely understanding. "They thought I was beautiful, and they made me feel beautiful. They never made me feel uncomfortable. If they couldn't understand what I was saying they would just ask me to repeat it. They never pressured me.

"But I could not go to my parents when I was having trouble with the children in the neighborhood, and that happened quite often. The kids were curious and would make me try to say words I couldn't pronounce clearly. There were times when they laughed at me. But I was taller than they were — so tall for my age that some of them would say I must be retarded — and I would beat them up. So their parents would come to my parents to complain that I had beaten their kids. But my parents stayed out of it. I stopped growing when I was 13 and I'm not taller than normal now. I'm just five feet five and a half.

"I didn't have any difficulty in school. My sister and I attended a private Montessori school taught by nuns. It was a little more selective with regard to its pupils. I was always good in school, so I guess that made up for other problems."

The palatal operation, done just before she entered school, also helped her classroom adjustment by improving her speech. "Before that I couldn't pronounce the hard sounds properly," she recalls. "My voice came out of my nose. By the age of nine or 10, however, I was having trouble with my teeth. The upper ones in front were so high that they would not close against my lower ones. My dentist tried to bring them down with braces and then considered removing them. However, he was afraid the whole bone in that part of the upper jaw would come out. Another operation was performed when I was 12, but a few years later I still needed more surgery, including plastic repair of the lip and nose."

In the summer of 1967, when Rita was 15, her mother, Marcella, a nurse, visited the exhibits at the International Congress of Plastic Surgery, in Rome, and stopped at the Lancaster Cleft Palate Clinic booth. "She was impressed by the results shown in the before-and-after pictures," Rita says. Her father, Danilo, then a chauffeur for the manager of an airline, got in touch with Harding and Mazaheri, who examined Rita and later made arrangements for her to come to Lancaster for the summer of 1968.

Examination at the H. K. Cooper Institute revealed that the premaxilla was displaced anteriorly, with the incisors so elevated as to produce a marked open bite. It was felt that it would be impossible to bring the upper teeth down for good occlusion, and the decision was therefore made to remove three of the teeth and replace them. Although this improved the occlusion, the upper lip still lacked adequate support, mainly because the lower lip protruded. In an operative procedure designed to improve her appearance, the surgeon transferred a wedge of tissue from her lower to her upper lip. The lips were sewed shut for about 18 days while the graft healed in the recipient site, after which it was severed from the donor site. Rhinoplasty was also performed to improve the nasal distortion.

Rita ruefully remembers this postsurgical period. "I had been looking forward to improving my English as soon as I got to the United States. I had studied it in school in Italy for several years, but it was British English and everything I said sounded a little weird. Unfortunately, I didn't have much chance to practice it during those first few weeks after the operation, with my mouth sewed shut. All I could do was watch and listen to others talk. Once my mouth was 'reopened,' I was able to join some other young people in a dormitory at the Millersville State College, where the Lancaster Clinic was conducting a summer program in speech therapy. Now I could talk, too."

Soon a speech appliance was constructed and with this and her speech lessons Rita made rapid strides, not only in speaking but in the English language. She went back to Italy in the fall of 1968, but returned for additional surgery in 1971, and she and her family have lived in the U.S. ever since.

A charming and industrious young woman who has been earning all of her own living and schooling expenses, Rita took a position as a governess after finishing high school and has had full-time jobs as an aide in a mental hospital and in a medical school laboratory. She has been in close touch with some of the research projects and is hoping to be admitted in a few years to medical school.

"As my speech and my English improve, I feel better," she says, in a voice almost totally free of the tones associated with cleft palate. "I have a little accent and for some people it is difficult to tell whether it is the accent or the cleft palate speech they are hearing. But I don't think the problem has interfered with my life at all. In fact it has been a boost for me because it has spurred me to do something."

Rita has strong opinions about the much discussed psychosocial effects of cleft anomalies. "Really, I think that if anybody is going to be permanently injured socially just because of a cleft palate and cleft lip—and I think this is highly unlikely—it must mean that something else is wrong with him. . . . It is partly a matter of fearing the stereotyped images. . . . People have to get used to the abnormal. I don't see my face. I see the others, and if it bothers them, it's their fault."

Her philosophy doubtless reflects the firm support she received as a child, which was quite unlike the reactions she sometimes witnessed in others. "I have known of women who were ashamed of their children with cleft lip or palate," she says. "They would stop my mother and me in our home town and ask about it, and I could see how they felt. I would like to emphasize the value of positive feedback from the parents. It is very important for this and for any problem which may have psychological overtones."

CASE NO. 5

David E. Arbogast (Figure 13–5) was born in West Virginia in 1933, with a unilateral cleft of the lip and palate. During infancy surgery was performed on the lip, and the palatal defect was partially closed, leaving an opening through the floor of the right nostril. When first seen at the Clinic in 1952, at the age of 19, David had a short palate, but his speech was quite good, with only slight nasality and a distortion of the S and S-blend sounds. His general articulation was good.

"What brought me to the Clinic was not my speech but a desire to get my lip fixed. I had gone around with a crooked lip all my life and I thought, boy, if I could just get it straightened out that would be the biggest thing that could happen to me.

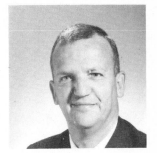

Figure 13–5 David Arbogast

"No, I don't think the lip or the palate had interfered with my social life. It was more my way of thinking about it rather than somebody else's reaction. I was probably much more conscious of it than other people were."

David Arbogast is a singer, a music teacher, and a piano tuner. He has been interested in music ever since he was in eighth grade, when he started on piano and began to play a trumpet.

"People would say, 'Why, you can't play a brass instrument,' meaning my lip would make it too difficult. But I would say, 'You just watch me!' If anybody told me I couldn't do something, it just turned me around and I did it. I soon changed to the baritone horn; the larger mouthpiece made it a little easier for me. But for some reason I never felt I had a handicap as other people might think of it. I believe a handicap is a state of mind, and I was not willing to let a handicap control me. I wanted to control it."

David's facial deformity was traumatic for his mother, however. He was the youngest of seven children, and two of his brothers were born with a cleft lip. "My mother told me that when she was pregnant with me she used to go out and walk up and down along the B & O tracks, near our house in Junior, West Virginia, almost frantic with fear that it would happen again. When I was born she had to feed me for some time with an eyedropper because I could not nurse with a bottle or at the breast. But she was a strong woman and when she died of cancer, in 1955, she was still a very happy and proud woman."

It was a sister of David who saw a magazine article about the Lancaster Clinic and brought it to her mother's attention. She got in touch with a friend in the West Virginia Division of Vocational Rehabilitation.

This division was at first opposed to providing financial assistance for treatment outside of the state, but one of its counselors persisted and succeeded in gaining this assistance not only for David Arbogast but for two girls with cleft lip, sisters who lived in the same part of the state.

He arrived in the spring of 1952 for a program that included surgical revision of the lip scar and extensive dental work, all of which greatly improved his appearance. The surgical notes state that the defect in the nostril floor was partly repaired by elevating mucoperiosteum flaps from the vomer and by bringing over nasal mucous membrane. With the addition of an appliance to complete the closure of the defect in the anterior part of the palate, and with speech lessons, an improvement was also brought about in his speech.

All this made a great difference in his life, David now says. As has happened with so many individuals, physical rehabilitation raised the educational sights for David Arbogast. Before coming to Lancaster he had no interest in college. After his high school graduation he did a brief stint in the coal mines, where his father had worked until "black lung" disease, miner's asthma, forced him to quit. There were a few years in a steel mill and a chemical plant. But at the Lancaster Clinic various psychological tests emphasized not only David's interest in music but his aptitude for it. And the West Virginia Division of Vocational Rehabilitation, recognizing his ability and his potential, offered him a four-year college scholarship if he would agree to remain in the state for four years of teaching in the public schools.

He had maintained his contact with music, conducting church choirs in his home town and taking voice lessons. "But what they did for me at the Clinic helped my singing voice tremendously," he says, "and the college scholarship gave me a new ambition." At Glenville State College he sang the tenor roles in musicals and upon graduation taught band for four years in the public schools of Clay County, West Virginia. Upon moving to Virginia he continued to teach band and choir, made recordings of several hymns, and became a member of the 80-voice Rockingham Male Chorus, in the Shenandoah Valley.

David Arbogast and his wife, Marty, who were high school sweethearts, adopted two teen-age children some years ago. "But we adopted them not because we were concerned about the possibility of giving birth to a child with a cleft, but simply because we could not have children of our own," he said.

"We probably would have wondered, if we were having a baby, whether it would or would not have a cleft. But I didn't really worry because we knew the Clinic was here, and so much can be done for children with this problem today. God has done a lot of good for humankind and one of the great things He did was to provide this clinic. It has afforded a livelihood for so many who were born with this defect and who might not otherwise have had such a successful life."

THE ROAD TO OTHER CAREERS

One could listen to the voices of many other patients to further illustrate the cleft palate individual's encounters with the social, psychological, and educational challenges of life. All of them have much to teach those who work with the handicapped.

Here is Dr. Phillip Achey (Figure 13–6), for example, left motherless at the age of three, but with a father who was determined to spare no effort or expense to help Phillip overcome the obstacles that a cleft lip and palate presented. Born on a farm near Lancaster, Phillip first came to the Lancaster Clinic in 1944 at the age of six, having previously undergone corrective surgery. He was fitted with a speech appliance and began a program of speech therapy. He is now an assistant professor of microbiology at the University of Florida, has no trouble speaking to classes of 150 students, and feels completely rehabilitated, although he returns to Lancaster at intervals for checkups and for dental work.

"The Clinic was the cornerstone, and without the highly competent

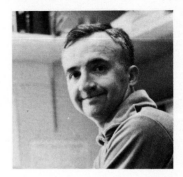

FIGURE 13-6   Phillip Achey

work of the staff and its total dedication to the patients' welfare, I doubt very much if I could have accomplished what I have and reached my current position in life. But the patient must work, too, and the family as well. My father and brothers were of tremendous importance. In that respect I was one of the fortunate ones."

Encouraging, too, is the story of a young woman we shall call Beatriz Avila, who came from her native Spain at the age of 17 with a wide open cleft of the palate for which nothing had been done. In spite of this handicap Beatriz went to school in this country for four years to learn English and acquire secretarial skills. She obtained her first job while still suffering from her speech impairment, but during her school years she visited several specialists hoping to find someone who could help her. Finally, after having received little benefit from most of these people, she was referred by one of them to the Lancaster Clinic.

Here a speech appliance was fitted for her and she began speech lessons on Saturday mornings, meanwhile continuing her full-time job. A very conscientious person, Beatriz would lock herself in her room and repeat over and over again the words and phrases assigned to her by the Clinic. A member of her family would sit with her and listen for errors or changes in the sounds and the pronunciation. "After several weeks of continuous practice with the prosthesis in place, all of a sudden it just happened," she recalled. "I began to pronounce words, especially those with plosive sounds, that I had never been able to master before. From there on it was success all the way, and by the end of the year my voice sounded as normal as anyone's."

"Not only did my voice change," Beatriz added. "My speech therapy was a tremendous help in perfecting my English pronunciation. To this day the greatest compliment I can receive is to be asked: 'Where did you learn to speak English so beautifully?' or, 'Are you English?'"

Beatriz Avila's personality also underwent a dramatic change, from that of a shy, reserved, and self-conscious girl to that of an outgoing young woman, full of life and eager to make up for lost time. She has held several jobs, from switchboard operator (where a clear voice was certainly essential) to top secretarial positions. She has traveled extensively, has worked for the U.S. government for several years here and abroad, and for the past few years has been affiliated with a top scientific organization in this country. She was recently married and writes she is very happy.

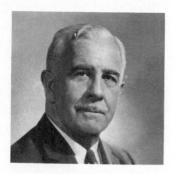

FIGURE 13-7   Daniel Test

Daniel Test, Jr. (Figure 13-7), a buoyant 70 years as this is written and a retired headmaster of a preparatory school, was born and spent his early years in the Pennsylvania Hospital in Philadelphia, but not as a patient. His father, Daniel Test, was superintendent of the hospital, the oldest in the United States, and the family occupied an apartment in the original Pine Street section, built in 1751. So Daniel grew up in a distinguished medical atmosphere. But not one of the three operations he underwent between the ages of two and six was very successful, as he recalls.

Although his speech had a nasal quality, he did not let it interfere with his educational progress. In school he received speech therapy, then called elocution. "I won an elocution contest at the Westtown school," he remembers, "although I won't say they didn't favor me. However, I did have some good competition."

Mr. Test became a teacher in the Williston Academy at East Hampton, Massachusetts, and while there he met John J. FitzGibbon, a leader in the development of modern speech prostheses, who prepared an appliance for him. In Philadelphia, where Mr. Test taught briefly at the Penn Charter school, he underwent further surgery of the palate, but again without gaining much improvement.

In the 1940s he visited the Lancaster Clinic, where Cooper made a new prosthesis for him. That, says Test, "has made possible the great life I have had." With his speech markedly improved, he took a personnel position in industry and later became headmaster at Westtown School, the Friends school near Philadelphia where he had won the speech contest years before. He retired several years ago.

Cooper and Robert Millard, the speech therapist, well remember the young man who hitch-hiked from western Wyoming after reading about the Clinic in a national magazine. He paced up and down outside the Clinic for several hours before getting up enough courage to come in. His problem was a bilateral cleft of the lip which early surgery had not satisfactorily corrected, and because of his appearance he had gone off by himself as a sheepherder. "I didn't have to talk to anyone out there on the ranch," he explained, "and there was no one to look at me or tease me."

A plastic surgeon affiliated with the Clinic reoperated upon the lip, and extensive dental work was carried out. These procedures, followed by several weeks of speech lessons in the Clinic's residency program, made a new man of the shy sheepherder. He was an intelligent, well-educated person (Cooper recalls that he knew a lot of Shakespeare) and a few years after returning to the West he became a banker and a member of the school board.

Another patient, helped by the fitting of a speech appliance, became a member of the cabinet in the Pennsylvania state government. This position required him to address gatherings of hundreds or thousands, which he did without the slightest hesitation or embarrassment. His speech was not perfect, but it was good enough to satisfy him, and as long as he had something to say and could make people understand him, he was happy. He was realizing his potential, and that, as we have repeatedly said, is the aim of the program.

Reference

1. Cooper, H. K.: Cleft palate: dentistry's opportunity. J. Am. Dent. Assoc., *42*:37, 1951.

INDEX